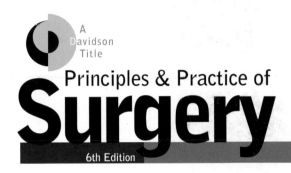

A
Davidson
Title

Principles & Practice of

Surgery

6th Edition

Commissioning Editor: *Laurence Hunter*
Senior Development Editor: *Ailsa Laing*
Project Manager: *Lucy Boon*
Illustration Manager: *Gillian Richards*
Illustrators: *Gillian Lee and Barking Dog Illustrators*

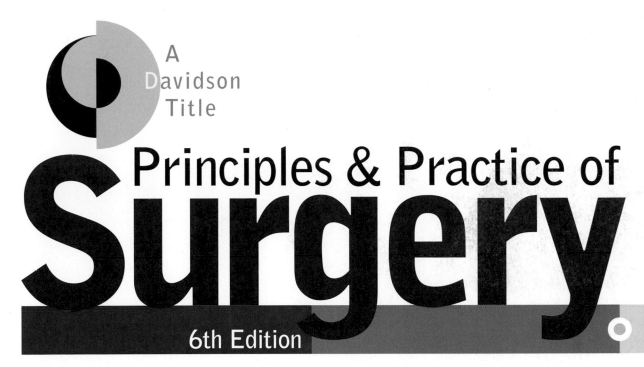

A Davidson Title

Principles & Practice of Surgery

6th Edition

Edited by

O. James Garden BSc MB ChB MD FRCS(Glas) FRCS(Ed) FRCP(Ed) FRACS(Hon) FRCSCan(Hon)
Regius Professor of Clinical Surgery, Clinical Surgery, University of Edinburgh;
Honorary Consultant Surgeon, Royal Infirmary of Edinburgh, UK

Andrew W. Bradbury BSc MB ChB MD MBA FRCS(Ed)
Sampson Gamgee Professor of Vascular Surgery and Director of Quality Assurance and
Enhancement, College of Medical and Dental Sciences, University of Birmingham;
Consultant Vascular and Endovascular Surgeon, Heart of England NHS Foundation Trust,
Birmingham, UK

John L.R. Forsythe MD FRCS(Ed) FRCS(Eng)
Consultant Transplant and Endocrine Surgeon, Transplant Unit, Royal Infirmary of Edinburgh;
Honorary Professor, Clinical Surgery, University of Edinburgh, UK

Rowan W. Parks MB BCh BAO MD FRCSI FRCS(Ed)
Professor of Surgical Sciences, Clinical Surgery, University of Edinburgh;
Honorary Consultant Hepatobiliary and Pancreatic Surgeon, Royal Infirmary of Edinburgh, UK

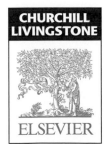

CHURCHILL LIVINGSTONE

ELSEVIER

Edinburgh   London   New York   Oxford   Philadelphia   St Louis   Sydney   Toronto   2012

ELSEVIER
CHURCHILL
LIVINGSTONE

First edition 1985
Second edition 1991
Third edition 1995
Fourth edition 2002
Fifth edition 2007
Sixth edition 2012
   Reprinted 2013, 2014

ISBN 978-0-7020-4316-1

British Library Cataloguing in Publication Data
A catalogue record for this book is available from the British Library

Library of Congress Cataloging in Publication Data
A catalog record for this book is available from the Library of Congress

 ELSEVIER your source for books, journals and multimedia in the health sciences
www.elsevierhealth.com

Working together to grow
libraries in developing countries

www.elsevier.com | www.bookaid.org | www.sabre.org

ELSEVIER   BOOK AID International   Sabre Foundation

The
Publisher's
policy is to use
**paper manufactured
from sustainable forests**

Printed in China

Contents

Preface

The sixth edition of *Principles and Practice of Surgery* continues to build on the success and popularity of previous editions and its companion volume *Davidson's Principles and Practice of Medicine*. Many medical schools now deliver undergraduate curricula which focus principally on ensuring generic knowledge and skills, but the continuing success of *Principles and Practice of Surgery* over the last 25 years indicates that there remains a need for a textbook which is relevant to current surgical practice. We believe that this text provides a ready source of information for the medical student, for the recently qualified doctor on the surgical ward and for the surgical trainee who requires an up-to-date overview of the management approach to surgical pathology. This book should guide the student and trainee through the key core surgical topics which will be encountered within an integrated undergraduate curriculum, in the early years of surgical training and in subsequent clinical practice.

We have striven to improve the format of the text and layout of information. Considerable effort has also been put into improving the quality of the radiographs and illustrations.

It is our intention that this edition is relevant to doctors and surgeons practising in other parts of the world. The four editors welcome the contributions of Professors Venkatramani Sitaram and Pawanindra Lal whose remit as co-editors on our associated *International Edition* is to ensure the book's content is fit for purpose in those parts of the world where disease patterns and management approaches may differ.

We remain indebted to the founders of this book, Professors Sir Patrick Forrest, Sir David Carter and Mr Ian Macleod who established the reputation of the textbook with students and doctors around the world. We are grateful to Laurence Hunter of Elsevier for his encouragement and enthusiasm and to Ailsa Laing for keeping our contributors and the editorial team in line during all stages of publication.

We very much hope that this edition continues the tradition and high standards set by our predecessors and that the revised content and presentation of the sixth edition satisfies the needs of tomorrow's doctors.

OJG, AWB, JLRF, RWP
Edinburgh and Birmingham, 2012

Contributors

Issaq Ahmed
MRCS BEng
Orthopaedic Registrar, Royal Infirmary of Edinburgh, UK

Derek Alderson
MB BS MD FRCS
Professor of Gastrointestinal Surgery and Barling Chair of Surgery, University Hospital Birmingham NHS Foundation Trust and University of Birmingham College of Medical and Dental Sciences, School of Cancer Sciences, Birmingham, UK

Andrew W. Bradbury
BSc MB ChB MD MBA FRCS(Ed)
Sampson Gamgee Professor of Vascular Surgery and Director of Quality Assurance and Enhancement, College of Medical and Dental Sciences, University of Birmingham; Consultant Vascular and Endovascular Surgeon, Heart of England NHS Foundation Trust, Birmingham, UK

Gordon L. Carlson
BSc MD FRCS
Consultant Surgeon, Salford Royal NHS Foundation Trust; Honorary Professor of Surgery, University of Manchester; Honorary Professor of Biomedical Science, University of Salford, UK

C. Ross Carter
MB ChB FRCS MD FRCS(Gen)
Consultant Pancreaticobiliary Surgeon, West of Scotland Pancreatic Unit, Glasgow Royal Infirmary, Glasgow, UK

Trevor J. Cleveland
BMedSci BM BS FRCS FRCR
Consultant Vascular Radiologist, Sheffield Vascular Institute, Sheffield Teaching Hospitals, Sheffield, UK

Andrew C. de Beaux
MB ChB MD FRCS
Consultant General and Oesophagogastric Surgeon; Honorary Senior Lecturer, University of Edinburgh, UK

J. Michael Dixon
BSc MBChB MD FRCS FRCS(Ed) FRCP
Consultant Surgeon and Honorary Professor, Edinburgh Breast Unit, Western General Hospital, Edinburgh, UK

Malcolm G. Dunlop
MB ChB FRCS MD FMedSci
Professor of Coloproctology, University of Edinburgh; Honorary Consultant Surgeon, Coloproctology Unit, Western General Hospital, Edinburgh, UK

Kenneth C.H. Fearon
MD FRCS(Gen)
Professor of Surgical Oncology, University of Edinburgh; Honorary Consultant Surgeon, Western General Hospital, Edinburgh

Steven M. Finney
MB ChB MD FRCS(Urol)
Consultant Urological Surgeon, Blackpool Victoria Hospital, Blackpool, UK

John L.R. Forsythe
MD FRCS(Ed) FRCS(Eng)
Consultant Transplant and Endocrine Surgeon, Transplant Unit, Royal Infirmary of Edinburgh; Honorary Professor, Clinical Surgery, University of Edinburgh, UK

O. James Garden
BSc MB ChB MD FRCS(Glas) FRCS(Ed) FRCP(Ed) FRACS(Hon) FRCSCan(Hon)
Regius Professor of Clinical Surgery, University of Edinburgh; Honorary Consultant Surgeon, Royal Infirmary of Edinburgh, UK

Savita Gossain
BSc MBBS FRCPath
Consultant Medical Microbiologist, Birmingham Health Protection Agency Laboratory, Heart of England NHS Foundation Trust, Heartlands Hospital, Birmingham, UK

Rachel H.A. Green
MB ChB BMed Biol FRCP FRCPath
Clinical Director, West of Scotland Blood Transfusion Centre at Gartnavel General Hospital, Glasgow, UK

Richard Hardwick
MD FRCS
Consultant Surgeon, Cambridge Oesophago-Gastric Centre, Addenbrookes Hospital, Cambridge, UK

Peter M. Hawkey
BSc DSc MB BS MD FRCPath

Professor of Clinical and Public Health Bacteriology and Honorary Consultant, Heart of England Foundation Trust and HPA West Midlands Regional Microbiologist, The Medical School, University of Birmingham, UK and Birmingham Health Protection Agency Laboratory, Heart of England NHS Foundation Trust, Heartlands Hospital, Birmingham, UK

Robert R. Jeffrey
FRCS(Ed) FRCP(Ed) FRCPS(Glas) FETCS

Consultant Cardiothoracic Surgeon, Aberdeen Royal Infirmary, Aberdeen, UK; Honorary Senior Lecturer, Department of Surgery, University of Aberdeen, UK

Thomas W.J. Lennard
MBBS MD FRCS

Head of School of Surgical and Reproductive Sciences, The Medical School, University of Newcastle upon Tyne, UK

Lorna P. Marson
MB BS MD FRCS

Senior Lecturer in Transplant Surgery, University of Edinburgh; Honorary Consultant Transplant Surgeon, Royal Infirmary of Edinburgh, UK

Colin J McKay
MD FRCS

Consultant Pancreaticobiliary Surgeon, West of Scotland Pancreatic Unit, Regional Upper GI Surgical Unit, Glasgow Royal Infirmary, Glasgow, UK

Stuart R. McKechnie
MB ChB BSc(Hons) PhD FRCA DICM

Consultant in Intensive Care Medicine and Anaesthetics, John Radcliffe Hospital, Oxford

Dermot W. McKeown
MB ChB FRCA FRCS(Ed) FCEM

Consultant in Anaesthesia and Intensive Care, Royal Infirmary of Edinburgh, UK

John C. McKinley
MB ChB BMSc(Hons) FRCS(Orth)

Consultant Orthopaedic Surgeon and Honorary Senior Clinical Lecturer, Department of Orthopaedics, Royal Infirmary of Edinburgh, UK

Douglas McWhinnie
MB ChB MD FRCS

Divisional Director of Surgery and Consultant General Surgeon, Milton Keynes Hospital, Milton Keynes, UK

Rachel E. Melhado
MD FRCS

Consultant Oesophago-Gastric and General Surgeon, Salford Royal Foundation Trust, Salford, UK

Lynn Myles
MB ChB BSc MD FRCP(Ed) FRCS(SN)

Consultant Neurosurgeon, Western General Hospital, Edinburgh, and Royal Hospital for Sick Children, Edinburgh, UK

Rowan W. Parks
MB BCh BAO MD FRCSI FRCS(Ed)

Professor of Surgical Sciences, Department of Clinical Surgery, University of Edinburgh; Honorary Consultant Hepatobiliary and Pancreatic Surgeon, Royal Infirmary of Edinburgh, UK

Simon Paterson-Brown
MB BS MPhil MS FRCS

Honorary Senior Lecturer, Clinical Surgery, University of Edinburgh; Consultant General and Upper Gastrointestinal Surgeon, Royal Infirmary of Edinburgh, UK

Mark A. Potter
BSc MB ChB MD FRCS(Gen)

Consultant Colorectal Surgeon, Western General Hospital, Edinburgh, UK

Colin E. Robertson
BA(Hons) MB ChB MRCP(UK) FRCP(Ed) FRCS(Ed) FFAEM

Honorary Professor of Accident and Emergency Medicine and Surgery, University of Edinburgh; Consultant, Accident and Emergency Department, Royal Infirmary of Edinburgh

Laurence H. Stewart
MB ChB MD FRCS(Ed) FRCS(Urol)

Consultant Urological Surgeon, Western General Hospital, Edinburgh, UK

Marc L. Turner
MB ChB MBA PhD FRCP(Ed) FRCP(Lon) FRCPath

Professor of Cellular Therapy, Edinburgh University and Associate Medical Director, Scottish National Blood Transfusion Service, Royal Infirmary of Edinburgh, UK

Timothy S. Walsh
MB ChB BSc MD MRCP FRCA

Consultant in Anaesthetics and Intensive Care, Royal Infirmary of Edinburgh, UK

James D. Watson
MB ChB FRCS(Ed) FRCS(Eng) FRCSG(Plast)

Consultant Plastic Surgeon, St John's Hospital, Livingston; Honorary (Clinical) Senior Lecturer in Surgery, University of Edinburgh, Edinburgh, UK

Ian R. Whittle
MB BS MD PhD FRACS FRCS(Ed) FRCP(Ed) FCS(HK)

Forbes Professor of Surgical Neurology, Department of Clinical Neurosciences, Western General Hospital, Edinburgh, UK

Janet A. Wilson
BSc MB ChB MD FRCS(Ed) FRCS

Professor of Otolaryngology, Newcastle University, Department of Head and Neck Surgery, Freeman Hospital, Newcastle upon Tyne, UK

SECTION 1

Principles of perioperative care

S.R. McKechnie
T.S. Walsh

01

Metabolic response to injury, fluid and electrolyte balance and shock

CHAPTER CONTENTS

THE METABOLIC RESPONSE TO INJURY

In order to increase the chances of surviving injury, animals have evolved a complex set of neuroendocrine mechanisms that act locoregionally and systemically to try to restore the body to its pre-injury condition. While vital for survival in the wild, in the context of surgical illness and treatment, these mechanisms can cause great harm. By minimizing and manipulating the metabolic response to injury, surgical mortality, morbidity and recovery times can be greatly improved.

Features of the metabolic response to injury

Historically, the response to injury was divided into two phases: 'ebb' and 'flow'. In the ebb phase during the first few hours after injury patients were cold and hypotensive (shocked). When intravenous fluids and blood transfusion became available, this shock was sometimes found to be reversible and in other cases irreversible. If the individual survived the ebb phase, patients entered the flow phase which was itself divided into two parts. The initial catabolic flow phase lasted about a week and was characterized by a high metabolic rate, breakdown of proteins and fats, a net loss of body nitrogen (negative nitrogen balance) and weight loss. There then followed the anabolic flow phase, which lasted 2–4 weeks, during which protein and fat stores were restored and weight gain occurred (positive nitrogen balance). Our modern understanding of the metabolic response to injury is still based on these general features.

Factors mediating the metabolic response to injury

The metabolic response is a complex interaction between many body systems.

The acute inflammatory response

Inflammatory cells and cytokines are the principal mediators of the acute inflammatory response. Physical damage to tissues results in local activation of cells such as tissue macrophages which release a variety of cytokines (Table 1.1). Some of these, such as interleukin-8 (IL-8), attract large numbers of circulating macrophages and neutrophils to the site of injury. Others, such as tumour necrosis factor alpha (TNF-α), IL-1 and IL-6, activate these inflammatory cells, enabling them to clear dead tissue and kill bacteria. Although these cytokines are produced and act locally (paracrine action), their release into the circulation initiates some of the systemic features of the metabolic response, such as fever (IL-1) and the acute-phase protein response (IL-6, see below) (endocrine action). Other pro-inflammatory (prostaglandins, kinins, complement, proteases and free radicals) and anti-inflammatory substances such as antioxidants (e.g. glutathione, vitamins A and C), protease inhibitors (e.g. α_2-macroglobulin) and IL-10 are also released (Fig. 1.1). The clinical condition of the patient depends on the extent to which the inflammation remains localized and the balance between these pro- and anti-inflammatory processes.

Table 1.1 Cytokines involved in the acute inflammatory response

Cytokine	Relevant actions
TNF-α	Proinflammatory; release of leucocytes by bone marrow; activation of leucocytes and endothelial cells
IL-1	Fever; T-cell and macrophage activation
IL-6	Growth and differentiation of lymphocytes; activation of the acute-phase protein response
IL-8	Chemotactic for neutrophils and T cells
IL-10	Inhibits immune function

(TNF = tumour necrosis factor; IL = interleukin)

The endothelium and blood vessels

The expression of adhesion molecules upon the endothelium leads to leucocyte adhesion and transmigration (Fig. 1.1). Increased local blood flow due to vasodilatation, secondary to the release of kinins, prostaglandins and nitric oxide, as well as increased capillary permeability increases the delivery of inflammatory cells, oxygen and nutrient substrates important for healing. Colloid particles (principally albumin) leak into injured tissues, resulting in oedema.

The exposure of tissue factor promotes coagulation which, together with platelet activation, decreases haemorrhage but at the risk of causing tissue ischaemia. If the inflammatory process becomes generalized, widespread microcirculatory thrombosis can result in disseminated intravascular coagulation (DIC).

Afferent nerve impulses and sympathetic activation

Tissue injury and inflammation leads to impulses in afferent pain fibres that reach the thalamus via the dorsal horn of the spinal cord and the lateral spinothalamic

tract and further mediate the metabolic response in two important ways:

1. Activation of the sympathetic nervous system leads to the release of noradrenaline from sympathetic nerve fibre endings and adrenaline from the adrenal medulla resulting in tachycardia, increased cardiac output, and changes in carbohydrate, fat and protein metabolism (see below). Interventions that reduce sympathetic stimulation, such as epidural or spinal anaesthesia, may attenuate these changes.

2. Stimulation of pituitary hormone release (see below).

The endocrine response to surgery

Surgery leads to complex changes in the endocrine mechanisms that maintain the body's fluid balance and substrate metabolism, with changes occurring to the circulating concentrations of many hormones following injury (Table 1.2). This occurs either as a result of direct gland stimulation or because of changes in feedback mechanisms.

Consequences of the metabolic response to injury

Hypovolaemia

Reduced circulating volume often characterizes moderate to severe injury, and can occur for a number of reasons (Table 1.3):

- Loss of blood, electrolyte-containing fluid or water.
- Sequestration of protein-rich fluid into the interstitial space, traditionally termed "third space loss", due to increased vascular permeability. This typically lasts 24–48 hours, with the extent (many litres) and duration (weeks or even months) of this loss greater following burns, infection, or ischaemia–reperfusion injury.

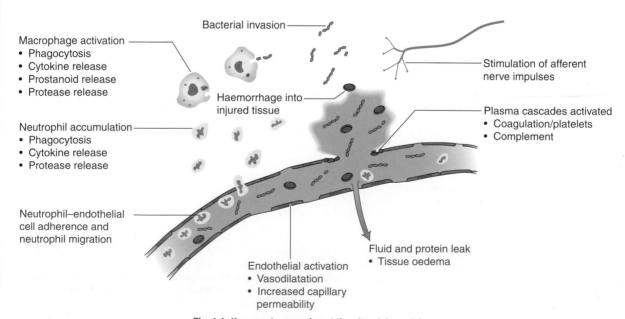

Macrophage activation
- Phagocytosis
- Cytokine release
- Prostanoid release
- Protease release

Bacterial invasion

Stimulation of afferent nerve impulses

Haemorrhage into injured tissue

Plasma cascades activated
- Coagulation/platelets
- Complement

Neutrophil accumulation
- Phagocytosis
- Cytokine release
- Protease release

Neutrophil–endothelial cell adherence and neutrophil migration

Endothelial activation
- Vasodilatation
- Increased capillary permeability

Fluid and protein leak
- Tissue oedema

Fig. 1.1 Key events occurring at the site of tissue injury.

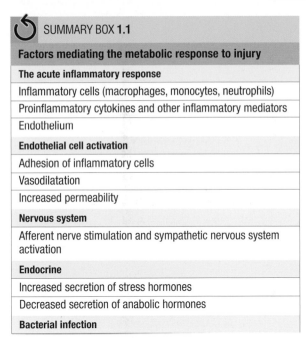

SUMMARY BOX 1.1

Factors mediating the metabolic response to injury

The acute inflammatory response

Inflammatory cells (macrophages, monocytes, neutrophils)

Proinflammatory cytokines and other inflammatory mediators

Endothelium

Endothelial cell activation

Adhesion of inflammatory cells

Vasodilatation

Increased permeability

Nervous system

Afferent nerve stimulation and sympathetic nervous system activation

Endocrine

Increased secretion of stress hormones

Decreased secretion of anabolic hormones

Bacterial infection

Table 1.3 Causes of fluid loss following surgery and trauma

Nature of fluid	Mechanism	Contributing factors
Blood	Haemorrhage	Site and magnitude of tissue injury Poor surgical haemostasis Abnormal coagulation
Electrolyte-containing fluids	Vomiting	Anaesthesia/analgesia (e.g. opiates) Ileus
	Nasogastric drainage	Ileus Gastric surgery
	Diarrhoea	Antibiotic-related infection Enteral feeding
	Sweating	Pyrexia
Water	Evaporation	Prolonged exposure of viscera during surgery
Plasma-like fluid	Capillary leak/sequestration in tissues	Acute inflammatory response Infection Ischaemia–reperfusion syndrome

Decreased circulating volume will reduce oxygen and nutrient delivery and so increase healing and recovery times. The neuroendocrine responses to hypovolaemia attempt to restore normovolaemia and maintain perfusion to vital organs.

Fluid-conserving measures

Oliguria, together with sodium and water retention – primarily due to the release of antidiuretic hormone (ADH) and aldosterone – is common after major surgery or injury and may persist even after normal circulating volume has been restored (Fig. 1.2).

Secretion of ADH from the posterior pituitary is increased in response to:

- Afferent nerve impulses from the site of injury
- Atrial stretch receptors (responding to reduced volume) and the aortic and carotid baroreceptors (responding to reduced pressure)

- Increased plasma osmolality (principally the result of an increase in sodium ions) detected by hypothalamic osmoreceptors
- Input from higher centres in the brain (responding to pain, emotion and anxiety).

ADH promotes the retention of free water (without electrolytes) by cells of the distal renal tubules and collecting ducts.

Aldosterone secretion from the adrenal cortex is increased by:

- Activation of the renin–angiotensin system. Renin is released from afferent arteriolar cells in the kidney in response to reduced blood pressure, tubuloglomerular feedback (signalling via the macula densa of the distal renal tubules in response to changes in electrolyte concentration) and activation of the renal sympathetic nerves. Renin

Table 1.2 Hormonal changes in response to surgery and trauma

	Pituitary	Adrenal	Pancreatic	Others
↑ secretion	Growth hormone (GH) Adrenocorticotrophic hormone (ACTH) Prolactin Antidiuretic hormone / arginine vasopressin (ADH/AVP)	Adrenaline Cortisol Aldosterone	Glucagon	Renin Angiotensin
Unchanged	Thyroid-stimulating hormone (TSH) Luteinizing hormone (LH) Follicle-stimulating hormone (FSH)	–	–	–
↓ secretion	–	–	Insulin	Testosterone Oestrogen Thyroid hormones

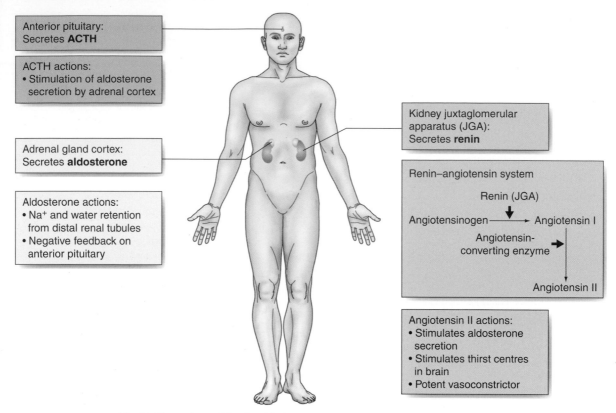

Fig. 1.2 The renin–angiotensin–aldosterone system. (ACTH = adrenocorticotrophic hormone)

converts circulating angiotensinogen to angiotensin (AT)-I. AT-I is converted by angiotensin-converting enzyme (ACE) in plasma and tissues (particularly the lung) to AT-II which causes arteriolar vasoconstriction and aldosterone secretion.

• Increased adrenocorticotropic hormone (ACTH) secretion by the anterior pituitary in response to hypovolaemia and hypotension via afferent nerve impulses from stretch receptors in the atria, aorta and carotid arteries. It is also raised by ADH.

• Direct stimulation of the adrenal cortex by hyponatraemia or hyperkalaemia.

Aldosterone increases the reabsorption of both sodium and water by distal renal tubular cells with the simultaneous excretion of hydrogen and potassium ions into the urine.

Increased ADH and aldosterone secretion following injury usually lasts 48–72 hours during which time urine volume is reduced and osmolality increased. Typically, urinary sodium excretion decreases to 10–20 mmol/24 hrs (normal 50–80 mmol/24 hrs) and potassium excretion increases to > 100 mmol/24 hrs (normal 50–80 mmol/24 hrs). Despite this, hypokalaemia is relatively rare because of a net efflux of potassium from cells. This typical pattern may be modified by fluid and electrolyte administration.

Blood flow-conserving measures

Hypovolaemia reduces cardiac preload which leads to a fall in cardiac output and a decrease in blood flow to the tissues and organs. Increased sympathetic activity results in a compensatory increase in cardiac output, peripheral vasoconstriction and a rise in blood pressure. Together with intrinsic organ autoregulation, these mechanisms act to try to ensure adequate tissue perfusion (Fig. 1.3).

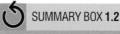
SUMMARY BOX **1.2**

Urinary changes in metabolic response to injury

↓ urine volume secondary to ↑ ADH and aldosterone release
↓ urinary sodium and ↑ urinary potassium secondary to ↑ aldosterone release
↑ urinary osmolality
↑ urinary nitrogen excretion due to the catabolic response to injury.

Increased energy metabolism and substrate cycling

The body requires energy to undertake physical work, generate heat (thermogenesis) and to meet basal metabolic requirements. Basal metabolic rate (BMR) comprises the energy required for maintenance of membrane polarization, substrate absorption and utilization, and the mechanical work of the heart and respiratory systems.

Although physical work usually decreases following surgery due to inactivity, overall energy expenditure may rise by 50% due to increased thermogenesis, fever and BMR (Fig. 1.4).

Thermogenesis: Patients are frequently pyrexial for 24–48 hours following injury (or infection) because pro-inflammatory cytokines (principally IL-1) reset temperature-regulating centres in the hypothalamus. BMR increases by about 10% for each 1°C increase in body temperature.

Basal metabolic rate: Injury leads to increased turnover in protein, carbohydrate and fat metabolism (see below). Whilst some of the increased activity might appear

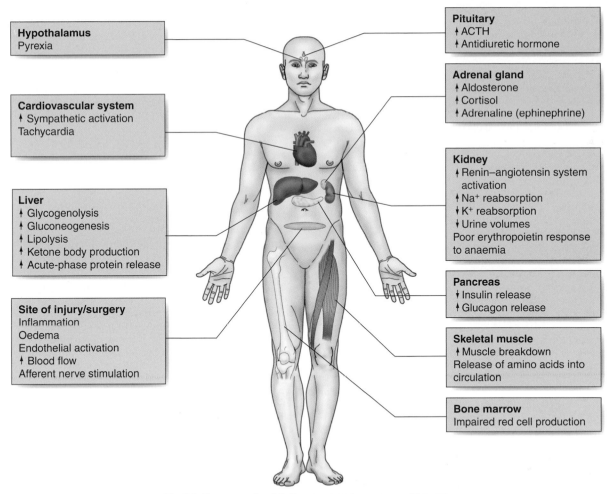

Fig. 1.3 Summary of metabolic responses to surgery and trauma.

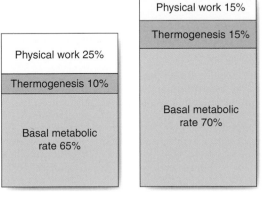

Healthy sedentary 70 kg man
- Total energy expenditure about 1800 kcal/day

24 hours following major surgery
- Total energy expenditure increased 10–30%
- Relative reduction in physical work due to inactivity
- Thermogenesis/heat energy increased by mild pyrexia
- Basal metabolic rate increased by raised enzyme and ion pump activity and increased cardiac work

Fig. 1.4 Components of body energy expenditure in health and following surgery.

metabolically futile (e.g. glucose–lactate cycling and simultaneous synthesis and degradation of triglycerides), it has probably evolved to allow the body to respond quickly to altering demands during times of extreme stress.

Catabolism and starvation

Catabolism is the breakdown of complex substances to their constituent parts (glucose, amino acids and fatty acids) which form substrates for metabolic pathways. Starvation occurs when intake is less than metabolic demand. Both usually occur simultaneously following severe injury or major surgery, with the clinical picture being determined by whichever predominates.

Catabolism

Carbohydrate, protein and fat catabolism is mediated by the increase in circulating catecholamines and proinflammatory cytokines, as well as the hormonal changes observed following surgery.

Carbohydrate metabolism

Catecholamines and glucagon stimulate glycogenolysis in the liver leading to the production of glucose and rapid glycogen depletion. Gluconeogenesis, the conversion of non-carbohydrate substrates (lactate, amino acids, glycerol) into glucose, occurs simultaneously. Catecholamines suppress insulin secretion and changes in the insulin receptor and intracellular signal pathways also result in a state of insulin resistance. The net result is hyperglycaemia and impaired cellular glucose uptake. While this provides glucose for the inflammatory and repair processes, severe hyperglycaemia may increase morbidity and mortality in surgical patients and glucose levels should be controlled in the perioperative setting.

Fat metabolism

Catecholamines, glucagon, cortisol and growth hormone all activate triglyceride lipases in adipose tissue such that 200–500 g of triglycerides may be broken down each day into glycerol and free fatty acids (FFAs) (lipolysis). Glycerol is a substrate for gluconeogenesis and FFAs can be metabolized in most tissues to form ATP. The brain is unable to use FFAs for energy production and almost exclusively metabolizes glucose. However, the liver can convert FFAs into ketone bodies which the brain can use when glucose is less available.

Protein metabolism

Skeletal muscle is broken down, releasing amino acids into the circulation. Amino acid metabolism is complex, but glucogenic amino acids (e.g. alanine, glycine and cysteine) can be utilized by the liver as a substrate for gluconeogenesis, producing glucose for re-export, while others are metabolized to pyruvate, acetyl CoA or intermediates in the Krebs cycle. Amino acids are also used in the liver as substrate for the 'acute-phase protein response'. This response involves increased production of one group of proteins (positive acute-phase proteins) and decreased production of another (negative acute-phase proteins) (Table 1.4). The acute-phase response is mediated by pro-inflammatory cytokines (notably IL-1, IL-6 and TNF-α) and although its function is not fully understood, it is thought to play a central role in host defence and the promotion of healing.

The mechanisms mediating muscle catabolism are incompletely understood, but inflammatory mediators and hormones (e.g. cortisol) released as part of the metabolic response to injury appear to play a central role. Minor surgery, with minimal metabolic response, is usually accompanied by little muscle catabolism. Major tissue injury is often associated with marked catabolism and loss of skeletal muscle, especially when factors enhancing the metabolic response (e.g. sepsis) are also present.

In health, the normal dietary intake of protein is 80–120 g per day (equivalent to 12–20 g nitrogen). Approximately 2 g of nitrogen are lost in faeces and 10–18 g in urine each day, mainly in the form of urea. During catabolism, nitrogen intake is often reduced but urinary losses increase markedly, reaching 20–30 g/day in patients with severe trauma, sepsis or burns. Following uncomplicated surgery, this negative nitrogen balance usually lasts 5–8

days, but in patients with sepsis, burns or conditions associated with prolonged inflammation (e.g. acute pancreatitis) it may persist for many weeks. Feeding cannot reverse severe catabolism and negative nitrogen balance, but the provision of protein and calories can attenuate the process. Even patients undergoing uncomplicated abdominal surgery can lose ~600 g muscle protein (1 g of protein is equivalent to ~5 g muscle), amounting to 6% of total body protein. This is usually regained within 3 months.

Starvation

This occurs following trauma and surgery for several reasons:

- Reduced nutritional intake because of the illness requiring treatment
- Fasting prior to surgery
- Fasting after surgery, especially to the gastrointestinal tract
- Loss of appetite associated with illness.

The response of the body to starvation can be described in two phases (Table 1.5).

Acute starvation is characterized by glycogenolysis and gluconeogenesis in the liver, releasing glucose for cerebral energy metabolism. Lipolysis releases FFAs for oxidation by other tissues and glycerol, a substrate for gluconeogenesis. These processes can sustain the normal energy requirements of the body (~1800 kcal/day for a 70 kg adult) for approximately 10 hours.

Chronic starvation is initially associated with muscle catabolism and the release of amino acids, which are converted to glucose in the liver, which also converts FFAs to ketone bodies. As described above, the brain adapts to utilize ketones rather than glucose and this allows greater dependency on fat metabolism, so reducing muscle protein and nitrogen loss by about 25%. Energy requirements fall to about 1500 kcal/day and this 'compensated starvation' continues until fat stores are depleted when the individual, often close to death, begins to break down muscle again.

Changes in red blood cell synthesis and coagulation

Anaemia is common after major surgery or trauma because of bleeding, haemodilution following treatment with crystalloid or colloid and impaired red cell production in bone marrow (because of low erythropoietin production by the kidney and reduced iron availability due to increased ferritin and reduced transferrin binding). Whether moderate anaemia confers a survival benefit following injury remains unclear, but actively correcting anaemia in non-bleeding patients after surgery or during critical illness does not improve outcomes.

Following tissue injury, the blood typically becomes hypercoagulable and this can significantly increase the risk of thromboembolism; reasons include:

- endothelial cell injury and activation with subsequent activation of coagulation cascades
- platelet activation in response to circulating mediators (e.g. adrenaline and cytokines)
- venous stasis secondary to dehydration and/or immobility
- increased concentrations of circulating procoagulant factors (e.g. fibrinogen)
- decreased concentrations of circulating anticoagulants (e.g. protein C).

Table 1.4 The acute-phase protein response

Positive acute-phase proteins (↑ after injury)
- C-reactive protein
- Haptoglobins
- Ferritin
- Fibrinogen
- α_1-Antitrypsin
- α_2-Macroglobulin
- Plasminogen

Negative acute-phase proteins (↓ after injury)
- Albumin
- Transferrin

Table 1.5 A comparison of nitrogen and energy losses in a catabolic state and starvation*

	Catabolic state	Acute starvation	Compensated starvation
Nitrogen loss (g/day)	20–25	14	3
Energy expenditure (kcal/day)	2200–2500	1800	1500

*Values are approximate and relate to a 70 kg man.

↻ SUMMARY BOX **1.3**

Physiological changes in catabolism

Carbohydrate metabolism

- ↑ Glycogenolysis
- ↑ Gluconeogenesis
- Insulin resistance of tissues
- Hyperglycaemia

Fat metabolism

- ↑ Lipolysis
- Free fatty acids used as energy substrate by tissues (except brain)
- Some conversion of free fatty acids to ketones in liver (used by brain)
- Glycerol converted to glucose in the liver

Protein metabolism

- ↑ Skeletal muscle breakdown
- Amino acids converted to glucose in liver and used as substrate for acute-phase proteins
- Negative nitrogen balance

Total energy expenditure is increased in proportion to injury severity and other modifying factors.

Progressive reduction in fat and muscle mass until stimulus for catabolism ends.

Factors modifying the metabolic response to injury

The magnitude of the metabolic response to injury depends on a number of different factors (Table 1.6) and can be reduced through the use of minimally invasive techniques, prevention of bleeding and hypothermia, prevention and treatment of infection and the use of locoregional anaesthesia. Factors that may influence the magnitude of the metabolic response to surgery and injury are summarised in table 1.6.

Anabolism

Anabolism involves regaining weight, restoring skeletal muscle mass and replenishing fat stores. Anabolism is unlikely to occur until the processes associated with catabolism, such as the release of pro-inflammatory mediators, have subsided. This point is often temporally associated with obvious clinical improvement in patients, who feel subjectively better and regain their appetite. Hormones contributing to this process include insulin, growth hormone, insulin-like growth factors, androgens and the 17-ketosteroids. Adequate nutritional support and early mobilization also appear to be important in promoting enhanced recovery after surgery (ERAS).

Table 1.6 Factors associated with the magnitude of the metabolic response to injury

Factor	Comment
Patient-related factors	
Genetic predisposition	Gene subtype for inflammatory mediators determines individual response to injury and/or infection
Coexisting disease	Cancer and/or pre-existing inflammatory disease may influence the metabolic response
Drug treatments	Anti-inflammatory or immunosuppressive therapy (e.g. steroids) may alter response
Nutritional status	Malnourished patients have impaired immune function and/or important substrate deficiencies. Malnutrition prior to surgery is associated with poor outcomes
Acute surgical/trauma-related factors	
Severity of injury	Greater tissue damage is associated with a greater metabolic response
Nature of injury	Some types of tissue injury cause a disproportionate metabolic response (e.g. major burns),
Ischaemia–reperfusion injury	Reperfusion of ischaemic tissues can trigger an injurious inflammatory cascade that further injures organs.
Temperature	Extreme hypo- and hyperthermia modulate the metabolic response
Infection	Infection is associated with an exaggerated response to injury. It can result in systemic inflammatory response syndrome (SIRS), sepsis or septic shock.
Anaesthetic techniques	The use of certain drugs, such as opioids, can reduce the release of stress hormones. Regional anaesthetic techniques (epidural or spinal anaesthesia) can reduce the release of cortisol, adrenaline and other hormones, but has little effect on cytokine responses

FLUID AND ELECTROLYTE BALANCE

In addition to reduced oral fluid intake in the perioperative period, fluid and electrolyte balance may be altered in the surgical patient for several reasons:

- ADH and aldosterone secretion as described above
- Loss from the gastrointestinal tract (e.g. bowel preparation, ileus, stomas, fistulas)
- Insensible losses (e.g. sweating secondary to fever)
- Third space losses as described above
- Surgical drains
- Medications (e.g. diuretics)
- Underlying chronic illness (e.g. cardiac failure, portal hypertension).

Careful monitoring of fluid balance and thoughtful replacement of net fluid and electrolyte losses is therefore imperative in the perioperative period.

Normal water and electrolyte balance

Water forms about 60% of total body weight in men and 55% in women. Approximately two-thirds is intracellular, one-third extracellular. Extracellular water is distributed between the plasma and the interstitial space (Fig. 1.5A).

The differential distribution of ions across cell membranes is essential for normal cellular function. The principal extracellular ions are sodium, chloride and bicarbonate, with the osmolality of extracellular fluid (normally 275–295 mOsmol/kg) determined primarily by sodium and chloride ion concentrations. The major intracellular ions are potassium, magnesium, phosphate and sulphate (Fig. 1.5B).

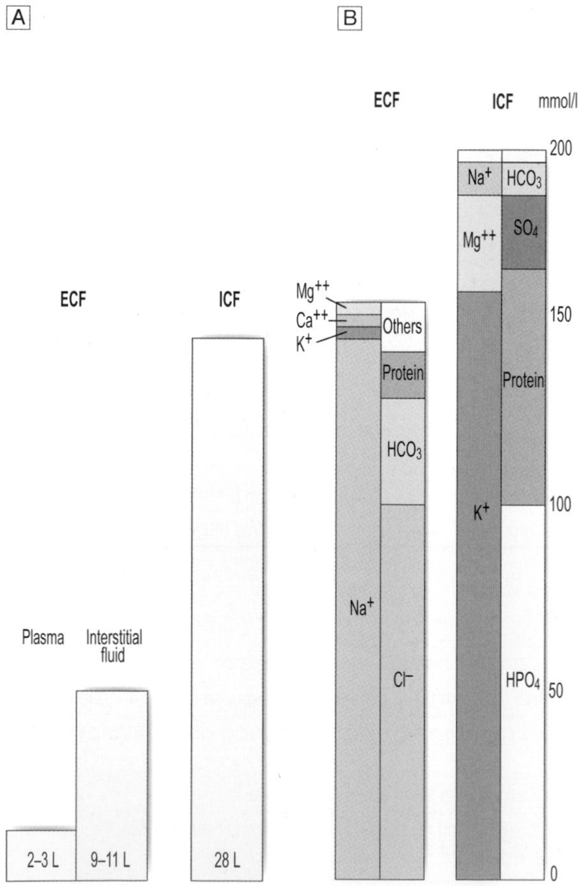

The distribution of fluid between the intra- and extravascular compartments is dependent upon the oncotic pressure of plasma and the permeability of the endothelium, both of which may alter following surgery as described above. Plasma oncotic pressure is primarily determined by albumin.

The control of body water and electrolytes has been described above. Aldosterone and ADH facilitate sodium and water retention while atrial natriuretic peptide (ANP), released in response to hypervolaemia and atrial distension, stimulates sodium and water excretion.

In health (Table 1.7):

- 2500 to 3000 ml of fluid is lost via the kidneys, gastrointestinal tract and through evaporation from the skin and respiratory tract
- fluid losses are largely replaced through eating and drinking
- a further 200–300 ml of water is provided endogenously every 24 hours by the oxidation of carbohydrate and fat.

In the absence of sweating, almost all sodium loss is via the urine and, under the influence of aldosterone, this can fall to 10–20 mmol/24 hrs. Potassium is also excreted mainly via the kidney with a small amount (10 mmol/day) lost via the gastrointestinal tract. In severe potassium deficiency, losses can be reduced to about 20 mmol/day, but increased aldosterone secretion, high urine flow rates and metabolic alkalosis all limit the ability of the kidneys to conserve potassium and predispose to hypokalaemia.

In adults, the normal daily fluid requirement is ~30–35 ml/kg (~2500 ml/day). Newborn babies and children contain proportionately more water than adults. The daily maintenance fluid requirement at birth is about 75 ml/kg, increasing to 150 ml/kg during the first weeks of life. After the first month of life, fluid requirements decrease and the '4/2/1' formula can be used to estimate maintenance fluid requirements: the first 10 kg of body weight requires 4 ml/kg/h; the next 10 kg 2 ml/kg/h; thereafter each kg of body requires 1 ml/kg/h. The estimated maintenance fluid requirements of a 35 kg child would therefore be:

$$(10 \times 4) + (10 \times 2) + (15 \times 1) = 75 \, \text{ml/h}.$$

The daily requirement for both sodium and potassium in children is about 2–3 mmol/kg.

Fig. 1.5 Distribution of fluid and electrolytes between the intracellular and extracellular fluid compartments. **A** Approximate volumes of water distribution in a 70 kg man. **B** Cations and anions.

Table 1.7 **Normal daily losses and requirements for fluids and electrolytes**

	Volume (ml)	Na⁺ (mmol)	K⁺ (mmol)
Urine	2000	80	60
Insensible losses from skin and respiratory tract	700	–	–
Faeces	300	–	10
Less water created from metabolism	300	–	–
Total	2700	80	70

Assessing losses in the surgical patient

Only by accurately estimating (Table 1.8) and, where possible, directly measuring fluid and electrolyte losses can appropriate therapy be administered.

Insensible fluid losses

Hyperventilation increases insensible water loss via the respiratory tract, but this increase is not usually large unless the normal mechanisms for humidifying inhaled air (the nasal passages and upper airways) are compromised. This occurs in intubated patients or in those receiving non-humidified high-flow oxygen. In these situations inspired gases should be humidified routinely.

Pyrexia increases water loss from the skin by approximately 200 ml/day for each 1°C rise in temperature. Sweating may increase fluid loss by up to 1 litre/hour but these losses are difficult to quantify. Sweat also contains significant amounts of sodium (20–70 mmol/l) and potassium (10 mmol/l).

The effect of surgery

The stress response

As discussed above, ADH leads to water retention and a reduction in urine volume for 2–3 days following major surgery. Aldosterone conserves both sodium and water, further contributing to oliguria. As a result, urinary sodium excretion falls while urinary potassium excretion increases, predisposing to hypokalaemia. Excessive and/or inappropriate intravenous fluid replacement therapy can easily lead to hyponatraemia and hypokalaemia.

'Third-space' losses

As described above, if tissue injury is severe, widespread and/or prolonged then the loss of water, electrolytes and colloid particles into the interstitial space can amount to many litres and can significantly decrease circulating blood volume following trauma and surgery.

Loss from the gastrointestinal tract

The magnitude and content of gastrointestinal fluid losses depends on the site of loss (Table 1.9):

- *Intestinal obstruction.* In general, the higher an obstruction occurs in the intestine, the greater the fluid loss because fluids secreted by the upper gastrointestinal tract fail to reach the absorptive areas of the distal jejunum and ileum.
- *Paralytic ileus.* This condition, in which propulsion in the small intestine ceases, has numerous causes. The commonest is probably handling of the bowel during surgery, which usually resolves within 1–2 days of the operation. Occasionally, paralytic ileus persists for longer, and in this case other causes should be sought and corrected if possible. During paralytic ileus the stomach should be decompressed using nasogastric

tube drainage, and fluid losses monitored by measuring nasogastric aspirates.
- *Intestinal fistula.* As with obstruction, fistulae occurring high in the gut are associated with the greatest fluid and electrolyte losses. As well as volume, it may be useful to measure the electrolyte content of the fluid lost in order to determine the fluid replacement required.
- *Diarrhoea.* Patients may present with diarrhoea or develop it during the perioperative period. Fluid and electrolyte losses may be considerable.

Intravenous fluid administration

When choosing and administering intravenous fluids (Table 1.10) it is important to consider:

- what fluid deficiencies are present
- the fluid compartments requiring replacement
- any electrolyte disturbances present
- which fluid is most appropriate.

Types of intravenous fluid

Crystalloids

Dextrose 5% contains 5 g of dextrose (D-glucose) per 100 ml of water. This glucose is rapidly metabolized and the remaining free water distributes rapidly and evenly throughout the body's fluid compartments. So, shortly after the intravenous administration of 1000 ml 5% dextrose solution, about 670 ml of water will be added to the intracellular fluid compartment (IFC) and about 330 ml of water to the extracellular fluid compartment (EFC), of which about 70 ml will be intravascular (Fig. 1.6). Dextrose solutions are therefore of little value as resuscitation fluids to expand intravascular volume. More concentrated dextrose solutions (10%, 20% and 50%) are available, but these solutions are irritant to veins and their use is largely limited to the management of diabetic patients or patients with hypoglycaemia.

Table 1.9 The approximate daily volumes (ml) and electrolyte concentrations (mmol/l) of various gastrointestinal fluids*

	Volume	Na+	K+	Cl-	HCO3-
Plasma	–	140	5	100	25
Gastric secretions	2500	50	10	80	40
Intestinal fluid (upper)	3000	140	10	100	25
Bile and pancreatic secretions	1500	140	5	80	60
Mature ileostomy	500	50	5	20	25
Diarrhoea (inflammatory)	–	110	40	100	40

*If gastrointestinal loss continues for more than 2–3 days, samples of fluid and urine should be collected regularly and sent to the laboratory for measurement of electrolyte content.

Table 1.8 Sources of fluid loss in surgical patients

	Typical losses per 24 hrs	Factors modifying volume
Insensible losses	700–2000 ml	↑ Losses associated with pyrexia, sweating and use of non-humidified oxygen
Urine	1000–2500 ml	↓ With aldosterone and ADH secretion; ↑ With diuretic therapy
Gut	300–1000 ml	↑ Losses with obstruction, ileus, fistulae and diarrhoea (may increase substantially)
Third-space losses	0–4000 ml	↑ Losses with greater extent of surgery and tissue trauma

Table 1.10 Composition of commonly administered intravenous fluids

	Na⁺ (mmol/l)	K⁺ (mmol/l)	Cl⁻ (mmol/l)	HCO₃⁻ (mmol/l)	Ca²⁺ (mmol/l)	Mg²⁺ (mmol/l)	Oncotic pressure (mmH₂O)	Typical plasma half-life	pH
5% dextrose	–	–	–	–	–		0	–	4.0
0.9% NaCl	154	0	154	0	0		0	–	5.0
Ringer's lactate (Hartmann's solution)	131	5	112	29*	1	1	0	–	6.5
Haemaccel (succinylated gelatin)	145	5.1	145	0	6.25		370	5 hours	7.4
Gelofusine (polygeline gelatin)	154	0.4	125	0	0.4	0.4	465	4 hours	7.4
Hetastarch	154	0	154	0	0		310	17 days	5.5
Human albumin solution 4.5% (HAS)	150	0	120	0	0		275	–	7.4

*The lactate present in Ringer's lactate solution is rapidly metabolized in the liver. This generates bicarbonate ions. Bicarbonate cannot be directly added to the solutions because it is unstable (tends to precipitate).

Sodium chloride 0.9% and Hartmann's solution are isotonic solutions of electrolytes in water. Sodium chloride 0.9% (also known as normal saline) contains 9 g of sodium chloride dissolved in 1000 ml of water; Hartmann's solution (also known as Ringer's lactate) has a more physiological composition, containing lactate, potassium and calcium in addition to sodium and chloride ions. Both normal saline and Hartmann's solution have an osmolality similar to that of extracellular fluid (about 300 mOsm/l) and after intravenous administration they distribute rapidly throughout the ECF compartment (Fig. 1.6). Isotonic crystalloids are appropriate for correcting EFC losses (e.g. gastrointestinal tract or sweating) and for the initial resuscitation of intravascular volume, although only about 25% remains in the intravascular space after redistribution (often less than 30–60 minutes).

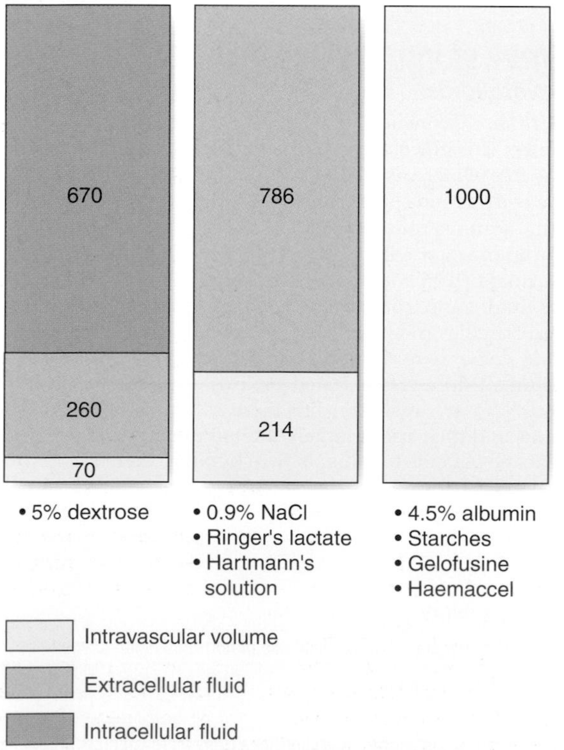

Balanced solutions such as Ringers lactate, closely match the composition of extracellular fluid by providing physiological concentrations of sodium and lactate in place of bicarbonate, which is unstable in solution. After administration the lactate is metabolised, resulting in bicarbonate generation. These solutions decrease the risk of hyperchloraemia, which can occur following large volumes of fluids with higher sodium and chloride concentrations. Hyperchloraemic acidosis can develop in these situations, which is associated with adverse patient outcomes and may cause renal impairment. Some colloid solutions are also produced with balanced electrolyte content.

Hypertonic saline solutions induce a shift of fluid from the IFC to the EFC so reducing brain water and increasing intravascular volume and serum sodium concentration. Potential indications include the treatment of cerebral oedema and raised intracranial pressure, hyponatraemic seizures and 'small volume' resuscitation of hypovolaemic shock.

Colloids

Colloid solutions contain particles that exert an oncotic pressure and may occur naturally (e.g. albumin) or be synthetically modified (e.g. gelatins, hydroxyethyl starches [HES], dextrans). When administered, colloid remains largely within the intravascular space until the colloid particles are removed by the reticuloendothelial system. The intravascular half-life is usually between 6 and 24 hours and such solutions are therefore appropriate for fluid resuscitation. Thereafter, the electrolyte-containing solution distributes throughout the EFC.

Synthetic colloids are more expensive than crystalloids and have variable side effect profiles. Recognized risks include coagulopathy, reticuloendothelial system dysfunction, pruritis and anaphylactic reactions. HES in particular appears associated with a risk of renal failure when used for resuscitation in patients with septic shock.

The theoretical advantage of colloids over crystalloids is that, as they remain in the intravascular space for several hours, smaller volumes are required. However, overall, current evidence suggests that crystalloid and colloid are equally effective for the correction of hypovolaemia (EBM 1.1).

670
260
70

786
214

1000

• 5% dextrose

• 0.9% NaCl
• Ringer's lactate
• Hartmann's solution

• 4.5% albumin
• Starches
• Gelofusine
• Haemaccel

Intravascular volume

Extracellular fluid

Intracellular fluid

Fig. 1.6 Distribution of different fluids in the body fluid compartments 30–60 minutes after rapid intravenous infusion of 1000 ml.

EBM **1.1 Crystalloid vs colloid to treat intravascular hypovolaemia**

'There is no evidence that resuscitation with colloids reduces the risk of death, compared to resuscitation with crystalloids, in patients with trauma, burns or following surgery.'

Perel P. et al., Cochrane Database Syst Rev. 2007 Oct 17;(4):CD000567

'The use of 4% albumin for intravascular volume resuscitation in critically ill patients is associated with similar outcomes to the use of normal saline.'

Finfer S. et al. The SAFE study. New Engl J Med 2004; 350:2247–2256.

Maintenance fluid requirements

Under normal conditions, adult daily sodium requirements (80 mmol) may be provided by the administration of 500–1000 ml of 0.9% sodium chloride. The remaining water requirement to maintain fluid balance (2000–2500 ml) is typically provided as 5% dextrose. Daily potassium requirements (60–80 mmol) are usually met by adding potassium chloride to maintenance fluids, but the amount added can be titrated to measured plasma concentrations. Potassium should not be administered at a rate greater than 10–20 mmol/h except in severe potassium deficiency (see section on hypokalaemia below) and, in practice, 20 mmol aliquots are added to alternate 500 ml bags of fluid.

An example of a suitable 24-hour fluid prescription for an uncomplicated patient is shown in Table 1.11; the process of adjusting this for a hypothetical patient with an ileus is shown in Table 1.12.

Table 1.11 Provision of normal 24-hour fluid and electrolyte requirements by intravenous infusion

Intravenous fluid	Additive	Duration (hrs)
500 ml 0.9% NaCl	20 mmol KCl	4
500 ml 5% dextrose	–	4
500 ml 5% dextrose	20 mmol KCl	4
500 ml 0.9% NaCl	–	4
500 ml 5% dextrose	20 mmol KCl	4
500 ml 5% dextrose	–	4

Table 1.12 Estimating fluid (ml) and electrolyte (mmol) requirements in a patient with ileus*

	Volume (ml)	Na$^+$	K$^+$
Urine	1500	80	60
Nasogastric aspirate	2000	240	20
Insensible loss	800	–	–
Minus endogenous water	–300	–	–
Net losses/requirements	4000	320	80

2 litres of normal saline would supply 300 mmol of Na$^+$.
2 litres of 5% dextrose would supply water.
The required 60–80 mmol of K$^+$ could be added as 20 mmol to alternate 500 ml bags.

*Assuming that the patient is in electrolyte balance and is losing 2 litres/day as nasogastric aspirate and 1.5 litres/day as urine, 24-hour losses can be calculated as shown.

In patients requiring intravenous fluid replacement for more than 3–4 days, supplementation of magnesium and phosphate may also be required as guided by direct measurement of plasma concentrations. The provision of parenteral nutrition should also be considered in this situation.

Treatment of postoperative hypovolaemia and/or hypotension

Hypovolaemia is common in the postoperative period and may present with one or more of the following: tachycardia, cold extremities, pallor, clammy skin, collapsed peripheral veins, oliguria and/or hypotension. Hypotension is more likely in hypovolaemic patients receiving epidural analgesia as the associated sympathetic blockade disrupts compensatory vasoconstriction. Intravascular volume should be rapidly restored with a series of fluid boluses (e.g. 250–500 ml) with the clinical response being assessed after each bolus (see below).

Specific water and electrolyte abnormalities

Sodium and water

Sodium is the major determinant of ECF osmolality (or tonicity) and so largely determines the relative ECF and ICF volumes. Hypo- and hypernatraemia reflect an imbalance between the sodium and, more often, water content of the ECF.

Water depletion

A decrease in total body water of 1–2% (350–700 ml) causes an increase in blood osmolarity and this stimulates brain osmoreceptors and the sensation of thirst. Clinically obvious dehydration, with thirst, a dry tongue and loss of skin turgor, indicates at least 4–5% deficiency of total body water (1500–2000 ml). Pure water depletion is uncommon in surgical practice, and is usually combined with sodium loss. The most frequent causes are inadequate intake or excessive gastrointestinal losses.

Water excess

For reasons explained above this is common in patients who receive large volumes of intravenous 5% dextrose in the early postoperative period. Such patients have an increased extracellular volume and are commonly hyponatraemic (see below). The increase in extracellular volume can be difficult to detect clinically as patients with water excess usually remain well and oedema may not be evident until the extracellular volume has increased by more than 4 litres. In patients with poor cardiac function or renal failure, water accumulation can result in pulmonary oedema.

Hypernatraemia

Hypernatraemia (Na$^+$ > 145 mmol/l) results from either water (or hypotonic fluid) loss or sodium gain. Water loss is commonly caused by reduced water intake, vomiting, diarrhoea, diuresis, burns, sweating and insensible losses from the respiratory tract. It is typically associated with a low extracellular fluid volume (hypovolaemia). In contrast, sodium gain is usually caused by excess sodium administration in hypertonic intravenous fluids and is typically associated with hypervolaemia.

Hypovolaemic hypernatraemia is treated with isotonic crystalloid to rapidly restore intravascular volume followed by the more gradual administration of water to correct the relative water deficit. The latter can be administered enterally (oral or nasogastric tube) or intravenously in the form of 5% dextrose. Cells, particularly brain cells, adapt to a high sodium concentration in extracellular fluid, and once this adaptation has occurred, rapid correction of severe hypernatraemia can result in a rapid rise in intracellular volume, cerebral oedema, seizures and permanent neurological injury. To reduce the risk of cerebral oedema, free water deficits should be replaced slowly with the sodium being corrected at a rate less than 0.5 mmol/h.

Hyponatraemia

Hyponatraemia ($Na^+ < 135$ mmol/l) can occur in the presence of decreased, normal or increased extracellular volume. The commonest cause is the administration of hypotonic intravenous fluids to replace sodium-rich fluid losses from the gastrointestinal tract or when excessive water (as intravenous 5% dextrose) is administered in the postoperative period. Other causes include diuretic use and the syndrome of inappropriate ADH secretion (SIADH). Co-morbidities associated with secondary hyperaldosteronism, such as cirrhosis and congestive cardiac failure, are potential contributing factors.

Treatment depends on correct identification of the cause:

- If ECF volume is normal or increased, the most likely cause is excessive intravenous water administration and this will correct spontaneously if water intake is reduced. Although less common in surgical patients, inappropriate ADH secretion promotes the renal tubular reabsorption of water independently of sodium concentration, resulting in inappropriately concentrated urine (osmolality > 100 mOsm/l) in the face of hypotonic plasma (osmolality < 290 mOsm/l). The urine osmolality helps to distinguish inappropriate ADH secretion from excessive water administration.
- In patients with decreased ECF volume, hyponatraemia usually indicates combined water and sodium deficiency. This is most frequently the result of diuresis, diarrhoea or adrenal insufficiency and will correct if adequate 0.9% sodium chloride is administered.

The most serious clinical manifestation of hyponatraemia is a metabolic encephalopathy resulting from the shift of water into brain cells and cerebral oedema. This is more likely in severe hyponatraemia ($Na^+ < 120$ mmol/l) and is associated with confusion, seizures and coma. Rapid correction of sodium concentration can precipitate an irreversible demyelinating condition known as central pontine myelinolysis and to avoid this, sodium concentration should not increase by more than 0.5 mmol/h. This can usually be achieved by the cautious administration of isotonic (0.9%) sodium chloride, occasionally combined with the use of a loop diuretic (e.g. furosemide). Hypertonic saline solutions are rarely indicated and can be dangerous.

Potassium

As about 98% of total body potassium (around 3500 mmol) is intracellular, serum potassium concentration (normally 3.5–5 mmol/l) is a poor indicator of total body potassium. However, small changes in extracellular levels do reflect a significant change in the ratio of intra- to extracellular potassium and this has profound effects on the function of the cardiovascular and neuromuscular systems.

Acidosis reduces Na^+/K^+-ATPase activity and results in a net efflux of potassium from cells and hyperkalaemia. Conversely, alkalosis results in an influx of potassium into cells and hypokalaemia. These abnormalities are exacerbated by renal compensatory mechanisms that correct acid–base balance at the expense of potassium homeostasis.

Hyperkalaemia

This is a potentially life-threatening condition that can be caused by exogenous administration of potassium, the release of potassium from cells (transcellular shift) as a

SUMMARY BOX 1.4

Aetiology of hyper- and hyponatraemia

Hypernatraemia

Hypovolaemic
- ↓ oral intake (e.g. fasting, ↓ conscious level) *
- Nausea and vomiting*
- Diarrhoea*
- ↑ Insensible losses (↑ sweating and/or ↑ respiratory tract losses)
- Severe burns*
- Diuresis (e.g. glycosuria, use of osmotic diuretics)

Euvolaemic
- Diabetes insipidus – central or nephrogenic

Hypervolaemic
- Excessive sodium load (hypertonic saline, TPN, sodium bicarbonate)
- ↑Mineralocorticoid activity (e.g. Conn's syndrome or Cushing's disease)

Hyponatraemia

Low extracellular fluid volume
- Diarrhoea*
- Diuretic use*
- Adrenal insufficiency
- Salt-losing renal disease

Normal extracellular fluid volume
- Syndromes of inappropriate ADH secretion (SIADH)
- Hypothyroidism
- Psychogenic polydipsia

Increased extracellular fluid volume
- Excessive water administration*
- Secondary hyperaldosteronism (cirrhosis, cardiac failure)
- Renal failure.

*Causes commonly encountered in the surgical patient are denoted with an asterisk.

result of tissue damage or changes in the Na^+/K^+-ATPase function, or impaired renal excretion.

Mild hyperkalaemia ($K^+ < 6$ mmol/l) is often asymptomatic, but as serum levels rise there is progressive slowing of electrical conduction in the heart and the development of significant cardiac arrhythmias. All patients suspected of having hyperkalaemia should have an ECG for this reason. Tall 'tented' T-waves in the precordial leads are the earliest ECG changes observed, but as hyperkalaemia progresses more significant ECG changes occur, with flattening (or loss) of the P waves, a prolonged PR interval, widening of the QRS complex and eventually, asystole. Severe hyperkalaemia ($K^+ > 7$ mmol/l) requires immediate treatment to prevent this (Table 1.13).

Hypokalaemia

This is a common disorder in surgical patients. Dietary intake of potassium is normally 60–80 mmol/day. Under normal conditions, the majority of potassium loss (> 85%) is via the kidneys and maintenance of potassium balance largely depends on normal renal tubular regulation. Potassium depletion sufficient to cause a fall of 1 mmol/l in serum levels typically requires a loss of ~100–200 mmol of potassium from total body stores. Potassium excretion is increased by metabolic alkalosis, diuresis, increased aldosterone release and increased losses from the gastrointestinal tract – all of which occur commonly in the surgical patient.

Table 1.13 Management of severe hyperkalaemia (K⁺ >7 mmol/l)

1. Identify and treat cause. Monitor ECG until potassium concentration controlled.	
2. 10 ml 10% calcium gluconate iv over 3 mins, repeated after 5 min if no response	Antagonizes the membrane actions of ↑ K⁺ reducing the risk of ventricular arrhythmias
3. 50 ml 50% dextrose + 10 units short-acting insulin over 2–3 mins. Start infusion of 10–20% dextrose at 50–100 ml/h	Increases transcellular shift of K⁺ of into cells
4. Regular salbutamol nebulizers	Increases transcellular shift of K⁺ of into cells
5. Consider oral or rectal calcium resonium (ion exchange resin)	Facilitates K⁺ clearance across gastrointestinal mucosa. More effective in non-acute cases of hyperkalaemia
6. Renal replacement therapy	Haemodialysis is the most effective medical intervention to lower K⁺ rapidly

SUMMARY BOX 1.5

Hyper- and hypokalaemia

Hyperkalaemia	Hypokalaemia
Consequences	
• Arrhythmias (tented T waves, ↓ HR, heart block, broadened QRS, asystole) • Muscle weakness • Ileus	• ECG changes (flattened T-waves, U-waves, ectopics) • Muscle weakness and myalgia
Causes	
Excess intravenous or oral intake	**Inadequate intake***
Transcellular shift – efflux of potassium from cells	**Gastrointestinal tract losses**
• Metabolic acidosis* • Massive blood transfusion* • Rhabdomyolysis (e.g. crush and/or compartment syndromes)* • Massive tissue damage (e.g. ischaemic bowel or liver)* • Drugs (e.g. digoxin, β-receptor antagonists)	• Vomiting* • Gastric aspiration/drainage* • Fistulae* • Diarrhoea* • Ileus* • Intestinal obstruction* • Potassium-secreting villous adenoma*
Impaired excretion	**Urinary losses**
• Acute renal failure* • Chronic renal failure • Drugs (ACE inhibitors, spironolactone, NSAIDs) • Adrenal insufficiency (Addison's disease).	• Metabolic alkalosis* • Hyperaldosteronism* • Diuretics* • Renal tubular disorders (e.g. Bartter's syndrome, renal tubular acidoses, drug-induced)
	Transcellular shift–influx of potassium into cells • Metabolic alkalosis* • Drugs* (e.g. insulin, β-agonists, adrenaline).

*Common causes in the surgical patient are denoted by an asterisk.

Oral or nasogastric potassium replacement is safer than intravenous replacement and is the preferred route in asymptomatic patients with mild hypokalaemia. Severe (K⁺ < 2.5 mmol/l) or symptomatic hypokalaemia requires intravenous replacement. While replacement rates of up to 40 mmol/h may be used (with cardiac monitoring) in an emergency, there is a risk of serious cardiac arrhythmias and rates exceeding 20mmol/h should be avoided. Potassium solutions should never be administered as a bolus.

Other electrolyte disturbances

Calcium

Clinically significant abnormalities in calcium balance in the surgical patient are most frequently encountered in endocrine surgery (See Chapter 24 of the 5th edition).

Magnesium

Hypomagnesaemia is common in surgical patients who have restricted oral intake and who have been receiving intravenous fluids for several days. It is frequently associated with other electrolyte abnormalities, notably hypokalaemia, hypocalcaemia and hypophosphataemia. Hypomagnesaemia appears to be associated with a predisposition to tachyarrhythmias (most notable torsades de pointes and atrial fibrillation), but many of the clinical manifestations of magnesium depletion are non-specific (muscle weakness, muscle cramps, altered mentation, tremors, hyper-reflexia and generalized seizures). As magnesium is predominantly intracellular, serum magnesium levels poorly reflect total body stores. Despite this limitation, serum levels are frequently used to guide (oral or parenteral) magnesium supplementation.

Phosphate

Phosphate is a critical component in many biochemical processes such as ATP synthesis, cell signalling and nucleic acid synthesis. Hypophosphataemia is common in surgical patients and if severe (< 0.4 mmol/l) causes widespread cell dysfunction, muscle weakness, impaired myocardial contractility and reduced cardiac output. Most hypophosphataemia results from the shift of phosphate into cells and most commonly occurs in malnourished and/or alcoholic patients commencing enteral or parenteral nutrition. The increased carbohydrate load leads to insulin secretion and this results in the rapid intracellular uptake of glucose and phosphate together with magnesium and potassium. For reasons that remain unclear, these changes are accompanied by fluid retention and an increase in ECF volume (refeeding syndrome). To avoid this syndrome, feeding should be established gradually and accompanied by regular measurement and aggressive supplementation of serum electrolytes (phosphate, magnesium and potassium). Micronutrient (notably B vitamin) deficiencies should also be corrected. Phosphate can be supplemented orally or by slow intravenous infusion.

Acid–base balance

There are two broad types of acid–base disturbance: acidosis ('acidaemia' if plasma pH < 7.35 or H^+ > 45) or alkalosis ('alkalaemia' if plasma pH > 7.45 or H^+ < 35). Both acidosis and alkalosis may be respiratory or metabolic in origin. While some meaningful data pertaining to acid–base balance can be derived from the analysis of venous blood, accurate assessment of acid–base disturbance relies on the measurement of arterial blood gases. This is frequently coupled with measurement of blood lactate concentration. Arterial blood gas analysis is a straightforward technique, with samples typically taken from the radial artery (Fig. 1.7) and rapidly analysed by near-patient or laboratory-based machines.

Common disturbances of acid–base balance encountered in the surgical patient are discussed below.

Metabolic acidosis

Metabolic acidosis is characterized by an increase in plasma hydrogen ions in conjunction with a decrease in bicarbonate concentration. A rise in plasma hydrogen ion concentration stimulates chemoreceptors in the medulla resulting in a compensatory respiratory alkalosis (an increase in minute volume and a fall in P_aCO_2).

Metabolic acidosis can occur as a result of increased production of endogenous acid (e.g. lactic acid or ketone bodies) or increased loss of bicarbonate (e.g. intestinal fistula, hyperchloraemic acidosis). The commonest cause encountered in surgical practice is lactic acidosis resulting from hypovolaemia and impaired tissue oxygen delivery (see section on shock). Treatment is directed towards restoring circulating blood volume and tissue perfusion. Adequate resuscitation typically corrects the metabolic acidosis seen in this context.

SUMMARY BOX **1.6**

Metabolic acidosis

Common surgical causes

Lactic acidosis
- Shock (any cause)
- Severe hypoxaemia
- Severe haemorrhage/anaemia
- Liver failure

Accumulation of other acids
- Diabetic ketoacidosis
- Starvation ketoacidosis
- Acute or chronic renal failure
- Poisoning (ethylene glycol, methanol, salicylates)

Increased bicarbonate loss
- Diarrhoea
- Intestinal fistulae
- Hyperchloraemic acidosis

Acid–base findings

Acute uncompensated
- H^+ ions ↑
- P_aCO_2 ↔
- Actual HCO_3^- ↓
- Standard HCO_3^- ↓
- Base deficit < −2

With respiratory compensation (hyperventilation)
- H^+ ions ↔ (full compensation) ↑ (partial compensation)
- P_aCO_2 ↓
- Actual HCO_3^- ↓
- Standard HCO_3^- ↓

Metabolic alkalosis

Metabolic alkalosis is characterized by a decrease in plasma hydrogen ion concentration and an increase in bicarbonate concentration. A rise in P_aCO_2 occurs as a consequence of the rise in bicarbonate concentration, resulting in a compensatory respiratory acidosis.

Metabolic alkalosis is commonly associated with hypokalaemia and hypochloraemia. The kidney has an enormous capacity to generate bicarbonate ions and this is stimulated by chloride loss. This is a major contributor to the metabolic alkalosis seen following significant (chloride-rich) losses from the gastrointestinal tract, especially when combined with loss of acid from conditions such as gastric outlet obstruction. Hypokalaemia is often associated with metabolic alkalosis because of the transcellular shift of hydrogen

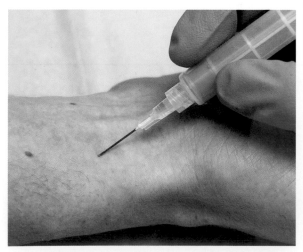

Fig. 1.7 A blood gas sample being taken from the radial artery under local anaesthesia.

ions shift into cells and because distal renal tubular cells retain potassium in preference to hydrogen ions.

The treatment of metabolic alkalosis involves adequate fluid replacement and the correction of electrolyte disturbances, notably hypokalaemia and hypochloraemia.

Respiratory acidosis

Respiratory acidosis is a common postoperative problem characterized by increased P_aCO_2, hydrogen ion and plasma bicarbonate concentrations. In the surgical patient, respiratory acidosis usually results from respiratory depression and hypoventilation. This is common on emergence from general anaesthesia and following excessive opiate administration. Occasionally, respiratory acidosis occurs in the context of pulmonary complications such as pneumonia. This is more usual in very sick patients or those with pre-existing respiratory disease. Patients with this cause of respiratory acidosis frequently require ventilatory support as the hypercapnia observed reflects inadequate respiratory muscle strength to cope with an increased work of breathing.

 SUMMARY BOX **1.7**

Metabolic alkalosis

Common surgical causes

Loss of sodium, chloride and water
- Vomiting
- Loss of gastric secretions
- Diuretic administration

Hypokalaemia

Acid–base findings

Acute uncompensated
- H^+ ions ↓
- P_aCO_2 ↔
- Actual HCO_3^- ↑
- Standard HCO_3^- ↑
- Base excess > + 2

With respiratory compensation (hypoventilation)
- H^+ ions ↔ (full compensation), ↓ (partial compensation)
- P_aCO_2 ↑
- Actual HCO_3^- ↑
- Standard HCO_3^- ↑

Respiratory alkalosis

Respiratory alkalosis is caused by excessive excretion of CO_2 as a result of hyperventilation. P_aCO_2 and hydrogen ion concentration decrease. Respiratory alkalosis is rarely chronic and usually does not need specific treatment. It usually corrects spontaneously when the precipitating condition resolves.

Mixed patterns of acid–base imbalance

Mixed patterns of acid–base disturbance are common, particularly in very sick patients. In this situation acid–base nomograms can be very useful in clarifying the contributing factors (Fig. 1.8).

SUMMARY BOX **1.8**

Respiratory acidosis

Common surgical causes

Central respiratory depression
- Opioid drugs
- Head injury or intracranial pathology

Pulmonary disease
- Severe asthma
- COPD
- Severe chest infection

Acid–base findings

Acute uncompensated
- H^+ ions ↑
- P_aCO_2 ↑
- Actual HCO_3^- ↔ or ↑
- Standard HCO_3^- ↔
- Base deficit < −2

With metabolic compensation (renal bicarbonate retention)
- H^+ ions ↔ (full compensation), ↑ (partial compensation)
- P_aCO_2 ↑
- Actual HCO_3^- ↑
- Standard HCO^- ↑↑

SUMMARY BOX **1.9**

Respiratory alkalosis

Common surgical causes

- Pain
- Apprehension/hysterical hyperventilation
- Pneumonia
- Central nervous system disorders (meningitis, encephalopathy)
- Pulmonary embolism
- Septicaemia
- Salicylate poisoning
- Liver failure

Acid–base findings

Acute uncompensated
- H^+ ions ↓
- P_aCO_2 ↓
- Actual HCO_3^- ↔ or ↓
- Standard HCO_3^- ↔
- Base excess > + 2

With metabolic compensation (renal bicarbonate excretion)
- H^+ ions ↔ (full compensation), ↓ (partial compensation)
- P_aCO_2 ↓
- Actual HCO_3^- ↓
- Standard HCO_3^- ↓

SHOCK

Definition

Shock exists when tissue oxygen delivery fails to meet the metabolic requirements of cells. An imbalance between oxygen delivery (DO_2) and oxygen demand can result from a

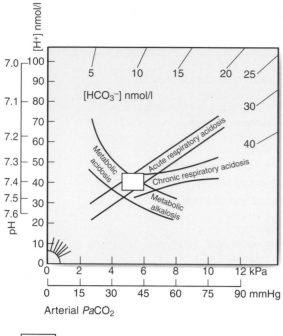

Normal range

95% Confidence limits

Fig. 1.8 Changes in blood [H⁺]. The rectangle indicates limits of normal reference ranges for [H⁺] and P_aCO_2. The bands represent 95% confidence limits of single disturbances in human blood in vivo. When the point obtained by plotting [H⁺] against P_aCO_2 does not fall within one of the labelled bands, compensation is incomplete or a mixed acid-base disturbance is present.

global reduction in oxygen delivery, maldistribution of blood flow, impaired oxygen utilization or an increase in tissue oxygen requirements. Left unchecked, shock will result in a fall in oxygen consumption (VO_2), anaerobic metabolism, tissue acidosis and cellular dysfunction leading to multiple organ dysfunction and ultimately death. Although shock is sometimes considered to be synonymous with hypotension, it is important to realise that tissue oxygen delivery may be inadequate even though the blood pressure and other vital signs remain normal.

Types of shock

Hypovolaemic shock

This is probably the commonest and most readily corrected cause of shock encountered in surgical practice and results from a reduction in intravascular volume secondary to the loss of blood (e.g. trauma, gastrointestinal haemorrhage), plasma (e.g. burns) or water and electrolytes (e.g. vomiting, diarrhoea, diabetic ketoacidosis) (Table 1.14).

 SUMMARY BOX **1.10**

Shock

Shock is an imbalance between oxygen delivery and oxygen demand. This results in cell dysfunction and ultimately cell death and multiple organ failure.

Table 1.14 Causes of haemorrhagic hypovolaemic shock

Gastrointestinal haemorrhage
- Oesophageal varices
- Oesophageal mucosal (Mallory–Weiss) tear
- Gastritis
- Gastric and duodenal ulceration
- Cancer
- Diverticula

Trauma
Ruptured aneurysm
Obstetric haemorrhage
- Ruptured ectopic pregnancy
- Placentia praevia
- Placental abruption
- Post-partum haemorrhage

Pulmonary haemorrhage
- Pulmonary embolus
- Cancer
- Cavitating lung lesions e.g. TB, aspergillosis
- Vasculitits

Major blood loss during surgery

Septic shock

Septic shock results from complex disturbances in oxygen delivery and oxygen consumption and can be defined as sepsis-induced hypotension (systolic BP < 90 mmHg, mean arterial blood pressure [MAP] < 70 mmHg) and/or tissue hypoperfusion (elevated lactate or oliguria) that persist despite adequate fluid resuscitation (~30 ml/kg) (Fig. 1.9).

Sepsis usually arises from a localized infection, with Gram-negative (38%) and (increasingly) Gram-positive (52%) bacteria being the most frequently identified pathogens. The commonest sites of infection leading to sepsis are the lungs (50–70%), abdomen (20–25%), urinary tract (7–10%) and skin.

Infection triggers a cytokine-mediated proinflammatory response that results in peripheral vasodilation, redistribution of blood flow, endothelial cell activation, increased vascular permeability and the formation of microthrombi within the microcirculation. Cardiac output typically increases in septic shock to compensate for the peripheral vasodilation. However, despite a global increase in oxygen delivery, microcirculatory dysfunction impairs oxygen delivery to the cells. Compounding disturbances in oxygen delivery, mitochondrial dysfunction blocks the normal bioenergetic pathways within the cell impairing oxygen utilization.

Cardiogenic shock

This occurs when the heart is unable to maintain a cardiac output sufficient to meet the metabolic requirements of the body (pump failure) and can be caused by myocardial infarction, arrhythmias, valve dysfunction, cardiac tamponade, massive pulmonary embolism, and tension pneumothorax.

Anaphylactic shock

This is a severe systemic hypersensitivity reaction following exposure to an agent (allergen) triggering the release of vasoactive mediators (histamine, kinins and prostaglandins) from basophils and mast cells. Anaphylaxis may be immunologically mediated (allergic anaphylaxis), when IgE, IgG or complement activation by immune complexes mediates the reaction, or non-immunologically mediated (non-allergic anaphylaxis). The clinical features of allergic

1

SUMMARY BOX 1.11

Sepsis – definitions

Systemic inflammatory response (SIRS)

SIRS is defined as 2 or more of the following criteria:
- Temperature > 38C° or < 36°C
- Heart rate > 90 beats per minute
- Respiratory rate > 20 per minute or P_aCO_2 < 4.5 kPa
- White cell count > 12 or < 4 × 10^9/l or > 10% immature neutrophils

Bacteraemia
- The presence of viable bacteria in the blood. The presence of other pathogens in the blood is described in a similar way i.e. viraemia, fungaemia and parasitaemia.

Sepsis
- The systemic response to infection. Defined as SIRS with confirmed or presumed infection.

Severe sepsis
- Sepsis with evidence of organ dysfunction.

Septic shock
- Sepsis-induced hypotension and/or tissue hypoperfusion (e.g. oliguria, lactic acidosis) despite adequate fluid resuscitation.

and non-allergic anaphylaxis may be identical, with shock a frequent manifestation of both. Anaphylactic shock results from vasodilation, intravascular volume redistribution, capillary leak and a reduction in cardiac output. Common causes of anaphylaxis include drugs (e.g. neuromuscular blocking drugs, β-lactam antibiotics), colloid solutions (e.g. gelatin containing solutions, dextrans), radiological contrast media, foodstuffs (peanuts, tree nuts, shellfish, dairy products), hymenoptera stings and latex.

Neurogenic shock

This is caused by a loss of sympathetic tone to vascular smooth muscle. This typically occurs following injury to the (thoracic or cervical) spinal cord and results in profound vasodilation, a fall in systemic vascular resistance and hypotension.

Pathophysiology

In clinical practice there is often significant overlap between the causes of shock; for example, patients with septic shock are frequently also hypovolaemic. Whilst differences can be detected at the level of the macrocirculation, most shock (exception neurogenic) is associated with increased sympathetic activity and all share common pathophysiological features at the cellular level.

Macrocirculation

When assessing a patient with shock, it is useful to remember that mean arterial blood pressure (MAP) is equal to the product of cardiac output (CO) and systemic vascular resistance (SVR) (Table 1.15).

Shock (inadequate tissue oxygen delivery) can occur in the context of a low, normal or high cardiac output.

In hypovolaemic shock there is catecholamine release from the adrenal medulla and sympathetic nerve endings, as well as the generation of AT-II from the renin–angiotensin system. The resulting tachycardia and increased myocardial contractility act to preserve cardiac output, whilst vasoconstriction acts to maintain arterial blood pressure and divert the available blood to vital organs (e.g. brain, heart and muscle) and away from non-vital organs (e.g. skin and gut). Clinically this manifests as pale, clammy skin with collapsed peripheral

Table 1.15 Haemodynamic and oxygen transport parameters

$$MAP = CO \times SVR$$

$$DO_2 \approx CO \times 1.34 \times [Hb] \times (SaO_2/100)$$

$$VO_2 = CO \times 1.34 \times [Hb] \times (SaO_2 - SvO_2)$$

MAP = mean arterial pressure; CO = cardiac output; SVR = systemic vascular resistance; DO_2 = oxygen delivery; [Hb] = haemoglobin concentration in g/dl; SaO_2 = arterial oxygen saturations; VO_2 = oxygen consumption; SvO_2 mixed venous oxygen saturations (sampled from pulmonary artery)

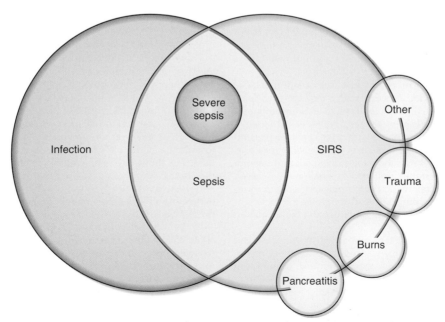

Fig. 1.9 The interrelationship between systemic inflammatory response syndrome (SIRS), sepsis and infection. Adapted from The American College of Chest Physicians and Society of Critical Care Medicine Consensus Conference Committee definitions for sepsis 1992.

veins and a prolonged capillary refill time. The resulting splanchnic hypoperfusion is implicated in many of the complications associated with prolonged or untreated shock.

In septic shock, circulating proinflammatory cytokines (notably TNF-α and IL-1β) induce endothelial expression of the enzyme nitric oxide (NO) synthetase and the production of NO which leads to smooth muscle relaxation, vasodilation and a fall in systemic vascular resistance. The (initial) cardiovascular response is a reflex tachycardia and an increase in stroke volume resulting in an increased cardiac output. Clinically this manifests as warm, well-perfused peripheries, a low diastolic blood pressure and raised pulse pressure. Fit young patients may compensate for these changes relatively well even though oxygen delivery and utilization is compromised at the cellular level. However, as septic shock progresses endothelial dysfunction results in significant extravasation of fluid and a loss of intravascular volume. Ventricular dysfunction also impairs the compensatory increase in cardiac output. As a result, peripheral perfusion falls and the clinical signs may become indistinguishable from those associated with the low-output state described above

In neurogenic shock, traumatic disruption of sympathetic efferent nerve fibres results in loss of vasomotor tone, peripheral vasodilation and a fall in systemic vascular resistance. Loss of cardiac accelerator fibres (T1–4) and anhydrosis as a result of loss of sweat gland innervation also frequently occur, with patients typically presenting with hypotension, bradycardia and warm, dry peripheries.

Cardiogenic shock typically presents with signs of a low-output state although, unlike hypovolaemic shock, circulating volume is typically normal or increased with increased circulating AT-II and aldosterone. If associated with left ventricular failure, there may be pulmonary oedema.

Microcirculation

Changes in the microcirculation (arterioles, capillaries and venules) have a central role in the pathogenesis of shock.

Arteriolar vasoconstriction, seen in early hypovolaemic and cardiogenic shock, helps to maintain a satisfactory MAP and the resulting fall in the capillary hydrostatic pressure encourages the transfer of fluid from the interstitial space into the vascular compartment so helping to maintain circulating volume. As described above, high vascular resistance in the capillary beds of the skin and gut results in a redistribution of cardiac output to vital organs.

If shock remains uncorrected, local accumulation of lactic acid and carbon dioxide, together with the release of vasoactive substances from the endothelium, over-ride compensatory vasoconstriction leading to pre-capillary vasodilatation. This results in pooling of blood within the capillary bed and endothelial cell damage. Capillary permeability increases with the loss of fluid into the interstitial space and haemoconcentration within the capillary. The resulting increase in blood viscosity, in conjunction with reduced red cell deformability, further compromises flow through the microcirculation predisposing to platelet aggregation and the formation of microthrombi.

In sepsis, there is up-regulation of inducible NO synthetase and smooth muscle cells lose their adrenergic sensitivity resulting in pathological arterio–venous shunting. Endothelial and inflammatory cell activation results in the generation of reactant oxidant species, disruption of barrier function in the microcirculation and widespread activation of coagulation. Microthombi occlude capillary blood flow and the consumption of platelets and coagulation factors leads to thrombocytopenia, coagulopathy and DIC (Fig. 1.10).

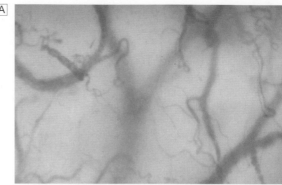

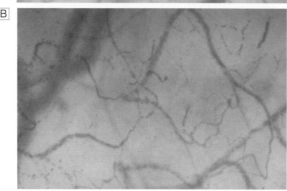

Fig. 1.10 The effect of septic shock on the microcirculation.
Photomicrograph from a video clip of the normal microcirculation [A] and the microcirculation in septic shock [B] Septic shock is associated with an increased number of small vessels with either absent or intermittent flow.

Cellular function

Under normal (aerobic) conditions, glycolysis converts glucose to pyruvate which is converted to acetyl-coenzyme-A (acetyl-CoA) and enters the Krebs cycle. Oxidation of acetyl-CoA in the TCA cycle generates nicotinamide adenine dinucleotide (NADH) and flavine adenine dinucleotide (FADH$_2$), which enter the electron transport chain and are oxidized to NAD$^+$ in the oxidative phosphorylation of adenosine diphosphate (ADP) to ATP.

The oxidative metabolism of glucose is energy efficient, yielding up to 38 moles of ATP for each mole of glucose, but requires a continuous supply of oxygen to the cell. Hypoxaemia blocks mitochondrial oxidative phosphorylation, inhibiting ATP synthesis. This leads to a decrease in the intracellular ATP/ADP ratio, an increase in the NADH/NAD$^+$ ratio and an accumulation of pyruvate that is unable to enter the TCA cycle. The cytosolic conversion of pyruvate to lactate allows the regeneration of some NAD$^+$, enabling the limited production of ATP by anaerobic glycolysis. However, anaerobic glycolysis is significantly less efficient, generating only 2 moles of ATP per mole of glucose and predisposing cells to ATP depletion (Fig. 1.11).

Under normal conditions, the tissues globally extract about 25% of the oxygen delivered to them, with the normal oxygen saturation of mixed venous blood being 70–75%. As oxygen delivery falls, cells are able to increase the proportion of oxygen extracted from the blood, but this compensatory mechanism is limited, with a maximal oxygen extraction ratio of about 50%. At this point, further reductions in oxygen delivery lead to a critical reduction in oxygen consumption and anaerobic metabolism, a state described as dysoxia (Fig. 1.12).

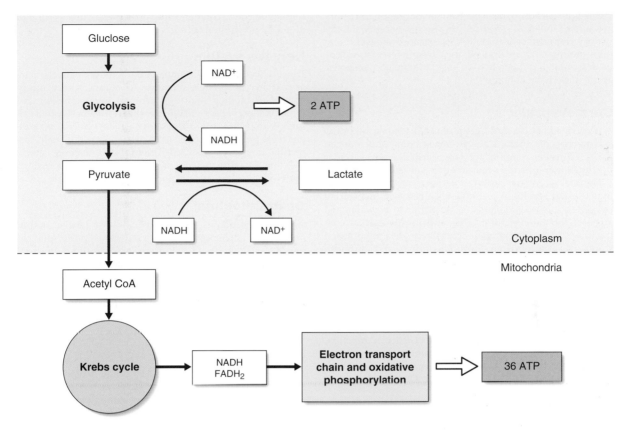

Fig. 1.11 Glycolysis. Simplified diagram illustrating glycolysis, the Krebs cycle and oxidative phosphorylation. Aerobic metabolism yields up to 38 moles of ATP per mole of glucose oxidized. Anaerobic metabolism is considerably less efficient yielding only 2 moles of ATP per mole of glucose.

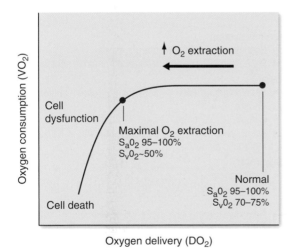

Fig. 1.12 The relationship between oxygen delivery, oxygen consumption and oxygen extraction (SaO_2–SvO_2). As oxygen delivery falls in shock, oxygen extraction increases until it reaches maximal oxygen extraction (45–50%). Further reductions in oxygen delivery result in a fall in oxygen consumption and tissue dysoxia. As ATP supply falls below ATP demand this leads to cell dysfunction and ultimately to cell death.

Anaerobic metabolism leads to a rise in lactic acid in the systemic circulation. Indeed, in the absence of significant renal or liver disease, serum lactate concentration may be a useful marker of global cellular hypoxia and oxygen debt. Similarly, a fall in mixed venous oxygen saturations may reflect increased oxygen extraction by the tissues and an imbalance between oxygen delivery and oxygen demand.

In septic shock, cell dysoxia and lactate accumulation may reflect a problem with both oxygen utilization and oxygen delivery. The increased sympathetic activity occurring in sepsis leads to increased glycolysis and an increase in pyruvate generation. Coupled with dysfunction of the enzyme pyruvate dehydrogenase, this leads to accumulation of pyruvate and (hence) lactate. In addition, sepsis is associated with significant mitochondrial dysfunction and marked inhibition of oxidative phosphorylation. The phrase 'cytopathic shock' has been used to describe this condition.

The movement of sodium against a concentration gradient is an active process requiring ATP. Reduction in ATP supply leads to intracellular accumulation of sodium, an osmotic gradient across the cell membrane, dilation of the endoplasmic reticulum and cell swelling. When combined with the failure of other vital ATP-dependent cell functions and the reduction in intracellular pH associated with the accumulation of lactic acid, the result is disruption of protein synthesis, damage to lysosomal and mitochondrial membranes and ultimately cell necrosis.

The effect of shock on individual organ systems

As described above, shock leads to increased sympathetic activity. This results in a rise in CO, SVR and MAP. Preservation and redistribution of cardiac output, coupled with intrinsic organ autoregulation, helps to maintain adequate perfusion and oxygen delivery to vital organs (brain, heart, skeletal muscle). However, these compensatory mechanisms have limits, and in the case of severe, prolonged and/or uncorrected shock ('decompensated' shock), the clinical manifestations of organ hypoperfusion become apparent.

Shock also leads to the up-regulation of pro-inflammatory cytokines (TNF-α, IL-1β and IL-6) and the systemic inflammatory response syndrome (SIRS), organ dysfunction and multiple organ failure. Indeed, the clinical presentation may be determined as much by this host inflammatory response as the underlying aetiology.

Cardiovascular

As described above, cardiogenic shock leads to a fall in CO and neurogenic shock leads to vasodilation and reduced SVR. However, significant myocardial and vascular dysfunction frequently occur in other causes of shock.

Despite coronary autoregulation, severe (diastolic) hypotension results in an imbalance between myocardial oxygen supply and demand and ischaemia in the watershed areas of the endocardium. This impairs myocardial contractility. Hypoxaemia and acidosis deplete myocardial stores of noradrenaline (norepinephrine) and diminish the cardiac response to both endogenous and exogenous catecholamines. Acid–base and electrolyte abnormalities, combined with local tissue hypoxia, increase myocardial excitability and predispose to both atrial and ventricular dysrhythmias. As described above, circulating inflammatory mediators implicated in the pathogenesis of sepsis and SIRS depress myocardial contractility and ventricular function, increase endothelial permeability (resulting in intravascular volume depletion) and cause widespread activation of both coagulation and fibrinolysis (leading to DIC).

Respiratory

Tachypnoea driven by pain, pyrexia, local lung pathology, pulmonary oedema, metabolic acidosis or cytokines is one of the earliest features of shock. The increased minute volume typically results in reduced arterial PCO_2 and a respiratory alkalosis as described above. Initially this will compensate for the metabolic acidosis of shock but eventually this mechanism is overwhelmed and blood pH falls.

In hypovolaemic states, there is reduction in pulmonary blood flow and this leads to underperfusion of ventilated alveolar units so increasing ventilation–perfusion (V/Q) mismatch. In cardiogenic shock, left ventricular failure and pulmonary oedema often compromises the ventilation of perfused alveolar units increasing the shunt fraction (Qs/Qt) within the lung. Increased V/Q mismatch and shunt fraction also occur in sepsis. The net result is hypoxaemia that may be refractory to increases in inspired oxygen concentration.

Sepsis and hypovolaemic shock are both recognized causes of acute lung injury and its more severe variant, the acute respiratory distress syndrome (ARDS). This is characterized by the influx of protein-rich oedema fluid and inflammatory cells into the alveolar air spaces and appears to be cytokine-mediated (notably IL-8, TNF-α, IL-1and IL-6).

Renal

As a result of the mechanisms discussed above, reduced renal blood flow results in the production of low volume (< 0.5 ml/kg/h), high osmolality and low sodium content urine. If shock is not reversed, hypoxia leads to acute tubular necrosis (ATN) characterized by oligo-anuria and urine with a high sodium concentration and an osmolality close to that of plasma. With a fall in glomerular filtration, blood urea and creatinine rise; hyperkalaemia and a metabolic acidosis are also usually present.

Renal failure occurs in about 30–50% of patients with septic shock. In addition to the mechanisms responsible for the simple pre-renal failure described above, there is an imbalance in pre- and postglomerular vascular resistance, mesangial contraction and microvascular injury leading to glomerular filtration failure.

Nervous system

Due to the increased sympathetic activity, patients may appear inappropriately anxious. As compensatory mechanisms reach their limit and cerebral hypoperfusion and hypoxia supervene, there is increasing restlessness, progressing to confusion, stupor and coma. Unless cerebral hypoxia has been prolonged, effective resuscitation will usually correct the depressed conscious level rapidly. In septic shock, the clinical picture may be complicated by the presence of an underlying (septic) encephalopathy and/or delirium.

Gastrointestinal

As described above, the redistribution of cardiac output observed in shock leads to a marked reduction in splanchnic blood flow. In the stomach, the resulting mucosal hypoperfusion and hypoxia predispose to stress ulceration and haemorrhage. In the intestine, movement (translocation) of bacteria and/or bacterial endotoxin from the lumen to the portal vein and then systemic circulation is thought to be a key mechanism underlying the development of SIRS and multiple organ failure.

Hepatobiliary

Despite its dual blood supply, ischaemic hepatic injury is frequently seen following hypovolaemic or cardiogenic shock. An acute, reversible elevation in serum transaminase levels indicates hepatocellular injury, and typically

---

 SUMMARY BOX **1.12**

Clinical effects of shock

Nervous system
- Restlessness, confusion, stupor, coma
- Encephalopathy and/or delirium common in sepsis

Renal
- Renal hypoperfusion → activation of rennin–angiotensin system
- Oliguria (< 0.5 ml/kg/h urine) → anuria
- Acute renal failure → ↑ urea, ↑ creatinine, ↑ K⁺ & metabolic acidosis

Respiratory
- Tachypnoea
- ↑ Ventilation/perfusion (V/Q) mismatch & ↑ shunt → hypoxia
- Pulmonary oedema (common in cardiogenic shock) → hypoxia
- Acute lung injury and acute respiratory distress syndrome → hypoxia

Cardiovascular
- ↓ Diastolic pressure → ↓ coronary blood flow
- ↓ Myocardial oxygen delivery → myocardial ischaemia → ↓ contractility & ↓ CO
- Acidosis, electrolyte disturbances and hypoxia predispose to arrhythmias
- Widespread endothelial cell activation → microcirculatory dysfunction

Gastrointestinal
- Splanchnic hypoperfusion → breakdown of gut mucosal barrier
- Stress ulceration
- Translocation of bacteria/bacterial wall contents into blood stream → SIRS
- Acute ischaemic hepatitis.

occurs 1–3 days following the ischaemic insult. Increases in prothrombin time and/or hypoglycaemia are markers of more severe injury. Significant ischaemic hepatitis is more frequent in patients with underlying cardiac disease and a degree of hepatic venous congestion.

Management

General principles

The management of shock is based upon the following principles:

- identification and treatment of the underlying cause
- the maintenance of adequate tissue oxygen delivery.

As with most clinical emergencies, treatment and diagnosis should occur simultaneously with the immediate assessment and management following an Airway, Breathing, Circulation (ABC) approach.

The early recognition and treatment of potentially reversible causes (e.g. bleeding, intra-abdominal sepsis, myocardial ischaemia, pulmonary embolus, cardiac tamponade) is essential and may be facilitated by a detailed history, a thorough clinical examination (Table 1.16) and focused investigations.

Whilst shocked patients may be more sensitive to the effects of opiates, there is no justification for withholding effective analgesia if indicated and this should be titrated intravenously (e.g. morphine in 1–2mg increments) to response during the initial assessment and treatment.

Most patients with shock will require admission to a high dependency (HDU) or intensive care unit (ICU).

Airway and breathing

Hypoxaemia must be prevented and, if present, rapidly corrected by maintaining a clear airway (e.g. head tilt, chin lift) and administering high flow oxygen (e.g. 10–15litres/min). The adequacy of this therapy can be estimated continuously using pulse oximetry (SpO_2), but frequent arterial blood gas analysis allows a more accurate assessment of oxygenation (P_aO_2), ventilation (P_aCO_2) and indirect measures of tissue perfusion (pH, base excess, HCO_3^- and lactate). In patients with severe hypoxaemia, cardiovascular instability, depressed conscious level or exhaustion, intubation and ventilatory support may be required.

Circulation

Initial resuscitation should be targeted at arresting haemorrhage and providing fluid (crystalloid or colloid) to restore intravascular volume and optimize cardiac preload. It is common practice to use blood to maintain a haemoglobin concentration > 10g/dl (haematocrit around 0.3) during the initial resuscitation of shock if there is evidence of inadequate oxygen delivery, such as a raised lactate concentration or low central venous saturations (measured from a central venous catheter). A reduction in tachycardia, increasing blood pressure, and improving peripheral perfusion and urine output in response to a series of 250–500ml fluid challenges indicate 'fluid responsiveness' and suggest that further fluid and optimization of preload may be required. Once parameters stop improving it is unlikely that further fluid will be beneficial, particularly if there is an associated fall in oxygen saturation and the development of pulmonary oedema. As resuscitation continues, more invasive monitoring allows the acid–base status, central venous pressure (CVP), pulmonary artery wedge pressure (PAWP), CO and mixed (S_vO_2) or central (Sc_vO_2) venous oxygen saturations to be used to further assess the response to fluid (Fig. 1.13).

If blood pressure remains low and/or signs of inadequate tissue oxygen delivery persist despite fluid resuscitation and the optimization of preload, then inotropes and/or vasopressors may be required. Although there is a degree of crossover in their mechanism of action, vasopressors (e.g. noradrenaline) cause peripheral vasoconstriction and an increase SVR while inotropes (e.g. dobutamine) increase myocardial contractility, stroke volume and cardiac output. The initial choice of inotrope or vasopressor therefore depends upon the underlying aetiology of shock and an understanding of the main physiological derangements (Table 1.17). Adrenaline, which has both vasopressor and inotropic effects, is a useful first line drug in the emergency treatment of shock. Vasoactive drug administration should be continuously titrated against specific physiological endpoints (e.g. blood pressure or cardiac output).

Hypovolaemic shock

The commonest cause of acute hypovolaemic shock in surgical practice is bleeding due to trauma, ruptured aortic aneurysm, gastrointestinal and obstetric haemorrhage (Table 1.14).

Normal adult blood volume is about 7% of body weight, with a 70kg man having an estimated blood volume (EBV) of around 5000ml. The severity of haemorrhagic shock is frequently classified according to percentage of EBV lost where class I (< 15%) represents a compensated state (as may occur following the donation of a unit of blood) and class IV (> 40%) is immediately life threatening (Table 1.18). The term 'massive haemorrhage' has a number of definitions

Table 1.16 Clinical assessment of shock

Conscious level	Restlessness, anxiety, stupor and coma are common features and suggest cerebral hypoperfusion
Pulse	Low volume, thready pulse consistent with low-output state; high volume, bounding pulse with high-output state
Blood pressure	Changes in diastolic may precede a fall in systolic blood pressure, with ↓ diastolic in sepsis and ↑ in hypovolaemic and cardiogenic shock
Peripheral perfusion	Cold peripheries suggest vasoconstriction (↑ SVR); warm peripheries suggest vasodilation (↓ SVR)
Pulse oximetry	Hypoxemia common association of all forms of shock and ↓tissue O_2 delivery
ECG monitoring	Myocardial ischaemia commonest cause of cardiogenic shock but common in all forms of shock
Urine output	< 0.5ml/kg/h suggestive of renal hypoperfusion
CVP measurement	Low CVP with collapsing central veins consistent with hypovolaemia
Arterial blood gas	Metabolic acidosis and ↑ lactate consistent with tissue hypoperfusion

In isolation, single measurements are not helpful. Measurements are far more useful when used in combination with the findings of a detailed clinical examination. Observation of trends over time, together with the response to therapeutic interventions (e.g. a fluid challenge) is key to the successful management of shock.

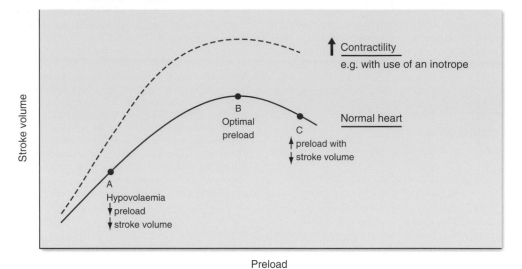

Fig. 1.13 Frank–Starling curve. Demonstrating the relationship between ventricular preload and stroke volume.

Table 1.17 Effects of commonly used vasoactive drugs

Drug	CO	SVR	Main effects
Adrenaline	↑	↑	α- & β-agonist; positive inotrope and vasopressor
Noradrenaline	↔/↓	↑	α-agonist; vasopressor
Dobutamine	↑	↓	β1-agonist; positive inotrope and systemic vasodilator
Dopamine	↑	↓	β1-agonist (at doses > 5 μg/kg/min); positive inotrope and systemic vasodilator
Dopexamine	↑	↓	β1-agonist; positive inotrope and systemic vasodilator
Levosimendan	↑	↓	Calcium sensitizer; positive inotrope and systemic vasodilator
Milrinone	↑	↓	Phosphodiesterase inhibitor; positive inotrope and systemic vasodilator
Glyceryl trinitrate	↑	↓	Nitric oxide-mediated vasodilatation

CO = cardiac output; SVR = systemic vascular resistance

Table 1.18 Estimated blood loss and presentation of hypovolaemic shock

	Class I	Class II	Class III	Class IV
Blood loss (ml)	< 750	750–1500	1500–2000	> 2000
Blood loss (% EBV)	< 15	15–30%	30–40%	> 40%
Pulse	< 100	> 100	> 120	> 140
Blood pressure	Normal	Decreased	Decreased	Decreased
Respiratory rate	14–20	20–30	30–40	> 35
Urine output (ml/h)	> 30	20–30	5–15	Negligible
CNS symptoms	Normal	Anxious	Confused	Lethargic

Adapted from Committee on Trauma: Advanced Trauma Life Support Manual

including: loss of EBV in 24 hours; loss of 50% EBV in 3 hours; blood loss at a rate ≥ 150 ml/min.

Arrest of haemorrhage and intravascular fluid resuscitation should occur concurrently; there is little role for inotropes or vasopressors in the treatment of a hypotensive hypovolaemic patient. As described above, fluid therapy should be titrated to clinical and physiological response.

In the emergency situation, before bleeding has been controlled, a systolic blood pressure of 80–90 mmHg is increasingly used as a resuscitation target (permissive hypotension) as it is thought less likely to dislodge clot and lead to dilutional coagulopathy. Once active bleeding has been stopped, resuscitation can be fine-tuned to optimize organ perfusion and tissue oxygen delivery as described above. It remains unclear whether permissive hypotension is appropriate for all cases of haemorrhagic shock but it appears to improve outcomes following penetrating trauma and ruptured aortic aneurysm.

Rapid fluid resuscitation requires secure vascular access and this is best achieved through two wide-bore (14- or 16-gauge) peripheral intravenous cannulae; cannulation of a central vein provides an alternative means.

As discussed above, the type of fluid used (crystalloid or colloid) is probably less important than the adequate restoration of circulating volume itself. In the case of life-threatening or continued haemorrhage, blood will be required early in the resuscitation. Ideally, fully cross-matched packed red blood cells (PRBCs) should be administered, but type-specific or O Rhesus-negative blood may be used until it becomes available. A haemoglobin concentration of 7–9 g/dl may be sufficient to ensure adequate tissue oxygen delivery in stable (non-bleeding) patients, but a haemoglobin target of > 10 g/dl may be more appropriate in actively bleeding patients. Massive transfusion can lead to hypothermia, hypocalcaemia, hyper- or hypokalaemia and coagulopathy.

The acute coagulopathy of trauma (ACoT) is well recognized and multifactorial. Dilution of clotting factors and platelets as a result of fluid resuscitation, combined with their consumption at the point of bleeding, results in clotting factor deficiency, thrombocytopaenia and coagulopathy. Hypothermia, metabolic acidosis and hypocalcaemia also significantly impair normal coagulation. Resuscitation strategies aggressively targeting the 'lethal triad' of hypothermia, acidosis and coagulopathy appear to significantly improve outcome following military trauma and observational studies support the immediate use of measures to prevent hypothermia, early correction of severe metabolic acidosis (pH < 7.1), maintenance of ionized calcium > 1.0 mmol/l and the early empirical use of clotting factors and platelets.

Where possible, correction of coagulopathy should be guided by laboratory results (platelet count, prothrombin time, activated partial thromboplastin time and fibrinogen concentration). Thromboelastography (TEG) or rotational thromboelastometry (ROTEM) provide near-patient functional assays of clot formation, platelet function and fibrinolysis and are also now widely used to guide the management of coagulopathy. Clotting factor deficiency is normally treated by the administration of fresh frozen plasma (FFP) (10–15 ml/kg), thrombocytopenia or platelet dysfunction by the administration of platelets (usually one 'pool' or adult dose containing $2–3 \times 10^{11}$ platelets). Fibrinogen deficiency (< 1.0 g/l) is best treated with fresh frozen plasma or cryoprecipitate (usually one 'pool' of 10 single donor units). The antifibrinolytic, tranexamic acid, can be used to inhibit fibrinolysis and has been shown to reduce mortality from bleeding when used early (< 3 hours) and empirically following major trauma. Early administration is important for its beneficial effect.

In the case of rapid haemorrhage, it is often not possible to use traditional laboratory results to guide the correction of coagulopathy because of the time delay in obtaining these results. This has lead to a formula-driven approach to the use of PRBC, FFP and platelets targeting the early empirical treatment of coagulopathy. Although the evidence for these strategies is still emerging, current military guidelines advocate the administration of warmed PRBC and fresh frozen plasma (FFP) in a 1:1 ratio as soon as possible in the resuscitation of major haemorrhage following trauma in conjunction with platelet transfusions to maintain platelets $> 100 \times 10^9$.

A recombinant form of activated factor VII (rVIIa) is approved for the management of bleeding in haemophiliacs with inhibitory antibodies to factors VIII or IX. Although rVIIa has been used effectively in the treatment of life-threatening haemorrhage in other patient groups, its use is associated with a significant rate of arterial thromboembolic events and it remains unclear whether its unlicensed use in these groups is justified.

Septic shock

The principles guiding the management of septic shock are:
- the identification and treatment of underlying infection
- early goal-directed therapy to optimize tissue oxygen delivery.

The Surviving Sepsis Campaign has published evidence-based guidelines on the management of severe sepsis and septic shock: http://www.survivingsepsis.org .

Early recognition of severe sepsis and septic shock is critical. This requires a high index of suspicion together with a detailed history and examination to identify signs of organ dysfunction and potential sources of infection. Hospital-acquired infection should always be considered as a cause of clinical deterioration in surgical patients.

As with all forms of shock, the initial assessment and management of septic shock should follow an A, B, C approach. However, in patients with septic shock there is evidence that protocolized early goal-directed therapy (EGDT) improves survival (EBM 1.2) and this should be started as soon as signs of sepsis-induced tissue hypoperfusion are recognized (hypotension, elevated lactate, low central venous saturations or oliguria). The widely accepted resuscitation goals for the first 6 hours of this strategy are:
- Central venous pressure (CVP) of 8–12 mmHg
- Mean arterial blood pressure ≥ 65 mmHg
- Urine output ≥ 0.5 ml/kg/h

- Central venous (superior vena cava) O_2 saturation (S_cvO_2) $\geq 70\%$ or mixed venous (pulmonary artery) O_2 saturation (SvO_2) $\geq 65\%$.

EBM 1.2 Early goal-directed therapy in severe sepsis

'Goal-directed therapy in the first six hours of resuscitation significantly reduces the mortality of patients with severe sepsis or septic shock.'

Rivers E, et al. N Engl J Med 2001; 345: 1368–1377.

As described above, septic shock is associated with both relative and absolute hypovolaemia as a result of profound vasodilation and extravasation of fluid from the intravascular space. Both crystalloid and colloid can be used to restore intravascular volume although HES solutions should probably be avoided because of concerns about inducing acute renal failure. Current guidelines suggest a target CVP of ≥ 8 mmHg and this frequently requires large volumes of fluid. Persistent hypotension (MAP < 65 mmHg) following restoration of circulating volume is best treated with a vasopressor such as noradrenaline in the first instance. While the titration of fluid and vasopressor to a MAP ≥ 65 mmHg should be sufficient to preserve tissue perfusion in most patients, this may not be the case in all patients (e.g. those with hypertension) and it is important to supplement these simple resuscitation end-points with additional markers of global tissue perfusion (lactate and central venous saturations) to determine whether oxygen delivery is adequate. If serum lactate is elevated (> 2 mmol/l) and central venous saturations are low (< 70%) in the context of septic shock this suggests inadequate tissue oxygen delivery with increased oxygen extraction from the blood and anaerobic metabolism. In this situation, oxygen delivery can be increased by transfusion of PRBC to achieve a haemoglobin concentration of about 10 g/dl (haematocrit around 0.3) and/or increasing cardiac output using an inotrope such as dobutamine.

In patients with hypotension unresponsive to fluid resuscitation and vasopressors, intravenous hydrocortisone has been shown to promote reversal of shock. However, this does not appear to translate into a mortality benefit and the use of corticosteroids is associated with an increased risk of secondary infections. Because of this, the use of corticosteroids in the treatment of refractory septic shock remains contentious.

Treatment of infection involves adequate source control and the administration of appropriate antibiotics. Source control includes the removal of infected devices, abscess drainage, the debridement of infected tissue and interventions to prevent ongoing microbial contamination such as repair of a perforated viscus or biliary drainage. This should be achieved as soon as possible following initial resuscitation and should be performed with the minimum physiological disturbance; where possible, percutaneous or endoscopic techniques are preferable to open surgery.

Intravenous antibiotics must be administered as soon as possible (EBM 1.3), preferably in discussion with a microbiologist. The choice depends on the history, the

EBM 1.3 Early administration of antibiotics

'In the presence of septic shock, each hour delay in the administration of effective antibiotics is associated with a measurable (~8%) increase in mortality.'

Kumar A, Roberts D, Wood KE, et al: Duration of hypotension prior to initiation of effective antimicrobial therapy is the critical determinant of survival in human septic shock. Crit Care Med 2006; 34:1589–1596.

likely source of infection, whether the infection is community- or hospital-acquired and local patterns of pathogen susceptibility. Covering all likely pathogens (bacterial and/or fungal) usually involves the use of empirical broad-spectrum antibiotics in the first instance, with these rationalized or changed to reduce the spectrum of cover once the results of microbiological investigations become available.

One or more (peripheral) blood cultures should be taken prior to the administration of antibiotics but this must not delay therapy. Culture of urine, cerebrospinal fluid, faeces and bronchoalveolar lavage fluid may also be indicated. Targeted imaging (CXR, ultrasound, computed tomography) may also help identify the source of infection.

In septic patients at high risk of death, most of whom will have an Acute Physiology and Chronic Health Evaluation (APACHE) II ≥ 25 or multiple organ failure, there is some evidence that the early use of recombinant activated protein C (rhAPC) reduces mortality. However, it is clear that the use of rhAPC is associated with a significant risk of serious bleeding complications and this risk may be higher in surgical patients. This expensive therapy should only be used under the supervision of an intensive care specialist.

Cardiogenic shock

The commonest cause of cardiogenic shock is acute (anterior) myocardial infarction. As with other forms of shock, the management of cardiogenic shock is based upon the identification and treatment of reversible causes and supportive management to maintain adequate tissue oxygen delivery. This involves active management of the four determinants of cardiac output: preload, myocardial contractility heart rate, and afterload.

Routine investigations to identify the cause of cardiogenic shock include serial 12-lead ECGs, troponin or creatinine kinase-MB (CK-MB) levels and a CXR. A transthoracic echocardiogram may provide useful information on (systolic and diastolic) ventricular function and exclude potentially treatable causes of cardiogenic shock such as cardiac tamponade, valvular insufficiency and massive pulmonary embolus.

General supportive measures include the administration of high concentrations of inspired oxygenation. In patients with cardiogenic pulmonary oedema, there is some evidence that continuous positive airway pressure (CPAP) improves oxygenation, reduces the work of breathing and provides subjective relief of dyspnoea. It remains unclear whether these advantages translate into a significant survival benefit.

For patients with acute myocardial ischaemia, intravenous opiates should be titrated cautiously to control pain and reduce anxiety. In addition to providing analgesia, opiates reduce myocardial oxygen demand and reduce afterload by causing peripheral vasodilation.

As with all forms of shock, correction of hypovolaemia and optimization of intravascular volume (preload) is of central importance in maximizing stroke volume, cardiac output and tissue oxygen delivery. However, the management of fluid balance in cardiogenic shock can be challenging. Patients with acute heart failure and cardiogenic shock are usually normovolaemic or relatively hypovolaemic as a result of intravascular fluid loss into the lungs and the development of pulmonary oedema. In contrast, patients with chronic heart failure are usually hypervolaemic as a result of long-standing activation of the renin–angiotensin system and salt and water retention. The key point is that some patients in cardiogenic shock are hypovolaemic and require fluid resuscitation. This is best achieved by careful titration of a fluid challenge and assessment of the clinical response in an appropriately monitored environment (see above). Once hypovolaemia has been corrected and cardiac preload optimized, refractory hypotension and/or signs of inadequate tissue perfusion may require treatment with vasoactive drugs. This frequently requires a careful balance of vasodilator, inotrope and vasoconstrictor.

The major derangements in cardiogenic shock are a reduction in cardiac output and a compensatory increase in systemic vascular resistance. The use of a vasodilator such as glyeryltrinitrate (GTN) may reduce SVR (afterload) and improve cardiac output, but vasodilation frequently results in a significant reduction in blood pressure compromising tissue perfusion. Adrenaline, an α- and β-agonist with both inotropic and vasoconstricting actions, is frequently used in the emergency management of cardiogenic shock, increasing both myocardial contractility and SVR. However, while adrenaline may increase blood pressure, it significantly increases myocardial workload, potentially worsening myocardial ischaemia and profound vasoconstriction further reduces already-compromised tissue perfusion. Frequently, the most appropriate choice of vasoactive drug in cardiogenic shock is one that has both inotropic and vasodilating properties such as the β-agonist dobutamine. Alternative ino-dilating agents include the calcium sensitizer levosimendan and the phosphodiesterase inhibitor milrinone. Noradrenaline is also an effective treatment for cardiogenic shock under some circumstances. Whenever a vasoactive drug is given the patient requires monitoring in a high dependency or critical care area.

The intra-aortic balloon pump (IABP) is increasingly used as an adjunct in the supportive management of cardiogenic shock. This device works by inflating a balloon in the thoracic aorta during diastole, with deflation occurring in systole. Inflation during diastole augments the diastolic blood pressure improving coronary perfusion and myocardial oxygen delivery; deflation in systole reduces afterload. While it still remains unclear which patient groups benefit from insertion of an IABP, they are generally used as a bridge to more definitive treatment such as percutaneous coronary intervention (PCI), coronary artery bypass grafting (CABG) or mitral valve repair.

Anaphylactic shock

The management of anaphylactic shock is illustrated in Table 1.19.

Table 1.19 The management of anaphylaxis

1. Stop administration of causative agent (drug/fluid)
2. Call for help
3. Lie patient flat, feet elevated
4. Maintain airway and give 100% O_2
5. Adrenaline (epinephrine)
   - 0.5–1.0 mg (0.5–1.0 ml of 1:1000) IM *or*
     If experienced using IV adrenaline
   - 50–100 µg (0.5–1.0 ml of 1:10 000) IV titrated against response
6. Intravascular volume expansion with crystalloid or colloid
7. Second-line therapy
   Antihistamine: Chlorphenamine 10–20 mg slow IV
   Corticosteroid: Hydrocortisone 200 mg IV

R.H.A. Green
M.L. Turner

02

Transfusion of blood components and plasma products

INTRODUCTION

Blood transfusion can be life-saving and many areas of surgery could not be undertaken without reliable transfusion support. However, as with any treatment, transfusion of blood and its components carries potential risks, which must be balanced against the patient's need. The magnitude of risk depends on factors such as the prevalence of infectious disease in the donor population, the resources and professionalism of the organization collecting, processing and issuing the blood and plasma products, and the care with which the clinical team administers these products.

BLOOD DONATION

In the UK, whole blood is donated by healthy adult volunteers over the age of 17 years with normal haemoglobin levels. The standard 480 ml donation contains approximately 200 mg of iron, the loss of which is easily tolerated by healthy donors. Blood components (red cells, platelets and plasma) can be separated from the donated blood or obtained from the donor as separate products by the use of a cell separator, in a process called apheresis.

Strict donor selection and the testing of all donations are essential to exclude blood that may be hazardous to the recipient, as well as ensuring the welfare of the donor. All donations are ABO-grouped, Rhesus (Rh) D-typed, antibody-screened, and tested for evidence of hepatitis B, hepatitis C, human immunodeficiency virus (HIV) I and II, human T-cell leukaemia virus (HTLV) I and II and syphilis, using tests for antibody to the virus, viral antigen or nucleic acid. Some donations are also tested for antibody to cytomegalovirus (CMV), so that CMV-negative blood can be provided for patients such as transplant recipients and premature infants. Dependent on epidemiology, other testing may be required, e.g. malaria, West Nile virus.

Due to concerns regarding transmission of variant Creutzfeldt–Jakob disease (vCJD) by transfusion, a number of new precautions have been introduced. Since 1999 all blood donated in the UK has been filtered to remove white blood cells (leucodepletion), UK plasma has been excluded from fractionation, and since April 2004 people who have received a blood or blood product transfusion in the UK after 1980 have been excluded from donating blood. Some countries currently exclude donations from individuals who resided in the UK during the time of the bovine spongiform encephalitis (BSE) epidemic. There is currently no blood test for vCJD.

BLOOD COMPONENTS

The components that can be prepared from donated blood are shown in Figure 2.1 and their descriptions follow.

Red blood cells in additive solution

Donated whole blood is collected into an anticoagulant (citrate) and nutrient (phosphate and dextrose) solution (CPD). Centrifugation removes virtually all of the

2

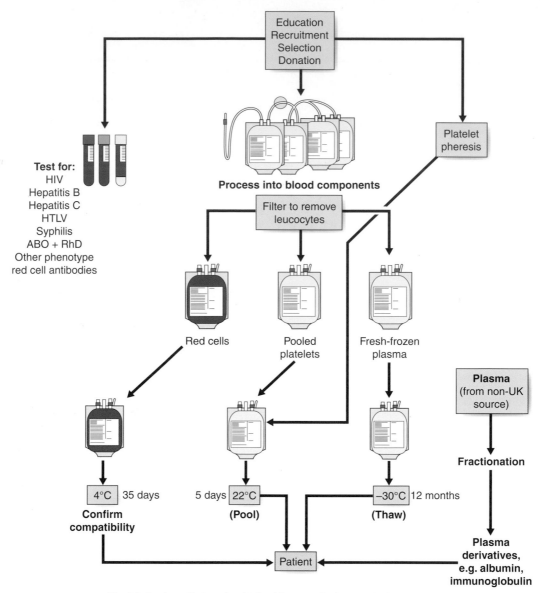

Test for:
HIV
Hepatitis B
Hepatitis C
HTLV
Syphilis
ABO + RhD
Other phenotype
red cell antibodies

Education
Recruitment
Selection
Donation

Platelet
pheresis

Process into blood components

Filter to remove
leucocytes

Red cells

Pooled
platelets

Fresh-frozen
plasma

Plasma
(from non-UK
source)

Fractionation

4°C 35 days

**Confirm
compatibility**

5 days 22°C

(Pool)

−30°C 12 months

(Thaw)

Patient

**Plasma
derivatives,
e.g. albumin,
immunoglobulin**

Fig. 2.1 Products that can be obtained from a unit of donated whole blood.

associated plasma, and a solution of saline, adenine, glucose and mannitol is then added to provide optimal red cell preservation. The red cell concentrate is then run through a leucodepletion filter to reduce the white cells to a concentration of less than $5 \times 10^6/l$. The final product has a haematocrit of 55–65% and a volume of approximately 300 ml. The blood cannot be sterilized, so that blood transfusion can transmit organisms not detected by donor screening. Red cell concentrates must be stored at +4°C ± 2°C.

Transfused blood must be ABO- and RhD-compatible with the recipient and transfused through a sterile blood administration set with an in-line macroaggregate filter, designed for the procedure. The set should be primed with saline and no other solutions transfused simultaneously. This product is indicated for acute blood loss and anaemia and is the most widely available form of red cells for transfusion.

Platelets

Platelet concentrates can be made either from centrifugation of whole blood or from an individual donor using apheresis. An adult dose is manufactured from four separate donations pooled together or one apheresis collection. In the UK it is advised that over 80% of platelets are procured by apheresis in order to minimize the number of donors a patient is exposed to. Platelets are currently concentrated in plasma rather than an optimal additive solution and carry a greater risk of bacterial contamination as they cannot be refrigerated but must be stored at 22°C ± 2°C. For this reason many platelet concentrates are now tested for bacterial contamination prior to release.

Platelets are infused through a standard blood-giving set over less than 30 minutes. As the concentrate contains some red cells and plasma, it should ideally be ABO- and RhD-compatible with the recipient. RhD-negative girls and women of child-bearing potential must receive RhD-negative platelets or, if only RhD-positive platelets are available, prophylactic RhD immunoglobulin should also be given. An adult dose should raise an adult platelet count by $20–40 \times 10^9/l$.

Platelet concentrates are indicated in thrombocytopenia, when platelet function is defective, and in patients receiving massive blood transfusions when there is microvascular bleeding (oozing from mucous membranes, needle puncture sites and wounds).

Fresh frozen plasma (FFP)

Some 200–300 ml of plasma can be removed from a unit of whole blood and stored frozen at −30°C. FFP contains albumin, immunoglobulins and, most importantly, all of the coagulation factors. FFP can be stored at −30°C for a year and is thawed to 37°C before issue. FFP must be ABO-compatible with the recipient and should be transfused within 4 hours of thawing. The average adult dose is 3–4 units. Imported, virally inactivated plasma (treated with methylene blue or solvent detergent) is available for use in children up to the age of 16 years and patients who require repeated exposure to FFP, such as patients undergoing plasma exchange for thrombotic thrombocytopenic purpura.

FFP is used when there are multiple coagulation factor deficiencies (e.g. disseminated intravascular coagulation, DIC) associated with severe bleeding. It may be indicated in selected patients who are over-anticoagulated with warfarin, but there are now prothrombin complex concentrates which should usually be used in preference for this purpose. In the case of massive blood loss arising during or after surgery, the decision whether to use FFP and, if so, how much to use, should be guided by timely tests of coagulation. FFP should not be used to correct prolonged clotting times in patients who are not bleeding or who are not about to undergo immediate surgery.

Cryoprecipitate

A single unit of cryoprecipitate can be removed from 1 unit of FFP after controlled thawing. After resuspension in 10–20 ml plasma, the cryoprecipitate is frozen once more to −30°C, in which condition it can be stored for up to a year. It is enriched in high molecular weight plasma proteins such as fibrinogen, factor VIII, von Willebrand factor, factor XIII and fibronectin. A normal adult dose is 10 units. ABO-compatible units should be given, and the product infused as soon as possible after thawing. Cryoprecipitate is used when fibrinogen levels are low, as in DIC. However the pooling required to manufacture cryoprecipitate does lead to high donor exposure per dose and many countries do not produce this product, preferring instead to use higher volumes of FFP or fibrinogen concentrates to reverse hypofibrinogenaemia.

PLASMA PRODUCTS

Fractionated products are manufactured from large pools (several thousand donations) of donor plasma that undergo some form of viral inactivation stage through the manufacturing process. Virus inactivation processes now mean that these products should not transmit HIV I and II or hepatitis B and C, but this may not apply to heat-resistant viruses that have no lipid envelope (e.g. hepatitis A) or to prions.

Human albumin

Albumin is prepared by fractionation of large pools of plasma that, at the end of processing, is pasteurized at 60°C for 10 hours. There are no compatibility requirements.

Solutions of 4.5 or 5% are used to maintain plasma albumin levels in conditions where there is increased vascular permeability, e.g. burns, and are sometimes used in acute blood volume replacement, although crystalloid or non-plasma colloid solution would be the recommended first-line volume expander. Randomized controlled trials on the use of albumin suggest that there is no clear advantage from the use of albumin solutions in the treatment of hypovolaemia over judicious use of saline or colloid solutions. Resuscitation with crystalloid requires volumes of fluid three times greater than with colloid (see chapter 7).

Twenty per cent albumin solutions can be used when hypoproteinaemia is associated with oedema or ascites which is resistant to diuretics (e.g. liver disease, nephrotic syndrome). Twenty per cent albumin is hyperoncotic, so that there is a risk of acutely expanding the intravascular space and precipitating pulmonary oedema.

Factor VIII and Factor IX concentrates

Factor VIII and IX concentrates have been widely used in the treatment of haemophilia. In the UK these have almost completely been replaced by recombinant products to reduce, inter alia, the vCJD transmission risk.

Prothrombin complex concentrates

These products contain factors II, IX and X, and may also contain factor VII (vitamin K-dependent clotting factors). Their use is indicated in the prophylaxis and treatment of bleeding in patients with single or multiple deficiencies of these factors, whether congenital or acquired. They are used to reverse the anticoagulant effect of warfarin when there is major bleeding. Care must be taken in patients with liver disease as this therapy may be thrombogenic.

Immunoglobulin preparations (90% IgG)

These are prepared from fractionation of large pools of plasma from unselected donors or from individuals known to have high levels of specific antibodies. Some products are administered intramuscularly. The indications for some of the more commonly used immunoglobulins are shown in Table 2.1 e.g. hyperimmune globulin against hepatitis B, herpes zoster, tetanus and RhD. Intravenous IgG was originally developed as replacement therapy for immunodeficiency states, but is also used to treat immune thrombocytopenia and other rare diseases such as Guillain–Barré syndrome.

Table 2.1 Indications and doses for the most commonly used specific immunoglobulins

Problem	Patients eligible for IgG	Preparation	Dose
Hepatitis B	Needle-stick or mucosal exposure victims Should also be immunized	Hepatitis B IgG	1000 iu for adults and 500 iu for children < 5 years
Tetanus-prone wounds	Non-immune patients with heavily contaminated wounds Toxoid should be administered with IgG	Tetanus IgG	250 iu routine prophylaxis 500 iu if > 24 h since injury or heavily contaminated wound

RED CELL SEROLOGY

The red cell membrane is a bilipid layer that contains over 400 red cell antigens that have been classified into 23 systems.

ABO antigens

Nearly all deaths from transfusion error are due to ABO-incompatible transfusion. ABO are carbohydrate antigens present on the majority of cells of the body. Their presence depends on the pattern of inheritance of genes encoding glycosyltransferases. Since carbohydrate antigens are widely expressed by other organisms including bacteria, individuals who lack A or B antigens will produce anti-A and anti-B antibodies, respectively. These are usually IgM antibodies (naturally occurring) and are present from the age of 3–6 months. ABO antibodies can react at body temperature and activate complement, and are of major clinical significance as a cause of rapid intravascular haemolysis. For example, transfusion of group A blood to a group B patient results in haemolysis of the transfused red cells because of the anti-A antibodies present in the recipient. Similarly, group O individuals have both anti-A and anti-B antibodies in their plasma that will react with any red cells apart from group O (Table 2.2). Group O blood (Universal donor) can be used in the majority of recipients because it will not be destroyed by anti-A or anti-B antibodies and because processing removes most of the plasma from the unit and hence reduces the donor antibodies contained within.

Rhesus antigens (RH)

Allelic genes at two closely linked loci on chromosome 1 code for this complex blood group system. Phenotypes termed Rhesus D positive or negative (complete absence of D expression), and biallelic C,c and E,e antigens exist. RhD is by far the most immunogenic of the Rhesus antigens and is the only one for which blood is routinely grouped. Individuals who are RhD-negative do not normally have anti-RhD in their plasma unless they have been immunized by previous transfusion or pregnancy. Antibodies to RhD are IgG antibodies do not activate complement, although they do cause extravascular haemolysis. RhD antibodies can cause transfusion reactions and haemolytic disease of the newborn (HDN). It is therefore essential that RhD-negative girls and women of child-bearing potential are not transfused with RhD-positive blood to avoid the stimulation of antibodies to RhD.

Other red cell antigens

Many different blood group antigens exist against which antibodies can be formed of varying clinical significance, depending on their propensity to cause intra- or extravascular haemolysis and HDN. The most important of these are those of the Kell, Kidd and Duffy systems.

PRETRANSFUSION TESTING

Pretransfusion testing consists of three steps:

1. *Blood grouping* involves determining the patient's ABO and RhD type. The donors' blood groups will already be determined by the Blood Service at the time of taking the donation.
2. *Antibody screening* involves the use of a panel of cells to screen a sample of the patient's serum for the presence of clinically significant antibodies. Around 2% of a patient population are likely to have red cell antibodies and where present the specificity of these is identified using further, more detailed, cell panels. The sample is then retained for up to 7 days.
3. *Cross-matching* involves checking the compatibility of the donor units with the patient's serum. This can take three forms:
   - If the patient has an antibody, donor blood negative for the offending antigen(s) is identified and an Indirect Antiglobulin Test (IAT) cross-match carried out. This process may take several hours, depending on the population incidence of the antigen(s) in question.
   - If the patient has no abnormal antibodies, then blood can normally be released much more quickly after a rapid-spin cross match which effectively only checks for ABO incompatibility.
   - Some laboratories are able to release blood by electronic issue where there is accurate patient identification, a historic blood group and antibody screen, no serum antibodies and a secure blood bank testing and computer system that can reliably select and issue blood of compatible type. These systems allow very rapid release of blood.

Maximal Surgical Blood Ordering Schedule (MSBOS)

Cross-matched units are then allocated to the individual patient and held in reserve for 48 hours either in the hospital blood bank or in a local blood fridge. The hospital MSBOS lists the number of units of blood routinely cross-matched preoperatively for elective surgical procedures. This surgical tariff is based on retrospective analysis of actual blood use. The aim is to correlate as closely as possible the number of units cross-matched to the numbers of units transfused. It does not account for individual differences in blood transfusion requirements of different patients undergoing the same procedure, nor does it identify over-transfusion.

Under electronic cross-match, it is often possible to release blood on an 'as required' basis, again either from the blood bank or from a 'remote issue' blood fridge. In this situation the MSBOS becomes redundant and blood wastage improves.

Table 2.2 **The antigens and antibodies of the ABO blood group system**

Blood group	Frequency (UK) %	Red cell antigen	Plasma antibody	Compatible donor blood
A	42	A	Anti-B	A or O
B	8	B	Anti-A	B or O
AB	3	AB	—	AB, A, B or O
O	47	—	Anti-A,B	O only

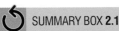

SUMMARY BOX 2.1

Ordering blood in an emergency

- Immediately take samples for cross-matching, ensuring that the sample and the request form are clearly and correctly labelled and are the same on subsequent requests. If the patient is unidentified, then some form of emergency admission number is the best identifier
- Inform the blood bank of the emergency, the volume of blood required, and where blood is to be delivered
- One individual should take responsibility for all communications with the blood bank, and should ensure that it is clear who will be responsible for blood delivery
- In cases of exsanguination, use emergency group O Rh(D)-negative blood
- Do not ask for cross-matched blood in an emergency.

In an emergency the laboratory must be told of the urgency and quantity of blood needed as soon as possible, and asked what they can provide in the time available. Group O RhD-negative blood is available in all hospitals for emergencies where the blood group of the patient is unknown. Patient samples can be rapidly ABO- and RhD-typed, and compatible blood released after a rapid test of ABO compatibility while the antibody screen is ongoing and group O RhD-negative blood is being transfused.

INDICATIONS FOR TRANSFUSION

The decision to transfuse is a complex one. Clinical judgment plays a vital role, as there is no consensus on the precise indications for red cell transfusion. The clinician prescribing any blood component should consider the risks and benefits of transfusion for each individual patient. Tolerance of anaemia is dependent on a number of factors, including the speed of onset, age, level of activity and co-existing disease. In chronic anaemia, fatigue and shortness of breath, although subjective, are still useful in determining the need for transfusion. In acute anaemia (usually secondary to blood loss), the effects of hypovolaemia need to be differentiated from those of anaemia. Healthy adults can tolerate significant blood loss (30–40% of circulating volume) without adverse effects and would not normally require transfusion. This is largely due to adaptive mechanisms such as a compensatory rise in cardiac output and peripheral vasodilatation, which act to maintain tissue oxygen delivery. The actual haemoglobin concentration is not a reliable clinical indicator in acute haemorrhage and does not in itself indicate a definite need for transfusion; however, it can act as a prompt for the clinician to seek other features that suggest transfusion is required. In a clinically stable situation, red cell transfusion is usually not required with a haemoglobin concentration of $\geq 100\,\text{g/l}$.

Generally, in healthy individuals, a transfusion threshold of 70–80 g/l is appropriate, as this leaves a margin of safety over the critical level of 40–50 g/l, at which point oxygen consumption becomes limited by the amount that the circulation can supply. For elderly patients or those with cardiovascular or respiratory disease, who may tolerate anaemia poorly, transfusion should be considered at a haemoglobin concentration of $\leq 80\,\text{g/l}$ to maintain a haemoglobin level of around 100 g/l. In the intensive care setting, some studies have shown that maintaining a lower haemoglobin threshold may be associated with better patient outcomes, at least

EBM 2.1 Red cell transfusion in the correction of a low haemoglobin in critically ill patients

'A single large RCT of red cell transfusion in patients in intensive care showed that patients who were maintained with an Hb in the range of 70–90 g/l had a lower mortality and morbidity compared to those with an Hb maintained in the range of 100–120 g/l. The former groups received approximately half the number of red cell units.'

Hebert PC, et al. with the Canadian Transfusion Requirements in Critical Care Group. N Engl J Med 2004; 340:409–417.

For further information: www.transfusionguidelines.org.uk
www.sign.ac.uk

in some patient groups. The best available evidence for this is the randomized, controlled TRICC trial (EBM 2.1), which compared a liberal transfusion strategy (Hb 100–120 g/l) with a restrictive one (Hb 70–90 g/l). Overall in-hospital mortality was significantly lower in the restrictive group, although the 30-day mortality rate was not significantly different. However, the 30-day mortality rate was significantly lower in the restrictive transfusion group for those patients who were less ill (APACHE < 20) or younger (< 55 years of age). These data show that a restrictive strategy is at least equivalent, and in some patient groups is superior, to a more liberal transfusion strategy.

BLOOD ADMINISTRATION

Avoidable errors in the requesting, supply and administration of blood lead to significant risks to patients. Multiple errors contribute to more than 50% of 'wrong blood' incidents reported to the UK Serious Hazards of Transfusion (SHOT) scheme. Of these, 70% occur in clinical areas and 30% occur in laboratories. Acute haemolytic transfusion reactions due to ABO incompatibility can be fatal and are most often caused by errors in identification of the patient at the time of blood sampling or administration (EBM 2.2).

The British Committee for Standards in Haematology has produced a guideline for the administration of blood and blood components and the management of transfused patients. This contains a number of recommendations that should be adhered to in order to minimize transfusion error. These include the following:

1. It is crucial that the identity of the patient is established verbally (if possible) *and* by checking the patient identification wristband before blood is taken. The sample must be labelled fully (in handwriting) before leaving the bedside. (Sample tubes must never be pre-labelled.)

EBM 2.2 Risks of fatal transfusion reactions–cases reported to national reporting systems

'In the UK between 1996 and 2000 there were 33 reports of death attributed to transfusion. During this period approximately 10 million units of blood components were supplied. The largest cause of major morbidity remains transfusion of the incorrect unit of blood, leading to an incompatible red cell transfusion reaction.'

Love EM, Soldan K. Serious hazards of transfusion, Annual report 1999–2000. Manchester: SHOT; 2009.

For further information: www.shotuk.org and www.transfusionguidelines.org.uk

2. The blood request form should be completed and should provide, as a minimum, the patient's full name, date of birth and hospital number. Each patient must have a unique identification number. The location of the patient, number and type of blood or blood components and time when required, the patient's diagnosis and the reason for the request are also essential.

3. Before transfusion is commenced, the following details must be checked by two individuals, at least one of whom must be a State Registered Nurse (SRN) or medical officer:

   a. Full patient identity on the patient wristband against the compatibility label on the unit of blood.

   b. ABO and Rh(D) type on the pack compatibility label.

   c. Donation number on the pack compatibility label.

   d. Expiry date of the pack.

   e. Examination of the pack to ensure that there are no leaks or evidence of haemolysis.

   If there are any discrepancies, the blood must not be transfused and the laboratory must be informed immediately.

4. As a minimum, the patient's pulse rate, blood pressure and temperature should be recorded prior to commencing the transfusion, 15 minutes after commencement of each unit (as this is when transfusion reactions are most likely), and on completion of the transfusion. The vital signs should be rechecked if the patient feels unwell during the transfusion.

5. A permanent record of the transfusion of blood and blood components and the administration of blood products must be kept in the medical notes. This should include the sheets used for the prescription of blood or blood components and those used for nursing observations during the transfusion. An entry should also be made in the case notes, documenting the date, the indication for transfusion, the number and type of units used, whether or not the desired effect was achieved, and the occurrence and management of any adverse effects.

SUMMARY BOX 2.2

Safety checks for blood administration

Before administering blood, two staff members (one of whom must be a doctor or trained staff nurse) must check:

- the patient's full identity (wristband, and verbally if possible)
- the blood pack, compatibility label and report form (noting donation number and expiry date)
- the blood pack for signs of haemolysis or leakage from the pack.

Any discrepancies mean that the blood must not be transfused and that the laboratory must be informed immediately.

ADVERSE EFFECTS OF TRANSFUSION

A voluntary anonymised reporting scheme for serious hazards of transfusion (SHOT) has been in place in the UK since 1996, and the incidence of reported hazards is shown in Figure 2.2. The greatest concern for most patients is the risk of transfusion-transmitted infection, but by far the most common risk is the transfusion of an incorrect blood component.

Transfusion reactions can be divided into those that occur early (acute transfusion reactions, or ATRs, occurring within 24 hours of commencing but usually during the transfusion) and those that occur late (delayed transfusion reactions, or DTRs, occurring more than 24 hours after commencing the transfusion and often once the patient has been discharged). Acute adverse reactions to blood transfusion require urgent investigation and management, as they may be life-threatening. The major acute causes frequently have similar symptoms and signs, and blind treatment may initially be necessary until the exact cause becomes apparent. Acute and delayed adverse effects of transfusion are listed in Tables 2.3 and 2.4, respectively. The risks of infection from blood transfusion are listed in Table 2.5. Management of acute transfusion reactions is illustrated in Figure 2.3.

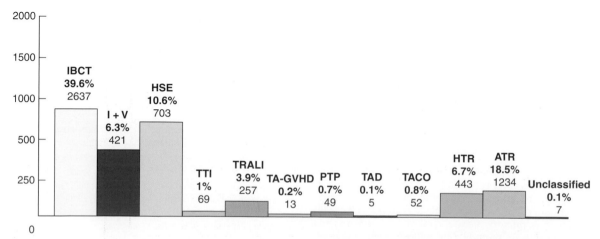

Fig. 2.2 SHOT report for 1996–2009 (*n* = 6653) showing the rate (%) of serious hazards of transfusion reported in the UK. (ATR = acute transfusion reaction; HTR = haemolytic transfusion reaction; IBCT = incorrect blood component transfused; TACO = transfusion associated circulatory overload; TAD = transfusion associated dyspnoea; PTP = post-transfusion purpura; TA-GVHD = transfusion-associated graft-versus-host disease; TRALI = transfusion-related acute lung injury; TTI = transfusion-transmitted infection; I&U = inappropriate and unnecessary transfusion; HSE = handling and storage errors)

Table 2.3 Acute transfusion reactions

	Cause	Implicated components	Clinical features
Immunological			
Acute haemolytic transfusion reaction	ABO-incompatible transfusion resulting in acute intravascular haemolysis	RCC Platelets FFP Cryo	Develops within minutes. Chills, fevers, rigors, chest tightness, infusion site pain, hypotension, shock, DIC and acute renal failure. May be fatal.
Transfusion-associated acute lung injury	HLA or neutrophil Abs in donor plasma react with recipient leucocytes	Any plasma-containing component (RCC, FFP, cryo, platelets)	Develops within 4 hours of transfusion. Dyspnoea, cough, fever, hypoxia, pulmonary infiltrates (ARDS). With supportive care, improvement over 2–4 days in 80% of patients.
Febrile non-haemolytic transfusion reaction	Neutrophil Ab in recipient plasma reacts with donor leucocytes	RCC Platelets FFP Cryo	Develops late in course of transfusion. Usually mild. Full recovery expected.
Allergic reactions	Reaction to plasma proteins	Any plasma-containing component	Urticaria/itch within minutes of start of transfusion. Occasionally severe with anaphylaxis. Usually full recovery with appropriate management.
Non-Immunological			
Bacterial contamination	Contamination during collection or storage. Rarely, bacteraemic donor	Platelets most commonly RCC	Symptoms/signs of sepsis develop early in course of transfusion. May be fatal.
Transfusion-associated circulatory overload	Over-transfusion	Any	Symptoms/signs of acute left ventricular failure. Resolves with appropriate management.

(Ab = antibody; Ag = antigen; ARDS = acute respiratory distress syndrome; Cryo = cryoprecipitate; DIC = disseminated intravascular coagulation; FFP = fresh frozen plasma; HLA = human leucocyte antigen; RCC = red cell concentrate)

Table 2.4 Delayed transfusion reactions

	Cause	Implicated components	Clinical features
Immunological			
Delayed haemolytic transfusion reaction	Patient has red cell Ab at undetectable level. Re-exposure to Ag results in secondary immune response and extravascular haemolysis	Red cells Platelets	May be asymptomatic or develop jaundice, fever and haemoglobinuria with a fall in haemoglobin. Seldom fatal but can result in significant morbidity if the patient is already unwell
Alloimmunization	Recipient forms Ab in response to donor Ag	Red cells	Usually not detected until subsequently grouped and saved or cross-matched
Post-transfusion purpura	Recipient has a platelet-specific Ab and develops secondary immune response on re-exposure, resulting in destruction of donor platelets and, through an unknown mechanism, recipient platelets	Platelets Red cells	Sudden development of severe thrombocytopenia associated with bleeding 5–12 days following transfusion. Complications are related to bleeding. Platelet count usually recovers with appropriate management, which includes i.v. immunoglobulin
Transfusion-associated graft-versus-host disease	Viable T lymphocytes transfused into immunocompromised recipient	Any cellular product	Fever, desquamating rash, abnormal LFTs and pancytopenia develop 1–4 weeks following transfusion. Mortality rate > 90%. Prevent by irradiation of cellular components in patients at high risk
Non-Immunological			
Transfusion-transmitted infection: Risks shown in Table 2.5 **Iron overload**: Chronic red cell transfusion leads to accumulation of iron in tissues, e.g. liver, heart, pancreas			

(Ag = antigen; Ab = antibody)

Table 2.5 Risks of a single red cell unit transmitting disease in the UK

Infection	Estimated risk (per unit transfused)
Hepatitis B	1:50 000–1:200 000
Hepatitis C	1:200 000
HIV	1:2 500 000
HTLV	1:10 000 – 100 000
vCJD	Unknown, not zero
Bacterial	1:2000–10 000

SUMMARY BOX **2.3**

Transfusion errors

- Almost all deaths from transfusion reaction are due to ABO incompatibility
- Errors in patient identification at the time of blood sampling or administration are the major cause (occurring in at least 1:1000–1:2000 transfusions)
- When taking the initial blood sample:
  Check the patient's identity verbally and on the wrist identification band
  Label the sample fully before leaving the bedside
  Make sure that the blood request form is clearly and accurately completed.

AUTOLOGOUS TRANSFUSION

As immunological and infective complications can result from donated blood, the use of the patient's own blood may be considered in certain situations to try to reduce the need for allogeneic blood.

Preoperative donation

Autologous blood can be collected from otherwise fit patients preoperatively and stored for 35 days preoperatively. These units are subject to the same testing and processing as allogeneic donations. There is no evidence to show a reduction in allogeneic transfusion in patients who have donated autologous blood and in fact some which may suggest that these individuals require more following autologous donation. This being the case, the use of autologous predeposit has diminished and UK guidance indicates it is really only of use in individuals where they are of such a rare blood type and it may be difficult to identify suitable donations.

Isovolaemic haemodilution

This technique is restricted to patients in whom significant blood loss (> 1000 ml) is anticipated. Following induction of anaesthesia, up to 1.5 litres of blood is withdrawn preoperatively into a clearly labelled blood pack containing a standard anticoagulant, and replaced by saline to maintain blood volume. The fall in haematocrit reduces the loss of red cells (and haemoglobin) during surgical bleeding while maintaining optimal tissue perfusion. The withdrawn blood can be re-infused, either during surgery or postoperatively, with transfusion complete before the patient leaves the responsibility of the anaesthetist. Blood is maintained at the point of care, minimizing the risk of administrative or clerical errors, although standard pre-transfusion checks should be carried out to ensure the correct pack(s) are re-infused.

Cell salvage

Blood can be collected from the operation site either directly during surgery or by the use of collection devices attached to surgical drains. During surgery, blood can be collected by suction, processed by a cell salvage machine in which it is anticoagulated while the cells are washed to remove clots and debris, and then returned to the patient. The process is contraindicated in patients with malignancy or sepsis, and is only appropriate when there is substantial blood loss. Several litres of blood can be salvaged intraoperatively, far more than with other autologous techniques. Postoperative drainage can be returned to the patient, most commonly not washed. This process does require some positive suction pressure, and in some circumstances this may lead to increased blood loss. The other main disadvantage is that salvaged blood is not haemostatically intact, as there may have been clotting in the wound leading to consumption of clotting factors and platelets. Cell salvage can significantly reduce the exposure of patients to allogeneic blood and is used extensively in cardiac surgery, trauma surgery and liver transplantation.

TRANSFUSION REQUIREMENTS IN SPECIAL SURGICAL SETTINGS

Massive transfusion

Massive transfusion denotes the transfusion of the equivalent of the circulating blood volume within a 24-hour period (i.e. 10–12 units in an adult). It is needed most often in severe trauma and in bleeding from the gastrointestinal tract or various obstetric disorders. Although massive transfusion restores circulating blood volume and oxygen-carrying capacity, it is frequently complicated by dilutional coagulopathy, which may be exacerbated by consumptional coagulopathy in patients with an underlying disorder such as liver disease or DIC. Table 2.6 outlines some of the complications of massive transfusion.

Cardiopulmonary bypass

Platelets and coagulation factors may be activated or lost in the extracorporeal circulation during cardiopulmonary bypass at open heart surgery, so that FFP and platelet transfusion may be needed to deal with postoperative bleeding. The platelet count may be normal but the platelets are likely to be dysfunctional, having been activated by the extracorporeal circuit. Platelet transfusion is indicated if there is microvascular bleeding, or if the bleeding cannot be corrected surgically after the patient is off bypass and once heparin has been reversed with an appropriate dose of protamine sulphate. Coagulation screens should be performed to assess required therapy prior to infusion of coagulation factors in all but life-threatening haemorrhage. Near-patient testing of coagulation, e.g. thromboelastography, may also guide decisions on the need for blood component therapy.

Aspirin is commonly administered to patients awaiting bypass surgery. This drug has a prolonged inhibitory effect on platelet function (5–7 days), and should therefore, where possible, be stopped 7 days before surgery and commenced immediately postoperatively, when it significantly helps graft patency.

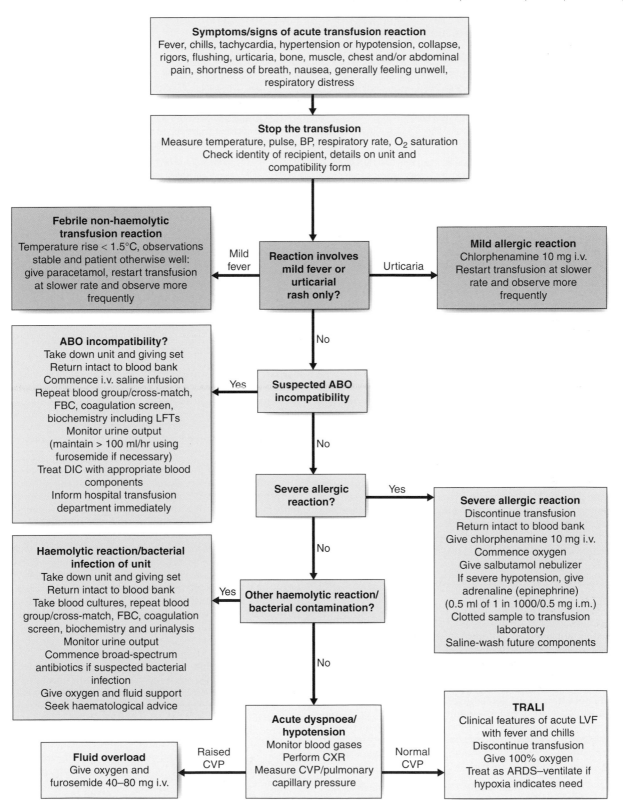

Fig. 2.3 Management of an acute transfusion reaction. (DIC = disseminated intravascular coagulation; LVF = left ventricular failure; TRALI = transfusion-related acute lung injury)

2

Table 2.6 **Complications of massive transfusion**

Complication	Mechanism	Management
Thrombocytopenia	Consumption/DIC Dilutional after 1.5–2.0 blood volumes replaced	In patients with acute bleeding, transfuse platelets to maintain count $> 50 \times 10^9/l$ ($> 100 \times 10^9/l$ if acute trauma or CNS injury)
Coagulopathy	Consumption/DIC Dilutional after 1.0 blood volume replaced	If continued blood loss and PT or APTT ratio $> 1.5 \times$ control levels, give FFP 10–15 ml/kg. If fibrinogen < 1.0 g/l, cryoprecipitate is also indicated
Hypocalcaemia	Citrate anticoagulant binds to ionized Ca, lowering plasma levels (only problematic in neonates and liver disease)	If ECG shows signs of hypocalcaemia, give 5 ml Ca gluconate (or equivalent paediatric dose) over 5 mins. Repeat if ECG remains abnormal
Hyper- or hypokalaemia	Red cell degeneration during storage increases plasma K^+. Following transfusion, red cells rapidly normalize Na/K equilibrium, which may lead to $\uparrow K^+$	Careful monitoring of K^+ levels in massive transfusion
Hypothermia	Transfusion of blood at 4°C lowers core temperature	Prevent by use of blood warmer when transfusion rate > 50 ml/kg/h in adults (15 ml/kg/h in children)
ARDS	Multifactorial	Minimize risk by maintaining tissue perfusion, correct hypotension and avoid over-transfusion

(APTT = activated partial thromboplastin time; ARDS = acute respiratory distress syndrome; DIC = disseminated intravascular coagulation; FFP = fresh frozen plasma; PT = prothrombin time)

METHODS TO REDUCE THE NEED FOR BLOOD TRANSFUSION

Large variations in transfusion practice are currently seen in the European Union. This is due to many factors, including differences in the patient populations treated, surgical and anaesthetic techniques, and attitudes to and availability of blood, as well as differences in pre- and postoperative care. Such differences in transfusion practice have not been shown to be associated with significant differences in mortality. These findings indicate that it may be possible to reduce blood transfusion through various interventions without impacting negatively on clinical outcomes.

Acute volume replacement

Non-plasma colloid volume expanders of large molecules, such as dextran, are a relatively inexpensive colloidal alternative to plasma in first-line management of patients who are volume-depleted as a result of bleeding.

In the initial resuscitation of patients with haemorrhagic shock, the adequacy of volume replacement is usually of much greater importance than the choice of fluid. A reasonable guide in adults is 1000 ml of crystalloid (0.9% saline or Ringer's lactate solution), followed by 1000 ml of colloid, and then replacement with red cells. In the elderly and those with cardiac impairment, red cell replacement should be started earlier to maintain oxygen-carrying capacity without causing fluid overload.

Mechanisms for reducing blood use in surgery

Preoperative

When surgery is elective, significant reductions in blood use can be made by ensuring that the patient has a normal haemoglobin and by correcting any pre-existing anaemia, e.g. iron or folic acid deficiency. Drugs that interfere with haemostasis, e.g. non-steroidal anti-inflammatory drugs, aspirin and warfarin, should be stopped where appropriate. An abnormal clotting screen or platelet count should be investigated and corrected prior to surgery. To ensure optimal management, these issues should be addressed 4–6 weeks prior to surgery at preoperative assessment clinics.

Intraoperative

The training, experience and competence of the surgeon performing the procedure are the most crucial factors in reducing operative blood loss. The importance of meticulous surgical technique, with attention to bleeding points, cannot be underestimated. Other techniques, such as posture, the use of vasoconstrictors and tourniquets, and avoidance of hypothermia, should always be considered, as these can have a significant impact on perioperative blood loss. Certain pharmacological agents, e.g. antifibrinolytics such as tranexamic acid, may significantly reduce the requirements for blood and are indicated in certain operative procedures.

Fibrin sealant mimics the final stage in the coagulation cascade, in which fibrinogen is converted to fibrin in the presence of thrombin, factor XIII, fibronectin and ionized calcium. Freeze-dried sterilized fibrinogen, fibronectin and factor XIII can be delivered from one barrel of a double-barrelled syringe while thrombin, calcium and aprotinin are delivered from the other. If the two mixtures meet at a surgical bleeding site the solution clots almost immediately, the clot resolving over a period of days. Fibrin sealant has been used in vascular, cardiac and liver surgery and in situations where even small amounts of bleeding can be problematic (e.g. middle ear surgery).

Acute normovolaemic haemodilution and intraoperative blood salvage are two of the autologous methods of blood conservation that can be employed during surgery to reduce exposure to transfusion. They are described in the section on autologous programmes.

Postoperative

Postoperative cell salvage (see above) can reduce the need for allogeneic transfusion.

The decision to transfuse postoperatively should depend on several factors (see 'Indications for transfusion'). Blood transfusion should be limited to the amount of blood required to raise the haemoglobin above the transfusion threshold and/or achieve clinical stability, even if this is only 1 unit. Appropriate use of antifibrinolytic drugs such as tranexamic acid and the routine prescribing of iron and folic acid also reduce postoperative transfusion. A reduction in transfusion has been shown to result from the introduction of simple protocols that give guidance on when the haemoglobin should be checked and red cells transfused.

BETTER BLOOD TRANSFUSION

In recent times, attention has been focused on blood transfusion practice for a number of reasons. These include concerns about the transmission of vCJD by blood transfusion, increased costs associated with new safety measures such as leucocyte depletion, documented variations in transfusion practice and recommendations arising from the SHOT scheme. Better Blood Transfusion (BBT) programmes have been established in many countries with the purpose of promoting the safe, efficient and appropriate use of blood components and plasma derivatives. The aims of BBT are to establish protocols and guidelines to nationally approved standards, implement accredited learning programmes, audit transfusion practice and achieve a reduction in inappropriate blood use.

FUTURE TRENDS

Whilst the demand for blood has fallen over the past few years, ever more stringent donor selection guidelines and social and economic changes are impacting negatively on the donor base. Furthermore it is predicted that demand will rise again over the next few decades as an increasingly elderly population requires more healthcare. This means that blood should be considered a scarce and valuable commodity that should be responsibly prescribed.

Although red cell substitutes are under development, fluorocarbon oxygen carriers have found limited clinical application and concerns have been raised around potential toxicity of haemoglobin solutions

Recombinant human erythropoietin raises haemoglobin levels in patients with chronic renal failure but its use in the wider clinical setting has been limited.

The objective in managing surgical patients should be to minimize anaemia and bleeding and hence the need for transfusion. Although it is clear that no patient should be transfused unnecessarily, it is equally certain that no patient should be allowed to exsanguinate because of concerns regarding blood safety.

3

K.C.H. Fearon
G.L. Carlson

Nutritional support in surgical patients

CHAPTER CONTENTS

INTRODUCTION

It goes without saying that without food there can be no life, that food is a basic human right, and that it behoves every doctor to pay attention to the nutritional needs of their patients. Nevertheless, approximately one-third of all patients admitted to an acute hospital will have evidence of protein-calorie malnutrition and two-thirds will leave hospital either malnourished or having lost weight. Against this background it is important to recognize that in Western Society there is now an epidemic of obesity. Whilst obese individuals generally have a matching increase in lean body mass, there is a subgroup with underlying muscle wasting (sarcopenic obesity) who are at high risk of metabolic syndrome and postoperative complications. Patients with sarcopenic obesity are difficult to recognize clinically due to the fact that their muscle wasting is obscured by overlying fat.

Malnutrition has damaging effects on psychological status, activity levels and appearance. Paradoxically, in the surgical patient a low body fat content may sometimes be viewed as an advantage, making technical aspects of surgery easier. There is, however, clear evidence that patients with severe protein depletion have a significantly greater incidence of postoperative complications, such as pneumonia and wound infection, and a prolonged hospital stay.

Nutritional disorders in surgical practice have two principal components. First, starvation can be initiated by the effects of the disease, by restriction of oral intake, or both. Simple starvation results in progressive loss of the body's energy and protein reserves (i.e. subcutaneous fat and skeletal muscle). Second, there are the metabolic effects of stress/inflammation; namely, increased catabolism and reduced anabolism. These result in a variety of changes, including a low serum albumin concentration, accelerated muscle wasting and water retention. Although malnutrition may be the result of starvation, in most surgical patients it results from a combination of reduced food intake and metabolic change (Fig. 3.1).

ASSESSMENT OF NUTRITIONAL STATUS

The main energy reserves in the body are found in subcutaneous and intra-abdominal fat. Loss of fat reserves does not usually impair function. In contrast, there are no true protein reserves in the body. Thus, in the face of starvation or stress, structural tissues such as skeletal muscle and the gut are autocannibalized to liberate amino acids, resulting in functional impairment that can eventually impede recovery.

The key elements of nutritional assessment include current food intake, levels of energy and protein reserves, and the patient's likely clinical course (Fig. 3.2). Patients who have not eaten for 5 days or more require nutritional support, and those with symptoms such as anorexia, nausea, vomiting or early satiety are at risk of a reduced food intake and hence undernutrition. Levels of energy reserves are most easily assessed by examining for loss of subcutaneous fat (skinfolds), whereas protein depletion is most commonly manifest as skeletal muscle wasting (Fig. 3.3). A history of weight loss of more than 10–15% is highly significant. Patients can also be assessed according to their body mass index – BMI = weight (kg)/height (m²). The normal BMI is 18.5–24.9. A value less than 18 is suggestive of significant protein-calorie undernutrition. Finally, it is important to recognize that in assessing the nutritional status of patients, knowledge of their likely clinical course is vital (Fig. 3.4). For example, if patients are well nourished, they should be able to withstand the brief period of fasting associated with major surgery. However, if patients are severely malnourished (e.g. weight loss of 15%, BMI 17), then even a short further period of starvation or catabolism may make them so critically undernourished that this may

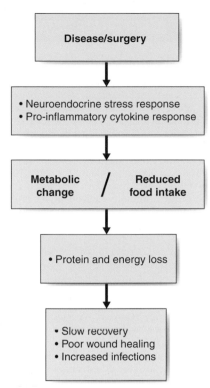

Fig. 3.1 Mechanisms linking the effects of disease/surgery on patient outcomes.

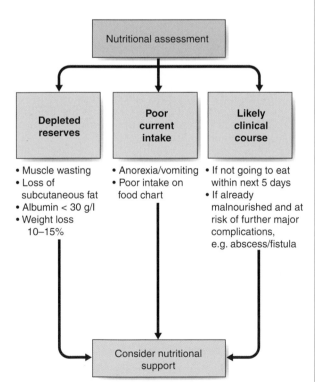

Fig. 3.2 Nutritional assessment in surgical patients.

become life-threatening in itself. Taken together, a patient's food intake, level of reserve and likely clinical course should alert the astute clinician to the need for nutritional support and should be part of the routine daily appraisal of every patient during a surgical ward round.

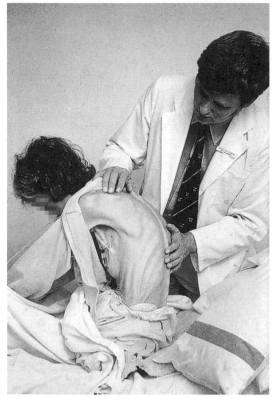

Fig. 3.3 Protein-energy malnutrition in a surgical patient, illustrating depleted muscle and subcutaneous fat stores.

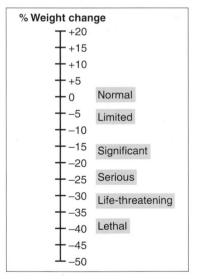

Fig. 3.4 Alterations in nutritional status associated with weight loss.

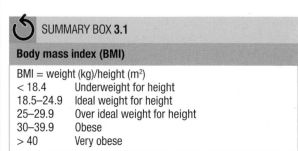

SUMMARY BOX 3.1

Body mass index (BMI)

BMI = weight (kg)/height (m²)

< 18.4	Underweight for height
18.5–24.9	Ideal weight for height
25–29.9	Over ideal weight for height
30–39.9	Obese
> 40	Very obese

ASSESSMENT OF NUTRITIONAL REQUIREMENTS

Energy and protein/nitrogen requirements vary, depending on weight, body composition, clinical status, mobility and dietary intake. For most patients, an approximation based on weight and clinical status is sufficient. Relevant values are given in Table 3.1. Few adult patients require more than 25–30 kcal/kg/day (approximately 1800–2200 kcal in an adult of average body mass). Additional calories are unlikely to be used effectively and may even constitute a metabolic stress. Particular caution must be exercised when refeeding the chronically starved patient because of the dangers of hypokalaemia and hypophosphataemia (notably cardiac dysrhythmias).

The most common method for assessing protein/nitrogen requirement is based on body weight (Table 3.1). Although more accurate assessment for patients receiving nutritional support can be derived from measurement of 24-hour urinary urea excretion, which can be converted to an estimate of 24-hour urinary nitrogen loss, this is seldom necessary in routine clinical practice.

Enteral diets will usually provide protein whereas parenteral nutrition provides the nitrogen (N) in the form of amino acids. The nitrogen equivalent of protein can be calculated by multiplying nitrogen requirement by a conversion factor of 6.25. In practice, nitrogen requirements are usually estimated based upon predicted calorie intake and the level of metabolic stress. Most patients will require 1gN per 200 kcal of energy provided daily (typically 10gN) in the absence of sepsis but this may increase to as much as 18–20g N in critically ill, catabolic and septic patients. Even if losses are in excess of this, more than 18 g nitrogen/day (equivalent to 112 g protein) is seldom given because it is unlikely to be used effectively. It is usually impossible to prevent substantial loss of protein reserves and lean body mass in critically ill patients and the aim of meeting requirements in such patients is primarily to limit losses resulting from catabolism.

Table 3.1 **Estimation of energy and protein requirements in adult surgical patients**

	Uncomplicated	Complicated/stressed
Energy (kcal/kg/day)	25	30–35
Protein (g/kg/day)*	1.0	1.3–1.5

*Grams of protein can be converted to the equivalent amount of nitrogen by dividing by 6.25.

CAUSES OF INADEQUATE INTAKE

The ideal way for surgical patients to take in enough nutrients is for them to eat or drink palatable food. Unfortunately, the catering budget is often far too low for the provision of appetizing food, and wastage of unwanted food can account for up to 40% of that served. Other reasons for a poor food intake include the patient being too weak and anorexic, or having a mechanical problem such as obstruction of the gastrointestinal tract. Patients with increased metabolic demands may have some difficulty in taking sufficient food to meet such demands. Patients with a normal functional gut may also have a reduced food intake due simply to the cumulative effects of repeated periods of fasting to undergo investigations such as endoscopy or radiology.

Some patients suffer from what is best described as 'intestinal failure', i.e. a state in which the amount of functioning gut is reduced below a level where enough food can be digested and absorbed for nourishment. Intestinal failure can be acute (when it is usually reversible) or chronic (when it is frequently permanent). Acute intestinal failure is relatively common, especially after abdominal surgery when it commonly results from the development of surgical complications, whereas chronic intestinal failure is comparatively rare. The principal causes of acute intestinal failure are mechanical intestinal obstruction and paralytic ileus, frequently associated with abdominal sepsis, as well as intestinal fistula formation, in which bowel content is lost externally or short-circuited (internal fistula) before it can be adequately digested and absorbed. Chronic intestinal failure may result from short bowel syndrome, following extensive small bowel resection, extensive small bowel disease, such as Crohn's disease, and motility disorders, such as chronic intestinal pseudo-obstruction. In some patients with short bowel syndrome, the remaining intestine may adapt over a period of months or years by a process of progressive dilatation and mucosal hyperplasia, allowing the patient to regain nutritional independence. Reconstructive surgery may also improve the function or even be employed to increase the functional length of remaining intestine in selected cases.

Specialized nutritional treatment is required in patients with intestinal failure if the patient is to remain adequately nourished. The provision of nutrition in many patients with acute intestinal failure is further complicated by the metabolic consequences of ongoing inflammation or sepsis. As a general rule, this results in increased energy requirements and impaired ability to utilize administered nutrients, rendering nutritional support less effective. The priority in providing effective nutritional support for such patients is therefore to simultaneously eliminate sepsis.

METHODS OF PROVIDING NUTRITIONAL SUPPORT

Nutrients can be given via the gastrointestinal tract, i.e. enteral nutrition, or intravenously, i.e. parenteral nutrition (Fig. 3.5). Parenteral nutrition is indicated only when enteral feeding is not feasible. Very few patients are not suitable for some form of enteral feeding, which is both safer and cheaper than parenteral nutrition (EBM 3.1). Certainly, all those who have a normal length of functioning gastrointestinal tract, and most of those who have a reduced amount, can be fed by this route. Furthermore,

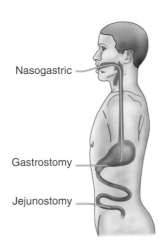

Fig. 3.5 Routes of enteral nutrition.

EBM 3.1 **Enteral vs parenteral nutrition in surgical patients**

'Enteral nutrition should be first choice for nutritional support in the critically ill surgical patient.'

Gramlich L, et al. Nutrition 2004; 20:843–848.

---

the ingestion of even suboptimal amounts of food may help maintain the gut function, which may have beneficial metabolic and immunological consequences. A flexible and pragmatic approach, which employs a combination of both enteral and parenteral nutrition, tailoring the route of nutrient provision to the patient's ability to tolerate and benefit from it, is desirable.

Enteral nutrition

Oral route

As stated previously, it is essential to provide warm, appetizing food on the wards, to make sure there are enough nursing and auxiliary staff available to help elderly/infirm patients take their food, and to encourage nursing staff to be aware of the nutritional needs of all patients. It is against this basic background of nutritional care that the need for artificial nutritional support should be considered.

Many patients suffer from early satiety (feeling full after a meal), and encouraging them to eat small amounts frequently or to sip an oral supplement between meals can help overcome this symptom. Oral supplements come in cartons of about 250 ml and each contains about 250 kcal and 10 g of protein. These should be available to all patients who require them. There is a range of flavours and the texture can be changed if chilled, for example. Most patients manage to take one or two cartons per day if required. However, fatigue with such supplements is commonplace and leads to reduced efficacy in the long run.

There are numerous reasons why surgical patients may suffer from anorexia (i.e. poor appetite) (Table 3.2). Before embarking on tube enteral feeding, it is important to manage actively any symptoms that can be treated (e.g. oral thrush with nystatin, nausea with anti-emetics, provision of adequate dental hygiene or artificial dentures) and thus boost spontaneous oral intake. For patients who are unable to swallow, or for those whose anorexia is resistant to other therapy, nasoenteral feeding via a fine-bore tube should be used.

Table 3.2 **Causes of anorexia in surgical patients**
• Intestinal obstruction
• Ileus
• Cancer anorexia
• Depression, anxiety, pain
• Drugs, e.g. opiates
• Oral ulceration/infection
• General debility/weakness

Methods of administration of enteral feeds

Nasogastric or nasojejunal tubes

If patients cannot drink or sip a liquid feed for mechanical reasons, or if they are unconscious or on a ventilator, enteral nutrition can be given by a fine-bore nasogastric or naso-enteric tube. The position of the tube tip should be checked radiologically, or by aspirating gastric content and confirming the presence of acid by litmus paper, before nutrients are infused. Patients who need prolonged enteral feeding can learn to pass a fine-bore tube each evening and feed themselves overnight. When carried out at home, this is known as home enteral nutrition.

Gastrostomy and jejunostomy

If nasogastric feeding is impossible due to disease or obstruction of the upper alimentary tract, nutrients may be given through a tube placed into the gastrointestinal tract below the lesion (Fig. 3.6). Thus a patient with pseudobulbar palsy or an oesophageal fistula can be fed through a gastrostomy, and a patient with a gastric or duodenal fistula can be fed through a jejunostomy.

Specially designed gastrostomy tubes can now be inserted by a combined percutaneous and endoscopic (PEG) method, and are particularly valuable for prolonged feeding when there is no impairment of gastric emptying (e.g. stroke patients). Feeding jejunostomy tubes can be inserted at the time of laparotomy if the surgeon anticipates that prolonged nutritional support will be needed postoperatively (e.g. in patients undergoing oesophagectomy and gastrectomy for cancer, or necrosectomy for severe pancreatitis).

Complications of enteral nutrition

Just because enteral feeds are administered directly into the gastrointestinal tract, it cannot be assumed that this technique is free from complications. Indeed, complications of enteral nutrition may be at least as common as with parenteral

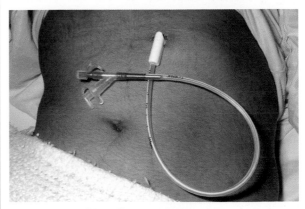

Fig. 3.6 Patient with feeding gastrostomy.

SUMMARY BOX 3.3

Enteral nutrition

- If patients cannot eat adequate amounts of food, they should be reviewed by the ward dietitian
- If oral supplements fail, a fine-bore tube can be used for supplemental or total enteral nutrition
- Most patients tolerate a whole-protein feed (1 kcal/ml), which can be escalated to 100 ml/hour and thus supply about 2400 kcal/day and 14 g nitrogen/day
- If a tube cannot be passed down the oesophagus, gastrostomy and jejunostomy feeding should be considered
- The main complications of enteral feeding relate to patient tolerance (nausea, vomiting and diarrhoea) and to the insertion site (gastrostomy or jejunostomy).

nutrition and can be equally life-threatening. Diarrhoea is more common with nasogastric than with nasoenteric feeding. It may be managed by reducing the rate of infusion and by ensuring the patient is not on broad-spectrum antibiotics. In some cases, selection of lower osmolarity feed (such as an elemental feed rather than semi-elemental or peptide feeds may help). Vomiting can be managed by reducing the rate of feeding and by the use of prokinetic drugs such as metoclopramide or erythromycin. Monitoring of fluid and electrolyte balance is important, at least in the acute phase of a patient's illness (for metabolic complications, see 'Parenteral nutrition'). It can be extremely difficult to monitor the adequacy of enteral feeding, particularly in the presence of diarrhoea and/or vomiting. A significant proportion of patients receiving enteral feeding are unable to tolerate the rate of calorie infusion required for effective nutritional support. Excessive infusion of nasogastric feed may cause marked abdominal bloating, resulting in splinting of the diaphragm and impaired respiratory function.

Complications also occur because of difficulty in placing the tubes. Examples include a fine-bore nasogastric tube inserted wrongly into the respiratory tract, or early accidental removal of a jejunostomy tube, with intraperitoneal leakage. The fixation of the jejunum to the abdominal wall required to minimize the risk of intraperitoneal leakage associated with feeding jejunostomy may in turn increase the risk of small bowel volvulus. As with other areas of nutrition supplementation, attention to detail is paramount.

Parenteral nutrition

Intravenous feeding is indicated when patients have intestinal failure (see above).

Parenteral nutrition can provide the patient's total needs for protein, energy, electrolytes, trace metals and vitamins, i.e. total parenteral nutrition (TPN). The need to restrict volume means that concentrated solutions are used. As such solutions are irritant and thrombogenic, they are usually administered through a catheter positioned in a large high-flow vein, such as the superior vena cava.

Indications for TPN

The chief indication for TPN is intestinal failure. TPN can be both effective and life-saving when postoperative complications develop, especially when these prevent enteral nutrition or are associated with infection. Situations in which TPN is invaluable include prolonged paralytic ileus, high

output proximal small intestinal fistula, abdominal sepsis, and in dealing with the increased metabolic demands that follow severe injury.

TPN should continue until intestinal function has recovered sufficiently to allow nutrition to be maintained by the oral or enteral route. In cases of high-output, proximal small bowel fistula, parenteral feeding is continued until the fistula has closed spontaneously or has been closed surgically.

Composition of TPN solutions

TPN is usually provided in pre-prepared all-in-one bags containing 3 litres or more. TPN is compounded in the pharmacy under strict sterile conditions, and its contents usually infused over 18–24 hours using a volumetric infusion pump. Most pharmacies have three or four standard regimens available for compounding, according to patient requirements. The solutions contain fixed amounts of energy and nitrogen, and typically provide 1400–2400 kcal (50% glucose, 50% lipid) and 10–14 g nitrogen.

Fluid and electrolyte needs are also catered for. Many patients on TPN need additional water, sodium and potassium because of excess loss from, for example, a high-output fistula. Trace elements and vitamins can also be incorporated, and the demands created by infection and excessive loss can be met. An example of a standard TPN regimen is given in Table 3.3.

Administration of TPN

TPN solutions are typically very hypertonic and acidic (because of the glucose and amino acid content). They therefore have to be infused relatively slowly into a vein with a high blood flow in order to prevent chemically induced thrombophlebitis and secondary venous thrombosis. Vascular access to the superior vena cava (SVC) is normally obtained directly through the internal jugular or subclavian vein, or indirectly via a peripherally inserted central (PIC) line. The catheter tip is usually sited, using radiological guidance, at the junction of the SVC and right atrium, as the blood flow is maximum at that point.

Cannulae are made of silastic or polyurethane and are of fine bore. For longer-term feeding, catheters are tunnelled subcutaneously to reduce the risk of infection. For very long term (including home) parenteral feeding a Hickman catheter is used; this type of silastic catheter has a Dacron cuff, which secures it in the subcutaneous fat. With good care, a correctly positioned Hickman catheter can remain in place for several months or years (Fig. 3.7).

Table 3.3 Standard parenteral nutrition regimen

Constituent	Quantity
Non-protein energy	2200 kcal
Nitrogen	13.5 g
Volume	2500 ml
Sodium	115 mmol
Potassium	65 mmol
Calcium	10 mmol
Magnesium	9.5 mmol
Phosphate	20 mmol
Zinc	0.1 mmol
Chloride	113.3 mmol
Acetate	135 mmol
(Adequate vitamins and trace elements)	

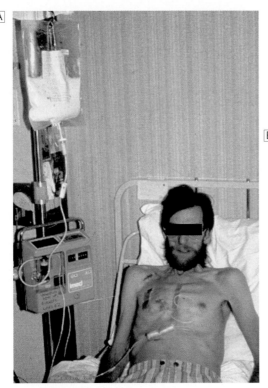

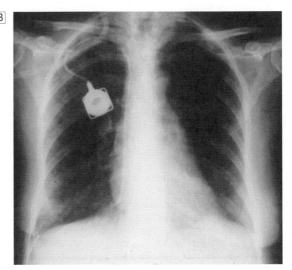

Fig. 3.7 **Total parenteral nutrition (TPN).** ⒶMalnourished patient receiving TPN. ⒷChest X-ray of patient with indwelling Portacath for long-term TPN. The subcutaneous catheter hub is accessed using a Huber needle.

Complications of TPN

Catheter problems

Percutaneous insertion of a catheter may damage adjacent structures and can cause pneumothorax, air embolus and haematoma. Catheter placement under ultrasound guidance helps avoid such problems. Incorrect catheter positioning is excluded by taking a chest X-ray prior to commencing infusion.

Thrombophlebitis

Thrombosis is common when long lines are used, when the catheter tip is not in an area of high flow, and when very hypertonic solutions are infused. The telltale signs are redness and tenderness over the cannulated vein, together with swelling of the whole limb and engorgement of collateral veins if the thrombosis is more proximal. Occasionally, a superior mediastinal syndrome develops in patients with superior vena cava thrombosis. If major vessel occlusion is suspected, the diagnosis is confirmed by venography and anticoagulation is commenced with heparin. If vascular access has to be maintained, an attempt can be made to lyse the clot with urokinase or plasminogen activator. If the clot cannot be dissolved, the cannula must be removed and a new one positioned in an unoccluded vein. The patient may need to remain on long-term anticoagulation.

Infection

Catheter related sepsis and blood stream infection are the most frequent complications of TPN. The usual offending organisms are coagulase-negative staphylococci, *Staphylococcus aureus* and coliforms, but the incidence of fungal infection is increasing, possibly because many of the patients requiring TPN are immunocompromised or receiving broad-spectrum antibiotics. Catheter infections are completely avoidable and almost always the result of poor line care, with infection usually introduced via the catheter hub

as a result of deficient aseptic technique. The insertion site must be protected with an occlusive dressing and should be cleansed on alternate days with an antiseptic agent. The line must only be used for infusion of nutrients and never for taking or giving blood or administering drugs. Great care is taken to avoid contamination when changing bags. A nutrition support nurse is invaluable in avoiding catheter sepsis and supervising all aspects of catheter care. If the patient receiving TPN develops pyrexia, the protocol outlined in Table 3.4 should be followed. While catheter related sepsis in short term TPN is generally managed by removing the catheter, an

---

Table 3.4 Detection and treatment of catheter related sepsis

If a pyrexia > 38°C develops, or there is a further rise in temperature if already pyrexial
- Stop parenteral nutrition and check for other sources of pyrexia (e.g. chest or urinary tract infection)
- Take peripheral and central line blood cultures
- Administer intravenous fluids
- Heparinize catheter
- Consult senior medical staff

If blood culture is negative
- Restart parenteral nutrition and continue to monitor for signs of sepsis

If blood culture is positive
- Remove catheter and send tip for bacteriological analysis
- Administer appropriate antibiotic therapy
- If necessary, replace catheter and restart parenteral nutrition within 24–48 hours

Where central access must be preserved
- Seek specialist advice from hospital nutrition team

attempt is usually made to salvage the catheter and treat the infection with antibiotics in patients receiving long term TPN via tunneled catheters, because repeated catheter removal eventually results in loss of venous access. Provided there is no evidence of septic shock, polymicrobial or fungal catheter infection (in which case the catheter is removed), the catheter is salvaged by 'locking it' twice daily for up to 14 days with a solution of vancomycin and urokinase, while intravenous antibiotics appropriate to the causative organism are continued. An alternative route for provision of TPN is employed until serial cultures confirm that the catheter infection has resolved.

Metabolic complications

Metabolic complications include under- or overhydration. Patients with co-existing medical conditions (e.g. cardiac failure) should be carefully monitored. There is a physiological upper limit to the amount of glucose that can be oxidized (4 mg/kg/min) and prolonged glucose infusion in excess of this rate may lead to hyperglycaemia and fatty infiltration of the liver with disordered liver function. Mildly abnormal liver enzymes in patients receiving TPN are common. However, severe and progressive abnormalities and, in particular, biochemical or clinical jaundice should lead to a prompt re-evaluation of the feeding regimen. Excessive administration of glucose may also aggravate respiratory failure as a consequence of the need to eliminate larger amounts of carbon dioxide consequent upon increased carbohydrate oxidation. Intolerance of glucose is particularly likely in sepsis and critical illness as a result of insulin resistance. Hyperglycaemia may require a reduction of the glucose load, concomitant infusion of insulin via a separate pump, or both.

Hypokalaemia and hypophosphataemia are common when severely malnourished patients are re-fed after a long period of starvation because of the large flux of potassium and phosphate into the cells; correction is by further supplementation. Abnormal liver function tests may occur in severely stressed or septic patients. If the changes are marked and progressive, the overall substrate load should be reduced and discontinuation of parenteral nutrition considered.

Peripheral venous nutrition

TPN solutions can be compounded specifically to facilitate administration via a peripheral vein, using lipid emulsions and less hypertonic solutions of amino acids. These solutions are less likely to provoke thrombophlebitis but are still usually suitable only for short term use and conventional techniques should be employed if long-term nutritional support is needed. Peripheral catheters require

SUMMARY BOX 3.4

Parenteral nutrition

- Parenteral feeding is indicated if the patient cannot be fed adequately by the oral or enteral route
- The need to restrict volume when using total parenteral nutrition (TPN) means that concentrated solutions are used, which may be irritant and thrombogenic. TPN is therefore infused through a catheter in a high-flow vein (e.g. superior vena cava)
- TPN is usually given in an 'all-in-one' bag with a mixture of glucose, fat and L-amino acids combined with fluid, electrolytes, vitamins, minerals and trace elements
- The major complications with TPN can be classed as catheter-related, septic or metabolic. A multidisciplinary approach to the management of TPN patients by a nutrition team will minimize such complications.

the same level of care as central catheters, and the patient must still be monitored for signs of infection or metabolic complications.

MONITORING OF NUTRITIONAL SUPPORT

Patients receiving nutritional support are monitored to detect deficiency states, assess the adequacy of energy and protein provision, and anticipate complications. Patients receiving enteral feeding require less intense monitoring but are prone to the same metabolic complications as those fed intravenously.

Pulse rate, blood pressure and temperature are recorded regularly, an accurate fluid balance chart is maintained (including insensible losses), and the urine is checked daily for glycosuria. Body weight is measured twice weekly.

Serum urea and electrolytes are measured daily, as are blood glucose levels if there is glycosuria. Full blood count, liver function tests, and serum albumin, calcium, magnesium and phosphate are monitored once or twice weekly. In patients where there is a concern about failure to respond to an apparently adequate nutritional regimen or there is ongoing electrolyte imbalance, urine may be collected over one or two 24-hour periods each week to measure nitrogen or electrolyte losses respectively. For patients on long-term enteral nutrition or TPN (i.e. longer than 2–3 weeks) less intense monitoring is appropriate once they are stable.

S. Gossain
P.M. Hawkey

04

Infections and antibiotics

IMPORTANCE OF INFECTION

In the latter half of the 19th century Louis Pasteur hypothesized that bacteria caused infection by being carried through the air (germ theory of disease). Aware of Pasteur's work, in 1865, Joseph Lister first used carbolic acid (phenol) as a spray in the operating theatre to successfully prevent and treat infection in compound fractures. In the early part of the 20th century, with the advent of sterilized instruments, surgical gowns and the first rubber gloves, antisepsis was replaced by modern aseptic surgical techniques which were championed by Birmingham surgeon Robert Lawson Tait. Penicillin was discovered by Alexander Fleming in 1928 and first used clinically in 1940 by Howard Florey. The prevention and treatment of surgical infection was further transformed by the many different classes of antibiotics that were discovered through the latter part of the 20th century. Nevertheless, control of infection in surgical practice remains an important and challenging issue due to the emergence of antibiotic-resistant organisms and the rise in the numbers of elderly, co-morbid and immunocompromised patients undergoing increasingly complex surgical interventions that frequently involve the use of implants. The risk of infection is related to the type of surgery (Table 4.1). Postoperative infections impact on patient outcomes and increase the length of hospital stay, which in turn increases the cost of surgery. In the UK, there is now a legal duty on hospitals to do all they can to minimize the risk of healthcare associated infections (HCAI) in patients.

BIOLOGY OF INFECTION

Many body surfaces are colonized by a wide range of micro-organisms, called commensals, with no ill effects (Fig. 4.1). However, once the normal defences are breached in the course of surgery, such as skin (e.g. *Staphylococcus aureus* and bowel (e.g. *Bacteroides* spp. and *Escherichia coli*) commensals can then cause infection. Infection is defined as the proliferation of micro-organisms in body tissue with adverse physiological consequences. The factors involved in the evolution of infection are shown in Figure 4.2.

Bacterial factors

The size of the inoculum is important with smaller numbers of bacteria being more easily removed by the host's immune response. Bacteria with greater pathogenic potential (virulence) in soft tissue (e.g. *Streptococcus pyogenes* versus *Escherichia coli*) will require a lower inoculum to establish infection. Pathogenic bacteria release a wide variety of exotoxins that can act locally, regionally and systemically having spread via the bloodstream, lymphatics and along nerves (e.g. tetanospasmin which causes tetanus). Other bacterial pathogenicity factors which are released include haemolysins which destroy red blood cells; streptokinase, elastase and hyaluronidase which damage connective tissues. Endotoxin (lipopolysaccharide, LPS), a component of the cell wall, is liberated when Gram-negative bacteria break up (lysis). LPS stimulates endothelial cells and macrophages to release cytokines which mediate the inflammatory response and produce septic shock. Lipoteichoic acid is the equivalent molecule in Gram-positive bacteria.

Host defence systems

Commensals limit the potential virulence of pathogens by depriving them of nutrients, preventing their adherence and by producing various cell signalling substances that interfere with their activities. Administration of broad-spectrum antibiotics can lead to the replacement of commensals with a pathogen; for example, *Clostridium difficile* in the colon which is a common cause of, potentially life threatening, diarrhoea in postoperative patients.

Table 4.1 Classification of operative wounds and infection risk with prophylaxis

	% Infection rate with prophylaxis*
Clean (e.g. non-traumatic wound, respiratory / gastrointestinal /genitourinary tracts intact)	0.8
Clean-contaminated (e.g. non-traumatic wound, respiratory / gastrointestinal /genitourinary tracts entered but insignificant spillage)	1.3
Contaminated (e.g. fresh traumatic wound from dirty source, gross spillage from gastrointestinal tract or infected urine/bile or major break in aseptic technique)	10.2

*Based on data from: Olson M, O'Connor M, Schwartz ML. Surgical wound infections. A 5-year prospective study of 20,193 wounds at the Minneapolis VA Medical Center. Ann Surg. 1984 Mar;199(3):253–259.

Man has evolved a wide range of defences that act at the interface with the surrounding environment. Skin provides a dry, inhospitable mechanical barrier to organisms and also secretes fatty acids in the sebum that kill or suppress potential pathogens. Tears and saliva contain a range of antibacterial substances such as lysozyme; and the low pH of gastric secretions kills many ingested pathogenic bacteria. Many mucosal surfaces are covered in secreted mucus which both acts as a physical barrier and binds bacteria via specific receptors.

Macrophages, neutrophils and complement provide innate immunity through phagocytosis and bacterial lysis. The complement system (a cascade of bioactive proteins) which is activated when required attracts the phagocytic cells, directly lyses pathogens and increases vascular permeability. Immunity can also be acquired through antibody and cell mediated mechanisms. There are two types of T-lymphocytes involved in cell mediated immunity; CD4 help macrophages kill phagocytosed bacteria and CD8 kill cells infected with intracellular pathogens, especially viruses. The five classes of antibody (IgA, IgM, IgG, IgD and IgE) are secreted by B-lymphocytes, usually following stimulation via T cells. Antibodies, with or without complement, bind to and opsonize, lyse or kill the pathogen.

Cytokines (small peptide molecules) are released by leucocytes and facilitate the interaction between immune cells. Over activation of this cytokine cascade leads to the Systemic Inflammatory Response Syndrome (SIRS). Typically, a patient presents with signs of severe infection but instead of improving with antibiotic treatment develops worsening fever, hypotension, tissue hypoxia, acidosis and multiple organ failure.

A number of host factors make infection more likely:

- Old age, obesity, malnutrition, cancer and immunosuppressive agents (e.g. steroids) and diabetes
- The presence of dead tissue; for example, burned flesh or haematoma provide a rich source of nutrients for bacteria and hamper the local immune response
- Poor vascularity; in the leg this is often associated with peripheral arterial disease and diabetes
- Foreign material present in tissues either as a result of trauma (e.g. broken glass, clothing, shrapnel) or surgical procedure (e.g. joint replacements, heart valves, vascular prostheses).

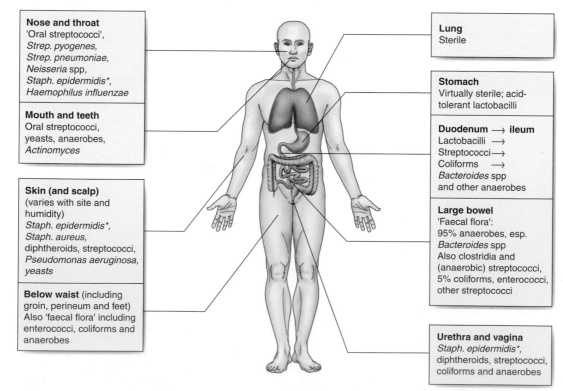

Nose and throat
'Oral streptococci',
Strep. pyogenes,
Strep. pneumoniae,
Neisseria spp,
Staph. epidermidis,*
Haemophilus influenzae

Mouth and teeth
Oral streptococci,
yeasts, anaerobes,
Actinomyces

Skin (and scalp)
(varies with site and humidity)
Staph. epidermidis,*
Staph. aureus,
diphtheroids, streptococci,
Pseudomonas aeruginosa,
yeasts

Below waist (including groin, perineum and feet)
Also 'faecal flora' including enterococci, coliforms and anaerobes

Lung
Sterile

Stomach
Virtually sterile; acid-tolerant lactobacilli

Duodenum ⟶ ileum
Lactobacilli ⟶
Streptococci⟶
Coliforms ⟶
Bacteroides spp
and other anaerobes

Large bowel
'Faecal flora':
95% anaerobes, esp.
Bacteroides spp
Also clostridia and
(anaerobic) streptococci,
5% coliforms, enterococci,
other streptococci

Urethra and vagina
Staph. epidermidis,*
diphtheroids, streptococci,
coliforms and anaerobes

Fig. 4.1 Distribution of normal adult flora. Mucosal or skin breaches may allow normal flora to infect usually sterile sites. Overgrowth by potentially pathogenic members of the normal flora may occur with changes in normal composition, e.g. after antimicrobial treatment, local changes in pH (vagina and stomach) or defective immunity (e.g. AIDS or immunosuppressive treatment). The most common yeast is *Candida albicans*. *Staphylococcus epidermidis* is the most common 'coagulase-negative staphylococcus' frequently found on skin. Density of colonization varies greatly with age and site.

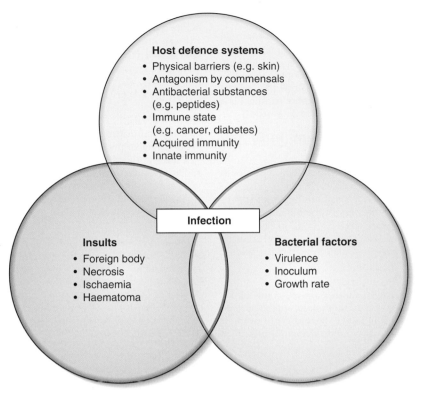

Host defence systems
- Physical barriers (e.g. skin)
- Antagonism by commensals
- Antibacterial substances
  (e.g. peptides)
- Immune state
  (e.g. cancer, diabetes)
- Acquired immunity
- Innate immunity

Infection

Insults
- Foreign body
- Necrosis
- Ischaemia
- Haematoma

Bacterial factors
- Virulence
- Inoculum
- Growth rate

Fig. 4.2 Factors important in the development of infection and their inter-relationship.

PREVENTING INFECTION IN SURGICAL PATIENTS

All UK hospitals now have infection prevention programmes which include measures to minimize risks to patients and staff from infections which may be acquired during and after surgery.

Preoperative MRSA screening

Since 2008 hospitals in England have been required to screen all elective surgical patients for methicillin-resistant *Staphylococcus aureus* (MRSA). Carriers receive decolonization treatment (nasal mupirocin cream and antiseptic skin wash) and appropriate antibiotic prophylaxis, usually a glycopeptide antibiotic (e.g. teicoplanin) prior to surgery. This policy reduces MRSA transmission in surgical wards (EBM 4.1). Screening for nasal carriage of *Staphylococcus aureus* followed by decolonization also reduces surgical wound infection (EBM 4.2). These hospitals now screen emergency admissions although the timing of available results will determine whether this has an impact on management and outcomes.

Aseptic technique

The term 'aseptic technique' refers to specific practices performed immediately before and during a surgical procedure to reduce postoperative infection. These include hand washing, surgical scrub, skin preparation of the patient, maintaining a sterile field and using safe operating practices.

EBM **4.1 Preventing MRSA transmission in surgical patients by rapid polymerase chain reaction (PCR) screening for MRSA**

'A prospective, cluster, two-period cross-over design trial where all MRSA positive patients were decolonized and isolated (only for 17% patients). Infection control practices were the same in both groups.

13 952 patient wound episodes included and results showed that patients on wards using conventional screening were 1.49 times (p = 0.007) more likely to acquire MRSA. It was concluded that rapid PCR screening and decolonization reduces transmission of MRSA.'

Hardy K, et al. Reduction in the rate of methicillin-resistant *Staphylococcus aureus* acquisition in surgical wards by rapid screening for colonization: a prospective, cross-over study. Clin Microbiol Infect. 2010; 16:333-9.

EBM **4.2 Preventing surgical site infections in nasal carriers of *Staphylococcus aureus***

'A randomized, double-blind, placebo-controlled, multicentre trial over 20 months where a total of 6671 patients were screened for S. aureus nasal carriage using PCR. The subgroup of surgical-site infections caused by S. aureus was reduced by 60% among those in the active treatment group (nasal mupirocin ointment plus chlorhexidine wash) as compared to those in the placebo group.'

Bode LG, et al. Preventing surgical-site infections in nasal carriers of *Staphylococcus aureus*. N Engl J Med. 2010; 362:9-17.

4

Hand decontamination

The operating team should wash their hands prior to each operation on the list using an aqueous antiseptic surgical solution, with a single-use brush for the nails. The 'six-step hand hygiene technique' is now widely adopted (Fig. 4.3). Hospitals will have policies for which antiseptic agents are used. Where hands are not soiled, alcohol hand gel is a suitable alternative for decontamination on the wards.

Personal protective equipment (PPE) for staff

The operating team should wear sterile gowns and gloves during the operation. Consideration should be given to wearing two pairs of gloves when there is a high risk of perforation and the consequences of contamination may be serious (e.g. in patients known or suspected to be infected with blood-borne viruses, (BBV)). Visors and goggles can be worn to protect from splash inoculation with body fluids.

Skin preparation

Although it is not possible to sterilize the skin, antiseptics such as chlorhexidine or povidone-iodine applied to the surgical site prior to incision reduce the number of resident organisms and so the risks of wound infection. Antiseptics

containing alcohol must be allowed to evaporate completely before using diathermy.

Surgical instruments

To prevent cross-infection only sterile instruments are used. Sterilization is usually undertaken in Sterile Services Departments (SSD) in hospitals.

Terminology

- Decontamination: a process which removes or destroys infectious or unwanted material
- Cleaning: the physical removal of soil and organic matter
- Disinfection: the removal or destruction of some micro-organisms but not bacterial spores
- Sterilization: the complete destruction of all micro-organisms including spores.

Used surgical instruments are first thoroughly washed in automated washer disinfectors which reach temperatures of 85–95°C (thermal disinfection), remove organic matter and kill most micro-organisms except spores. Instruments can then be packed and processed in a steam sterilizer or autoclave to destroy any remaining micro-organisms and their spores. Pressures above atmospheric are used so that higher temperatures can be achieved (e.g. 121°C for 20 minutes; 134°C for 5 minutes).

Wet hands under warm running water, apply soap, then follow this procedure

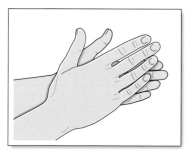

1. Rub palm-to-palm

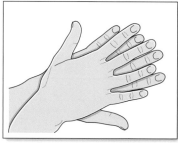

3. Rub the back of both hands
   (right palm over left back
   and then *vice versa*)

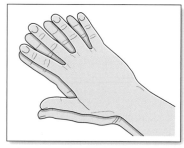

3. Rub palm-to-palm
   interlacing the fingers

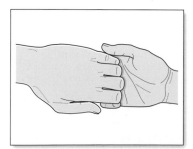

4. Rub the backs of fingers
   by interlocking the hands

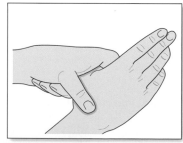

5. Rub the thumbs
   (rotational rubbing of right thumb
   clasped in the left palm, and
   then *vice versa*)

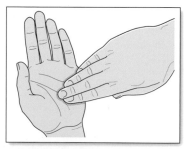

6. Rub palms with fingertips
   (rotational rubbing of right fingers
   on left palm, and then *vice versa*)

Rinse the hands under running water, and dry thoroughly

Technique based on that of Ayliffe *et al* (1978)

Fig. 4.3 Six-step hand hygiene technique.

Creutzfeldt–Jakob disease (CJD) and other prion diseases

These normal decontamination processes do not destroy prions (infectious agents composed only of protein) and so patients known to have, or at risk of, CJD must be identified prior to surgery. Wherever possible, disposable surgical instruments are used. Whether disposable or not, all instruments used on such patients must be subsequently destroyed by incineration.

 SUMMARY BOX 4.1

Prevention of infection

- Preoperative screening of patients for MRSA, and subsequent decolonization of carriers, is now an integral part of surgical care in UK hospitals
- The routine practices of hand washing, surgical scrub, skin preparation of the patient and maintaining a sterile field are collectively known as 'aseptic technique'
- The practice of aseptic technique is an important component in preventing surgical site infections
- Sterility of surgical instruments is critical to preventing cross-infection. This may be achieved by decontamination of instruments in SSDs or by using sterile, disposable instruments.

PROPHYLACTIC USE OF ANTIBIOTICS

Antibiotic prophylaxis is defined as their use before, during, or after a diagnostic, therapeutic, or surgical procedure to prevent infectious complications. The evidence base and guidance can be found at www.sign.ac.uk/pdf/sign104.pdf and in the *British National Formulary* (BNF).

Timing and dose

The aim is to achieve high concentrations of drug at the surgical site from the time of incision. In most situations this involves a single parenteral dose at induction. If the surgery is prolonged or blood loss high then a second intraoperative dose may be advised.

Antibiotic choice

The antibiotic chosen must cover the expected pathogens for that operative site. Most hospitals have policies that take into account local resistance patterns. In recent years, co-amoxiclav has largely replaced cefuroxime because of the latter's propensity to cause *C. difficile* infection. Information on antibiotic prophylaxis in special circumstances e.g., prevention of endocarditis; joint prostheses and dental treatment may be found in the BNF.

Carriage of resistant organisms and prophylaxis

This should be recognized as a risk factor for surgical site infection following high risk operations, especially when a surgical implant is being used, e.g., vascular graft, prosthetic joint, etc. Where carriage of MRSA or Extended Spectrum Beta Lactamase (ESBL)-producing *Escherichia coli* is known or suspected, appropriate antibiotics should be used for prophylaxis; if in doubt, seek expert advice from a microbiologist.

Prophylaxis for immunosuppressed patients

The choice of agent will depend on individual circumstances and expert microbiological help should be sought. Splenectomized patients are at increased risk of infection with encapsulated bacteria and protozoa and should be:

- commenced on lifelong antibiotic prophylaxis with penicillin or amoxicillin
- immunized against pneumococcus, *Haemophilus influenzae* type b (Hib), Group C meningococcus.

For elective splenectomy, the vaccines should be given 2–4 weeks prior to the procedure and for emergency procedures, 2–4 weeks after. In addition, travellers to areas endemic for meningococcus groups A, W135 or Y infection or for malaria should take expert advice.

 SUMMARY BOX 4.2

Prophylactic antibiotics

- Antibiotic prophylaxis in surgical practice aims to prevent infection by achieving high concentrations of antibiotic at the incision and site of operation during surgery
- The choice of antibiotic must cover the likely pathogens for the operation site
- A single dose of antibiotic is usually adequate for prophylaxis, although during prolonged procedures or where there is excessive blood loss, a second dose may be required
- In some circumstances, e.g. colonization with multi-resistant bacteria or immunocompromised patients, the antibiotic choice may need to be modified and expert advice should be sought.

MANAGEMENT OF SURGICAL INFECTIONS

Surgical infections are of two types; those that occur in patients who:

- have undergone a surgical procedure
- present with sepsis and require surgery as part of their management.

Diagnosis

Infections in the early postoperative period (< 48 hours) are most likely to be respiratory or urinary; wound infections usually becoming evident later. Implant-related infections may not be evident for weeks, months or even years. Leakage of a gastrointestinal anastomosis usually presents after 5–6 days with low grade pyrexia and abdominal symptoms and signs; there may also be leakage of bowel content from surgical drains. Questioning for cough, dysuria and abdominal pain is important. Tachycardia, tachypnoea and pyrexia are all indicators of infection. Should hypotension and signs of septic shock be present, urgent resuscitation and assessment by the critical care unit outreach team is required. Whenever possible, the focus of infection should be identified (e.g. plain x-ray, ultrasound, computed tomography, (CT), or magnetic resonance imaging, (MRI)) and

4

cultures taken (e.g. urine, sputum) before commencing antibiotic treatment. Aspiration of pus from deep seated infections (e.g. subphrenic abscess) followed by Gram staining to guide empirical therapy is helpful. Intravenous lines should be removed and cultured together with blood in any patient suspected of having bacteraemia. If indicated, urine and sputum should also be cultured. Serious sepsis in the surgical patient often arises from intra-abdominal infections (IAI). Approximately 30% of patients admitted to the ICU with IAI die, and if peritonitis develops mortality rises to 50%. Early diagnosis and treatment is essential but clinical examination is often unreliable, even misleading. CT, or MRI, preferably with contrast, should be performed to detect peritoneal leaks and collections of pus and can be life-saving. An integrated and logical approach to patient management should be followed as described in the surviving sepsis guidelines which are summarized in Tables 4.2 and 4.3.

Antibiotic therapy

Antibiotics are almost inevitably an adjunct to surgical treatment in surgical infections e.g. drainage of abscesses, debridement, excision of infected tissue or lavage of a serous cavity.

- Antibiotic policies – each hospital has its own antibiotic formulary and this should be consulted. The principles behind such policies are shown in Table 4.4.
- Specimens for culture and sensitivity testing should always be obtained if possible and then specific antibiotics used as suggested in Table 4.5. It is not always possible to await these results if the patient is

seriously ill and empirical therapy should be started immediately according to Table 4.6.
- When using some antibiotics such as gentamicin and vancomycin, therapeutic drug monitoring is needed to (i) establish adequate serum concentrations and (ii) identify toxic concentrations before renal or neurological damage develops. Specific protocols are available from microbiology/pharmacy departments at individual hospitals.
- Advice should be sought early about antibiotic treatment regimens from microbiologists/infectious diseases specialists, particularly when the diagnosis is not certain and/or the patient is critically ill.

Table 4.3 Severe sepsis care pathway

1. **Oxygen:** high flow 15 l/min via non-rebreathe mask. Target saturations > 94%
2. **Blood cultures:** take at least one set plus all relevant blood tests e.g. FBC, U&E, LFT, clotting, glucose Consider urine/sputum/swab samples.
3. **IV antibiotics** as per hospital guidelines
4. **Fluid resuscitate:** if hypotensive give boluses of 0.9% saline or Hartmann's 20 ml/kg up to a max of 60 ml/kg
5. **Serum lactate** and **haemoglobin (Hb):** Ensure Hb > 7g/dl
6. **Catheterize** and commence fluid balance chart

PLUS

a. Call Outreach Team if appropriate
b. Discuss with Consultant

http://www.survivingsepsis.org/

Table 4.2 Screening for sepsis and severe sepsis

Are any two of the following present?	
• Temperature < 36 or > 38.3°C • Heart rate > 90bpm • WCC > 12 or < 4 × 10⁹/l	• Respiratory rate > 20/min • Acutely altered mental state • Hyperglycaemia in the absence of diabetes

If yes:

Does the patient have a history or signs suggestive of a new infection?	
• Cough/sputum/chest pain • Abdominal pain/distension/diarrhoea • Line infections	• Dysuria • Headache with neck stiffness • Cellulitis/wound infection/septic arthritis

If yes, patient has **SEPSIS**

Are there any signs of organ dysfunction?	
• SBP < 90 mmHg or MAP < 65 mmHg • Urine output < 0.5 ml/kg/hr for 2 hrs • INR > 1.5 or APTT > 60s • Bilirubin > 34 mmol/l	• Lactate > 2 mmol/l • New need for oxygen to keep SpO₂ > 90% • Platelets < 100 × 10⁹/l • Creatinine > 177 mmol/l

NO: Treat for SEPSIS:	**YES: Patient has SEVERE SEPSIS**
• Oxygen • Blood cultures • IV antibiotics • Fluid therapy • Reassess for SEVERE SEPSIS with hourly observations	Start SEVERE SEPSIS CARE PATHWAY (Table 4.3)

WCC, white cell count; MAP, mean arterial pressure, SBP systolic blood pressure; INR, international normalized ratio; APTT, activated partial thromboplastin time. http://www.survivingsepsis.org/

Table 4.4 Principles underlying antibiotic policy

- Antibiotics should be avoided in self-limiting infections and due consideration should be given to expense, toxicity and the need to avoid the emergence of resistant strains
- Choice of therapy is determined positively by knowledge of the nature and sensitivities of the infecting organism(s). Therapy may be initiated on clinical evidence, but must be reviewed in the light of culture/sensitivity reports
- Restrict the use of antibiotics to which resistance is developing (or has developed)
- Single agents are preferred to combination therapy, and narrow-spectrum agents are preferred to broad-spectrum agents whenever possible
- Adequate doses must be given by the recommended route at correct time intervals
- Antibiotics that are used systemically must not be used topically
- Antibiotics used for prophylaxis are not used for treatment
- The side effects of antibiotics should be known by the prescriber and monitored
- Expensive antibiotics are not used if equally effective and cheaper alternatives are suitable
- With few exceptions (e.g. lung abscess), antibiotics should not be used to treat abscesses unless adequate surgical or radiological drainage has been achieved
- Policies may include automatic 'stop' orders

SPECIFIC INFECTIONS IN SURGICAL PATIENTS

Surgical site infection (SSI)

All surgical wounds are contaminated by microbes but in most cases infection does not develop because of innate host defences. A complex interplay between host, microbial, and surgical factors ultimately determines whether infection takes hold and how it progresses (Fig. 4.2, EBM 4.3 and see Table 4.1).

4

EBM 4.3 SSI classification

'Superficial incisional SSI: *Infection involves only skin and subcutaneous tissue of incision.*

Deep incisional SSI: *Infection involves deep tissues, such as fascial and muscle layers. This also includes infection involving both superficial and deep incision sites and organ/space SSI draining through incision.*

Organ/space SSI: *Infection involves any part of the anatomy in organs and spaces other than the incision, which was opened or manipulated during operation.'*

Horan TC, et al. CDC definitions of nosocomial surgical site infections, 1992: a modification of CDC definitions of surgical wound infections. Infect Control Hosp Epidemiol. 1992; 13:606-8.

Table 4.5 Antibiotics in surgery: suggestions for specific therapy

Organism	First choice	Alternative
Methicillin-sensitive *Staphylococcus aureus (MSSA)*	Flucloxacillin	Clarithromycin
Methicillin-resistant *Staphylococcus aureus* (MRSA) *	Vancomycin	Linezolid Daptomycin
Coagulase-negative staphylococci	Vancomycin	Linezolid Daptomycin
Streptococcus pneumoniae	Benzylpenicillin	Clarithromycin
Streptococcus pyogenes (group A β-haemolytic streptococcus)	Benzylpenicillin Clindamycin	Clarithromycin
Enterococci	Amoxicillin	Vancomycin
Bacteroides species	Metronidazole	Co-amoxiclav

Escherichia coli
  1. Sepsis, including bacteraemia
  2. Urinary tract infection
	
	Piperacillin-Tazobactam
	Trimethoprim
		
		Meropenem
		Co-amoxiclav

Haemophilus influenzae	Amoxicillin	Co-amoxiclav
Klebsiella spp	Co-amoxiclav	Meropenem
Proteus species	Co-amoxiclav	Meropenem
Pseudomonas aeruginosa	Piperacillin-Tazobactam	Meropenem
Clostridium spp	Benzylpenicillin + metronidazole	Metronidazole
Clostridium difficile	Stop predisposing antibiotic Metronidazole	Vancomycin, oral, re-treat relapse

These suggestions should be considered in the light of local epidemiology, sensitivities, drug availability, site and severity or infection.
*Gould FK et al. Guideline (2008) for the prophylaxis and treatment of methicillin-resistant *Staphylococcus aureus* (MRSA) infections in the UK. J. Antimicrobial Chemotherapy 2009;63:849-861

Table 4.6 Empirical therapy for acute infections

Type of Infections	Antimicrobial	Alternative
Chest infection		
Uncomplicated	Amoxicillin	Clarithromycin
Community-acquired pneumonia	Benzyl penicillin + clarithromycin	Levofloxacin + clarithromycin
'Aspiration' pneumonia	Co-amoxiclav	Levofloxacin + metronidazole
Hospital-acquired/postoperative	Piperacillin-tazobactam	Meropenem + vancomycin
Urinary tract infection		
'Lower' infection	Trimethoprim	Amoxicillin
Acute pyelonephritis	Co-amoxiclav	Gentamicin
Prostatitis	Ciprofloxacin	
Wound infection		
Cellulitis	Penicillin + flucloxacillin	Clarithromycin
Abscess	Drain collection	Flucloxacillin
Intra-abdominal sepsis	Amoxicillin + metronidazole + gentamicin	Meropenem
Cholecystitis-cholangitis	Co-amoxiclav	Meropenem
Pelvic inflammatory disease	Azithromycin + metronidazole + gentamicin	Doxycycline + piperacillin-tazobactam
Amputations and gas gangrene	Benzylpenicillin + metronidazole	Metronidazole
Septicaemia and septic shock	Amoxicillin + metronidazole + gentamicin/ciprofloxacin	Piperacillin-tazobactam, meropenem
Severe ***Pseudomonas*** infections	Piperacillin-tazobactam + gentamicin	Meropenem ± gentamicin
Candida sepsis	Fluconazole	Caspofungin

Note The suggestions are for occasions when immediate treatment is necessary. Amendments may be necessary in the light of local epidemiology.

Diagnosis

Superficial SSIs can be identified by pyrexia, local erythema, pain and excessive tenderness, and sometimes discharge. Deeper infection may present more insidiously with pyrexia, leucocytosis, and organ dysfunction such as prolonged postoperative ileus. Diagnosis may require radiological imaging and sometimes exploratory laparotomy.

Treatment

Cellulitis can be treated with antibiotics but an abscess will require drainage as antibiotics will not penetrate pus. Drainage may involve simply laying open the wound and healing by secondary intention. Deeper, more complex collections will need formal drainage either radiologically (under ultrasound or CT guidance) or by means of open surgery.

Prevention

The risks of SSI can be reduced by:
- Careful surgical technique to minimize tissue damage, bleeding and haematoma
- Appropriate antibiotic prophylaxis
- Avoidance of infective surgical complication e.g. anastomotic leak.

Urinary tract infections (UTI)

These are common and may range from simple cystitis to pyelonephritis or even perinephric abscess. Catheterized patients are at increased risk of infection. The most common organisms are *Escherichia coli*, *Klebsiella* species, *Enterococcus faecalis* and *Pseudomonas aeruginosa*. Multi-resistant organisms such as ESBL-producing *E. coli* and MRSA are increasingly being seen and can be difficult to treat. Symptoms include dysuria, fever and, in patients who are not catheterized, frequency and nocturia. Cystitis may not give rise to any clinical signs. Pyelonephritis is typically associated with rigors, renal angle pain and tenderness. Urine samples must be sent for microscopy and culture. In catheterized patients the urine frequently contains organisms but not white cells. This does not require antibiotics unless there are signs of systemic illness. The urine will not become sterile until the catheter is removed. Trimethoprim, gentamicin and co-amoxiclav are reasonable antibiotic choices until sensitivities become available. Fluoroquinolones (e.g. ciprofloxacin) may be used although *C. difficile* infection is a risk particularly in elderly patients. Expert advice should be sought in the case of multi-drug resistant pathogens. Aseptic introduction and meticulous care of the urinary catheter helps to prevent bacteria entering the urinary tract (Fig. 4.4).

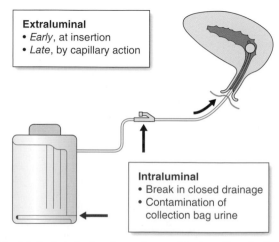

Extraluminal
- *Early*, at insertion
- *Late*, by capillary action

Intraluminal
- Break in closed drainage
- Contamination of collection bag urine

Fig. 4.4 Routes of entry of uropathogens into the catheterized urinary tract.

Respiratory tract infections

This comprises upper and lower respiratory tract infection, lung abscess and empyema. The commonest causes are *Streptococcus pneumoniae* and *Haemophilus influenzae*. Gram-negative organisms (e.g. *Escherichia coli*, *Pseudomonas aeruginosa*) and MRSA can be implicated, especially during and after mechanical ventilation. Symptoms include fever, tachypnoea, cough, increased respiratory secretions, breathlessness and confusion. Diagnosis is made on the basis of history, examination, arterial blood gases, chest X-ray, cultures (blood, sputum and bronchial washings) and sometimes specialist radiology (e.g. CT). A positive sputum culture without clinical symptoms and signs of infection does not automatically merit antimicrobial therapy. Antibiotic treatment should follow the local hospital policy; penicillin plus clarithromycin is a typical choice until sensitivities becomes available. Abscess or empyema should be drained. Physiotherapy, early mobilization and adequate pain relief in the postoperative period will help prevent respiratory infection.

Clostridium difficile infection (CDI)

This occurs when the normal colonic microflora is disturbed by the administration of antibiotics in patients either pre-colonized with or exposed after antibiotic treatment to *C. difficile* (an anaerobic spore-forming bacillus). Some antibiotics are particularly prone to cause CDI: clindamycin (the first identified in 1978), cephalosporins and fluoroquinolones. The disease is much more common in the elderly and in hospitals with poor cleaning. The bacterium produces two cytotoxins A and B (some strains only produce B) that destroy the colonic mucosal cell cytoskeleton. A spectrum of disease is seen ranging from abdominal discomfort to profuse watery diarrhoea (one of the commonest features), severe abdominal cramps and rarely toxic dilatation of the colon leading to rupture. At colonoscopy characteristic yellow plaques, bleeding mucosa and islands of normal tissue are seen, which is called pseudomembranous colitis. Surgical patients can acquire CDI as a consequence of antibiotic treatment or prophylaxis. Infrequently patients with severe CDI may require urgent surgical referral. Emergency colectomy in patients with fulminant colitis can be life saving although mortality is high. Diagnosis of CDI is by identification of the toxins in faeces by enzyme immunoassay (EIA) or the more sensitive and specific PCR detection of the toxin genes. Treatment of mild/moderate disease is with oral metronidazole, with severe disease responding better to oral vancomycin. Control is aimed at isolating patients with diarrhoea, reducing the environmental burden of spores by cleaning with bleach solutions and reducing the selective pressure from high risk antibiotics by antibiotic stewardship. Current UK guidelines are available in the document '*Clostridium difficile* – how to deal with the problem' (www.dh.gov.uk); (www.hpa.org.uk).

Fungal infections

These are increasing in incidence; the main risk factors include: immunocompromise (e.g. leukaemia, HIV infection), prolonged ICU stay, gastrointestinal tract surgery, central venous catheters and use of total parenteral nutrition (TPN), and prolonged use of multiple or broad spectrum antibiotics. The most common organism is *Candida albicans*. Nystatin can be given orally to treat infections of the oropharynx. Fluconazole, voriconazole and caspofungin are available for treatment of systemic infection.

Infections of prosthetic devices

In many fields of surgery the use of implants has become routine and affords huge clinical benefit. Nevertheless, there is a small risk of device-related infection which can be catastrophic for the patient. Bacteria, often commensals such as coagulase-negative staphylococci can be introduced at the time of surgery and form a biofilm of extracellular material (glycocalyx) around the device which is resistant to the body's defences and the penetration of some antibiotics. Alternatively, the implant can be 'seeded' via the bloodstream months, even years, later from a bacteraemia arising from another source e.g. *Staphylococcus aureus* skin sepsis or *E. coli* UTI. Antibiotics alone are often unsuccessful and removal of the device is frequently necessary to eradicate the sepsis. Such surgery may be difficult and associated with significant morbidity and mortality.

SUMMARY BOX 4.3

Management of surgical infection

- The risk of surgical site infection rises in direct proportion to the degree of microbial contamination of the wound
- Whenever possible, the focus of infection should be identified by careful history-taking, clinical examination, imaging and microbiological culture
- Collections of pus should be drained
- In many surgical infections, antibiotics are often an adjunct to surgical treatment, e.g. drainage of abscesses, debridement, excision of infected tissue or lavage of a serous cavity
- Tetanus immunization status of patients must be determined prior to elective surgery or following trauma.

INFECTIONS PRIMARILY TREATED BY SURGICAL MANAGEMENT

Abscess

This is a localized collection of pus containing neutrophils, dead tissue and organisms that can develop anywhere in the body. The commonest pathogen is *Staphylococcus aureus*. Abscesses in the abdomen or pelvis often contain a mixture of gut bacteria e.g. *E. coli*, enterococci and anaerobic bacteria. Abscesses close to the skin are often painful and the overlying skin will be raised, red and hot to the touch. Large or multiple skin abscesses may cause systemic upset. Deeper abscesses may present with a 'swinging' pyrexia, systemic upset and symptoms relating to pressure on surrounding tissues. The pus must be drained and sent for microscopy and culture. This can be achieved through needle aspiration (e.g. breast), radiologically under ultrasound or CT guidance (e.g. subphrenic), or via open surgery (e.g. perianal). Antibiotics do not usually penetrate into abscesses but may be required for treatment if the patient is systemically unwell or for prophylaxis if a surgical wound is being made in the course of drainage.

Necrotizing fasciitis

This is an uncommon but severe, life-threatening infection of skin and subcutaneous tissues characterized by necrosis of deep fascia (Fig. 4.5). There are two main types depending on causative organisms.

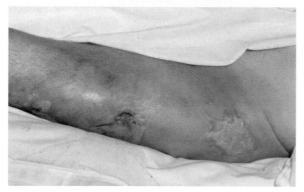

Fig. 4.5 Necrotizing fasciitis of the lower limb. (Courtesy of the Medical Microbiology Dept., University of Edinburgh.)

- Type I: Polymicrobial aetiology which is also known as synergistic bacterial gangrene; Fournier's gangrene is a special type affecting the perineal area
- Type II: Single organism infection, usually by β-haemolytic Group A streptococci (*Streptococcus pyogenes*).

The infection usually starts at a site of (often minor) trauma and can spread very quickly as bacterial exotoxins and enzymes lead to necrosis of fat and fascia and eventually overlying skin. The patient is usually febrile, toxic and in severe pain. Initially, the overlying skin may appear deceptively normal but as the infection progresses there is oedema, discoloration and crepitus (due to gas production). Urgent surgical debridement of all necrotic tissue is essential and several visits to theatre may be required. Initial antibiotic choice is usually empirical with a combination of broad-spectrum agents against likely pathogens e.g. carbapenems, clindamycin and metronidazole. Antibiotic therapy can later be tailored according to the results of pus and tissue cultures.

Diabetic foot infections

Infections involving the feet in diabetic patients range from cellulitis to complex skin and soft tissue infection to chronic osteomyelitis. Clinical diagnosis is based on the presence of cellulitis, purulent discharge, pain, tenderness and gangrene. Signs of systemic toxicity may be present in severe infection. Microbiological diagnosis is best achieved by culture of tissue and bone biopsy samples as culturing surface swabs merely indicates which microorganisms are colonizing the ulcer/wound. Radiological investigation for osteomyelitis includes plain X-rays and MRI. Antibiotic therapy is usually the first line of treatment although a multidisciplinary team approach including vascular and general surgeons may be invaluable. Surgical involvement is required for debridement, drainage of abscess and/or amputation in chronic osteomyelitis.

Gas gangrene

This is rarely seen in civilian practice and is typically associated with the battlefield. *Clostridium perfringens*, a spore-forming anaerobic bacterium normally found in soil and faeces, is the main cause; other species include *Clostridium novyi* and *Clostridium septicum*. Patients become rapidly and profoundly septic as exotoxins lead to rapidly spreading muscle necrosis with overlying skin discolouration,

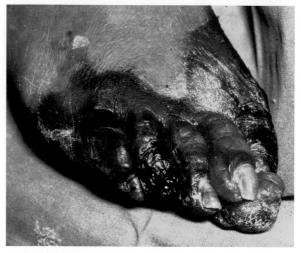

Fig. 4.6 Gangrene developing in the foot of a diabetic. (Courtesy of Mr A.S. Whyte FRCS.)

oedema and crepitus (Fig. 4.6). Even with urgent wide surgical excision of all necrotic tissue and high-dose antibiotics (penicillin and metronidazole) the disease still carries a high mortality.

Infections following trauma

Risk of infection will be related to the amount of tissue damage and contamination with extraneous material (e.g. soil, clothing, etc). Heavily contaminated wounds need thorough cleaning and debridement of all non-viable tissue; failure may lead to severe infections including gas gangrene. A short course of broad spectrum antibiotics have been shown to reduce the incidence of early infection in open limb fractures. It is essential to determine the patient's tetanus immunization status.

Tetanus

This is caused by *Clostridium tetani*, a spore-forming anaerobic organism which enters the body through soil or animal faecal contamination of a wound, injury or burn and then multiplies anaerobically in tissues, if the wound is not adequately cleaned or debrided. The incubation period varies from 4 to 21 days. Tetanospasmin (a neurotoxin) spreads along nerves from the site of infection and causes generalized rigidity and spasm of skeletal muscles. The muscle stiffness usually involves the jaw (lockjaw) and neck and then becomes generalized. The mortality ranges from 10 to 90%, being highest in infants and the elderly. Antibiotic treatment is with penicillins or, for penicillin allergic patients, clarithromycin but is only an adjunct to correct surgical care of wounds and further specialized medical treatment. Tetanus can be prevented by immunization. In the UK, all young children are offered the tetanus vaccine as part of the routine NHS childhood vaccination programme (www.nhs.uk/conditions/Tetanus); current advice is to have five doses over a life time. For non-immune individuals who have suffered a tetanus-prone injury, Human Tetanus Immunoglobulin (HTIG) is given to provide immediate protection together with wound debridement, active immunization and antibiotic treatment.

HEALTHCARE ASSOCIATED INFECTIONS (HCAI)

In 2006 a survey of 190 acute hospitals in England showed that 8.2% of patients had developed a HCAI (previously known as a nosocomial infection), most commonly SSI, GI infections, UTI, and pneumonia. The UK Health Act of 2006 (revised 2008) places a legal duty on hospitals to do all they can to minimize the risk of HCAI. The hospital infection control team are most closely involved in the design and delivery of the HCAI programme and will liaise with the microbiology laboratory to ensure that infections caused by important pathogens are identified at an early stage and that trends in antibiotic resistance are monitored. However, all staff members and students have a duty to take responsibility for this very important aspect of patient care. In recent years, there has been a national focus on reducing MRSA and *C. difficile* infections in England using a multi-faceted approach; Figure 4.7 shows the successful reduction in England of MRSA bloodstream infections (bacteraemia) from 2006 to 2010 but continuing high levels of MSSA bacteraemia. Monitoring SSI is also an important quality indicator. The Nosocomial Infection National Surveillance Service (NINSS), a national programme of SSI surveillance, was established in the UK in 1997. Participation in the scheme is voluntary (except for orthopaedic surgery) but provides hospitals with useful benchmarking data for the main types of surgery. This systematic collection of infection data (surveillance) is by nurse follow-up of all patients who have undergone surgery during a given period. Surveillance nurses will inspect surgical wounds for any signs of infection and often also follow-up the patient once discharged home to detect infection. This enables the early identification of increased incidences of infection so that measures can be taken to prevent further infections. These measures could include suspension of further surgery; deep cleaning of theatres; change in antibiotic treatments and isolation of infected patients.

SUMMARY BOX 4.4

Healthcare associated infection (HCAI)

- All hospitals must have effective programmes for prevention and control of HCAI
- The hospital infection control team design and deliver the HCAI programme, but all staff working in healthcare must take responsibility for preventing HCAI
- Monitoring for trends in surgical site infection is an important indicator of the quality of patient care.

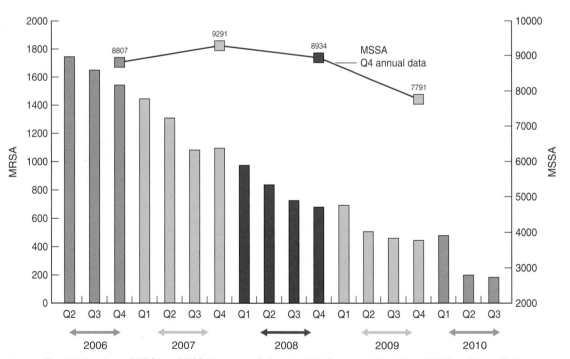

Fig. 4.7 Numbers of MRSA and MSSA bacteraemia (quarterly) in England, derived from HPA Surveillance Data.

5

R.E. Melhado
D. Alderson

Ethics, preoperative considerations, anaesthesia and analgesia

CHAPTER CONTENTS

This chapter encompasses the wide ranging area of perioperative care, from ethical issues surrounding consent, to preoperative preparation and optimization, as well as strategies for the management of postoperative pain. An overview of anaesthesia is included with particular emphasis on its impact on preoperative preparation and selection of patients for surgical intervention.

ETHICAL AND LEGAL PRINCIPLES FOR SURGICAL PATIENTS

The level of trust invested in surgeons by patients when they submit to a surgical procedure is unique in society, as is the potential for harm and exploitation. It is paramount therefore that the practice of surgery is subject to ethical and legal principles that enshrine the rights of patients and the duties of surgeons within the context of varying societal expectations. Medical ethics is a complex area, particularly with the challenges that advances in bioethics and new technologies bring, and there should be sufficient latitude within the framework of medical ethics to accommodate differing views in resolving ethical dilemmas. In the United Kingdom, ethical standards are upheld by regulatory bodies such as the General Medical Council and the Surgical Royal Colleges (Table 5.1).

Medical ethics is not just an abstract subject but a practical and rigorous discipline that applies on a daily basis to surgical practice. Its importance cannot be overestimated. This section seeks to give an overview of medical ethical and legal principles with the exception of the ethics surrounding transplantation which is discussed in the chapter on transplantation.

Principles in surgical ethics

Surgeons regularly need to make decisions that involve a broad understanding of medical ethics. Obtaining fully informed consent is probably the most common example, but surgeons are often involved in ethical dilemmas in acute situations involving unconscious and critically injured patients. Ethical issues are also encountered in surgical research and in the world of surgical publication. The information below cannot cover every prevailing philosophy relating to medical ethics, but is intended to provide guidance that can be applied to most situations that the surgeon is likely to encounter.

Principalism

Principalism is a widely adopted approach to medical ethics. Championed by Beauchamp and Childress, it judges all possible actions in a particular ethical dilemma against four principles. These are autonomy, beneficence, non-malfeasance and justice (Summary Box 5.1). Each is considered in more detail below and while addressed separately, it becomes apparent that the principles are linked and do not simply cover four unrelated issues. Protagonists of this approach to bioethics suggest that it provides a practical framework for working through ethical dilemmas, allowing identification of important issues and is universally applicable with its four principles widely acceptable irrespective of culture or religious beliefs. The principles can be applied to most surgical clinical scenarios and if each element is given due consideration it is unlikely that the resulting decision will be unethical.

Autonomy

Autonomy is a basic aspect of humanity – a right to determine how we live with fundamental respect for dignity, integrity and authenticity. Central to this is the principle

Table 5.1 The duties of a doctor registered with the General Medical Council

Patients must be able to trust doctors with their lives and health. To justify that trust you must show respect for human life and you must:	
Make the care of your patient your first concern	
Protect and promote the health of patients and the public	
Provide a good standard of practice and care	Keep your professional knowledge and skills up-to-date
	Recognize and work within the limits of your competence
	Work with colleagues in the ways that best serve patients' interests
Treat patients as individuals and respect their dignity	Treat patients politely and considerately
	Respect patients' right to confidentiality
Work in partnership with patients	Listen to patients and respond to their concerns and preferences
	Give patients the information they want or need in a way they can understand
	Respect patients' right to reach decisions with you about their treatment and care
	Support patients in caring for themselves to improve and maintain their health
Be honest and open and act with integrity	Act without delay if you have good reason to believe that you or a colleague may be putting patients at risk
	Never discriminate unfairly against patients or colleagues
	Never abuse your patients' trust in you or the public's trust in the profession
You are personally accountable for your professional practice and must always be prepared to justify your decisions and actions.	

that the doctor should never impose treatment upon an individual, except where necessary to prevent harm to others. Autonomy respects the individual's right to opinions, make choices and act on personal values and beliefs. For example, if a competent Jehovah's Witness declines a life-saving blood transfusion based on strongly held beliefs, this should be upheld even if it seems foolish to those treating them. Autonomy does not, however, give the patient the right to treatment on demand.

Beneficence: doing good

This encompasses the moral obligation surgeons have to their patients, to do them good in treating or attempting to cure their diseases. This invites the question as to whose definition of 'good' is used. Historically, the surgeon made the judgement, with little input from the patient as to what was in their best interest. Nowadays, the course of action which will result in the most patient good is agreed following a discussion between the patient and surgeon in which patient preferences and medical advice are both taken into account. The principle of beneficence dictates that surgeons are well placed to do good by being competent, keeping up-to-date, performing audit and undergoing accreditation and revalidation as part of an assurance to the patients and society that they serve.

Non-malfeasance: avoiding harm

This important principle, *primum non nocere* ('first do no harm') has been enshrined in medical practice since the Hippocratic Oath. Of course, many treatments have inherent risks with real complications where harm can result. As long as the risk is in proportion to the potential benefit of a proposed treatment from the competent patient's perspective and consent to that treatment has been given on the basis of reasonable information, then the principle of non-malfeasance is not violated.

Justice: promoting fairness

The principles that healthcare should be fair and available to all is topical, particularly as treatments become more sophisticated and expensive. As long as demand outstrips supply and exceeds what society can afford, debate on this subject will continue. The resulting process of rationing requires a system of justice that does not discriminate on the basis of race, sex, age, gender or religion to administer resources. It is beyond the scope of this chapter to cover the broad issue of resource allocation. Such issues inevitably refer to large cohorts rather than the individual patient within such a group. The focus for the surgeon is more likely to involve individual patients and how their interests should be prioritized: for example, when managing a waiting list for surgery. Resources may be allocated on clinical grounds such as threat to life or degree of pain. These perceptions of clinical need consider the timeliness of intervention to achieve a favourable outcome (e.g. emergency surgery), or the severity of the condition and its consequences if left untreated (e.g. cancer, abdominal aortic aneurysm).

SUMMARY BOX 5.1

Four tenets of principalism

1. Autonomy – Respecting the individual's right to self determination.
2. Beneficence – The surgeon's obligation to do good.
3. Non-malfeasance – The surgeon's obligation to avoid harm.
4. Justice – Treating all patients equally.

Informed consent

General considerations

Informed consent is central to the practice of surgery, and has to be obtained for surgical procedures, other treatment modalities, investigations, screening tests and prior to patient participation in research. Informed consent is not only ethically correct but also a legal riht and should be respected even if the patient's wishes are at variance with the surgeon's opinion. Informed consent can only be obtained from patients with 'capacity'. This should be assumed for all conscious adults unless there is evidence to the contrary. The patient's views must be respected and upheld after an information sharing process that conveys all the information the patient needs and wants in order to make a decision. The surgeon must maximize the opportunity for patients to consent and facilitate the process wherever possible.

Capacity exists if a patient can:

- understand and retain the information presented
- weigh up the implications, including risk and benefit of the options
- communicate their decision.

Circumstances where the capacity to consent may not exist:

- children
- mental illness
- fluctuating or irreversible loss of cognitive function
- patients subject to undue coercion.

Other important considerations in obtaining consent relate to who should obtain consent and when, and what information should be shared/withheld and in what format. In general terms, the surgeon performing the procedure has responsibility to obtain consent but this can be delegated provided the person to whom it is delegated:

- is suitably trained and qualified
- has sufficient knowledge of the proposed procedure including risks
- understands the process of consent (in the UK as laid out by the GMC).

The information that should be shared with a patient to obtain consent should start from a mutual understanding by both doctor and patient of the medical condition, as well as the patient's views, beliefs and prior knowledge. All treatment options should be detailed, including the option of no treatment alongside the risks, side effects, potential benefits and burdens and the risk that the treatment will be unsuccessful. All potential serious adverse outcomes, no matter how rare should be discussed, along with more frequent minor complications. Risks and benefits should, wherever possible be quantified in percentage terms. These figures should derive from audited local/personal practice and not simply plucked from the literature. It is acceptable for the surgeon to give the patient advice; but, in such circumstance, any conflict of interest must be declared.

If a patient expresses the wish that they do not want the information required for informed consent and understands the potential consequences, then information can be withheld on the basis of non-malfeasance, but only when serious psychological harm might ensue and not simply because the patient may be upset or refuse treatment. This is called 'therapeutic privilege'. The provision of procedure specific patient information sheets can supplement the process of informed consent, but does not negate the doctor's responsibility to ensure patient's understanding of the procedure.

Consent may be implied or explicit. Implied consent is considered adequate for routine interventions with negligible risks where patient consent is implied by their cooperation (e.g. venepuncture). The majority of interventions require explicit consent; this may be oral or written. It is perhaps surprising that although written consent is obtained for the majority of procedures, it is only a legal requirement for organ donation and fertility treatment in the UK. Nevertheless, the existence of a written, dated form of consent provides evidence that a consultation covering specific issues was likely to have taken place.

Increasingly in the UK patients may not have sufficient English to enable the process of informed consent. In such circumstances it is tempting to conduct the consultation and consent process via a family member or friend acting as an informal interpreter. However, best practice is to use the services of an official translator. Similarly, written information should in the appropriate language; if this is not possible the translator should read it out to the patient who then has an opportunity to ask questions back through the translator. It goes without saying that the medical records should clearly document that this process has taken place.

SUMMARY BOX 5.2

Informed consent

- Establish patient's capacity
- Gather information on the patient's views, attitudes and wishes regarding their health
- Provide information on treatment options (including no treatment) and the risks and benefits of each and their likely outcomes
- Respect the patient's decision.

Consent in specific circumstances
Children

Children should be involved in the discussions surrounding their treatment wherever possible. In the UK, patients aged 16 years and over are presumed to be competent to consent with legal frameworks guiding treatment of 16 and 17 year olds who do not have capacity to consent. In children under the age of 16, their mental ability to understand, retain, weigh up and use information as well as communicate their decision is more important than their age in determining their capacity to consent. It should be borne in mind that while capacity may exist for simple procedures this does not necessarily translate into the ability to weigh up more complex treatments. For those that lack capacity, treatment can be provided with the consent of parents or the courts in the United Kingdom. Where either a competent child or the parents refuses life saving treatment, or where disagreement exists between parents, legal advice should be sought. Procedures undertaken on cultural or religious grounds, such as circumcision, are usually permissible if it is in the patient's best interests taking psychological, cultural and social benefits into account.

Mental illness

Patients with mental illness may retain the capacity to consent. In emergency or urgent situations, treatment may be provided with their compliance if the patient lacks capacity to consent. Although treatment may be administered compulsorily for the treatment of mental illness, treatment for other medical disorders must not be imposed even where mental illness means that the patient lacks capacity. Legal advice is frequently needed in this setting.

Transient / irreversible cognitive impairment

The emergency situation is relatively straightforward; life saving treatment and intervention necessary to prevent deterioration may be provided in the patient's best interests. In general, the patient's involvement in treatment decisions

Table 5.2 Sources of further information on ethics

Publications
- Guidelines published by the General Medical Council (also available on-line) include:
  - Good Medical Practice, 2006
  - 0–18 years: guidance for all doctors, 2007
  - Consent: patients and doctors making decisions together, 2008
  - Confidentiality, 2009
  - Treatment and care towards the end of life, 2010
  - Good practice in research and consent to research, 2010
- Jonathan Herring. Medical Law and Ethics. 2nd edition, Oxford University Press, 2008
- Margaret Brazier and Emma Cave. Medicine, Patients and the Law. Penguin, 2007

Websites
- www.gmc-uk.org/guidance
- Human Tissue Act: www.hta.gov.uk/ legislationpoliciesandcodesofpractice/codesofpractice.cfm
- Research governance: www.dh.gov.uk/prod_consum_dh/ groups/dh_digitalassets/@dh/@en/documents/digitalasset/ dh_4122427.pdf
- Declaration of Helsinki: www.cirp.org/library/ethics/helsinki/
- Declaration of Geneva: www.cirp.org/library/ethics/geneva/

should be maximized and in making a treatment decision, the surgeon should take into account their own knowledge of the patient's beliefs, views and previously expressed preferences and advanced directives, as well as those close to the patient, those with legal authority over the patient, appointed representatives and the views of those the patient wishes to be considered. Decisions should always be taken in the patient's best interest, should maximize the patient's future options and be consensual, involving all relevant parties listed previously. If a consensus cannot be reached then legal advice should be sought or the case referred to the courts to decide.

Confidentiality

Confidentiality is a central element in the doctor–patient relationship. There are exceptions where confidentiality can and should be breached for the protection of others (e.g. notifiable diseases such as tuberculosis). In the context of multidisciplinary team working, only information necessary to enable treatment by a third party should be divulged. When patients are discussed for the purposes of teaching or publication, patient identity must be concealed. Confidentiality is not just an important principle, it may be legally enforceable, for example by the Data Protection Act.

See Table 5.2 for important sources of information regarding ethics in medicine.

Specific topics

Euthanasia and 'end-of-life' issues

Euthanasia is described as a deliberate intervention undertaken with the express intention of ending life, to relieve intractable suffering due to an incurable, progressive disease. It is usually requested by the patient and is illegal in the UK, as is assisted suicide.

Other 'end-of-life' issues such as withholding and withdrawing futile treatments or any treatments at the request of a competent patient are separate issues and should not be confused with euthanasia. Where treatment with 'double effect' is used, such as opiate analgesia (relieves pain and anxiety while shortening life), this is acceptable because the primary intention was to relive pain, distinguishing it from euthanasia.

Abortion

In the UK, legal abortion is permitted under the terms of the Abortion Act 1967; amended by the Human Fertilisation and Embryology Act 1990 that reduced the gestational age at which abortion could be carried out from 28 to 24 weeks. The conditions for performing abortion up to 24 weeks of gestation are that continuing the pregnancy would cause greater risk of injury to the mental or physical health of the woman, or any existing children of her family. Abortion can be carried out after the 24th week of pregnancy if it is necessary to save the mother's life, if there is grave risk of permanent injury to the mental or physical health of the woman by continuing the pregnancy, or if there is substantial risk that the child would have severe physical or mental problems that would render them seriously handicapped. In all cases, two registered medical practitioners have to agree the criteria and appropriateness of the abortion. While a doctor has no obligation in UK law to be involved in abortion if he/she has a conscientious objection, they must refer the patient to a doctor who is. This conscientious objection does not extend to emergency situations where the life or health of the mother is endangered. Although surgeons are only infrequently involved in decisions around abortion, understanding the law is important, especially in the context of trauma or acute abdominal pain in the early stages of pregnancy.

Negligence

In order for a surgeon to be found negligent three prerequisites must be fulfilled. Firstly, it must be demonstrated that the surgeon owed the patient a duty of care (this is usually assumed), secondly, it must be shown that that the doctor breached that duty of care; and, thirdly that, on the balance of probabilities (more likely than not), the breach of duty resulted directly in harm (causation). Medical negligence can relate to diagnosis, treatment and the failure to warn a patient of risks that would have resulted in the patient refusing an intervention. The standard against which a doctor's performance is measured was established in case law in 1957 (the Bolam case). This states that a doctor is not guilty of negligence if he has acted 'in accordance with a practice accepted as proper by a responsible body of medical men skilled in that particular area'. In practice, Bolam defends a doctor's practice if a body of medical opinion can be found to support that doctor's actions. It facilitates the defence of minimal acceptable practice rather than ideal practice. A subsequent House of Lords ruling went further stating that, 'the court has to be satisfied that the exponents of the body of opinion relied on can demonstrate that such an opinion has a logical basis … that the experts have directed their minds to the question of risks and benefits and have reached a defensible conclusion'. This updated ruling (Bolitho) provides the legal basis for most complaints that result in an allegation of negligence. Several professional organizations in the UK offer advice and support to doctors including the British Medical Association, the General Medical Council, and medical defence organizations.

Human Tissue Act

The Human Tissue Act 2004 replaced the Human Tissue Act 1961, the Anatomy Act 1984 and the Human Organ Transplants Act 1989, in England and Wales. A similar

5

act was passed in Scotland in 2006. This was in response to inadequacies in preceding legislation brought to light by inquiries into the storage of human tissue in the Alder Hey and Bristol inquiries. The Human Tissue Act places consent as the fundamental principle in the storage of human tissue, whether from living patients or the deceased and issues legislation and guidance regarding the removal, storage and use of human tissue.

Completion of a death certificate

Following the death of a patient, it is a legal requirement that a death certificate be completed before the body is released for cremation or burial. Death certification must be completed by the doctor who has attended the deceased during their last illness and includes a record of the patient's name and age, as well as the date, time and place of death. The cause of death has to be recorded, as well as any contributing conditions that have led directly to the cause of death and significant conditions that contributed to the death but are unrelated to the disease causing it. In certain situations a death has to be referred as a legal requirement to the coroner's office in England, Wales and Northern Ireland or to the Procurator Fiscal in Scotland for consideration of a post mortem examination to establish the cause of death. These include: recent surgery, where death may be due to abortion, accidental death, death in suspicious/violent/unnatural circumstances, death due to suspected poisoning, self neglect, negligence or suicide, death occurring in prison or police custody, where the death may be due to industrial disease or related to the deceased person's employment, where the cause of death is unknown; and unexpected death.

Where cremation is requested, a separate cremation form has to be completed by a doctor who attended the deceased during their last illness and a second doctor who is at least five years full registration. Care must be taken to identify the presence of pacemakers and other potential explosive devices in the body. The cremation of foetal remains of less than 24 weeks gestation does not require a cremation certificate.

Post-mortem examination

A post mortem is carried out in two situations. There may be a legal requirement to establish the cause of death prior to a death certificate being issued as detailed above. This mandatory Coroners' post mortem does not require the consent of the deceased person's family. Alternatively, the deceased person's next of kin, relatives or doctors may request a post mortem to provide information about the deceased's illness or cause of death. In this instance consent from the next of kin should be obtained to proceed with post mortem examination and should include details of the possible outcomes of post mortem. The Human Tissue Act provides specific recommendations for the handling and storage of tissues and organs removed at post mortem. Further detail is beyond the scope of this chapter.

Research governance

Research governance serves to improve research quality and safeguard the public by enhancing ethical and scientific quality, promoting good practice, reducing adverse incidents and ensuring lessons are learned, and preventing poor performance and misconduct. All of this is be achieved through a broad range of regulations, principles and standards of good practice, originally enshrined in the Declaration of Helsinki in 1964 (for more information see

version 6, released in 2008). Research governance applies to everyone involved in medical research whether as chief investigator, care professional, researcher, the employing institution or sponsor. This governance safeguards participants, protects researchers and investigators, minimizes risk, and enables the monitoring of practice and performance. Surgical journals place great emphasis on research governance. Work that does not demonstrate adherence to satisfactory ethical and quality standards is likely to be rejected.

Ethics committees

Research on human subjects is necessary to advance medical knowledge and treatment. Ensuring that it is carried out in a safe and ethical way is the remit of the ethics committee. The Declaration of Helsinki sets out the principles of ethical research. All clinical trials involving human subjects or tissue must receive ethical approval prior to commencing recruitment. For information on how ethical approval is obtained in the UK see the National Research Ethics Service which is part of the National Patient Safety Agency (http://www.nres.npsa.nhs.uk/). The composition of ethics committees is important and should reflect societal diversity in terms of age, gender, ethnicity and disability and embody a broad range of experience and expertise so that the scientific, clinical and methodological aspects of a research proposal can be reconciled with the welfare of the research participants.

Ethics committees take into consideration a whole range of aspects of a research proposal before giving approval. Their primary consideration is to safeguard the rights, safety and wellbeing of research subjects. They examine the recruitment process, including informed consent, the quality of information given to subjects, payments to subjects, the risks of the research protocol including safety measures and information, compensation procedures and indemnity. The likelihood and capability of the trial design to answer the research questions is considered as well as adequacy of resources, plans for data processing, storage and protection.

PREOPERATIVE ASSESSMENT

Careful preoperative assessment is fundamental to achieving good surgical outcomes. The same principles apply to both emergency and elective situations, the only difference usually being the extent to which preoperative assessment must be compromised when an emergency condition requires urgent intervention.

Assessment of operative fitness and perioperative risk

In the elective surgical setting, preoperative assessment takes place in several stages beginning at the point of referral. A good referral letter should include details not only of the presenting complaint but also of the patient's general health, co-morbidities and current medication. The first contact with the surgical team is usually in the out-patient clinic and this consultation may lead to a decision to offer surgery. In reaching such a decision, the surgeon should consider not only the physical fitness of the patient to withstand the proposed surgery, but also the likely impact on their social and emotional wellbeing. When making the decision to operate, the risks and potential benefits of surgery should be weighed against those of alternative or no treatment. The purpose of preoperative assessment is to prepare the patient for surgery, identify co-morbid conditions, estimate and perioperative risk by optimizing the patient's physical condition. The majority of preoperative assessment for elective surgery takes place in the preoperative assessment clinic one to two weeks before surgery, and culminates in the admission immediately prior to, increasingly in the UK on the morning of, surgery.

The first priority is to establish the severity and extent of the condition requiring surgery by employing appropriate imaging and other investigations. For example, it is important to know that both recurrent laryngeal nerves are functional prior to thyroid surgery as damage is a recognized complication of this type of operation, on the other hand malignant conditions require appropriate staging to establish the disease extent. The second objective is to identify co-morbid conditions through careful clinical assessment and through optimization, minimize perioperative risk. Figure 5.1 details the areas of potential perioperative risk and Figure 5.2 shows a logical sequence of preoperative assessment. Details of previous operations and anaesthetics should be sought, as well as drug, alcohol and smoking history, specific allergies and concerns. Investigations to assess the surgical condition, co-morbid conditions and general health should be arranged as soon as possible to minimize surgical delay. Thorough and timely preoperative assessment is essential to avoid the expense and delay of cancelled or delayed surgery. Good quality assessment and appropriate optimizations prior to admission mean that many patients can be admitted on the day of surgery.

An anaesthetic review should be requested prior to admission where there is increased risk, fitness for surgery is in doubt or there are specific anaesthetic issues requiring input. Other specialist input may be required, including cardiology, respiratory and haematology.

On the morning of surgery, both the surgeon and anaesthetist should reassess the patient and identify outstanding issues and any changes in their condition. Care should be taken to ensure that all investigation results are available as well as necessary blood products and special equipment. Details of the anaesthetic should be discussed, and

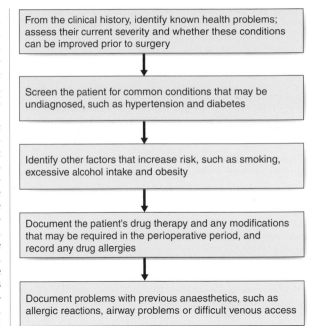

From the clinical history, identify known health problems; assess their current severity and whether these conditions can be improved prior to surgery

↓

Screen the patient for common conditions that may be undiagnosed, such as hypertension and diabetes

↓

Identify other factors that increase risk, such as smoking, excessive alcohol intake and obesity

↓

Document the patient's drug therapy and any modifications that may be required in the perioperative period, and record any drug allergies

↓

Document problems with previous anaesthetics, such as allergic reactions, airway problems or difficult venous access

Fig. 5.2 A logical approach to assessing perioperative and anaesthetic risk.

postoperative analgesic strategies, taking into account patient preferences wherever possible.

In the emergency situation this process is condensed. Judging the timing of surgery is crucial. The surgeon must determine which interventions will optimize the patient's condition while avoiding deterioration due to unnecessary delay progression of the acute surgical problem.

Oxygen delivery in minimizing operative risk

A number of important studies have demonstrated that postoperative morbidity and mortality are related to inadequate oxygen delivery to the tissues, resulting in hypoxia. Oxygen delivery (DO_2) is dependent on cardiac output (CO) and the oxygen content of arterial blood (CaO_2).

$$DO_2 = CO \times CaO_2$$

The arterial oxygen content in turn depends on the delivery of oxygen to the alveoli, its efficient transfer from alveoli into blood, adequately functioning haemoglobin, the arterial partial pressure of oxygen and arterial haemoglobin oxygen saturation. In an average resting adult an oxygen requirement of approximately 250 ml/min is exceeded by delivery of around 1000 ml/min, resulting in considerable reserve. When oxygen demand increases, cardiac output may rise and tissue oxygen extraction may increase to up to 50–60% in order to compensate. If this does not meet tissue oxygen demand, hypoxia with anaerobic metabolism ensues. If uncorrected this can cause local and remote organ damage, dysfunction, multiple organ failure and ultimately death. It has been shown that the duration of oxygen debt correlates with the presence and magnitude of postoperative complications and mortality. It therefore follows that patients with poor cardiovascular and respiratory reserve or anaemia, and who are less able to increase oxygen delivery, are at higher perioperative risk and that measures taken to optimize their condition and oxygen delivery will help to minimize that risk.

Direct surgical risk
Technical problems with surgery and anaesthesia
Surgical complications, e.g. wound infection
Can be measured from audit of practice or from published data

Physiological stress of surgery
Mostly involves the cardiovascular and respiratory systems
Often difficult to predict. Depends on the nature of the surgery, the technical success of surgery, and the physiological fitness or reserve of the patient

Psychological
Anxiety in relation to proposed surgery and anaesthesia
Sources of anxiety may be unexpected; for example, a patient may have little concern about the surgery itself but be terrified of postoperative nausea or of being 'aware' during the operation

Fig. 5.1 Areas of perioperative risk.

5

Goal directed measures to optimize cardiac index, oxygen delivery, mixed venous oxygen saturation and minimize anaerobic metabolism using intraoesophageal Doppler probes, pulmonary artery catheters, intravenous fluid loading, blood transfusion, supplemental oxygen and inotropes have all been shown to improve outcomes.

Systematic preoperative assessment

Cardiovascular system

The severity of cardiovascular disease is assessed and signs of undiagnosed or inadequately treated disease sought. Angina and previous myocardial infarction indicate significant coronary artery disease although bypass grafting, angioplasty and coronary artery stenting may ameliorate their associated risks. Exertional dyspnoea, orthopnoea and paroxysmal nocturnal dyspnoea may indicate left ventricular failure, whilst significant dependent oedema could signify right sided heart failure. The drug history is important and may alert to the presence and severity of cardiovascular disease. Blackouts and dizzy spells may be a sign of arrhythmias, carotid artery or valvular heart disease. Clinical examination should detect arrhythmias, carotid artery, heart murmurs, hypertension and signs of cardiac failure. Antiplatelet agents and anticoagulants are widely prescribed in the general population and may need to be stopped or modified prior to surgery (see below).

Respiratory system

A history of new or increased cough, sputum production, and shortness of breath or wheeze may indicate unsuspected respiratory disease or an exacerbation of pre-existing pulmonary disease. In patients with asthma, chronic obstructive pulmonary disease (COPD) or fibrotic lung disease, purulent sputum may indicate an infective exacerbation. In asthmatics, previous ITU and hospital admissions as well as steroid dependency indicate severe disease. Functional respiratory reserve is best assessed by exercise tolerance, for example how far a patient can walk on the flat, up an incline, or how many stairs they can climb before needing to rest because of shortness of breath. Significant dyspnoea should be investigated with pulmonary function tests.

Patients with features of acute viral respiratory illness should have surgery postponed where possible. This is due to the increased risk of bronchospasm and susceptibility of the respiratory epithelium to postoperative bacterial pneumonia which is compounded by the effect of general anaesthesia which depresses ciliary activity, reducing the clearance of secretions and pathogens.

Smoking

All patients should be offered support to quit smoking, particularly once the decision to operate has been made. The benefits of preoperative smoking cessation are listed in Table 5.3 and should be explained to the patient. Some of the benefits occur within hours (reduced circulating nicotine and carboxyhaemoglobin) while others take weeks, months, or even years. Despite the significant advantages in the perioperative period, many patients are unable or unwilling to stop smoking prior to and after their surgery. Referral to specialist services that support patients to stop smoking may help.

Preoperative exercise

Interest in preoperative exercise has resulted from surgical enhanced recovery programs which aim to reduce the length of hospital stay following surgery and expedite

Table 5.3 Benefits of preoperative smoking cessation

- Reduced airway hyper-reactivity / bronchospasm
- Reduced sputum production reduces the risk of atelectasis
- Improved ciliary function results in increased sputum clearance, helping to protect against infection
- Reduced carboxyhaemoglobin increases oxygen carrying capacity of blood
- Reduced nicotine related systemic and coronary vasoconstriction

return to normal activity. In addition, it has been hypothesized that preoperative exercise may reduce perioperative morbidity by improving cardio-respiratory performance. Some early studies investigating preoperative exercise programs, particularly in the field of orthopaedic surgery showed improved preoperative functional status and muscle strength which resulted in reduced inpatient rehabilitation requirements. However, results have been conflicting and this remains an active area of research.

Alcohol

It is important to obtain an accurate history as significant alcohol consumption can impact surgical planning. In chronic alcohol abuse, liver enzymes are induced, increasing hepatic drug metabolism. Consequently, increased doses of hepatically metabolized drugs, including anaesthetic agents are required to achieve therapeutic effect. Conversely, in acute alcohol intoxication reduced anaesthetic doses are required. In addition, the risk of aspiration pneumonia should be anticipated and preventive measures taken. The risk of alcohol withdrawal should also be anticipated and prevented in habitual alcohol consumers with use of detoxification protocols. In patients with a significant alcohol history, the risk of alcohol related liver and cardiac disease and coagulopathy should be anticipated.

Nutritional status

All patients should have their height and weight measured and BMI (body mass index) calculated. A history of weight loss should be sought and quantified as a percentage of the patients starting weight. It is important to look for signs of malnutrition such as low BMI, bodyweight < 90% predicted, > 20% weight loss, hypoproteinaemia and hypoalbuminaemia as they have all been related to increased rates of postoperative complications (particularly infective and pulmonary) as well as delayed anastamotic and wound healing. Pre-existing hypoalbuminaemia compounded by perioperative fasting and haemodilution results in oedema which may delay recovery. For these reasons, it is important to treat malnutrition preoperatively if time permits. The use of nutritional support should be considered in conjunction with dieticians.

Obesity

Obese patients are at increased risk from surgery and anaesthesia and special equipment may be required. Obese patients are at risk of major associated co-morbidities (e.g. diabetes, obstructive sleep apnoea, degenerative joint disease and cardiovascular disease). Table 5.4 details some of the technical difficulties, perioperative risks and comorbid conditions associated with obesity. If the risks of surgery are outweighed by its potential benefits, surgery may be postponed. In practice, the majority of patients cannot lose weight without support and referral to the GP and dietician for weight loss programmes, including supervised exercise, may be beneficial.

Table 5.4 Significance of obesity in the perioperative period

Cardiovascular system
- Hypertension and ischaemic heart disease more common
- Accurate blood pressure measurement difficult
- Increased risk of right-sided heart failure associated with obstructive sleep apnoea

Respiratory system
- Airway management more difficult
- Reduced lung volumes
- Increased incidence of obstructive sleep apnoea
- Increased risk of perioperative hypoxia
- Increased risk of atelectasis, pneumonia and pulmonary embolism

Surgical
- Surgical access difficult
- Increased wound infection and dehiscence

Other
- Venous access difficult
- Increased incidence of diabetes mellitus
- Increased risk of hiatus hernia and aspiration pneumonia

Drug therapy

A comprehensive drug history should be recorded prior to admission for surgery. In general patients should take their routine medication right up to the time of surgery. The perioperative management of diabetes mellitus and patients on anticoagulation is considered separately. Drugs that require special consideration in the perioperative period are discussed below.

Long-term steroid therapy

Increased circulating cortisol is an important part of the metabolic response to surgical stress. Long-term steroid therapy may result in hypoadrenalism and the inability to mount an effective response to surgical stress. It is therefore important that patients receive steroid therapy throughout the perioperative period. An increased steroid dose is usually necessary to counter surgical stress for all but minor procedures. High doses (100 mg hydrocortisone every 6 hours) may be needed if the risk of hypoadrenalism is compounded further by postoperative complications including infection. Signs of hypoadrenalism include hypotension/ shock, hyponatraemia and hyperkalaemia and should be sought in any steroid-dependent patient who is unwell in the postoperative period. Urgent steroid treatment is needed to avoid an Addisonian crisis.

Antiplatelet therapy and anticoagulants

Antiplatelet therapy with aspirin, clopidogrel and dipyridamole is common. The risk of thromboembolic events, particularly myocardial infarction, if antiplatelet therapy is withdrawn should be weighed against the risk of surgical haemorrhage if treatment is continued. In general, aspirin should be continued. Clopidogrel, commonly used after coronary and peripheral stenting, should not be withdrawn prior to stent endothelialization which takes up to 6 months. Where possible, surgery should be postponed and antiplatelet agents withdrawn only after consultation with a cardiologist or vascular surgeon.

Anticoagulation with warfarin, commonly for prevention of embolic events in atrial fibrillation, and for treatment of deep vein thrombosis and pulmonary embolism is also frequently encountered. The risk of a thromboembolic event with anticoagulant suspension has to be balanced against the risk of bleeding in an anticoagulated patient undergoing surgery. The use of bridging anticoagulation should be considered and is discussed in more detail in the section on abnormal coagulation (see below).

Oral contraceptives and hormone replacement therapy

Depending on the type of surgery being planned and the patient's other risk factors for venous thromboembolism, it may be advisable to discontinue oestrogen-containing drugs (combined oral contraceptive pills [OCP] and hormone replacement therapy [HRT]) 4–6 weeks beforehand. However, opinions on this vary and the decision taken has to balance the possible increased risk of thromboembolism against those of unwanted pregnancy and side-effect (OCP) and side-effects (HRT).

Psychiatric drugs

Concurrent use of lithium, monoamine oxidase inhibitors (MAOI), tricyclic antidepressants and phenothiazines can all complicate general anaesthesia. Tricyclic antidepressants (TCA) and phenothiazines can both cause hypotension and TCAs are also associated with increased risks of arrhythmia. In the case of phenothiazines, the risk of stopping the medication outweighs the potential benefits but the anaesthetist should be aware of the potential complications. It is not essential that tricyclic antidepressants be stopped preoperatively, but the anaesthetist should be alerted. Lithium should be stopped 24 hours prior to surgery as it mimics sodium, potentiating the action of neuromuscular blocking agents. Monoamine oxidase inhibitors interact with opiates and vasopressor agents with the potential of neurological and cardiovascular complications. Ideally, they should be stopped 2–3 weeks prior to surgery, but in an emergency opiates and pressor agents should be avoided.

Allergies

Adverse and idiosyncratic reactions to drugs and other substances should be recorded and steps taken to avoid the allergen as a second exposure may result in a life-threatening hypersensitivity reaction. Common examples in the surgical realm include antibiotics, iodine, adhesive dressings and latex. Full-blown anaphylactic reactions to latex are rare but some degree of latex sensitivity is common. Special care has to be taken to clear the patient environment of latex for those with severe allergic responses as it is common in gloves and other surgical and anaesthetic equipment.

Pregnancy

Elective surgery should be avoided in the first and third trimesters of pregnancy. The risk of miscarriage and potential teratogenicity is high in the first trimester and this is usually encountered in relation to surgery for an acute abdomen at this stage. Third trimester surgery is associated with significant maternal risks and premature labour (see Table 5.5). If surgery is necessary, it is best undertaken in the second trimester in conjunction with the obstetric team. Surgery in pregnancy is usually an emergency or related to the pregnancy. Early involvement of the anaesthetist is essential as much of the excess risk relates to the general anaesthesia.

Previous operations and anaesthetics

Details of previous anaesthetics including complications, side effects and reactions should be sought. Previous anaesthetic charts are a useful source of information and should alert the anaesthetist to potential anaesthetic challenges including a difficult endotracheal intubation. Previous

5

> **Table 5.5 Perioperative risks associated with surgery in pregnant patients**
>
> - Spontaneous abortion or premature labour
> - Hypotension on supine position (inferior vena caval compression in second and third trimesters)
> - Gastro-oesophageal reflux (increased risk of aspiration)
> - Hypoxia (due to high metabolic rate and reduced lung functional residual capacity)
> - Teratogenic effects of drugs (particularly in first trimester)
> - Pre-eclampsia/eclampsia
> - Amniotic fluid embolism

major anaesthetic complications or a suspicious family history should alert to the possibility of a rare inherited abnormality. Pseudocholinesterase deficiency is an inherited enzyme abnormality also known as scoline apnoea and is characterized by prolonged apnoea requiring prolonged ventilation in response to short acting, depolarizing muscle relaxants such as suxamethonium chloride. Diagnosis is confirmed by demonstrating decreased plasma cholinesterase activity. Malignant hyperpyrexia is an inherited autosomal dominant condition characterized by life-threatening hyperpyrexia as a result of abnormal muscle metabolism after exposure to volatile anaesthetic agents or suxamethonium. Diagnosis is complex and investigations should be carried out in specialist centres.

The most common complaint after general anaesthesia is postoperative nausea and vomiting (PONV). This causes significant patient distress, delays recovery and discharge following day case procedures. Steps to minimize PONV include the use of short-acting anaesthetic agents and potent centrally-acting antiemetic drugs (e.g. ondansetron), as well opiate avoidance.

> **SUMMARY BOX 5.3**
>
> **Key factors in the anaesthetic history**
>
> - Adverse drug reactions
> - Difficult intubation (more common in patients with restricted neck movement, limited mouth opening, a short neck or a receding chin)
> - Damaged/loose teeth, crowns, poor dentition
> - Previous postoperative nausea or vomiting
> - Previous postoperative pain problems
> - Needle or mask phobia
> - Family history of adverse reactions to anaesthetics.

Preoperative investigations

Preoperative investigations are undertaken to assess fitness for anaesthetic and identify problems amenable to correction prior to surgery. Preoperative investigations commonly include haematological, biochemical, radiological, cardiovascular and respiratory tests. Most surgical units will have local protocols guiding the use of preoperative investigations.

Haematology

Full blood count

The majority of patients undergoing surgery will have a preoperative full blood count. The oxygen carrying capacity of blood (haemoglobin concentration) is of paramount

> **SUMMARY BOX 5.4**
>
> **Preoperative investigation**
>
> Preoperative investigations should be tailored appropriately to avoid unnecessary tests and comprise of both those assessing the patient's fitness for surgery and those specific to the condition requiring surgical intervention
>
> **Haematological** full blood count (FBC), coagulation screen, cross match / group and save
>
> **Biochemistry** urea and electrolytes (U&E), liver function tests (LFTs)
>
> **Microbiology** Sputum, MRSA screen, virology (patients at high risk of blood borne viruses e.g. HIV)
>
> **Radiological** Plain X ray, ultrasound scan, computed tomography, magnetic resonance imaging, contrast and radionucleotide studies
>
> **Respiratory** Pulmonary function tests, arterial blood gases.
>
> **Cardiovascular** ECG, echocardiogram, exercise testing, thallium scan, CPEX (cardiopulmonary exercise testing).

importance but the platelet and white cell count are also important considerations in terms of haemostatic capacity and where sepsis is suspected. Any patients undergoing surgery with the potential for significant blood loss should have a full blood count, as should those with signs or symptoms of anaemia, patients with significant cardiorespiratory disease that may compromise oxygen delivery to the tissues and those with overt or suspected blood loss (for example gastrointestinal tract symptoms).

Wherever possible, anaemia should be corrected preoperatively to optimize oxygen delivery to the tissues. Preoperative blood transfusion should only be considered for haemoglobin concentrations below 8 g/dl unless the patient is at increased risk of tissue hypoxia due to significant cardiorespiratory disease, especially severe ischaemic heart disease or severe intraoperative bleeding (EBM 5.1). (http://www.transfusionguidelines.org.uk) The threshold for transfusion should be higher (because lower haemoglobin concentrations are tolerated) in patients with chronic anaemia (such as renal failure patients) where compensatory mechanisms such as increased red blood cell 2,3-diphosphoglycerol and reduced blood viscosity increase oxygen delivery.

> **EBM 5.1 Red cell transfusion trigger**
>
> 'A multicentre randomized controlled trial in 838 critically ill patients with a haemoglobin of < 9 g/dl randomized to a restrictive (haemoglobin < 7 g/dl) or liberal transfusion policy (haemoglobin < 10 g/dl) showed no increase in mortality and an increase in hospital survival in the restrictive transfusion group.'
>
> Herbert PC, et al. New Engl J Med 1999; 340(6): 409–417.

An abnormally elevated white cell count may indicate infection or haematological disease and should be investigated preoperatively. Thrombocythaemia increases the risk of thromboembolism and prophylactic measures should be taken. Thrombocytopenia may need to be corrected to reduce the risk of bleeding. The UK blood transfusion service recommends transfusing to a platelet count of $50 \times 10^9/l$ for lumbar puncture, epidural anaesthesia, endoscopy with biopsies and surgery in non-critical sites and to $100 \times 10^9/l$ for more major surgery including critical sites such as neurosurgery or ophthalmic surgery. Advice from a haematologist may be helpful.

Coagulation screen

The indications for coagulation studies are shown in Table 5.6 and include suspected abnormal clotting, anticoagulation treatment and consideration of epidural anaesthesia. When disseminated intravascular coagulation (DIC) is suspected, such as in sepsis, fibrinogen, fibrinogen degradation products (FDP) and D-dimers should be measured. The surgical implications of selected disorders of coagulation are considered below.

Cross matching

Most hospitals have local policies that govern the indications for group and save and cross matching, as well as the number of units required for a given procedure. These policies reflect local resources and availability of blood and blood products in the elective and emergency settings. For rare blood groups and patients with known antibodies, it is important to allow adequate time for cross matching as blood may not be available locally. Blood transfusion and blood products are discussed in more detail in Chapter 2.

Biochemistry

Urea and electrolytes

Analysis of urea and electrolytes (U&E) is not necessary in young patients presenting for minor surgery. Elderly patients and those presenting for major surgery, as well as patients with renal dysfunction, cardiovascular disease, fluid balance problems including dehydration and patients on diuretic therapy or any drug therapy that may affect electrolyte balance or renal function should all have routine blood chemistry analysis. Potassium homeostasis is of particular concern as both hypo- and hyperkalaemia can cause arrhythmias. Abnormalities in electrolyte concentrations and renal function should be corrected preoperatively. A detailed discussion of fluid and electrolyte disorders can be found in Chapter 1X.

Liver function tests

All patients with known liver disease, significant alcohol consumption or signs of liver disease should have liver function tests measured.

Cardiac investigations

Electrocardiography (ECG) is of very limited value in predicting the risk of ischaemic events and generally should only be performed in the elderly (over 65 years), to detect occult rhythm disorders or signs of previous cardiac events. In younger patients ECG should be restricted to those with signs of, or known, cardiovascular disease and those with risk factors for ischaemic heart disease. Routine chest X-ray should only be performed in the context of cardiovascular assessment where congestive cardiac failure is suspected. Echocardiography is used to assess cardiac function (left ventricular ejection fraction in particular) and may be indicated prior to major surgery and in patients with suspected valvular disease and heart failure. A 24-hour ECG is useful in patients with a history suggestive of paroxysmal arrhythmias or heart block – usually syncopal attacks. Tests of cardiovascular physiological reserve include exercise ECG, thallium scan, stress echocardiography and cardiopulmonary exercise tests (CPEX). CPEX is a dynamic test of cardiopulmonary reserve that is used selectively to help select patients for high risk surgery such as thoracic, vascular and cardiac surgery. This measures VO_2 max (maximum oxygen consumption) and carbon dioxide excretion under exercise conditions, which is related to overall fitness, as well as the anaerobic threshold (the point at which respiration switches from aerobic to anaerobic metabolism). There is some controversy regarding its value in predicting the risk of an adverse outcome for an individual patient or for specific operations, but it may aid the decision-making process.

In general, the involvement of a cardiologist is advisable if anything more than basic cardiac evaluation is required. The significance of common arrhythmias is listed in Table 5.7. The perioperative management of patients with pacemakers is discussed below.

Table 5.6 Indications for preoperative coagulation studies

Patient factors
- Liver disease, including jaundice and excess alcohol consumption
- Haematological disease affecting coagulation
- Anticoagulant therapy
- Shock, risk of disseminated intravascular coagulation e.g. sepsis
- Suspected coagulopathy: excessive bleeding or bruising
- Suspected prothrombotic disorder: history of thromboembolic events

Surgical factors
- Major hepatobiliary surgery
- Surgery involving anticoagulation: cardiopulmonary bypass, major vascular surgery
- High risk of major blood loss
- Consideration of epidural anaesthesia

Table 5.7 Significance of common arrhythmias in the perioperative period.

Arrhythmia	Significance
Uncontrolled atrial fibrillation	May compromise cardiac output Exclude metabolic causes, e.g. electrolyte abnormality, and thyrotoxicosis Ventricular rate should be controlled prior to surgery
Controlled atrial fibrillation	Rarely causes severe perioperative problems unless associated with other significant heart disease Patient may be on anticoagulants; if not, consider thromboprophylaxis
Ventricular extrasystoles	Usually of little significance May indicate ischaemia in patients with ischaemic heart disease
First-degree heart block, asymptomatic bi- or trifascicular block or asymptomatic second-degree heart block	Little significance. Previously considered an indication for temporary pacemaker insertion Now usually managed by careful monitoring in the perioperative period
Third-degree heart block	Requires pacemaker insertion prior to anaesthesia

5

> ### SUMMARY BOX 5.5
>
> **History, symptoms and signs associated with elevated perioperative cardiovascular risk**
>
> - Myocardial infarction within the past 6 months
> - Poor left ventricular function
> - Poorly controlled cardiac failure
> - Resting diastolic blood pressure > 110 mmHg
> - Poorly controlled/untreated arrhythmia
> - Age > 75
> - Significant aortic stenosis.

Respiratory investigations

Patients with purulent sputum suspected of having a chest infection should have sputum culture and antibiotic sensitivity performed. Preoperative chest X-ray is a useful baseline in patients with known or suspected pulmonary disease, and may demonstrate consolidation, atelectasis and pleural effusions. Routine chest X-ray is not indicated, having poor sensitivity to detect new respiratory disease.

Pulmonary function tests are useful to gauge severity and reversibility of the obstructive component of respiratory disease and may help guide therapy to optimize function.

Pulmonary function tests are indicated in pre-existing significant pulmonary disease, patients with significant respiratory symptoms, and in patients undergoing thoracic surgery. Table 5.8 lists the commonly performed pulmonary function tests. Although commonly used, the evidence that preoperative pulmonary function tests are predictive of postoperative complications is not convincing. Indications for preoperative arterial blood gas analysis are given in Table 5.9.

The high risk patient

Blood borne viruses (hepatitis B, C and HIV) all pose risk to the surgical team and precautions should be taken to minimize the risk of inoculation. Similar precautions are also recommended for patients with a known or suspected diagnosis of Creutzfeldt–Jacob Disease (CJD) or vCJD (variant CJD) and patients at increased risk of hepatitis B, C or HIV where their viral status is not known. High risk patients include intravenous drug users (IVDUs), recipients of multiple blood transfusions and blood products, including haemophiliacs and those from HIV endemic areas, particularly sub-Saharan Africa. The adoption of universal precautions for all patients is recommended and helps minimize the risk of inoculation injury to the surgical team.

Table 5.8 Respiratory function tests commonly carried out preoperatively

Respiratory function test	Significance
FEV1	Forced expire volume. Volume of air forcibly expelled in one second
FVC	Forced vital capacity. Volume of air forcibly expelled from full inspiration to maximal expiration.
FEV1/FVC ratio	**Restrictive** lung disease (fibrosing alveolitis or scoliosis): the FEV1 and FVC are reduced proportionately with an unchanged FEV1/FVC ratio **Obstructive** pulmonary disease (asthma and COPD): the FEV1 is reduced by a greater extent than the FVC resulting in a reduced FEV1/FVC ratio A ratio of < 70% indicates obstructive pulmonary disease and bronchodilator therapy is indicated.
PEFR	Peak expiratory flow rate. Maximum speed of expiration. PEFR < 70% of expected indicates poorly controlled obstructive lung disease.
Gas transfer factor	An estimate of the lungs' ability to transfer gases. Usually performed by inhaling a gas mixture containing a small amount of carbon monoxide Reduced in conditions that reduce the surface area available for gas transfer (emphysema), conditions that thicken the alveolar membrane (fibrosis), interstitial lung disease, asbestosis and anaemia Increased in polycythaemia (some laboratories adjust for haemoglobin concentration)

Table 5.9 Indications for blood gas analysis in the preoperative period

Surgical presentation	Useful features
Elective surgery Chronic respiratory disease: Moderate to severe COPD Fibrotic lung disease Bronchectasis and cystic fibrosis Severe chest wall deformity e.g. ankylosing spondylitis Lung malignancy	Degree of hypoxaemia (respiratory failure) Distinguish type I (characterized by normocapnia) from type II (characterized by hypercapnia) respiratory failure Detect degree of compensation of hypercapnia (uncompensated, acute hypercapnia results in respiratory acidosis)
Emergency surgery As above. Acute respiratory disease: pneumonia, pleural effusion, ARDS, pneumo- or haemothorax, suspected pulmonary embolism Dyspnoea, decreased SaO$_2$ Shock	As above Document acid–base disturbance including the presence and degree of metabolic acidosis indicating inadequate tissue perfusion and to guide resuscitation

COPD = chronic obstructive pulmonary disease; ARDS = acute respiratory distress syndrome

All members of the surgical team should be immunized against hepatitis B. All blood exposure incidents should be reported to occupational health according to local protocol for assessment and consideration of post-procedure prophylaxis. Theatre staff should be notified of high risk patients. Precautions include wearing goggles, waterproof gowns and protective footwear, double gloving and the use of disposable surgical and anaesthetic equipment where possible. Meticulous surgical technique is important with minimal sharps handling and avoidance of direct tissue contact with hands. Stapling devices should replace sutures where possible and sharp needles replaced by blunt ones where practicable. Specimens from high risk patients should be appropriately labelled and transported separately.

Where patient testing for blood borne viruses is indicated, i.e. post blood exposure incident or in high risk patients where viral status is not known, it should be performed only after appropriate consent and counselling.

Preoperative MRSA screening

Infection with methicillin resistant *Staphylococcus aureus* (MRSA) can have devastating clinical consequences, causing significant in-hospital morbidity and mortality, prolonging hospital stay and increasing cost. Preoperative MRSA screening has been shown to be an effective strategy to decrease MRSA infection rates by identifying asymptomatic carriers and allowing decolonization treatment prior to hospital admission which reduces the risk of transmission and clinical infection (see chapter 4). Preoperative MRSA screening involves swabbing the areas (nostrils, perineum and axillae) regularly colonized by *Staphylococcus aureus*. MRSA carriers should then undergo preoperative decolonisation using daily antibacterial shampoo, body wash and nasal cream three times daily for five days. Although this regime is only 50–60% effective, in the remainder, reduced bacterial shedding reduces the risk of transmission and infection. Where possible, MRSA positive emergency admissions should be nursed in single room isolation until decolonization is complete.

Assessment of the patient for emergency surgery

The principles of assessment, investigation and preparation of patients for elective surgery apply equally to the emergency setting but may be curtailed by a lack of time and information. As a result, emergency surgery is often associated with increased morbidity and mortality compared to elective surgery. Emergency patients often require resuscitation prior to surgery and a stepwise approach to airway, breathing and circulation should be followed. Particular care should be taken to restore circulating volume wherever possible prior to surgery, with the exception of life threatening haemorrhage or where haemodynamic stability cannot be maintained. This is because anaesthesia is associated with attenuation of normal cardiovascular compensatory mechanisms and significant hypotension can result.

Over–zealous attempts to restore biochemistry, haematology and coagulation to normal at the expense of a marked delay in surgery are to be avoided. This is particularly the case in the timing of surgery for sepsis, where the risk of progression of the septic process may outweigh small benefits associated with interventions that delay surgery (e.g. the correction of modest hyperglycaemia in the diabetic patient with peritonitis).

The preoperative ward round

The purpose of the preoperative ward round is to ensure that the patient has been adequately assessed and prepared for surgery and involves both surgeon and anaesthetist. Consideration should be given to the appropriate administration of drugs in the perioperative period as well as a comprehensive, multidisciplinary approach to the perioperative period. Patient questions should be addressed and full explanations of the surgical procedure, anaesthesia, postoperative analgesia, as well as the use of catheters, drains and postoperative monitoring should be given.

 SUMMARY BOX 5.6

Principles of perioperative management

Preoperative
- Optimization of chronic conditions
- Optimization of acute physiological disturbances
- Information sharing / psychological preparation / informed consent
- Surgical strategy / planning / investigations specific to surgical indication.

Intra-operative
- Patient safety – monitoring and positioning
- Equipment – available and functioning
- Operative team – expertise correct.

Postoperative recovery
- Analgesia
- Nutrition
- Physiotherapy / mobilization
- Rehabilitation / occupational therapy
- Further treatment planning.

Drug-management considerations
- DVT prophylaxis
- Antibiotic prophylaxis
- Preoperative anxiolytics
- Continuation of regular medication including route of administration
- Glycaemic control
- Reversal of anticoagulation
- Analgesia
- Fluid and electrolyte requirements.

Nutrition
Where there is going to be a prolonged period of reduced oral intake, enteral or parenteral nutrition should be considered.

Venous thromboembolism prophylaxis

In the United Kingdom, 25 000 people die each year from venous thromboembolism (VTE): many of these deaths are preventable (EBM 5.2). A substantial proportion of these

EBM 5.2 **Venous Thromboembolism**

'Each year, it is estimated that 25 000 die from venous thromboembolism in the UK.

Mechanical methods of prevention are effective.

Pharmacological prophylaxis is cost effective.'

NICE Clinical Guideline 92: Venous thromboembolism – Reducing the risk. (2010).
SIGN Clinical Guideline 122: Prevention and management of venous thromboembolism. (2010).

5

are surgical patients. In addition to death from pulmonary embolism (PE), deep vein thrombosis (DVT) causes substantial morbidity which may persist to cause the chronic health problems of post-thrombotic syndrome with leg ulceration and swelling with huge health care costs.

All patients should have their risk of VTE assessed prior to, or on, admission to hospital to enable prophylactic measures to be taken. The patient's risk of bleeding should be taken into consideration and balanced against the risk of DVT when deciding on thromboprophylaxis. The magnitude of the risk of DVT relates to patient and operative factors as shown in Table 5.10. Measures should be taken to reduce the risk of VTE, in addition to thromboprophylaxis; these include maintaining hydration, encouraging mobility and in patients at very high risk of VTE the use of an inferior vena caval filter. Women should consider stopping oestrogen-containing contraceptives and hormone replacement therapy four weeks prior to surgery.

Mechanical and pharmacological thromboprophylaxis is available (Table 5.11). All surgical patients with increased risk of VTE should be offered mechanical VTE prophylaxis at admission and pharmacological VTE prophylaxis if the risk of bleeding is low. Thromboprophylaxis should be continued until mobility is not significantly reduced, usually for 5–7 days with the exception of orthopaedic lower limb surgery where it should be continued for 2–4 weeks after surgery.

Table 5.10 Patients at risk of venous thromboembolism

Medical patients
- Significantly reduced mobility ≥ 3 days or
- Expected ongoing reduced mobility with a VTE risk factor.

Surgical patients
- Total anaesthetic + surgical time > 90 mins **or**
- Pelvic or lower limb surgery with total anaesthetic + surgical time > 60 mins **or**
- Acute surgical admission with inflammatory or intra-abdominal condition **or**
- Reduced mobility expected **or**
- Any VTE risk factor.

VTE risk factors
- Active cancer or cancer treatment
- Age > 60 years
- Intensive care admission
- Dehydration
- Known thrombophilia
- BMI > 30kg/m^2
- Presence of significant medical comorbidity (heart disease, metabolic, endocrine or respiratory pathology, acute infectious or inflammatory conditions)
- Personal history of or first degree relative with VTE
- Hormone replacement therapy
- Oestrogen containing contraceptives
- Varicose veins with phlebitis

Pregnancy
- Women admitted during pregnancy or up to 6 weeks post partum
- If surgery is planned mechanical plus pharmacological VTE prophylaxis
- Surgery not planned, use mechanical VTE prophylaxis and consider pharmacological prophylaxis if VTE risk factors present

Adapted from: Venous thromboembolism: reducing the risk. NICE clinical guideline 92, 2010.

Table 5.11 Thromboprophylaxis

Mechanical
- Anti-embolism stockings (knee or thigh length)
- Foot impulse devices
- Intermittent pneumatic compression devices (knee or thigh length)

Pharmacological
- Low molecular weight heparin (LMWH)
- Unfractionated heparin (renal failure)
- Fondaparinux

Antibiotic prophylaxis

Antibiotic prophylaxis refers to the use of antibiotics perioperatively to reduce the incidence of surgical site infections (EBM 5.3). Surgical site infections (SSI) refer to infections of the wound, tissues involved in the surgery or devices where surgery involves the insertion of implants or surgical devices (see Chapter 4). Prevention of SSI is important because they are responsible for approximately 16% of hospital acquired infections and cause considerable morbidity, prolonged hospital stay and increased costs. Every surgical patient should be assessed for the risk of SSI and its potential severity and appropriate prophylactic antibiotics selected. The risk of SSI depends on patient and operative risk factors, including the wound class (Table 5.12), SSI risk should be balanced against the risks of antibiotic prophylaxis such as allergy and increasing the prevalence of resistant bacteria and infection

---

EBM 5.3 Antibiotic prophylaxis

'A single therapeutic dose of antibiotic is sufficient in most circumstances with enough half life to achieve activity throughout the operation.
Prophylactic antibiotics should be given intravenously.
Intravenous prophylactic antibiotics should be given ≤ 30 mins before the skin is incised.
The choice of antibiotic should cover the expected pathogens for that operative site.'

SIGN Clinical Guideline 104: Antibiotic prophylaxis in surgery – principles (2008).

Table 5.12 Degree of contamination

Class	Definition
Clean	Operations in which no inflammation is encountered and which do not breach the respiratory, alimentary or genitourinary tracts. Operating theatre technique is continuously aseptic
Clean–contaminated	Operations which breach the respiratory, alimentary or genitourinary tracts but without significant spillage
Contaminated	Operations where acute inflammation is encountered or where the wound is visibly contaminated, e.g. gross spillage from a hollow viscus or compound injuries less than 4 hours old
Dirty	Operations in the presence of pus, a perforated hollow viscus or a compound injury more than 4 hours old

with organisms like *Clostridium difficile*. In general a single dose of intravenous antibiotics is adequate provided the half-life permits activity throughout the operation.

Preoperative anxiolytic medication

The use of preoperative anxiolytics is at the anaesthetist's discretion. The aim is for the patient to arrive in the anaesthetic room in a relaxed, pain-free state. This can often be achieved by adequate explanation of the planned procedure and reassurance. Very anxious patients may require an anxiolytic. Oral benzodiazepines are commonly used as they have a relatively long duration of action meaning accurate timing of administration with regard to anaesthetic induction is not required.

Preoperative fasting

The purpose of fasting preoperatively is to try to ensure an empty stomach and minimize the risk of regurgitation and aspiration during induction of anaesthesia. Where possible, patients should be starved of food for 6 hours and of clear fluids for 2 hours (EBM 5.4). This may not be possible in the emergency setting in which case anaesthetic technique is adjusted to minimize the risk of aspiration. There are situations where an empty stomach cannot be guaranteed despite fasting. These include pregnancy, gastric outlet or bowel obstruction and any condition that causes a functional gastroparesis (autonomic neuropathy with delayed gastric emptying is common in long-standing diabetes). In such patients a nasogastric tube may be indicated.

EBM 5.4 Perioperative fasting

'Water and drinks without milk allowed up to 2 hours prior to induction of anaesthesia.

In children, breast milk allowed up to 4 hours prior to induction of anaesthesia.

Food, including sweets and drinks containing milk up to 6 hours prior to anaesthesia.

Chewing gum not permitted on the day of surgery.

Routine medication continued, can be taken with 30 ml fluid or 0.5 ml/kg in children.'

Perioperative fasting in adults and children, Royal College of Nursing 2005.

Perioperative implications of chronic disease

Some of the more important and common chronic diseases are discussed below.

Cardiovascular disease

Ischaemic heart disease

Ischaemic heart disease is common; increases with age; and significant number of patients with significant coronary artery disease are asymptomatic. Preoperative assessment therefore should focus not only on documented ischaemic heart disease but also on the diagnosis and investigation of occult or undiagnosed disease, especially in high-risk groups (Table 5.13).

Myocardial infarction

In patients with previous myocardial infarction (MI), the risk of a perioperative MI decreases with time from infarction (Table 5.14), but overall is approximately 6%. This contrasts

Table 5.13 Factors indicating increased risk of ischaemic heart disease

- Family history
- Smoking
- Hypertension
- Diabetes mellitus
- Obesity
- Hypercholesterolaemia

Table 5.14 Risk of postoperative myocardial infarction according to time elapsed after previous myocardial infarction.

Time elapsed after MI	Incidence of postoperative MI (%)
> 6 months	5
4–6 months	10–20
< 3 months	20–30

with patients without a history of MI whose risk is around 0.2%. The mortality of perioperative MI is approximately 50% greater than that of non-perioperative MI. In general, a delay of six months for elective surgery is recommended with three months delay for more urgent surgery, although individual patient factors need to be considered, taking the risks of delayed surgery into account. Post-infarction coronary artery angioplasty, stenting and bypass surgery may reduce the risk of perioperative MI meaning that surgery may be safely carried out sooner. Advice from cardiologists may be helpful in planning the timing of surgery following MI to minimize risk and optimise medical treatment.

Postoperative MI may be difficult to diagnose due to atypical or silent presentations, particularly in diabetics. In addition, thrombolysis is often contraindicated because of the risk of postoperative bleeding. Advice from a cardiologist should be sought early once the diagnosis is suspected.

Angina

The risk of perioperative myocardial infarction increases with symptom severity in patients with angina. This should be assessed by the frequency of angina symptoms, duration of attacks and precipitating factors. In particular, the limitation on everyday activities (walking, stair climbing etc.) by angina is a good guide to disease severity. Results of previous cardiac investigations, including coronary angiography taking into account the time elapsed since they were performed may help gauge disease severity. Cardiology input may help to optimize the patient for general anaesthetic.

Unstable angina, despite maximal medical therapy represents a very high risk situation with the risk of perioperative MI around 25% and the patient should be referred to a cardiologist for investigation and management. Risk of perioperative MI may be reduced by preoperative coronary artery bypass, angioplasty or stenting. The decision to proceed with surgery depends upon the indication, weighing the risk of perioperative MI against that of delaying or cancelling surgery.

Coronary artery bypass graft (CABG), percutaneous angioplasty and stenting

Patients may present for surgery after coronary artery bypass grafting, percutaneous angioplasty or stenting. The risk of perioperative MI in these patients may be reduced significantly, even to that of a patient without a history of MI, but is dependent on the success of the procedure. These patients should be assessed in the same manner as a patient with angina. Most will be on an antiplatelet drug or an anticoagulant (see above).

Congestive cardiac failure

The commonest cause of congestive cardiac failure is ischaemic heart disease but the exact cause should be determined where possible as it may influence treatment. Cardiac failure is associated with a number of complications as a result of either poor pump function or underlying cardiac disease (Table 5.15). Uncontrolled heart failure indicated by peripheral oedema, paroxysmal nocturnal dyspnoea or orthopnoea

is associated with very high perioperative risk and should be controlled prior to elective surgery.

Valvular heart disease

The severity of valvular heart disease should be assessed by clinical evaluation and echocardiography. Associated arrhythmias and cardiac failure should be excluded. An algorithm for the preoperative work-up of these patients in shown in Figure 5.3. Antibiotic prophylaxis guided by local protocol will depend on the risk of bacterial endocarditis according to the surgical procedure and the presence and type (metallic or bioprosthesis) of prosthetic heart valve.

Pacemakers

Pacemaker function may be affected by anaesthetic equipment and diathermy. It is important to establish the indication for pacemaker insertion, the date of insertion and last check, as well as the pacemaker type prior to surgery. Advice from the pacemaker clinic may need to be sought. Referral may be necessary for preoperative device reprogramming or a check if more than three months have elapsed since the last check. Monopolar diathermy should be avoided. Bipolar diathermy or ultrasonic energy devices are preferred. If monopolar diathermy cannot be avoided, care should be taken when placing the patient return electrode to direct the electrical current away from the pacemaker.

Table 5.15 Increased perioperative risk in patients with cardiac failure.

Mechanism	Complication
Poor 'pump function'	Pulmonary oedema
	Cardiogenic shock
	Renal failure
	Organ ischaemia, e.g. bowel ischaemia
	Deep venous thrombosis
Cardiac disease	Arrhythmias
	Myocardial infarction
	Venous thromboembolism

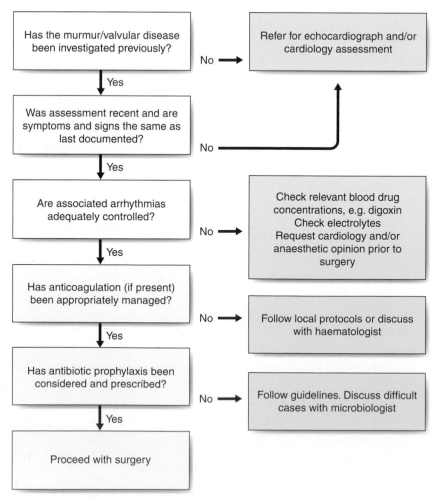

Fig. 5.3 An algorithm for managing patients with known or suspected valvular heart disease.

Hypertension

Uncontrolled hypertension increases the risk of perioperative myocardial infarction and cerebrovascular accident. A diagnosis of hypertension requires repeated, accurate blood pressure measurements which should be interpreted with respect to the patient's age. An elevated diastolic pressure is of greater significance than the systolic pressure, contributing most of the excess risk. Organ blood flow is tightly regulated over a range of blood pressures; in hypertensive patients, this range is elevated rendering them vulnerable to organ hypoperfusion even with modest intra-operative hypotension during anaesthesia.

Hypertension should be controlled in the elective setting for a few weeks prior to surgery. This is to enable the autoregulatory mechanisms that control organ blood flow to reset and maintain organ perfusion at the lower blood pressure, a process that takes several days. Elective surgery should usually be postponed when the diastolic pressure exceeds 110 mmHg. In the emergency situation a modest reduction in blood pressure to minimize cardiovascular risk whilst maintaining adequate organ perfusion can be achieved intraoperatively by careful titration of antihypertensives. Regional anaesthetic techniques offer an alternative approach in the emergency setting, by avoiding the potentially large swings in blood pressure associated with general anaesthesia that may cause dysregulation of organ perfusion.

Perioperative management of patients with cardiovascular disease

Drug therapy

In general, cardiac medications should be taken right up to the time of surgery and re-introduced as soon as possible postoperatively. Where the oral route is not available postoperatively, an alternative should be found. The following two classes of drug merit further consideration:

Beta-blockers. Although it has been suggested that the perioperative use of β-blockers may reduce cardiovascular morbidity and mortality, the evidence is inconclusive and somewhat conflicting. Patients already established on a β-blocker should continue because of the risk of rebound tachycardia increasing myocardial oxygen demand with increased risk of myocardial ischaemia.

Angiotensin-converting enzyme (ACE) inhibitors. These drugs are commonly used to treat cardiac failure and hypertension. Due to the significant risk of intra- and postoperative hypotension with these drugs, the anaesthetist should decide whether to omit them perioperatively.

Cardiovascular management

The principle of perioperative cardiovascular management is to protect against myocardial ischaemia by:

Minimizing myocardial oxygen demand. Cardiac output can be increased by increasing preload, reducing afterload, and increasing heart rate and contractility. The most efficient way of increasing cardiac output, whilst minimizing myocardial oxygen demand is by fluid loading to increase preload. Peripheral vasoconstriction, tachycardia and sympathetic activation all increase myocardial oxygen consumption and should be avoided.

Maximizing myocardial oxygen supply. Blood supply to the left ventricle occurs during diastole and depends on the coronary perfusion pressure (diastolic blood pressure minus left ventricular end diastolic pressure). Left ventricular blood supply is therefore optimal when tachycardia is avoided, the duration of diastole is maximal and diastolic blood pressure high.

In order to optimize and monitor myocardial oxygen supply and demand closely, patients with significant

Table 5.16 Monitors of cardiovascular status during the perioperative period.

Monitor	Information given
Arterial catheter	Continuous measurement of blood pressure
Central venous catheter	Central venous pressure (estimate of cardiac preload with important exceptions)
Pulmonary artery catheter	Pulmonary capillary wedge pressure (a measure of left atrial pressure) and cardiac output (by thermodilution)
Oesophageal Doppler	Cardiac output

EBM 5.5 Optimizing high-risk patients using invasive monitoring and resuscitation targets

'A significant number of RCTs have compared standard perioperative management to one that involved invasive cardiovascular monitoring and the use of fluids and adrenergic drugs to achieve resuscitation targets during the perioperative period. A recent review of these trials concluded that optimization regimens in high-risk surgical patients, many of whom have cardiorespiratory disease, reduce mortality and morbidity.'

Davies SJ, Wilson RJT. Br J Anaesth 2004; 93(1):121–128.

cardiovascular and respiratory disease may benefit from invasive perioperative monitoring (Table 5.16 and EBM 5.5).

Respiratory disease

Patients with significant respiratory disease require close monitoring, preferably in a high dependency or intensive care unit, particularly after thoracic or major abdominal surgery where hypoventilation, atelectasis and pneumonia are common. It is essential that adequate analgesia is provided to enable the clearance of secretions and avoid atelectasis by coughing to avoid hypoxia and pneumonia. It is also important to remember that a small proportion of patients with chronic hypercarbia rely on hypoxic drive for ventilation and that high concentrations of inspired oxygen may cause hypoventilation and respiratory failure. These patients walk a tightrope between the increased postoperative complications associated with hypoxia and respiratory failure where hypoventilation ensues from excess supplemental oxygen therapy. They are particularly vulnerable to postoperative complications such as respiratory failure and pneumonia requiring respiratory support including ventilation. The perioperative management of patients with respiratory disease is discussed below.

Anaesthetic technique

General anaesthesia is associated with a risk of respiratory complications in part due to altered respiratory function caused by general anaesthesia. This is of particular concern in patients with pre-existing respiratory disease and reduced respiratory reserve. Where possible, general anaesthesia should be avoided through the use of regional anaesthetic techniques in this patient group.

Postoperative analgesia

Effective postoperative analgesia is important to maintain adequate cough, sputum clearance and ventilation, particularly in patients who have undergone thoracic and major abdominal surgery in order to avoid atelectasis, chest infection and hypoxia. Regional anaesthetic techniques, including spinal and epidural analgesia are effective in this regard. Parenteral opiates are effective analgesics but care should be taken not to cause respiratory depression or obtund the conscious level.

Physiotherapy

Pre- and postoperative chest physiotherapy is particularly important in patients with respiratory disease. Manoeuvres that facilitate maximal inspiratory effort and the use of incentive spirometry are particularly useful in minimizing the risk of atelectasis and guarding against hypoxia and pneumonia.

Postoperative ventilation

Postoperative ventilation may be indicated for respiratory failure as a result of insufficient respiratory reserve or complications such as pneumonia. Meticulous attention to analgesia and regular chest physiotherapy may avoid the need for ventilation. The duration of endotracheal intubation should be minimized because it also increases the risk of pneumonia. The use of non-invasive respiratory support with either non-invasive ventilation (NIV) or continuous positive airway pressure (CPAP) via a face mask may avoid the need for ventilation and be a useful bridge whilst weaning a patient from ventilatory support.

Diabetes mellitus

The increased perioperative risk associated with diabetes mellitus is attributable to related co-morbidities and poor glycaemic control which is exacerbated by surgical stress.

Diabetic comorbidity

Vascular disease
Diabetics develop both a specific microangiopathy (typified by diabetic retinopathy and nephropathy) and macrovascular disease with accelerated atherosclerosis that results in increased risk of ischaemic heart disease, cerebrovascular accident, peripheral vascular disease, renovascular disease, hypertension and delayed wound healing.

Renal disease
Diabetes is the single commonest cause of chronic renal failure in the UK. Due to a lack of renal reserve, diabetics are particularly vulnerable to acute renal failure resulting from hypotension, nephrotoxic drugs, radiological contrast agents and sepsis. A significant proportion of patients developing postoperative renal failure will remain dialysis dependent. It is therefore imperative that care is taken to protect against further kidney insult.

Neuropathy
Diabetic neuropathy has a number of manifestations. It is most commonly encountered by the vascular surgeon in association with limb ischaemia as a component of non-healing ulceration. Autonomic neuropathy should be anticipated and can result in delayed gastric emptying with risk of aspiration during induction of anaesthesia. A lack of sympathetic cardiovascular compensation to anaesthetic induced hypotension or bleeding can result in severe hypotension.

Infection
Diabetic patients are at increased risk of infective complications particularly if glycaemic control is poor.

Effect of surgical stress on diabetic control
Part of the metabolic response to surgery involves glucose mobilization and lipolysis with increased circulating insulin levels to maintain homeostasis and normoglycaemia. The net result in diabetics is a tendency towards hyperglycaemia and ketoacidosis following surgery, which is exaggerated if complications such as sepsis develop. Glycaemic control should be monitored closely and insulin or oral hypoglycaemic drug doses titrated accordingly. The metabolic response to surgery is discussed in more detail in chapter 1.

Principles of perioperative diabetes management
The aim of perioperative diabetic management is to maintain stable circulating glucose levels, ensuring an adequate supply to the cells. A circulating glucose concentration of 6–10 mmol/l is a reasonable target range. As hypoglycaemia is more dangerous to the patient than hyperglycaemia, moderate hyperglycaemia is acceptable. Care should be taken to administer sufficient potassium when insulin is administered as insulin increases cellular potassium uptake, with a tendency towards hypokalaemia. The approach used to achieve perioperative glycaemic control depends on a number of factors including:
- whether the diabetes is usually diet, tablet or insulin controlled
- the magnitude of the surgical stress
- the presence of sepsis or other complications
- whether the patient is 'nil by mouth'.

In practice, many units have protocols for the perioperative management of diabetes, which can be tailored to the individual patient. Table 5.17 gives examples of the typical approach to diabetic control.

Methods of insulin administration
For patients with poor glycaemic control or not established on their usual diabetic medication because normal dietary intake has not been established, sliding scale insulin is normally administered. Sliding scale insulin regimens consist of intravenous insulin, glucose and potassium that can be given as a single mixed infusion (the Alberti regimen) (Table 5.18) or as separate infusions of insulin and glucose with potassium. Single mixed infusions are simple, cheap and safer, with less risk of hypoglycaemia, but at the expense of greater flexibility and tight glycaemic control that can be achieved with separate insulin and glucose infusions.

Chronic renal failure

Patients with chronic renal failure are at increased risk of complications in the perioperative period (Table 5.19). Management of fluid balance and specific arrangements for dialysis should be undertaken in conjunction with a nephrologist.

Dialysis dependent patients
Considerations in dialysis dependent patients include:
- Fluid balance. The majority of these patients are anuric and depend on dialysis to remove excess water. Intravenous fluid should be administered with extreme caution.
- Access for dialysis. Patients will either have venous access for haemodialysis (fistulae or large intravenous cannulae) or peritoneal dialysis catheters. Care should be taken to protect this life preserving access. An arterio-venous or dialysis access graft fistula should never be used for intravenous access or phlebotomy.

Table 5.17 Typical scenarios for diabetic patients presenting for surgery.

Patient	Procedure	Management
Diet-controlled diabetic	Elective laparoscopic cholecystectomy (moderate stress response)	Monitor blood glucose until eating
Patient on oral hypoglycaemics	Hernia repair (minor stress response)	Omit oral hypoglycaemic on morning of surgery Monitor preoperatively for hypoglycaemia Monitor postoperatively until eating normally Restart oral hypoglycaemics when on normal diet
Normally well-controlled	Elective aortofemoral bypass (major stress response)	Omit oral hypoglycaemic on morning of surgery Monitor perioperatively for hypo- or hyperglycaemia If blood glucose > 10 mmol/l, commence glucose/insulin/potassium infusion
Normally poorly controlled blood sugar > 10 mmol/l	Emergency aortofemoral bypass (major stress response)	Commence glucose/insulin/potassium infusion prior to surgery Stop oral hypoglycaemics perioperatively
Insulin-dependent diabetic Well-controlled	Cataract surgery (minor stress response)	Omit morning insulin Monitor blood sugar for hypoglycaemia Restart regular insulin when eating
Normally well-controlled	Elective coronary artery bypass graft (major stress response)	Convert to glucose/insulin/dextrose *prior* to surgery Monitor blood sugar perioperatively Convert to subcutaneous short-acting insulin and then regular insulin as diet reintroduced
Blood sugar > 20 mmol/l or ketones in urine	Emergency laparotomy for diverticular abscess (major stress response)	Treat as diabetic ketoacidosis and stabilize prior to surgery Ensure adequate volume resuscitation Continue glucose/insulin/potassium infusion perioperatively Convert to intermittent short-acting and then normal insulin as diet reintroduced

Table 5.18 The Alberti Regimen

- 500 ml 10% dextrose *plus* 10 U short-acting soluble insulin *plus* 10 mmol KCl
- Run 500 ml every 4–6 hours via a controlled infusion pump
- Check blood glucose every 2–6 hours (depending on stability) and potassium 1–2 times daily
- On average, give 250 g glucose daily (1000 kcal) and 50 U insulin
- Adjust insulin and potassium according to results

Table 5.19 Risk factors in patients with renal failure undergoing surgery.

Cardiovascular
- Frequently have ischaemic heart disease
- Hypertension
- Left ventricular dysfunction

Respiratory
- Pulmonary oedema and fluid overload (impaired water clearance)

Gastrointestinal
- Delayed gastric emptying

Biochemical
- Electrolyte disturbance (especially hyperkalaemia)

Haematological
- Anaemia
- Impaired coagulation (platelet dysfunction)

Miscellaneous
- Malnutrition
- Multiple drug therapies
- Abnormal drug metabolism
- Vascular access

- Electrolyte imbalance, particularly hyperkalaemia is common. Frequent monitoring should be undertaken.
- Timing of dialysis. This should be decided after liaison with a nephrologist. Preoperative dialysis may be advised to optimize the patient for surgery.

Non-dialysis dependent patients

This group of patients have adequate renal function but have minimal functional reserve. They are at risk during the perioperative period of deteriorating renal function that renders them dialysis dependent. The risk of further deterioration in renal function can be reduced by:

- optimizing fluid balance directed by central venous pressure monitoring
- avoiding nephrotoxic drugs and radiological contrast agents
- treating sepsis aggressively
- protecting renal perfusion by avoiding hypotension.

The avoidance of renally excreted drugs that may accumulate is also important (e.g. morphine metabolites can build up causing oversedation and respiratory depression).

Jaundice

Preoperative diagnosis of the cause of jaundice is important because it will impact management. Pre-hepatic jaundice is usually due to haemolysis (e.g. massive transfusion and burns) or a defect in bilirubin conjugation (e.g. Gilbert's disease). Intrahepatic jaundice covers all of the abnormalities that may occur in the bilirubin conjugation process as well as its uptake by and secretion from the hepatocyte. Post-hepatic (surgical) jaundice is caused by posthepatic biliary obstruction. The risks of surgery in jaundiced patients relate to the following factors:

Hepatitis

The possibility of hepatitis B or C should be considered in patients with elevated aminotransferases or cirrhosis. Patients at increased risk of blood borne viruses such as hepatitis B and C include patients who have received multiple blood transfusions, intravenous drug abusers, those engaged in high risk sexual activity, as well as travel from an endemic area. Their viral status should be ascertained after appropriate consent in order to take appropriate measures to protect the healthcare staff.

Coagulopathy

Patients with obstructive jaundice and hepatocellular dysfunction are at risk of coagulopathy due to a lack of vitamin K and synthetic capacity. Adequate vitamin K depends on the presence of bile salts in the gut lumen for absorption. As a result, production of vitamin K dependent coagulation factors, II, VII, IX and X is reduced with a prolonged prothrombin time and a bleeding tendency. Clotting should be corrected preoperatively by the administration of vitamin K or fresh frozen plasma if urgent.

Acute renal failure

Acute renal failure commonly accompanies jaundice, and is referred to as the hepatorenal syndrome. Although the pathogenesis of renal failure in jaundice is not completely understood it is thought to be caused by sepsis complicating obstructive jaundice, the nephrotoxicity of conjugated bilirubin and dehydration. Prevention and treatment is with fluid loading using physiological crystalloids.

Cirrhosis

Cirrhotics have significantly increased perioperative morbidity and mortality which is related to the degree of hepatic decompensation and type of surgery. Non-alcoholic steatohepatitis is increasingly recognized, is associated with obesity and has been demonstrated to convey an excess risk for postoperative morbidity and mortality in patients undergoing major liver resection. A number of algorithms have been used to estimate postoperative mortality in this patient group including the Child–Turcotte–Pugh (CTP) score. This stratifies prothrombin time, albumin, the presence of ascites, encephalopathy and bilirubin to generate a score. CTP scores of A, B and C are associated with perioperative mortalities of 10, 30 and 80% for abdominal surgery. If the balance of risk favours surgery, hepatic function should be optimized. Postoperatively the patient will require intensive care monitoring.

Abnormal coagulation

Patients with abnormal coagulation fall into three categories.

Anticoagulant therapy

Patients receiving oral anticoagulants may require reversal of anticoagulation, bridging anticoagulation to cover the perioperative period and re-anticoagulation. Advice from a haematologist or cardiologist may be helpful. In general, warfarin should be stopped 4–5 days before surgery to achieve an INR < 2 for minor surgery and < 1.5 for major surgery. The risk of thromboembolism during the perioperative period without anticoagulation should be assessed (Table 5.20). Where the risk is high or medium, bridging anticoagulation with intravenous unfractionated heparin or low molecular weight heparin should be administered. Bridging anticoagulation is not required for patients at low risk of thromboembolism. Oral anticoagulation should be reintroduced as soon as the risk of haemorrhage has subsided and the patient is tolerating oral medication. Bridging anticoagulation should only be stopped once the INR is therapeutic.

Vitamin K can be used to reverse warfarin anticoagulation in patients requiring urgent surgery; it takes 24–48 hours to reverse anticoagulation. Where more rapid correction of coagulation is required, fresh frozen plasma and prothrombin complex concentrates are indicated. The use of prothrombin complex concentrates usually requires the approval of a haematologist. Protamine can be used to reverse the effects of heparin if urgent reversal is required (coagulation normalizes without treatment 4–6 hours after heparin cessation).

Inherited disorders of coagulation

The most common inherited disorder of coagulation is haemophilia A (factor VIII deficiency), followed by haemophilia B (factor IX deficiency) and Von Willebrand's Disease (Von Willebrand factor deficiency). These patients require factor infusions to achieve haemostatic levels at the time of surgery and throughout the immediate postoperative period until the risk of bleeding subsides. This should be organised in close collaboration with a haematologist.

Acquired coagulopathy

Acquired coagulopathy may herald the onset of disseminated intravascular coagulation (DIC) with associated thrombocytopenia. The triggers for DIC which leads include sepsis, malignancy, surgery, trauma, burns, anaphylaxis and blood transfusion reactions. DIC is characterized by microvascular coagulation, intense fibrinolysis, tissue ischaemia and the consumption of clotting factors and platelets. The diag-

Table 5.20 Risk stratification of conditions requiring consideration of continuous perioperative anticoagulation

High risk	Intermediate risk	Low risk
• Older mechanical mitral valve • Recently placed mechanical heart valve • Atrial fibrillation plus mechanical heart valve • Atrial fibrillation with history of thromboembolism • Recurrent arterial or idiopathic venous thromboembolic events • Venous or arterial thromboembolism in preceding 3 months • Hypercoagulable state	• Newer mitral mechanical valve • Older aortic mechanical valve • Cerebrovascular disease with multiple ischaemic episodes • Atrial fibrillation with risk factors for cardiac embolism • Venous thromboembolism > 3, < 6 months ago	• Atrial fibrillation without risk factors for thromboembolism • Remote venous embolism > 6 months ago • Cerebrovascular disease without recurrent ischaemic events • New model prosthetic aortic valve
Bridging anticoagulation required	**Bridging anticoagulation may be required**	**Bridging anticoagulation not required**

nosis is based on clinical and laboratory findings. The typical laboratory findings include thrombocytopenia, elevated prothrombin time (PT) and activated partial thromboplastin time (APTT), low fibrinogen, elevated fibrin and fibrinogen degradation products and D-dimers. Management is complex and centres around the treatment of the underlying cause; further treatment depends on whether bleeding or thrombosis predominate and should involve a haematologist.

Anaemia

The type and cause of anaemia should be ascertained, enabling preoperative correction where possible. Iron deficiency anaemia commonly encountered in surgical practice is usually as a result of gastrointestinal blood loss or menorrhagia. Where anaemic patients are scheduled for surgery with the potential for blood loss requiring transfusion, consideration should be given to blood-conserving surgical techniques such as cell salvage.

Musculoskeletal disease

Careful handling and positioning of the unconscious, anaesthetized patient is mandatory in order to avoid injury. Patients with deformity, rheumatoid arthritis and those with proven spinal instability or with a potentially unstable spine demand special attention. Atlanto-axial subluxation can result in an unstable cervical spine in rheumatoid patients leading to spinal cord damage if not protected. Plain cervical spine radiographs should be taken as a minimum requirement and the anaesthetist informed so that excessive neck movements during intubation can be avoided. The use of a neck collar can be used to highlight the potential danger to theatre staff.

Miscellaneous conditions

There are many other diseases with particular considerations in the perioperative period that are beyond the scope of this chapter for detailed discussion, Table 5.21 gives an overview of some of these.

ANAESTHESIA AND THE OPERATION

Prior to the induction of anaesthesia a preoperative check should be completed by the ward nursing and theatre staff, anaesthetist and surgeon. This is to guard against incorrect and wrong site surgery, prevent poor planning and adverse events.

Recent introduction of the World Health Organization (WHO) Surgical Safety Checklist has formalized this process. The preoperative check covers patient identity, proposed surgery and site (including marking), availability of clinical records, investigation results, consent and patient allergies, as well as equipment availability and anaesthetic concerns.

General anaesthesia

The aims of general anaesthesia are to produce a safe, reversible loss of consciousness, optimize the physiological response to surgery and provide good operating conditions. General anaesthesia has three components: loss of consciousness, analgesia, and muscle relaxation.

Local anaesthetic agents

Local anaesthetic agents such as lignocaine and bupivacaine exert their effect by causing a local, reversible blockade of nerve conduction by reducing nerve membrane sodium permeability. They are non-specific and act on autonomic, motor and sensory nerves equally. Their duration of action depends on the local anaesthetic agent used, dose, whether adrenaline has been co-administered and the proximity of local anaesthetic to the nerve.

Maximum local anaesthetic doses are shown in Table 5.22. A patient receiving large doses of local anaesthetic should be monitored with ECG, pulse oximetry and non-invasive blood pressure measurement. Local anaesthetic toxicity as a result of inadvertent injection into the blood stream or overdose may be heralded by perioral tingling and can result in arrhythmias and convulsions (Table 5.23). Intravascular

Table 5.22 Safe maximum doses of commonly used local anaesthetics

Drug	With adrenaline (epinephrine) (mg/kg)	Without adrenaline (epinephrine) (mg/kg)
Lidocaine	6	2
Bupivacaine	2	2
Prilocaine	Maximum 600 mg	

Table 5.23 Signs of local anaesthetic toxicity

Early
- Numbness/tingling of the tongue
- Perioral tingling
- Anxiety
- Lightheadedness
- Tinnitus

Late
- Loss of consciousness
- Convulsions
- Cardiovascular collapse
- Apnoea

Table 5.21 Relevance of some medical conditions in the perioperative period.

Condition	Considerations
Rheumatoid arthritis	Neck may be 'unstable', careful positioning necessary, complex drug therapy, associated chronic diseases, e.g. renal failure, lung disease
Multiple sclerosis	Reduced respiratory reserve; stress of surgery can cause relapse or worsening of disease
Epilepsy	Drugs may interact with anaesthetics; surgical stress and some drugs may precipitate seizures
Scoliosis or spondylitis	Can significantly reduce respiratory reserve; difficult endotracheal intubation
Myasthenia gravis	Risk of respiratory failure or aspiration; anaesthetic technique needs modifying
Sickle-cell anaemia	Stress of surgery, hypoxia, hypothermia can all precipitate sickle-cell crisis

injection should be avoided by aspirating on the needle prior to injection. Treatment of toxicity is supportive; the airway should be secured, ensuring adequate ventilation and the circulation supported with intravenous fluid and antiarrhythmics if necessary. Seizures should be controlled with small increments of intravenous benzodiazepines.

Local anaesthetics can be used to provide surgical anaesthesia and postoperative analgesia in a variety of techniques which are discussed in more detail below. Patients undergoing major surgery under regional anaesthesia should always be fasted as for a general anaesthetic in case sedation is required or conversion to general anaesthetic.

Spinal and epidural anaesthesia

Spinal anaesthesia

Spinal anaesthetic is defined by the introduction of local anaesthetic, usually lidocaine or bupivacaine into the subarachnoid space to block the spinal nerves before they exit the intervertebral foramina (Fig. 5.4). To protect against damage to the spinal cord, spinal anaesthesia is administered below L2, either at the L3/4 or L4/5 level. At this level, the cauda equina nerves acquire their perineural coverings and myelin sheath as they exit the dura making them exquisitely sensitive to the effect of local anaesthetic. As a result, 2–4 ml of local anaesthetic produces a dense block up to T6 level, with a rapid onset of action, giving 2–3 hours of surgical anaesthesia. The addition of 6–8% glucose increases the density of the spinal anaesthetic solution making it easier to control the level of the block using gravity. Aspiration of subarachnoid fluid confirms the correct site of the spinal needle.

Epidural anaesthesia

Both spinal and epidural anaesthesia block spinal cord sympathetic outflow. Rapid vasomotor paralysis with peripheral vasodilatation is an early sign of a successful spinal or epidural anaesthetic due to the rapid onset of blockade in these small unmyelinated fibres. Conversely, the resulting peripheral vasodilatation can be a nuisance with unwanted hypotension requiring treatment with intravenous fluids, vasoconstrictors, or reduction in the rate of the epidural infusion.

Epidural anaesthesia involves the injection of local anaesthetic into the epidural space which extends along the entire vertebral canal between the ligamentum flavum and dura mater (Fig. 5.5). Local anaesthetic spreads cranio-caudally penetrating the meningeal sheaths containing the nerve roots causing an anaesthetic block affecting several dermatomes. The level of epidural anaesthetic is therefore dictated by the proposed site of surgery and the dematomes involved. The nerve roots are fully covered and myelinated as they traverse the epidural space and therefore a larger volume (10–20 ml) of local anaesthetic, compared to spinal anaesthesia, is required to achieve anaesthesia. The technique by which a needle is introduced into the epidural space depends on sensing a loss of resistance as the needle passes through the ligamentum

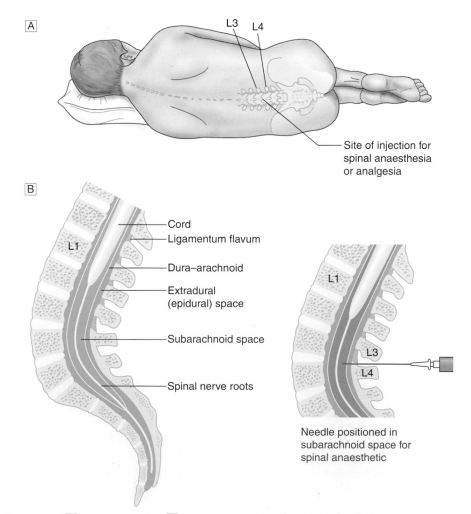

A

L3 L4

Site of injection for spinal anaesthesia or analgesia

B

Cord
Ligamentum flavum

L1

Dura–arachnoid

Extradural (epidural) space

Subarachnoid space

Spinal nerve roots

L1

L3
L4

Needle positioned in subarachnoid space for spinal anaesthetic

Fig. 5.4 Spinal anaesthesia. **A** Position of the patient. **B** The anatomy of the lumbar spine and position of the needle in the subarachnoid space as for spinal anaesthesia.

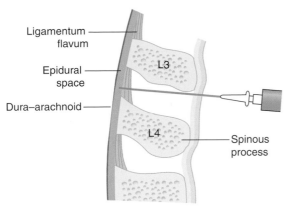

Fig. 5.5 Epidural anaesthesia.

flavum; aspiration ensures that the needle is not advanced too far into the subarachnoid space, termed a 'dural tap'. An ongoing CSF leak following a dural tap can lead to loss of CSF volume and headache. As well as adequate hydration, the CSF leak may be managed by the use of a blood patch. This involves using the patient's own blood injected into the epidural space to seal the leak. If a dural tap goes undetected with the injection of local anaesthetic into the subarachnoid space, a profound block of all spinal nerves will result, with the potential of respiratory arrest and profound hypotension. A catheter is often left in the epidural space to provide access for ongoing analgesia. Table 5.24 details some common complications of epidural anaesthesia. Both spinal and epidural anaesthesia block spinal cord sympathetic outflow. Rapid vasomotor paralysis with peripheral vasodilatation is an early sign of a successful spinal or epidural anaesthetic due to the rapid onset of blockade in these small unmyelinated fibres. Conversely, the resulting peripheral vasodilatation can be a nuisance with unwanted hypotension requiring treatment with intravenous fluids, vasoconstrictors, or reduction in the rate of the epidural infusion.

Peripheral nerve block

Peripheral nerve blockade requires a detailed working knowledge of the target nerve's surface anatomy, adjacent structures, as well as the cutaneous area supplied by it. Use of a nerve stimulator and insulated block needle can improve the accuracy of placement of the nerve block catheter. A list of commonly performed nerve blocks and their indications are detailed in Table 5.25.

Table 5.24 Complications of epidural anaesthesia and analgesia

Complication	Steps to avoid complication
Epidural abscess (0.015–0.05%)	Avoid if skin or systemic sepsis
Epidural haematoma (0.01%)	Correct coagulopathy, reverse anticoagulation and avoid in patients who have received recent heparin
Respiratory depression	Avoid high epidural block, (C3–5 innervate diaphragm)
Cardiac depression	Avoid mid-thoracic epidural, blocking cardiac sympathetic outflow. The loss of positive chrontropic and inotropic innervation results in cardiovascular instability and hypotension

Table 5.25 Commonly performed peripheral nerve blocks

Block	Indication
Axillary or supraclavicular	Upper limb surgery
Interscalene	Shoulder and upper limb
Femoral	Lower limb surgery
Sciatic	Lower limb surgery
Intercostal nerves	Thoracotomy, fractured ribs
Ilio-inguinal/ iliohypogastric	Inguinal hernia
Penile	Circumcision

Local infiltration

Local anaesthetics can be used to infiltrate the surgical field, either as the sole anaesthetic to allow minor surgery to be performed or as an adjunct to provide postoperative analgesia. Their effectiveness is impaired in inflamed or infected tissues due to increased pH and increased absorption due to vasodilatation and alternative anaesthetic techniques may be necessary. Local anaesthetics may be co-administered with adrenaline which prolongs their action by causing vasoconstriction resulting in decreased systemic absorption. Local anaesthetic with adrenaline should never be used at a site that has an end arterial supply i.e. digits or penis, as ischaemia and gangrene may ensue.

Topical anaesthesia

Due to the mucosal and to a lesser extent, cutaneous absorption of local anaesthetics, topical anaesthesia has a role in procedures involving the oral cavity, pharynx, larynx, urethra and conjunctiva. Cutaneous anaesthesia can also be achieved in children and needle-phobic adults prior to cannulation or venepuncture; tetracaine (Ametop) and prilocaine/lidocaine (Emla) creams are available for this purpose. Lignocaine is the most commonly used topical anaesthetic and is available as gel, ointment, cream or spray. The use of cocaine as a topical anaesthetic in otolaryngology has been largely phased out due to the intense sympathomimetic effect.

Postoperative analgesia

Good postoperative analgesia is essential in ensuring surgical success by minimizing psychological and physiological morbidity, enabling early mobilization and optimizing respiratory function. Despite this, approximately 20% of postoperative patients will have inadequate analgesia. Successful postoperative analgesia requires preoperative planning, taking into account the nature of the proposed surgery, patient factors and preferences and their comorbidity. Knowledge of pain physiology, assessment, analgesic drugs, including routes of delivery and pharmacology is essential. The pain pathway is illustrated in Figure 5.6. Many hospitals have acute pain teams involving doctors and specialist nurses to deliver improved patient analgesia.

Pain assessment

Adequate analgesia requires regular assessment of pain and the adequacy of analgesia. The patient's own subjective experience of pain should always be used. The method of pain assessment varies between institutions. Examples include non-linear scales such as no pain, mild, moderate or severe pain and linear scales where a pain score out of ten or a visual analogue scale (1–100 mm) is used.

5

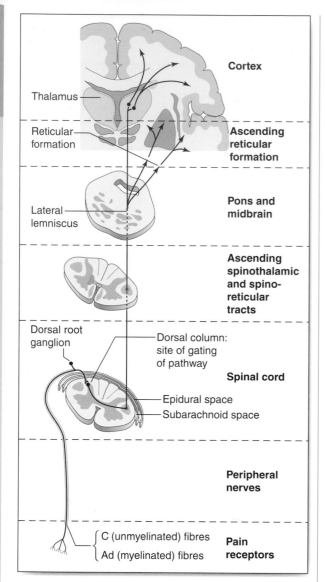

Fig. 5.6 The pain pathway.

Postoperative analgesic strategy

There is good evidence to guide postoperative analgesia. Multimodal analgesia, utilizing several analgesics that act at different parts of the pain pathway is more effective than the use of single agents and reduces the dose required of individual analgesics, minimizing side effects. Epidural analgesia and patient controlled parenteral opiate analgesia are commonly used for major surgery. Limb surgery lends itself to the use of postoperative peripheral nerve blocks. Subcutaneous or oral morphine regimens may be sufficient for less major surgery. In all cases paracetamol and non-steroidal anti-inflammatory drugs (NSAIDs), where appropriate, should be used alongside opiate analgesia. A step-down regimen should be in place to minimize the use of potent opioid analgesia as the requirement for them lessens as time elapses from surgery. Individual analgesic techniques are discussed below.

Epidural analgesia

Epidural analgesia is commonly achieved by a continuous infusion of local anaesthetic, usually in combination with an opiate, into the epidural space. A typical regimen of 0.1% bupivacaine with 2 mg/ml fentanyl running at a rate of up to 16 ml/hour is used for thoracic, abdominal and major lower limb surgery. Inserted prior to surgery, an epidural catheter can safely remain in place for up to five days. Pain relief is superior to parenteral opiates but careful patient monitoring in an appropriate environment by trained staff is needed. There is a rate of epidural failure due to misplacement, displacement, inadequate analgesia or intolerable side effects which should be managed with timely epidural replacement or substitution with another analgesic technique. In addition to the complications discussed above as per epidural anaesthesia, permanent neurological damage (0.005–0.05%) is a devastating but rare complication. Respiratory depression due to cephalad spread of opiates may also occur.

Patient-controlled analgesia (PCA)

Patient controlled analgesia (PCA) involves the use of a pre-programmed pump to deliver a small, pre-determined dose of drug, usually an opiate, with a minimum time period between doses (lock-out period). The lock-out period allows the patient to feel the effect of the opiate bolus before administering a subsequent dose, minimizing the amount of opiate consumed and the risk of respiratory depression which occurs in up to 11.5% of patients. A typical regimen would involve 1 mg morphine at 5-minute intervals, although this may vary according to patient size, age and history of opiate exposure. Background opiate infusions are not routine due to the increased risk of respiratory depression but may be useful in chronic opioid users. Similar to epidurals, PCA requires expensive pumps and to be successful, the patient must understand how it works and have the manual dexterity to use the pump. Care must be taken in correct pump programming and in delivering the correct concentration of opiates as deaths from respiratory depression have been reported.

Parenteral and oral opioid regimens

Strong opioids

Examples of strong opioids include buprenorphine, fentanyl, oxycodone and pethidine as well as morphine. In the absence of evidence of superiority of one strong opioid over another, morphine is the most commonly used, particularly in the postoperative period. Strong opioids, either oral or parenteral, are used as the primary analgesia for more minor surgery and on stepping down from an epidural or PCA in order to avoid an analgesic gap. Typical regimens of 10 mg morphine, either subcutaneously or orally, as required at one hour intervals are used although the dose should take the age, size and history of opiate use into account. Typical opioid side effects include respiratory depression, dysphoria, constipation, nausea and vomiting, pruritis, urinary retention and depressed conscious level. Opioids can be reversed with naloxone, an opioid antagonist.

Weak opioids

Examples of weak opioids, useful in the management of mild pain, include codeine, dihydrocodeine and tramadol. Codeine and dihydrocodeine are also available in preparation with paracetamol as cocodamol and codydramol respectively. Dihydrocodeine is not an effective analgesic, being equivalent to placebo in 30 mg dose and inferior to ibuprofen at 60 mg dose. In addition to being an opioid agonist, tramadol inhibits serotonin and noradrenaline re-uptake and is effective in neuropathic pain as well as in the acute pain setting.

Paracetamol, NSAIDs and selective Cox-2 inhibitors

Paracetamol is effective in the management of postoperative pain and can be administered by the oral, intravenous and rectal routes. Regular use has been shown to reduce opioid requirements by 20–30% and in combination with NSAIDs, the combination is more effective than NSAIDs alone. Paracetamol should therefore be prescribed to all postoperative patients except in the rare instance of contraindications.

NSAIDs are also an important component of multimodal postoperative analgesia. In combination with opioids, NSAIDs increase analgesia and have an opioid sparing effect, reducing consumption, postoperative nausea and vomiting and sedation. Their use is limited by their side effect profile, including renal impairment, impaired platelet function with the potential for increased postoperative bleeding, peptic ulceration and bronchospasm in individuals at risk. Asthma is not an absolute contraindication and previous use without adverse effects permits their use.

Selective cyclo-oxygenase (COX)-2 inhibitors such as celecoxib, parecoxib and etoricoxib are as effective as NSAIDs in the management of postoperative pain and have an opioid sparing effect. Their potential advantage is an improved side effect profile compared with NSAIDs, with no impairment of platelet function, reduced gastrointestinal complications and no associated bronchospasm. The use of COX-2 inhibitors is limited by their association with a small increased risk of thrombotic events (myocardial infarction and stroke) and therefore they should not be used except where NSAIDs are contraindicated and after assessing cardiovascular risk. COX-2 inhibitors are contraindicated in ischaemic heart disease, cerebrovascular and peripheral arterial disease and moderate to severe cardiac failure. They should also be used with caution in patients with risk factors for these conditions.

Neuropathic pain

Acute neuropathic pain in the postoperative period occurs in at least 1–3% of patients and is probably underestimated. It is a risk factor for chronic neuropathic pain which may be reduced by early intervention. Expert advice should be sought to advise on the management as neuropathic pain does not respond well to conventional analgesia regimes. Because it does not respond well to conventional analgesic regimes expert advice should be sought. There is evidence that intravenous lidocaine infusions and gabapentin reduce pain and

reduce opioid requirements. Tricyclic antidepressants are also used on the basis that they are effective in chronic neuropathic pain although their efficacy in reducing acute neuropathic pain has not been proven.

SUMMARY BOX 5.7

Postoperative pain control

Parenteral analgesia
- Epidural analgesia
- Patient controlled analgesia (PCA)
- Opiates (morphine/pethidine), paracetamol

Oral analgesia
- Paracetamol
- Non-steroidal anti-inflammatory drugs
- Weak opiates (tramadol, codeine)
- Strong opiates (morphine)

Neuropathic pain
- Tri-cyclic antidepressants
- Gabapentin
- Lidocaine.

Postoperative nausea and vomiting

Postoperative nausea and vomiting (PONV) is common affecting 20–30% of patients for whom it is very distressing. It is also a significant factor in causing delayed discharge from day case surgical units. Certain risk factors for PONV have been identified, these include female sex, type of surgery (e.g. gynaecological and laparoscopic surgery), being a non-smoker, a history of previous PONV or motion sickness and opioid use. Anaesthetic technique is also important as, inhalational anaesthetic agents, especially nitrous oxide are associated with PONV whereas intravenous anaesthesia with propofol has a lower incidence. Management of PONV centres on identifying high risk patients and instituting preventative measures. Ondansetron and dexamethasone are particularly effective in the prophylaxis and treatment of PONV.

5

M.A. Potter

Principles of the surgical management of cancer

THE BIOLOGY OF CANCER

A neoplasm or new growth consists of a mass of transformed cells that does not respond in a normal way to growth regulatory systems. These transformed cells serve no useful function and proliferate in an atypical and uncontrolled way to form a benign or malignant neoplasm. In normal tissues, cell replication and death are equally balanced and under tight regulatory control. However, when a cancer arises, this is generally due to genomic abnormalities that either increase cell replication or inhibit cell death (Fig. 6.1). The mechanisms by which this abnormal growth activity is induced (carcinogenesis) are complex and can be influenced in many ways: for example, inherited genetic make-up, residential environment, exposure to ionizing radiation or carcinogens, viral infection, diet, lifestyle and hormonal imbalances. These cellular insults give rise to alterations in the genomic DNA (mutations) and it is these mutations that lead to cancer. Mutations can lead to disruption of the cell replication cycle at any point and lead to either activation or over-expression of oncogenes, or the inactivation of tumour suppressor genes, or a combination of the two (Table 6.1). Defining which genes have been mutated in the primary and metastatic cancers may ultimately help predict prognosis. For example the amplification and over expression of *C-erbB-2* oncogene can give an indication of the aggressiveness of breast cancer. Scientists have now been able to sequence the entire human genome. This will allow identification of new genes and hence proteins involved in the formation of cancer that will eventually lead to a greater understanding of the development of cancer, and new treatments.

Changes within the cellular genome occur frequently and do not necessarily result in cancer. Natural protective mechanisms repair errors in DNA replication; similarly, immune surveillance, simple wastage (i.e. loss of cells from the surface) and programmed cell death (apoptosis) destroy mutant cells before they proliferate. For persistence of growth and hence cancer formation, these protective mechanisms must break down (e.g. failure of mismatch repair due to mutations in genes such as *MLHI* and *MSH2*,

or failure of apoptosis). The host's internal environment may also have a role in the 'promotion' of tumour growth. Good examples are the 'hormone-dependent' cancers of the breast, prostate and endometrium, which require a 'correct' balance of hormonal secretion from the endocrine glands of the host for their continued growth. The natural history of a tumour is also related to its growth rate, which in turn is determined by the balance between cell division and cell death. Some tumours are slow-growing (e.g. prostate) and years may pass before deposits reach a size that threatens normal organ function. Others grow rapidly as a result of a high rate of cell proliferation, and some expand rapidly (despite a relatively normal rate of cell proliferation) if cell death is slow to occur.

 SUMMARY BOX **6.1**

Factors leading to loss of cell cycle regulation

Growth of a cancer is due to loss of cell cycle regulation, which is dependent on:
- Increased cell proliferation
- Decreased programmed cell death (apoptosis)
- A combination of the two.

The adenoma–carcinoma progression

Neoplasms may be benign or malignant; the essential difference is the capacity to invade and metastasize. The cells of benign tumours do not invade surrounding tissues but remain as a local conglomerate. Malignant tumours are invasive and their cells can directly invade adjacent tissues or enter blood and lymphatic channels, to be deposited at remote sites. This malignant genotype develops as a result of the progressive acquisition of cancer mutations (by point mutation, chromosomal loss or translocation). This progressive accumulation of mutations may lead to the formation of cancer stem cells. In a similar manner to

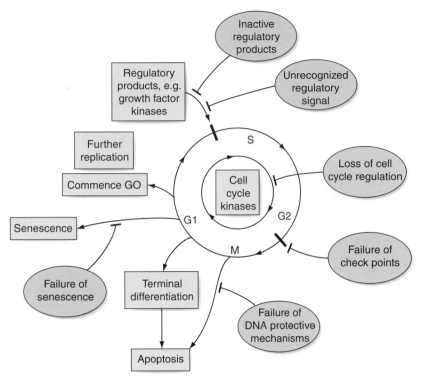

Fig. 6.1 Cell replication and cancer formation. Normal cell replication is under tight regulation by endogenous growth factors (green boxes). Mutations that result in abnormal growth factor proteins can lead to cancer formation (yellow elipses).

Table 6.1 Examples of gene mutations that can lead to cancer formation

Gene	Point of action in cell cycle
p16, CDK4, Rb	Cell cycle check point
MSH2, MLH1	DNA replication and repair
p53, fas	Apoptosis
E cadherin	Cellular adhesion
erb-A	Cellular differentiation
Ki-ras, erb-B	Regulatory kinases
TGF-β	Growth factors

other stem cells these cancer stem cells are pleuripotent (i.e. have the ability to give rise to more than one cell type). It is proposed they produce cells that form the epithelial, structural, and vascular components needed for cancer formation. However the cells arising from a cancer stem cell lack the normal response to the normal cell cycle controls and are, therefore, tumour forming. Such cancer stem cells could explain why cancers can relapse or metastasize. The acquisition of the malignant phenotype can be recognized histologically as a tumour develops from a benign adenoma through to a dysplastic lesion, and finally into an invasive carcinoma (Fig. 6.2). The concept of tumour progression from a benign to malignant phenotype provides the rationale behind screening and early detection programmes; i.e. if benign or pre-invasive lesions are removed, this will prevent invasive disease.

Invasion and metastasis

Benign tumours rarely threaten life but may cause a variety of cosmetic or functional abnormalities. In contrast, malignant tumours invade and relentlessly replace normal tissues, destroying supporting structures and disturbing function; they can spread to distant tissues (metastasize), eventually causing death. Metastases are cancer deposits similar in cell type to the original cancer found at remote (secondary) sites in the body.

The process of invasion and metastasis is complex (Fig. 6.3) and is dependent on the biology of the tumour. For metastases to occur it would appear that further mutations need to occur in the cancer cells. These extra mutations can be called the metastatic signature. Some tumours metastasize earlier in their clinical course than others. This variation may depend on the tissue of origin of the primary tumour, but can also vary widely according to the phenotype of individual tumours. For example, cancer of the breast is thought to metastasize early, and micrometastases are often present but not detectable when the patient first presents. Some patients with apparently localized colorectal cancer are cured by radical surgery, but others receiving the same treatment deteriorate rapidly with metastatic disease.

The mechanisms that control invasion and metastasis are obscure (Fig. 6.4). Local pressure effects from the expanding tumour and the increased motility of tumour cells may play a role in local invasion. Malignant cells secrete a number of factors that may determine their biological behaviour and promote growth at both primary and metastatic sites. The matrix metalloproteinases (MMPs) are endoproteinases with enzymatic activity directed against components of the extracellular matrix. Their action facilitates tumour cell invasion and metastasis by degrading extracellular collagens, laminins and proteoglycans. Other proteases, such as urokinase, plasminogen-activating factor and the cathepsins, are also involved in metastasis formation. Clumps of cancer cells can then embolize to distant tissues and form metastases. The location for the development of metastases could be a simple mechanical property with organs that have fine capillary beds, such as liver and lung, trapping circulating malignant cells which then develop into metastases. The

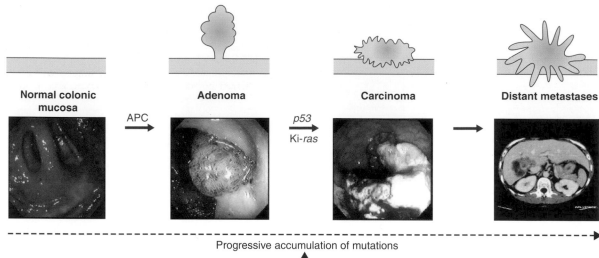

Fig. 6.2 Colorectal adenoma-carcinoma progression. By the progressive acquisition of genetic mutations, normal colorectal epithelium forms a benign polyp, which can progress to an invasive or metastatic cancer.

survival of metastatic deposits depends on angiogenesis, which is mediated by an imbalance between positive and negative regulatory molecules released by the tumour cells and surrounding normal cells. Negative factors, such as angiostatin or endostatin, will inhibit new vessel formation. Positive factors, such as vascular endothelial growth factors or fibroblast growth factors, will enhance metastasis. Cancer cells also secrete prostaglandins, which can induce osteolysis and may promote the development of skeletal deposits.

Natural history and estimate of cure

Calculations based on an exponential model of tumour growth suggest that three-quarters of the lifespan of a tumour is spent in a 'pre-clinical' or occult stage, and that the clinical manifestations of the disease are limited to the final quarter. For cure, every malignant cell must be eradicated. There

should be no recurrent tumour during the patient's lifetime, or evidence of residual tumour at death. This rigid definition of cure is rarely attainable. Instead, a normal duration of life without further clinical evidence of disease is generally accepted as evidence of cure, even though microscopic deposits of tumour may still be present.

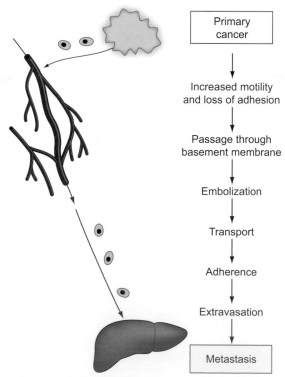

Fig. 6.3 Invasion and metastasis. Cancers invade adjacent tissues by direct infiltration. Spread to distant sites (metastasis) is via the bloodstream or lymphatics, or across body cavities (transcoelomic spread). Following initial growth, cancer cells lose local adherence and invade blood vessels. They are then transported via the bloodstream to adhere in distant organs and grow into secondary tumours.

Fig. 6.4 Metastasis. Following initial growth, cancer cells lose local adherence and invade blood vessels. They are then transported via the bloodstream to adhere in distant organs and grow into secondary tumours.

Measuring and comparing the outcome(s) of cancer treatment can be a difficult exercise. Cancer survival data is not normally distributed but skewed with many events happening early in the study period. Survival data is generally expressed as a time from a predefined starting point (e.g. time of surgery) to a similarly defined end point (e.g. disease relapse). Other time points may also be used and so a careful and precise definition of the time period used is essential. In addition, not all patients will have experienced the defined end point by the end of the study period. This phenomenon is known as censoring and mean survival time will be unknown for a subset of the study group. Other confounding factors such as age and the stage of disease also need to be considered. Hence special methods of data interpretation are required. These various statistical methods of cancer data interpretation and comparison are termed survival analysis.

Measures used in survival analysis include, survival and hazard probabilities, Kaplan–Meier equations and graphs (Fig 6.5), Cox's proportional hazard models, univariate and multivariate analysis. Survival is the probability that a subject survives from the starting point to the end point of the study period. Hazard is the probability that the subject has a specified event at one particular moment in time. 'Cure' rates of individual cancers are assessed by survival rates at various times after treatment. Conventionally, 5- and 10-year intervals are used. Cure rates vary according to the aggressiveness of the disease and the success of treatment. In some patients with cancer (e.g. stomach and lung), metastases grow rapidly and cause death within a few years of clinical presentation. In others (e.g. cancer of the breast and melanoma), many years may elapse before metastatic spread becomes evident and, even when metastases have occurred, life may be long. It is for this reason that 5-year survival rates cannot provide a satisfactory estimate of cure for all tumours.

THE MANAGEMENT OF PATIENTS WITH CANCER

The goals of treating cancer can be broadly grouped as follows: prevention, cure and palliation. Prevention seeks to modify behaviour to prevent cancer formation. For example, the avoidance of smoking or direct sunlight may prevent the formation of lung or skin cancer. Taking a small dose of aspirin on a regular basis may protect against colorectal cancer (chemoprevention). When a cancer has formed, treatment is aimed at cure for early-stage disease. When a cancer is locally advanced or has metastasized, the chance of cure reduces. In cancers that are felt to be incurable, treatment is then aimed at palliation of troublesome symptoms.

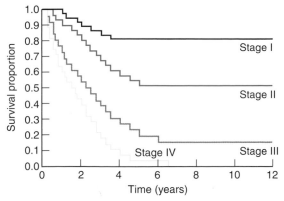

Fig. 6.5 Kaplan–Meier survival curve.

Screening

If cancer can be detected before it causes symptoms, then it is generally smaller, has less chance of having metastasized and is therefore more amenable to cure. Detecting benign lesions with malignant potential, pre-invasive cancer, and invasive malignancy before it becomes symptomatic is called screening (Fig. 6.6). Screening is expensive and its effectiveness in relation to cost must be critically evaluated before routine use (EBM 6.1). Screening is most effective when targeted at specific risk groups and when the screening test has a high level of acceptability to the target population. For successful screening, the test used must be able to detect the cancer at a stage when earlier treatment will lead to fewer deaths from the cancer. In any given population, the likelihood of a cancer being present is generally low (< 1%); hence, the test must be sensitive in order to detect these relatively rare lesions. The test must also be specific (i.e. have a low false-positive rate); otherwise, individuals will undergo unnecessary investigation or even inappropriate treatment. Finally, the proposed treatment of a cancer patient detected by a screening programme must be effective. In the UK, cervical cytology is offered to women on a 3-yearly basis until the age of 60, and mammographic screening (Fig. 6.7) is offered to women between 50 and 64 years on a 3-yearly basis. Other tumour types that might be amenable to screening are listed with their relevant screening tests in Table 6.2.

Screening for inherited cancer

Some forms of cancer can be inherited; for example, about 5% of patients with colorectal cancer develop the disease because of an autosomal dominant inherited mutation either in the *APC* gene (polyposis coli) or in the mismatch repair genes such as *MSH2* and *MLH1* (hereditary non-polyposis

---

EBM 6.1 **Recent screening trials**

'Studies in Sweden in the late 1980s established that screening for breast cancer allowed for early detection and improved cancer-specific survival. Recent studies have shown that these benefits can be achieved in the context of national screening programmes and for other cancers such as colorectal cancer.'

Blanks RG, et al. Br Med J 2000; 321:665–669.
Further reading on the breast cancer screening debate: US Preventative Services Task Force. Ann Intern Med 2009;151:716-726 and related articles pp 727 and 738.

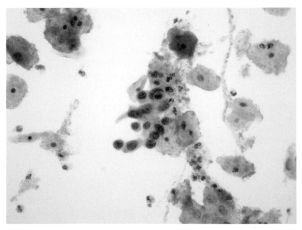

Fig. 6.6 Cervical cytology. A group of severely dyskaryotic squamous cells in a ThinPrep liquid-based cytology preparation (Courtesy of Dr A.R.W. Williams, Senior Lecturer/Honorary Consultant in Pathology, University of Edinburgh).

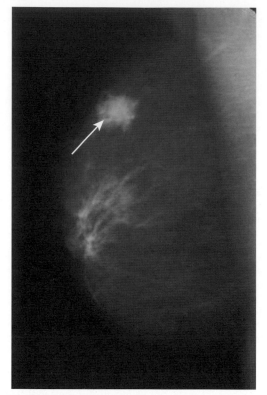

Fig. 6.7 Single mammogram showing malignancy (arrow) in peripheral breast tissue. (Courtesy of Mr M. Barber, Consultant Breast Surgeon, Western General Hospital, Edinburgh).

Table 6.2 Examples of cancer types that are or could be the subject of screening programmes

Cancer	Screening test
Breast	Mammography
Cervix	Smear cytology
Colon	Faecal occult blood test and flexible sigmoidoscopy Colonoscopy
Prostate	Prostate-specific antigen (PSA)

colorectal cancer, or HNPCC). Alternatively, about 5% of women develop breast cancer as a result of an autosomal dominant inherited mutation on the *BRCA1* or *BRCA2* genes. In these instances, closely related family members should be offered the appropriate tests to detect these specific mutations. Carriers of the mutation can then be offered prophylactic surgery, e.g. bilateral mastectomy (for *BRCA1* and *BRCA2* carriers) or restorative proctocolectomy (for *APC* carriers) in an attempt to eliminate subsequent cancer development.

 SUMMARY BOX 6.2

Criteria for screening programmes (http://www. screening.nhs.uk/screening)

A test for use in cancer screening must:
- Be sensitive
- Be specific
- Be acceptable
- Detect cancer at a stage when early treatment is beneficial
- Be cost-effective.

The cancer patient's journey

The management of cancer frequently involves surgery, be it radical for cure or palliative to relieve distressing symptoms. Because of the complexity of modern cancer management, cancer services in a hospital are currently organized around a multidisciplinary team approach. The team commonly includes surgeons, oncologists (radiotherapy/ chemotherapy), radiologists, pathologists and clinical nurse specialists (Table 6.3).

Good communication with the patient and between team members forms the basis of optimal patient care. There are several key stages in the management of the patient with cancer, which can be regarded as a journey from the onset of symptoms to definitive treatment and subsequent follow-up (Fig. 6.8). The exact sequence of events may differ from one patient to the next. For example, it may be necessary to remove the tumour to obtain full information on staging before an adequate treatment plan can be evolved. Patients usually begin their 'cancer journey' by deciding that a symptom or symptoms they have developed are serious enough to merit consultation with their GP. These symptoms may be a result of local or systemic effects of the cancer.

Symptoms that may initiate a patient's 'cancer journey'

Local effects

A tumour that lies on the surface of the body may become visible, change in shape or pigmentation, bleed, or discharge mucus or pus. A hollow viscus or duct may be obstructed by a tumour, e.g. a bronchus (causing pulmonary collapse), a segment of bowel (causing intestinal obstruction) or the bile duct or pancreatic duct (causing jaundice, or pancreatitis). A tumour within a closed space may cause pressure symptoms. For example, increased intracranial pressure may complicate intracerebral tumours, and paraplegia may arise from a spinal cord tumour. Invasion of an organ by a tumour may compromise its normal functions and cause organ failure. Invasion of tissues such as the pancreas, bone

Table 6.3 Multidisciplinary team involved in cancer care

Medical staff
- Surgeon
- Physician
- Radiologist
- Oncologist
- Radiotherapist
- Palliative care physician
- General practitioner

Nursing staff
- Ward nurse
- Chemotherapy nurse
- Clinical nurse specialist
- Hospice nurse

Paramedical staff
- Oncology dietitian
- Physiotherapist
- Occupational therapist
- Clergy

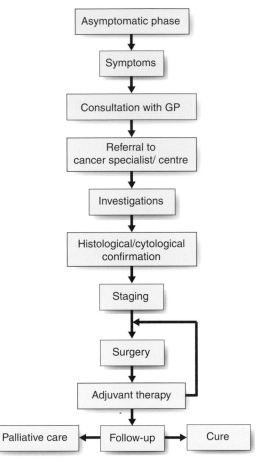

Fig. 6.8 The patient's cancer journey. During the patient's management, several key stages are encountered, from symptoms to diagnosis and treatment.

or nerves can cause severe pain. A cancer can also mimic the pain of benign disease: for example, dyspeptic symptoms in stomach cancer.

Systemic effects

Weight loss is often the key symptom that alerts both patients and their doctor to the possibility of malignant disease. A proportion of patients become so emaciated that they appear to die of starvation. This syndrome is known as cancer cachexia, and is clinically characterized by anorexia, severe weight loss, lethargy, anaemia and oedema.

The secretory products of some tumours can produce characteristic clinical syndromes. These products may be appropriate to the organ of origin. Thus, a tumour of the adrenal cortex may secrete excess corticosteroid and cause Cushing's syndrome; a parathyroid tumour may secrete excess parathormone and cause hypercalcaemia; and an islet cell tumour of the pancreas may secrete excess insulin and cause hypoglycaemia. On the other hand, secretory products may be inappropriate to the site of a tumour. Such 'ectopic' secretion occurs predominantly in tumours of neuroendocrine origin, and produces a variety of endocrine syndromes.

Consultation with the GP

Distressing or dramatic presenting symptoms such as rectal bleeding quite rightly produce a prompt referral from the GP to a hospital specialist. Frequently, however, the initial

presenting complaint of a patient with cancer is nonspecific, e.g. general malaise. Other symptoms, such as epigastric pain, are common complaints encountered by the GP and are usually associated with benign disease. These symptoms are more challenging to the GP and it can be difficult to decide which patient needs an urgent referral and which does not. Cancer patients presenting with such nonspecific symptoms may consult their GP on more than one occasion. Persistence of such nonspecific symptoms should raise the index of suspicion towards neoplastic disease and lead to specialist referral.

> ### SUMMARY BOX 6.3
>
> **Symptoms that should initiate investigation**
>
> - Weight loss
> - Rectal bleeding/melaena
> - Haemoptysis/persistent cough
> - Haematuria
> - Breast lump
> - Dysphagia/dyspepsia
> - Persistent headache
> - Persistent non-specific symptoms.

Referral to a specialist/cancer centre

Patients with a suspected diagnosis of cancer are often referred to the surgical outpatient clinic appropriate to the probable site of origin of the tumour. At the initial consultation, it is important to spend time taking a full and detailed history and examination. It is also important to spend time addressing any patient anxieties and in providing the patient with a clear view of any investigations that are planned. It is here that other members of the multidisciplinary team, such as the clinical nurse specialist, can help enormously. Increasingly, 'one-stop' clinics are being provided, allowing the initial consultation and investigations to be performed at one clinic attendance. This approach is particularly suited to the diagnosis of breast cancer.

Investigations

Investigations serve two main purposes. First, they are aimed at histological or cytological confirmation of the diagnosis of cancer. Second, they are used to assess the extent of the primary disease (local invasion) and to look for evidence of metastatic spread. This is known as 'staging' the disease.

Diagnostic investigations

Initial investigations to make the diagnosis should proceed in a logical order, starting with simple blood tests (e.g. tumour markers) and progressing through more complex imaging investigations, with the ultimate aim of obtaining histological or cytological confirmation of the diagnosis (Table 6.4). Plain radiology may demonstrate a soft tissue tumour, e.g. tumours of the lung or bone, but for tumours of the stomach or intestine, contrast studies are necessary. For some deep-seated tumours, e.g. those of the pancreas or brain, other methods of imaging are needed. These include angiography, radioactive scintigraphy and ultrasonography (US), CT (Fig. 6.9), MRI and positron emission

Table 6.4 Investigations for the diagnosis of cancer

Blood tests
- *Haematology* FBC
- *Biochemistry* LFTs, tumour markers

Radiology
- Plain X-rays, CXR
- Contrast-enhanced, barium enema
- Ultrasound, including endoscopic ultrasound
- CT
- CT PET
- MRI

Endoscopy
- Upper GI endoscopy
- Colonoscopy
- Endoscopic retrograde cholangiopancreatography (ERCP)

Cytology/histology
- Body fluids, e.g. sputum and urine
- Fine-needle aspiration (FNA), e.g. breast and thyroid cancer
- Radiologically guided FNA
- Endoscopic brushings or biopsy

Operative
- Examination under anaesthetic and biopsy
- Excision biopsy, e.g. lymph node
- Diagnostic laparoscopy and biopsy
- Laparoscopic ultrasound

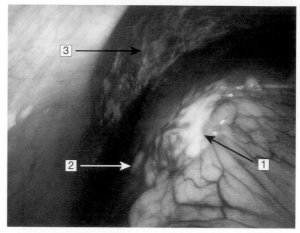

Fig. 6.10 Diagnostic laparoscopy showing primary gallbladder cancer invading the omentum (1), a liver metastasis (2) and peritoneal metastases (3).

Staging investigations

Staging investigations will depend on the site of the primary cancer and the relevant common sites of metastasis. Local invasion can be assessed – for example, in oesophageal cancer – by endoscopic ultrasound. CT or MRI scans can also be usefully employed to assess local invasion. Metastatic spread can be determined by a variety of investigations, e.g. bone scans, CT, PET scan and laparoscopy. When combined with CT, PET can be a particularly powerful way to detect metastatic disease (Fig. 6.11). Often, staging investigations will have been undertaken as part of the diagnostic process, e.g. CT scans.

The aim of staging is to define the extent of the disease, assess its likely prognosis, and permit the development of an appropriate treatment plan by the multidisciplinary team. Preoperative staging techniques continue to improve and provide evermore information. The use of MRI scanning for example in the treatment of rectal cancer allows for meticulous planning of preoperative treatment. This allows careful selection of patients for preoperative radiotherapy and can minimize the associated co-morbidity. The International Union against Cancer (Union Internationale Contre le Cancer, or UICC) has described a system of staging (TNM) in which three components are assessed. These are the extent of the primary tumour (T), the presence and

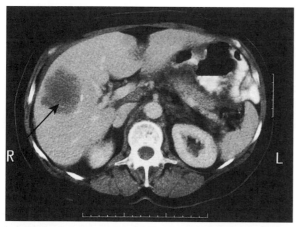

Fig. 6.9 Staging CT of the abdomen showing a large solitary liver metastasis (arrow) in a patient with colorectal cancer.

tomography (PET). Neoplastic disease can be confirmed cytologically, e.g. by the demonstration of malignant cells in secretions, in washings from hollow viscera, or in needle aspirates. Biopsies obtained at either upper or lower gastrointestinal endoscopy can provide material for histology, as can ultrasound or CT-guided Tru-cut needle biopsies. In some instances, it may be necessary to perform an examination under anaesthetic or diagnostic laparoscopy (Fig. 6.10) to obtain suitable diagnostic material. In general, a treatment plan for the management of a patient cannot be formulated until a histological or cytological diagnosis has been made. However, there are circumstances in which this is not possible (e.g. in certain patients with pancreatic cancer), and then clear radiological evidence may be used instead.

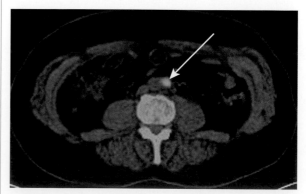

Fig. 6.11 CT/PET scan highlighting metastatic para aortic lymph node (arrow). Fused CT/PET image clearly showing metastatic node (courtesy of Dr J Brush, Consultant Radiologist, Western General Hospital, Edinburgh).

extent of metastases in regional lymph nodes (N), and the presence of distant metastases (M). The addition of numbers to each component indicates the extent of the disease within that category. The bigger the number, the more advanced the disease.

In the initial TNM system, only clinical, radiological and endoscopic investigations were used. Such clinical staging is still important in defining the extent of disease and may be used to plan the initial management of a patient. However, without histological confirmation, such clinical staging can sometimes be highly inaccurate. For example, the palpability of regional lymph nodes is a poor indicator of their involvement by tumour. Impalpable nodes may still contain metastases, whereas palpable nodes may be the seat of reactive hyperplasia (sinus histiocytosis) rather than tumour. Small deposits of tumour in viscera and bones cannot be detected by routine radiology, and thus many patients who on clinical and radiological grounds appear to have localized disease have in fact unrecognized widespread microscopic tumour deposits. For this reason, the TNM system has now been modified to include not only a pre-treatment clinical classification, but also a post-surgical pathological classification, denoted as pTNM. Excision of regional lymph nodes is one way to provide such information. In some melanomas and skin tumours, and in cancer of the bladder and large bowel, histological assessment of the depth of tumour penetration provides important information about the extent and prognosis of the disease. It must be recognized that all staging has its limitations and that microscopic tumour deposits may not be detected, particularly in terms of distant metastases. These staging systems are therefore used to provide a 'best-guess' scenario upon which to base the patient's treatment.

Prognosis is also affected by the biological characteristics of a tumour. For example, its degree of nuclear and cellular atypia and the extent of lymphocytic infiltration, inflammatory response, and perineural and vascular invasion all influence outcome. These factors, as well as biochemical indices (e.g. oestrogen receptor status in breast cancer), can all be used in the planning of a patient's treatment.

 SUMMARY BOX 6.4

Purpose of staging

- Define the extent of disease
- Assess likely prognosis
- Allow the development of a treatment plan.

Treatment

Following the initial diagnosis and staging, the patient may be discussed by the multidisciplinary team or may proceed to surgery, where the primary tumour, surrounding tissue and locoregional lymph nodes are excised and then sent for histopathology. Thus, the clinical staging is translated into histopathological staging; the multidisciplinary team can then discuss further aspects of management with the maximum amount of information available. The greater use of more sensitive staging investigations, the ongoing progress in chemotherapy agents and regimens and improvements in surgical techniques mean that treatment can be offered to patients with more advanced disease with increasing improvement in survival.

Benign tumours

Provided sufficient surrounding tissue is excised to ensure its complete removal, a benign tumour is cured by local excision. Some benign tumours, e.g. pleomorphic adenomas of the parotid, extend beyond their apparent macroscopic limits. Removal of the involved segment of the gland or organ is then the only sure way to cure.

Malignant tumours

A radical cancer operation implies complete removal of the tissue bearing the tumour, together with a margin of unaffected surrounding tissue. In some tumours, there is sequential spread, first locally, then to lymph nodes, and then to distant organs such as the liver and lungs. In this situation, careful local removal, along with the locoregional lymph nodes (known as 'en bloc resection'), can be curative. Often, however, the spread of a tumour may be more unpredictable and in essence the removal of local lymph nodes is simply to provide information for the stage of the cancer, rather than being of true therapeutic benefit. The management of regional lymph nodes thus depends on the site and type of the tumour. With some tumours, e.g. those of the gastrointestinal tract, regional lymph nodes are routinely resected on the basis that sequential spread may have occurred. In other tumours (e.g. breast cancer), lymph node sampling or sentinel node biopsy may be more appropriate, especially if en bloc lymph node resection may be associated with significant morbidity: for example, limb lymphoedema.

Complete radical excision, which is confirmed by histological examination with no evidence of lymph node metastasis, carries a high chance of surgical cure. A good example is the regional lymphadenectomy performed for colon cancer (Fig. 6.12). During any operation for cancer, care is taken to try to avoid the spillage of malignant cells which may cause cancer recurrence. In some sites (e.g. testis), it is usual to ligate the main vessels draining the area before the tumour is mobilized, so that further malignant cells are not shed into the circulation. Overall, a careful and meticulous approach to all aspects of the operation is vital. Attention to each detail improves the outcome of surgery.

There are data to suggest that surgery performed in specialist centres where surgeons are regularly performing radical operations produces better survival rates than surgery in non-specialist centres. Hence, surgeons are increasingly sub-specialized and concentrate on performing selected operations (EBM 6.2). One of the recent advances in surgical techniques is minimally invasive surgery. Using minimally invasive surgery the trauma related to surgery can be significantly reduced which can enhance the postoperative recovery. These techniques are being increasingly employed in the treatment of cancer. Early results suggested there might be an increase in metastases to the surgical wounds using these techniques, however, it is now recognised that minimally invasive surgical techniques can be used in the treatment of patients with cancer with no detriment to their outcome (EBM 6.3).

Adjuvant treatment

As mentioned previously, the most accurate staging of a patient with cancer is generally available after pathological evaluation of the resected specimen. Once this information is available, the patient can be discussed by the multidisciplinary team with a view to the need for further therapy.

Clearly, it is sometimes not possible to remove all the local disease. Moreover, early systemic dissemination may have occurred. Thus, an adjuvant to surgery is needed to provide both local and systemic control. For example, adjuvant

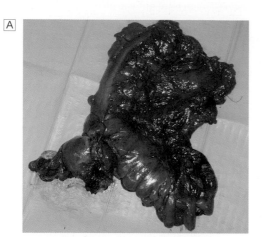

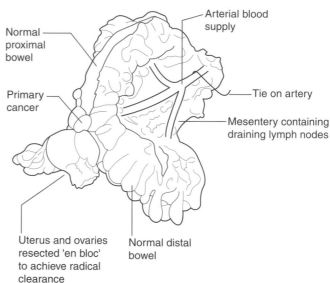

Fig. 6.12 Sigmoid cancer. A Operative specimen. B The diagram shows the structures that have been removed with this en bloc resection.

chemotherapy may help prevent both local recurrence and distant metastasis, and this is commonly used in patients with colorectal or breast cancer and who have lymph node involvement. However, surgical excision must be adequate, and adjuvant radiotherapy or chemotherapy must not be regarded as a safety net for careless surgical practice. In some cancers, such as ovarian cancer, transcoelomic spread occurs early and a radical operation is impossible. Here surgical reduction of the tumour burden may contribute to the success of systemic treatment, which is aimed at controlling the disease as a whole.

Achieving a balance between the relief of symptoms and the morbidity induced by radical cancer therapy is often difficult, and it is important to remember that the quality of life is as important as the duration of survival. Chemotherapy is potentially toxic; morbidity and quality of life must always be considered before undertaking this form of treatment.

The success of adjuvant chemotherapy varies from one histological type of cancer to another. In general, drugs are given in combination over a period of 6–12 months. Toxicity, such as mouth ulcers, diarrhoea, weakness and alopecia, is common but in general tolerable. Results in colorectal and breast cancer suggest that the likelihood of death from recurrent cancer is reduced by about 20–30% in patients with evidence of lymph node metastasis.

Because of the localized nature of radiotherapy, it is administered to reduce the chances of local recurrence rather than of distant metastasis. Radiotherapy may be given prior to surgery to try to 'down-stage' or shrink a bulky and fixed tumour (e.g. rectal cancer) and thus make surgery easier to perform. Sometimes radiotherapy is given to rectal cancers preoperatively, even if the cancer is surgically resectable, to improve subsequent local recurrence rates; this is termed neoadjuvant radiotherapy. Alternatively, it may be given to the postoperative patient in whom the chances of local recurrence are thought to be high (e.g. a patient in whom the margins at the edge of the resection specimen are involved with tumour). When tumours are relatively radiosensitive, radiotherapy can reduce the need for radical surgery and a more cosmetically acceptable conservative operation is then possible (e.g. lumpectomy and radiotherapy, as opposed to mastectomy in breast cancer).

The impact of intensive chemo- and radiotherapy on growth in children with malignant disease can be significant. The potential for cure, which is possible in many childhood malignancies, has to be balanced against the long-term morbidity of growth failure as a side effect of such treatment.

Other modes of adjuvant therapy include less toxic therapies, such as administration of the antioestrogen tamoxifen in women with breast cancer. Experimental models have shown that monoclonal antibodies, synthetic peptides, antisense oligonucleotides and soluble adhesion molecules can inhibit tumour growth. Gene therapy carries the potential to restore the function of altered tumour suppressor molecules. MMP inhibitors and angiogenesis inhibitors offer other potential avenues for novel anticancer therapy.

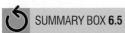

SUMMARY BOX 6.5

Principles of surgery for cancer

- Multidisciplinary team approach
- Accurate pre- and post-operative staging
- En bloc radical surgery
- Appropriate pre- and post-operative adjuvant therapy
- Good communication with patient and relatives
- Audit of results.

Surgery for metastases

Although the numbers are small (around 10–20% of patients with metastases), due to advances in surgical technique and improved chemotherapeutic agents, patients with metastatic disease are more likely to be offered surgical treatment for their cancer than previously. Surgical resection of colorectal liver metastases is eminently possible and has been shown to improve survival in patients that previously had a very poor prognosis giving this highly selected group of patients a potential 40% 5-year survival. Following discussion in the setting of a multidisciplinary team, surgeons are now increasingly prepared to offer liver resection and lung resection for the treatment of metastatic disease, often in conjunction with second- and third line chemotherapy regimens. The decision to operate, the timing of surgery and the type of chemotherapy agents used require careful consideration.

Follow-up

In most patients with tumours amenable to surgical treatment, it is important to check subsequently that there is no local recurrence of disease and that the patient is symptom-free (EBM 6.4). In general, patients are seen more frequently in the early months after surgery, as this is the period when recurrence is most likely; it is also the period when it is necessary to detect and treat non-cancer-related postoperative complications. The nature of the surgery will influence the follow-up strategy; patients undergoing palliative surgery will have different follow-up requirements from those undergoing curative surgery. However, it is often difficult to detect recurrence or metastasis in the asymptomatic postoperative patient, and some would question the value of routine sophisticated investigations in the detection of metastatic disease in such cases. Current evidence suggests that, in some cases, once the primary therapy has been undertaken, patients may be discharged back to their GP for follow-up with re-referral to the multidisciplinary team as necessary.

EBM 6.4 Need for follow-up

'The value of "aggressive" follow-up of postoperative cancer patients is controversial. Some have shown that systematic postoperative follow-up using a variety of techniques such as tumour markers, regular radiology and endoscopy can increase the number of patients with recurrence that is amenable to further surgery with curative intent.'

Castells A, et al. Dis Colon and Rectum 1998; 41(6):213–714. Lewis RA Br J General Practice 2009; 59:525-532.

Palliation of advanced cancer

The management of patients with incurable disease involves the relief of distressing symptoms (palliative care). This is a specialist branch of medicine in its own right, and the palliative care physician and the associated team play an important part in the overall management of the cancer patient. The terminal stages of malignancy can be prolonged, and pain and other distressing symptoms are common. Effective palliation is achieved by a variety of means. Local and/or systemic adjuvant therapy can be used to induce tumour regression: for example, to reduce the pressure effects of cerebral metastases. Surgery can be employed to resect symptomatic metastases or bypass a malignant obstruction. When a palliative operation is performed, the patient and his or her relatives should understand that its object is to prevent additional suffering, and not to attempt cure. Medical treatments are used to relieve symptoms such as pain, nausea, depression, infections etc. A wide range of analgesic and narcotic drugs is available to relieve pain. The choice depends on the type of pain, its severity, and the stage of the illness. The aim is to achieve complete analgesia without impairing mental clarity or inducing side effects. It is essential never to let the patient wait for the next dose of analgesic. The psychological and social aspects of care for both the patient and the family should also be addressed.

Prognosis and counselling

Honesty is the basis of the doctor–patient relationship and it is almost always best to tell patients that they have cancer. However, in doing so one should reveal as much of the truth as the patient wishes to have or can understand. In some cultures this may be difficult; close relatives may want to shield the patient from distressing information. Tact is required to ensure patient autonomy. When therapy is undertaken with curative intent, it is most important to emphasize that this is the goal in mind. Radical cancer surgery followed by radiotherapy or chemotherapy can be very arduous, and maintenance of morale is essential. When palliation is the objective, it is important not to remove the patient's hope, as 'the end of hope is the beginning of death'. It is usually best to speak to patients in a quiet, private room with one of the nursing staff present.

Care of the dying

Death from malignant disease is usually a gradual process of withdrawal. A sympathetic doctor can greatly help patients and their relatives. A dying patient must never feel abandoned in a surgical ward, and doctors and nursing staff must be prepared to spend time to help the patient die with dignity. In general, however, most patients die either at home (with support from palliative care nurses etc.) or in a hospice, where the level of quiet and care is appropriate to the situation. Early involvement of the hospice/palliative care team helps allay patient fears and optimize the control of distressing symptoms.

Palliative care of children with terminal malignant disease is becoming increasingly available in the UK. A number of children's hospices have now been established which offer this service and they have proven to be of great support, not only to affected children, but also to their parents and families.

C.E. Robertson
D.W. McKeown

7

Trauma and multiple injury

CHAPTER CONTENTS

TRAUMA EPIDEMIOLOGY

The most common cause of death from birth to the fourth decade, and the fourth most common cause overall, is trauma. For individuals between 15 and 24 years, trauma leads to three times as many deaths as any other cause. On average, for individuals of working age, heart disease and cancer result in the loss of 10 years of potential life, but road traffic accidents (RTAs) alone cause the loss of 30–35 years. The economic cost is staggering. Patients with trauma occupy 10% of hospital beds and, globally, trauma accounts for 1–2% of gross national product.

However, experience of trauma cannot be extrapolated from other countries to predict events or outcomes. For example, in the UK, RTAs, falls and interpersonal violence account for the majority of major trauma (Fig. 7.1). Fewer than 1 in 10 patients with major trauma have penetrating injury, and this is usually caused by knives. In the USA, approximately 20% of the population owns a gun, and RTA deaths are matched by firearm injuries. Staggeringly, having a gun in the home increases the risk of homicide three-fold, and that of suicide five-fold; and for 15–24-year-olds, these figures increase by a factor of 10. A recent UK study found that the total number of homicides over a 2-year period for a population of 0.8 million was similar to that seen in a single day among the same-sized population of many American cities. In so-called developed countries, annually, 1 person in 50 will be involved in an RTA. Of these, 1% will die, 10% will need hospital treatment and 25% will be temporarily disabled.

It is often quoted that trauma deaths have a trimodal distribution. The first 'peak', representing deaths occurring immediately after or within a few seconds of injury, contributes up to 50% of the total. The second 'peak', up to 4 hours after injury, accounts for 30% of deaths, and the final 20% take place (usually in an intensive care unit) days or weeks after the event. Much significance has been placed upon this alleged temporal relationship, particularly the second peak. On the basis that interventions for the second group of patients offered great potential for preventing unnecessary deaths, the provision and nature of prehospital and hospital trauma services in the USA and the UK were changed profoundly. Unfortunately, the 'second peak' is a myth, at least in the UK, where the vast majority of deaths occur immediately after or within a very few minutes of injury. Furthermore, the subsequent deaths do not cluster into peaks. So, although attempts to improve care for those who initially survive must continue, the overwhelming message is that trauma prevention is far more important than any other aspect.

Trauma is a common cause of death and morbidity in children. After the first year of life, it is the most common cause of death in the paediatric population. The most common causes of serious injury seen in children are RTAs and falls. Non-accidental injury accounts for a significant number of the remainder.

The pattern of injury seen in children differs from that in adults. The small mass of the child is less able to disperse the kinetic energy of impact; as a consequence, multi-system injury is more common. The large paediatric head (in proportion to the rest of the body) means that head injuries are common. The larger body surface area to body mass found in infants and children results in increased heat loss after injury. There are often significant psychological sequelae to major trauma in children. It has been estimated that as many as 60% of such children are left with behavioural or learning difficulties after a serious accident.

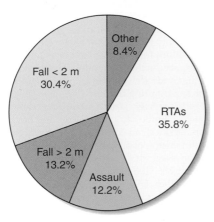

Fig. 7.1 Relative proportions of causes of trauma deaths. (Data kindly provided by the Scottish Trauma Audit Group 1992–1997.)

INJURY BIOMECHANICS AND ACCIDENT PREVENTION

To anticipate the injuries from any given trauma event, the clinician must understand the biomechanics involved. An accurate history can identify or predict the great majority of an individual patient's injuries.

The magnitude of injury is related to the energy transferred to the victim during the event, the volume/area of tissue involved, and the time taken for the interaction. Tissue characteristics, such as elasticity, plasticity and fluid content, are also important. These factors are summarized in the formula:

$$\text{Injury magnitude} \propto C \times (E/TV)$$

where E = energy transfer, T = time, V = volume of tissue, and C = tissue factors (a constant).

Kinetic energy, the energy of motion, is proportional to the mass of the object but to the square of its velocity. This can have unexpected effects. For example, a pedestrian struck by a car of mass 700 kg travelling at 100 km/h receives over three times more destructive energy than if hit by a heavy lorry of mass 5000 kg travelling at 40 km/h. If the car travels at 160 km/h, over 10 times the energy is involved. The longer the time frame during which the kinetic energy is transferred to the body, the less the acceleration/deceleration force sustained and the less the trauma that results.

These physical principles underpin strategies of accident prevention and protection. Obviously, reducing the chance of direct contact helps; separating pedestrians and traffic is the single most important factor in reducing pedestrian injury rates. This is illustrated by the fact that, in the US, less than 2% of traffic fatalities are pedestrians, whereas in the UK they account for 36% of the total. In a similar fashion, the central reservation barriers on motorways dramatically reduce the chances of high-speed head-on collisions (Fig. 7.2).

If impact does occur, then limitation of the velocities involved is the most important determinant in reducing injury. One in 10 drivers involved in RTAs has been travelling inappropriately fast. Even a 1 mph (1.6 km/h) reduction in *average* road speed reduces fatal accidents by 8%. The 20 mph (32 km/h) zones in residential areas, together with traffic calming measures, significantly reduce deaths and serious injuries, in particular to children and the elderly.

Contact factors can be minimized by vehicle design: crumple zones, energy-absorbing materials, preventing

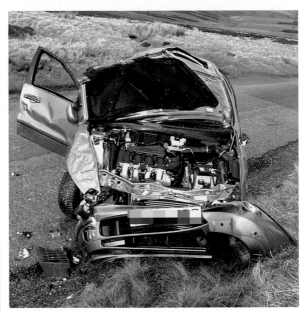

Fig. 7.2 Car involved in a high-speed, head-on collision, showing the magnitude of structural damage.

the ejection of passengers from the vehicle and reducing intrusion into the passenger compartment. For the occupants, seatbelts, airbags, collapsible steering columns and soft fascia compartments enable contact deceleration to take place over a longer time period, reducing the potential for injury (Fig. 7.3). Properly used, seatbelts reduce the risk of death/serious injury by 45%. Airbags further reduce the risk of death by 10% for belted drivers, and by 20% for unbelted front-seat passengers, but may not provide protection from side-impact events, or if the vehicle rolls over.

These devices can also modify the patterns of injury, particularly if they are incorrectly positioned. Seatbelts and airbags do reduce deaths overall but certain injuries, e.g. sternal fractures and soft-tissue neck injuries, may be associated with their use. If lap belts alone are used, pancreatic, renal, splenic and liver injuries are relatively more common and hyperflexion of the trunk over the belt can produce anterior compression fractures of the vertebrae. Finally, seatbelts are only protective when used. A recent study showed that 90% of all injured rear-seat passengers were unrestrained. These passengers increase the severity of their own injuries, as well as causing injury to restrained individuals in the front seats.

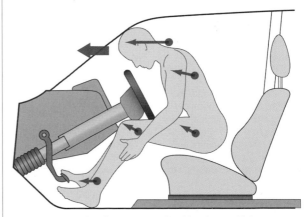

Fig. 7.3 Impact sites in an unrestrained head-on collision.

SUMMARY BOX 7.1

Accident features associated with major trauma

- Death of another individual in the same accident
- High-velocity impact, e.g. pedestrian or cyclist (motor or pedal) struck at > 30 kph, or vehicle occupants in collisions with closing speeds > 60 kph
- Entrapment in, or intrusion into, the passenger compartment of the vehicle
- Ejection from a vehicle
- Falls from heights > 3 m
- Penetrating injury of the chest, abdomen or neck.

ALCOHOL AND DRUGS

The message is often unwelcome, but few episodes of trauma are without direct human failing or causation. There is, for instance, a four-fold increase in the risk of being involved in an RTA while using a mobile telephone, even if hands free, a level similar to that seen when driving with a blood alcohol level at the UK legal limit (blood: 80 mg alcohol/ 100 ml of blood; breath: 3g mcg/100 ml breath).

The combination of youthful over-confidence, incompletely developed motor skills, and ready availability of high performance vehicles accounts for an extraordinarily high rate of accidents. These rates decline with age and experience, but at the other end of the spectrum, the elderly have a disproportionately high incidence of trauma because of co-existing medical conditions and visual/motor impairments that affect judgement.

At all ages, alcohol is the major causal factor for all types of trauma; 60% of individuals sustaining trauma in assaults have consumed alcohol. For burns, homicides and drowning, alcohol is implicated in 30–50% of events. Its combination with young males and road vehicles is particularly lethal; in this group, one-third of all fatalities, and 10% of all injuries, involve alcohol consumption. Drink-driving laws do reduce the proportion of fatal crashes involving intoxicated drivers, but high-risk behaviour remains common. Although death rates from alcohol-related events have fallen, the risk of being involved in an accident with a blood alcohol at the current UK driving limit is twice that for an individual with no alcohol in their blood. At higher levels, the risk dramatically increases even further. About 20% of RTA deaths are thought to be related to drug or substance misuse, but the difficulties of testing and the involvement of prescribed medications such as sedatives may mean that this is a considerable underestimate.

WOUNDS

Classification and production

- *Abrasions or grazes.* These are caused by the tangential application of blunt force. Dirt is often ingrained in the surface layers of skin, with the risk of short-term infection and, if untreated, later permanent 'tattooing'. The abrasion's site and nature may give useful clues as to the direction and magnitude of injury forces.
- *Contusions, ecchymoses or bruises.* These result from blunt force disrupting superficial capillaries. The overlying skin is intact. When small blood vessels are involved, a large collection of blood (haematoma) may develop. It is impossible to tell the age of a bruise accurately by

its colour, but if it is yellow (caused by breakdown of haemoglobin pigment to biliverdin and bilirubin), the bruise is likely to be at least 18 hours old.
- *Lacerations.* Blunt forces tear, shear or crush skin and soft tissues, producing lacerations. The wound edges are irregular and often abraded, contused and crushed, as are the surrounding tissues.
- *Incised wounds or 'cuts'.* These are produced by sharp edges, such as knives or glass shards, and have characteristically clean edges with clear margins. The greatest dimension of an incised wound is its length (cf. puncture wound).
- *Puncture wounds.* Sharp points or edges produce puncture wounds, in which the greatest dimension is the depth. When the wound pierces a body cavity, it is 'penetrating'; if it passes through a viscus, it is 'perforating'.

Gunshot wounds

Gunshot wound data (Fig. 7.4) highlight the gulf between UK and US practice. In the US, deaths from gunshot wounds are the fourth leading cause of years of potential life lost before the age of 65. Guns are used in over 60% of suicides and 70% of all homicides. Non-fatal gunshot wounds outnumber fatal ones two- to three-fold.

As with other injury, the exchange of energy is crucial. Low-velocity missiles cause local injury, involving tissue tearing and compression. When velocities exceed 500–600 m/s, cavitation injury – a temporary space torn in tissues at right angles to the direction of travel – is also produced. This process develops in microseconds and, depending upon the body tissues involved and their elasticity, can involve a volume many times the diameter of the bullet itself. The wounding potential can be further magnified by features specifically designed to increase the area of injury and the release of energy; examples include bullets that tumble in tissues and others designed to deform or fragment on impact (dum-dum or semi-jacketed bullets).

Shotgun events are relatively more common in the UK than handgun or rifle injuries (http://www.crimeandjustice. org.uk/). The muzzle velocity of these weapons is relatively high, but dissipation of the shot and air resistance on the pellets quickly decrease their velocity and limit the wounding potential (Fig. 7.5). These weapons are lethal at close range but, unless 'choked', are relatively less wounding at greater distances, where they tend to cause superficial injury to skin and subcutaneous tissues.

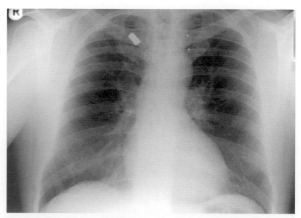

Fig. 7.4 Chest X-ray showing a bullet to the right of the upper mediastinum. (Courtesy of Miss Kate Wilson.)

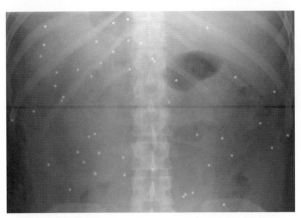

Fig. 7.5 X-ray of the lower chest and upper abdomen, showing pellets from a shotgun injury. Note the wide dissipation of the pellets.

FALLS

The major determinant of injury and the chance of death is directly proportional to the height fallen, as the accelerating force of gravity is constant. For practical purposes, the velocity at impact (v) is given by the equation:

$$v = \sqrt{2gh}$$

where g = gravitational constant (9.8 m/s) and h = height fallen in meters

Thus a body falling two storeys (10 m) has an impact velocity of around 50 kph. At impact, the deceleration forces are determined by the individual's mass, the nature of the landing surface and the body's orientation on landing. Surfaces such as mud, snow, soft earth and, to a lesser extent, water can permit an increased duration of impact, reducing deceleration forces and hence injury. For an 'average' man, a 5 m fall on to a concrete surface produces a deceleration force of approximately 700 g; if the landing is a soft, yielding surface, the stopping distance may be several centimetres, decreasing the force 10–20-fold.

The body's position during landing affects the contact area and the propagation of energy since, if the same force is dissipated over a larger area, there is less force per unit area and hence less damage (Figs 7.6 and 7.7). Feet-first falls involve a relatively small area of contact, but deceleration forces can be reduced by flexing the knees and hips. Regardless of the position on landing, however, for falls > 5 m there is a high incidence of deceleration injuries to intrathoracic and intra-abdominal structures, particularly where these are relatively immobile or tethered: for example, the aortic root and the mesenteric arteries. Overall, falls on to an unyielding surface from 15–20 m are associated with a greater than 50% mortality. Nevertheless, bizarre descriptions of survival from high falls do exist. There are well documented accounts of individuals surviving after falling from aircraft onto trees and deep snow. Clothing may also play a role in slowing the rate of fall: in 1885, Miss Sarah Ann Henley survived after a fall from the Clifton suspension bridge (~75 m) as her hooped crinolines acted as a parachute and the tide was out so that the landing surface was thick mud.

INJURY SEVERITY ASSESSMENT

Audit of trauma patients, both individually and as a group, is essential. To allow objective comparison between systems or hospitals, injury classifications have become standardized.

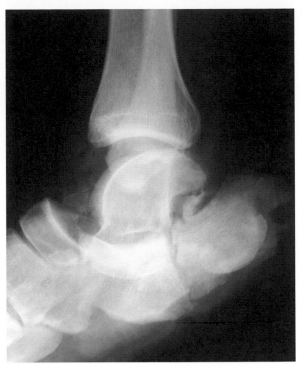

Fig. 7.6 Lateral view of ankle and grossly comminuted fracture of calcaneum, involving the subtalar joint. The mechanism of injury was a fall on to the feet from 15 metres.

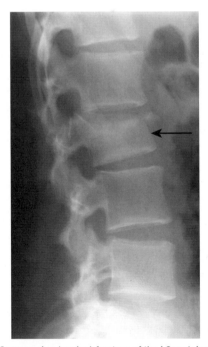

Fig. 7.7 Compression (wedge) fracture of the L2 vertebral body (arrow), caused by a fall from height.

Two types of classification are used. The first measures the severity of anatomical injury. The most commonly used system is the Abbreviated Injury Scale (AIS). Once the patient's injuries have all been identified (this may only be possible at discharge or autopsy), each separate

Table 7.1 Glasgow Coma Scale

Eyes open	
• Spontaneously	4
• To verbal command	3
• To pain	2
• No response	1
Best motor response	
To verbal command	
• Obeys verbal command	6
To painful stimulus	
• Localizes pain	5
• Flexion withdrawal	4
• Abnormal flexion (decorticate rigidity)	3
• Extension (decerebrate rigidity)	2
• No responses	1
Best verbal response	
• Orientated and converses	5
• Disorientated and converses	4
• Inappropriate words	3
• Incomprehensible sounds	2
• No response	1
Total number of points (minimum 3, maximum 15)	

injury is assessed from a scoring 'dictionary' and awarded a numerical score. The Injury Severity Score (ISS) is then derived from the three highest AIS scores within six body areas (head and neck, abdomen and pelvic contents, bony pelvis and limbs, face, chest and body surface). ISS provides an internationally recognized objective evaluation of anatomical injury.

The second type of classification is physiological. The best-known physiological scoring system is the Glasgow Coma Scale (Table 7.1), which is used to assess the neurological state of injured patients objectively, and which also has prognostic value. The Glasgow Coma score (GCS), in conjunction with two other physiological recordings, systolic blood pressure and respiratory rate, can be used to produce the 'Revised Trauma Score'. Although widely used, physiological scoring systems have intrinsic problems. Some patients with severe injury may not be identified initially, usually because the assessment has been performed before detectable physiological compromise has had time to occur. The system may also overestimate injury severity if physiological changes occur (due, for example, to alcohol) that are not reflected in the measured parameters, or which modify these factors. In addition, no allowance is made for factors such as comorbid features e.g. underlying cardiac or pulmonary disease or medications.

The combination of anatomical and physiological scoring systems allows comparisons between predicted and actual patient outcomes; age, and factors such as whether the injury was blunt or penetrating, can also be incorporated. This permits meaningful audit between hospitals and trauma systems. It must be stressed that these comparisons are valid for patient populations and have much less validity if applied to individual cases.

PREHOSPITAL CARE AND TRANSPORT

The objective of prehospital care is to prevent further injury, initiate resuscitation and transport the patient safely and rapidly to the most appropriate hospital. The size and demo-

graphics of the population served, along with geographical constraints, affect this directly.

In the USA, basic trauma care is often provided by fire and police services. Emergency medical technicians and paramedics supply advanced care, with direct communication links to the receiving hospital. If their injuries are several or severe, or if there is a significant mechanism of injury, patients may bypass the nearest hospital and be taken directly to a designated trauma centre.

In the UK and Europe, ambulance services, augmented by physician-led teams, often transport the patient to the nearest hospital. Paramedics can provide techniques such as tracheal intubation, peripheral intravenous access, and the administration of intravenous fluids and drugs. Intuitively, the use of such skills by ambulance paramedics at the scene of injury or en route to hospital should improve outcome for injured patients, but controlled studies have not demonstrated this. There are two main reasons for this. First, paramedic treatment may increase prehospital time, delaying definitive care. Such delay is closely related to increases in mortality. Second, the techniques used may themselves have intrinsically adverse effects. For example, intravenous fluids given to patients in whom bleeding cannot be controlled (e.g. intra-peritoneal bleeding, major vascular disruption, pelvic or long bone fractures) can precipitate additional blood loss by increasing blood pressure. Except for situations in which unavoidable delays will occur for a prehospital patient (usually entrapment or impalement, or rural or inaccessible locations), advanced pre-hospital techniques are probably inappropriate and time-wasting.

Transport from accident locus to hospital must be safe and rapid, with constant communication. In the UK, land-based ambulance service vehicles perform this, with additional support from helicopters and fixed-wing aircraft. Much experience has been obtained with helicopters in military medical environments, and in the USA and Australia; they dramatically increase costs and have additional risks for both patient and crew. Despite the potential to reduce journey times, the types of helicopter used in the UK have major operational difficulties with poor visibility, night-time flying, high winds and urban environments. Recent audit in an urban environment in the UK failed to show an improvement in response times, with longer on-scene times and no increase in survival for trauma patients. There is a clear justification for helicopter use in offshore and mountain rescue and in certain rural incident situations, but the majority of patients will continue to be transported by land ambulances.

TRAUMA CENTRES

A trauma patient should be provided with definitive surgical and intensive care facilities as soon as possible after injury. The problem is how to deliver this standard. In the 1970s and 1980s, trauma centres were introduced in the USA and a few European cities, where they unequivocally reduced preventable, in-hospital trauma deaths. Some of the results were remarkable, with 'avoidable' deaths reduced 5–10-fold for patients taken directly to a level 1 centre. The key elements in these systems were: transfer of patients from the accident scene directly to the centre; reception by senior staff on a 24-hour basis; the availability of all appropriate specialties on the same site; and a high throughput of patients.

Independent evaluation of the pilot trauma centre in England, however, failed to show a reduction in death

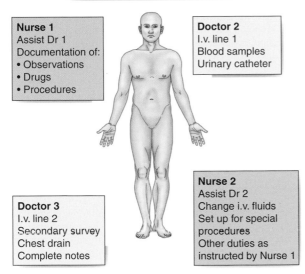

Doctor 1
Overall charge of case
Airway plus cervical spine control
Ventilation
Dictates order of priorities
Decides referral

Nurse 1
Assist Dr 1
Documentation of:
• Observations
• Drugs
• Procedures

Doctor 2
I.v. line 1
Blood samples
Urinary catheter

Doctor 3
I.v. line 2
Secondary survey
Chest drain
Complete notes

Nurse 2
Assist Dr 2
Change i.v. fluids
Set up for special
procedures
Other duties as
instructed by Nurse 1

Fig. 7.8 Trauma team organization.

rates. Two facts may explain this disappointing result. The first is the difference in trauma epidemiology, in relation to both the nature of the trauma and the volume of patients presenting. Secondly, despite having run for several years, the centre was not fully integrated into a comprehensive regionalized system (EBM 7.1). For the foreseeable future in the UK, the provision of care will be by a trauma team approach (Fig. 7.8), although reorganization and regionalization of trauma services in some UK areas is developing aspects of trauma centre care (http://www.rcseng.ac.uk/publications/docs/provision-of-trauma-care-1).

EBM 7.1 **Efficacy of trauma centres**

'Trauma systems are less developed in the UK than in North America. Designating, equipping and staffing a 'trauma centre' is only one component in developing an integrated trauma system. Mortality as a sole endpoint is a crude estimate of efficacy. Primary and secondary accident prevention are effective ways of cutting trauma deaths.'

Nicholl J, Turner J. BMJ 1997; 315:1349–1354.

RESUSCITATION IN THE EMERGENCY DEPARTMENT

The first 10 minutes

The receiving department should have advance warning from ambulance control to permit an appropriate manpower and resource response. Advance information required by the trauma team includes:

• estimated time of arrival
• number, age and sex of patients

• nature of the incident and any special features, e.g. associated chemical/radioactive contamination, helicopter transportation etc
• brief details of injuries, treatment given at the scene/in transit and current condition.

The resuscitation room must have all the equipment that will be needed for at least the first 1–2 hours of resuscitation. A calm, ordered approach is essential. Compliance with universal precautions for the disposal of sharps/instruments, and the use of gloves, face/eye protection and protective clothing is mandatory. All personnel must be appropriately immunized for hepatitis B.

If the number and severity of injured patients exceeds the facilities immediately available, the hospital's major incident plan may need to be activated. In this event, patients are triaged on arrival according to their priority for treatment.

During reception, a concise, relevant history is obtained from the ambulance crew and other emergency personnel, noting factors associated with an increased likelihood of severe injury. Digital camera images taken at the accident scene can help the receiving trauma team assess the mechanisms and forces involved and predict likely injuries.

A trauma team, consisting of 4–5 experienced doctors and nurses, is used for the patient's initial assessment and treatment (Fig. 7.8). Each team member has a pre-assigned role and performs this, unless directed otherwise by the team leader, who must have sufficient seniority and competence to direct and control the entire resuscitation process. The team members must be entirely familiar with the tasks required of them and perform them with minimal delay or questioning.

The patient's clothing is removed completely (cut off, if necessary, to avoid patient movement), allowing adequate access for examination and to avoid missing an occult external injury. Injured patients lose their normal thermo-regulatory ability, so they must then be kept warm and excessive exposure for examination or practical procedures should be avoided.

A traditional surgical approach, with history taking, clinical examination, investigation and treatment, is inappropriate in major trauma patients. An 'ABC' approach is logical and easy to remember, but although the steps are presented here sequentially, the trauma team performs and constantly reassesses all of these aspects *simultaneously*.

⟳ SUMMARY BOX **7.2**

The primary survey

• Airway with cervical spine control
• Breathing with ventilation
• Circulation with haemorrhage control
• Neurological disability and pupils
• Exposure and environment.

Airway

The patency of the airway is first assessed by direct inspection, identifying and removing obstructions. Loose-fitting dentures or dental plates are removed. Noisy breathing, snoring or stridor implies airway obstruction. A rigid suction catheter, used carefully to avoid stimulation of the sensitive pharynx, will remove blood, vomit, secretions and other debris from the mouth and oropharynx. Larger items, e.g. lumps of food, are extracted with forceps under direct vision.

The most common cause of airway obstruction is a reduced conscious level, with the tongue falling back and blocking the oropharynx. Airway clearance, together with the 'chin-lift' or 'jaw-thrust' manoeuvres, will correct this in the majority of cases. The airway is then constantly re-assessed by looking (to see the chest rise and fall), listening (for abnormal airway sounds) and feeling (for the patient's exhaled breath, using the side of the cheek or hand).

Assessment of conscious level helps in airway assessment. A patient speaking in complete sentences does not have an immediate airway problem (although one may develop later). The Glasgow Coma Scale can identify patients with established or potential problems and, if the score is < 8/15, usually mandates early definitive airway intervention, as the protective gag and swallow airway reflexes are likely to be absent or compromised. In the majority of cases, the upper airway is secured with simple positioning, regular suction and the use of basic adjuncts such as oro- or nasopharyngeal airways.

Control of the cervical spine

Irrespective of the airway control technique used, the cervical cord is constantly protected by manual in-line cervical control with the neck in the neutral position, or by using a carefully fitted semi-rigid neck collar, bolsters and tape.

Orotracheal intubation is the advanced airway technique of choice (Fig. 7.9). It protects the airway from aspiration of vomit or blood, and allows ventilation with controlled levels of oxygen and airway suctioning to remove debris. It does, however, require expertise in using anaesthetic and neuromuscular paralyzing agents. Prior to intubation, the patient is pre-oxygenated and must be carefully monitored throughout the process. A 'surgical' airway is extremely rarely needed; if one is required, a percutaneous cricothyrotomy is the simplest, safest and quickest surgical approach (see chapter 8).

Advanced airway techniques

These are required when:

- protective airway reflexes are absent (usually caused by altered consciousness)
- basic techniques are unable to cope with current or predicted airway compromise (e.g. major facial or burns/inhalation injury)
- there is a need for controlled ventilation (e.g. head and/ or chest injury).

Breathing

Optimal ventilation requires a patent upper and lower airway and effective function of the thoracic wall, lungs and diaphragm. Clinical assessment is extremely helpful. Respiratory compromise is characterized by tachypnoea or bradypnoea, the use of accessory muscles of respiration, and paradoxical (see-saw) movement of the chest and abdomen, indicating failure of normal diaphragmatic function. Hypoxia may be manifest by restlessness, tachycardia, confusion, agitation, pallor or sweating. Cyanosis is rare and difficult to detect clinically, particularly if hypovolaemia is present.

Concern about oxygen toxicity in the initial phase of resuscitation is unnecessary. Until the patient is stable and adequate tissue oxygen delivery has been confirmed, the highest possible concentration of oxygen should be administered. Pulse oximeters can detect arterial desaturation, but readings are unreliable in hypovolaemic, shocked patients, in limbs with vascular injury, or if abnormal haemoglobins (including carboxyhaemoglobin) are present. Pulse oximetry does not replace arterial blood gas analysis, as hypercapnoea can occur with normal SpO_2 levels.

Clinical inspection, palpation and auscultation of the neck and chest (including the back) should detect immediately life-threatening injuries such as flail segment, penetrating wounds, tension or open pneumothoraces, major haemothorax and cardiac tamponade. These conditions need immediate treatment, e.g. needle thoracocentesis for tension pneumothorax, or the insertion of an intercostal drain for haemothorax. Open or sucking chest wounds (Fig. 7.10) are rare but, if present, allow equalization of atmospheric and intrathoracic pressures. With large defects, atmospheric air passes through the wound into the intrathoracic space with each inspiration, and the lung collapses. To prevent this, the open wound is covered with a sterile occlusive dressing, taped on three sides. This acts as a flutter valve, and formal tube thoracostomy is then performed at a separate site from the open wound.

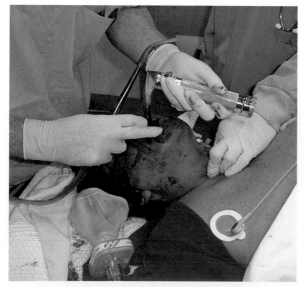

Fig. 7.9 Rapid-sequence intubation in a trauma patient: note cricoid pressure being applied to prevent regurgitation of stomach contents.

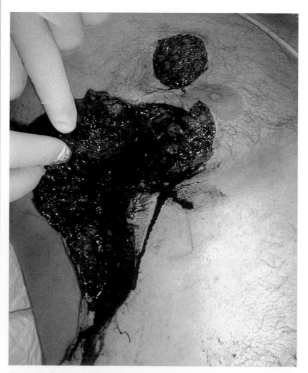

Fig. 7.10 Open (sucking) chest wound from a fall on to a metal stake.

Table 7.2 Clinical features of tension pneumothorax
• Cardiorespiratory distress (tachycardia, hypotension)
• Distended neck veins
• Asymmetric chest wall movement
• Hyper-resonant percussion note on affected side
• Absent or reduced breath sounds on affected side

Repeated arterial blood gas analyses are needed to ensure that hypoxia is not present and that alveolar ventilation is sufficient to prevent hypercapnoea. For patients who are intubated and ventilated, additional problems may develop. Positive-pressure ventilation may reduce cardiac output (manifest initially by tachycardia ± hypotension) because of decreased venous return to the heart, resulting from increased intrathoracic pressure during the 'inspiratory' phase of ventilation. The risk of pneumothorax (Table 7.2) in patients with coexisting chest injuries is markedly increased by positive-pressure ventilation. If a pneumothorax is already present, tension may be induced. For these reasons, tube thoracostomy is mandatory if a pneumothorax is present and positive-pressure ventilation, for whatever reason, is to be undertaken.

For patients in whom positive-pressure ventilation is instituted, the aim is to ensure adequate oxygenation (P_aO_2 levels > 12 kPa) and alveolar ventilation (P_aCO_2 levels ~ 4 kPa). Controlled ventilation is particularly important in patients with head injury, as hypercarbia causes dilatation of the cerebral vessels and increased intracranial pressure, whereas hypocarbia produces cerebrovascular vasospasm, compromising cerebral perfusion.

The drugs needed to permit intubation and controlled ventilation may themselves obscure important clinical features, particularly of neurological or abdominal injury. Before any drugs are used, the patient's neurological status must be recorded. Additional imaging, such as computed tomography (CT), will be required if there is any suspicion of associated head injury. Abdominal injury is commonly missed in patients with altered consciousness of whatever cause. Clinical signs are modified or absent in paralyzed and sedated patients, and so additional investigations, such as ultrasound, CT or diagnostic peritoneal lavage, are important (see below).

SUMMARY BOX 7.3

Common causes of breathing and ventilation problems

- Airway obstruction
- Tension pneumothorax
- Massive haemothorax
- Flail chest
- Open (sucking) chest wound
- Cardiac tamponade.

Gastric dilatation is common in trauma patients. It results from a combination of factors, including air-swallowing (in conscious patients), bag-mask ventilation (where the airway pressure exceeds the gastro-oesophageal closing pressure), and the effects of sympathetic nervous system overactivity and electrolyte disturbance on gastric peristalsis. A distended stomach full of air, fluid and food in a patient with compromised airway protective reflexes is a situation ripe for regurgitation and potentially fatal aspiration. In addition, the distended stomach will restrict diaphragmatic movement and impair respiration. To prevent these problems, a nasogastric tube is routinely inserted and suction applied; if there is any suspicion of an anterior cranial fossa fracture, an *oro*gastric tube is used.

Circulation

The clinical detection of blood loss and the resulting haemodynamic effects is crude and non-specific. Pulse rate, cuff blood pressure and peripheral perfusion (assessed by capillary refill time) are routinely noted every 5–10 minutes in the initial stages, but these recordings have major limitations. Homeostatic mechanisms in previously fit healthy adults mean that, depending upon the rate and site of blood loss, 20% or more of total circulating blood volume can be lost without a measurable change in these recordings. Isolated readings are especially misleading. Trends in pulse rate and blood pressure are of much greater value. A rising pulse rate combined with a falling blood pressure strongly suggests uncontrolled, often occult, blood loss.

Absence of these features does not necessarily mean that all is well. The patient may not be able to respond to hypovolaemia by increasing the heart rate because of age, pre-existing cardiac disease or medications such as β-blockers or calcium channel blockers. In addition, an individual's 'normal' values need to be considered. A blood pressure of 110/60 mmHg may represent severe hypotension if the patient's normal value is 190/120 mmHg, but may be normal for a healthy young adult. Unfortunately, this knowledge is rarely available in the early stages of resuscitation, and a high index of suspicion, bearing in mind the mechanism of injury, is therefore imperative.

To reduce blood loss is essential. External haemorrhage can invariably be controlled by simple direct pressure. Haemostasis from the sometimes profuse bleeding of scalp wounds is best achieved with carefully applied sutures or staples. Splinting of long-bone fractures reduces blood loss from fracture sites by up to 50%, makes the patient more comfortable, and reduces analgesic requirements (Fig. 7.11). In contrast, blood loss into the peritoneal cavity, thorax or pelvis is usually concealed, can be life-threatening, and cannot be simply controlled. Patients with major pelvic fractures pose a difficult management problem, as conventional splintage is impossible and massive and uncontrollable blood loss may result (Fig. 7.12). The optimal approach is the application of external fixator devices in the resuscitation phase, followed, if required, by angiographic embolization.

SUMMARY BOX 7.4

Situations where blood loss may be misappreciated

- The elderly
- Patients on concurrent drug therapy (e.g. β-blockers, antihypertensives, anti-anginals)
- Patients with a pacemaker
- Athletes
- Pregnancy
- Hypothermia.

The next priority is to insert and secure two large-bore (12–14 G) intravenous cannulae. The forearms or antecubital fossae are the most accessible peripheral sites, but the nature and location of the injuries may require alternative sites, such as the femoral or external jugu-

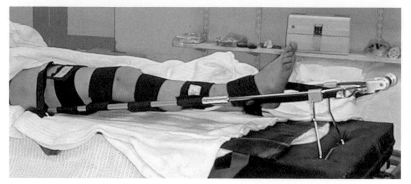

Fig. 7.11 Right lower limb in a traction device to provide splintage.

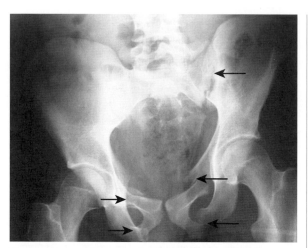

Fig. 7.12 X-ray of the pelvis, showing bilateral upper and lower pubic rami fractures (upper arrow), with 'butterfly' fragment and shearing injury affecting the left sacroiliac joint (lower arrows).

The choice of fluids for the replacement of traumatic blood loss is controversial and poorly understood. Intravenous volume replacement is begun with infusion of an isotonic crystalloid such as 0.9% saline or Ringer's lactate. In the UK, after 1000–2000 ml of crystalloid, a colloid is commonly given prior to, or together with, blood. Theoretically, colloids (such as albumin solutions, gelatins, starches or dextrans) might be expected to be more effective, but there is no good evidence to suggest this in clinical practice (EBM 7.2).

EBM 7.2 **Resuscitation fluid choice**

'There is no evidence from RCTs that volume resuscitation with colloids reduces the risk of death, compared to resuscitation with crystalloids, in patients with trauma.'

Perel P, Roberts I. Colloids versus crystalloids for fluid resuscitation in critically ill patients. Cochrane Database of Systematic Reviews 2011, Issue 3. Art. No.: CD000567. DOI: 10.1002/14651858.CD000567.pub4.

---

lar veins, to be used. Central venous cannulation is difficult and potentially hazardous in shocked hypovolaemic patients, so if percutaneous access cannot be obtained, a surgical cut-down at the saphenofemoral junction is preferable, although more time-consuming. Intraosseous access to long bones in the adult is a viable alternative for initial resuscitation. At the time of cannulation, initial venous blood samples should be taken, carefully labelled and sent for analysis, the laboratories having previously been alerted.

The effective resuscitation of the injured child requires an appreciation of the physiological differences that exist between children and adults. The normal cardiovascular and respiratory parameters vary with age. For example, the normal heart rate of a newborn infant is 160 beats/minute; the normal respiratory rate of a 1-year-old is about 30 breaths per minute. A knowledge of what is normal is required to allow the confident identification of the abnormal.

Suitable equipment is essential to resuscitate children of different ages and weights safely. Cuffed tracheal tubes are not used in small children. Small intravenous cannulae may be necessary and intraosseous needles can be used for vascular access in children. Different-sized cervical collars, oxygen face masks, laryngoscopes and other equipment should be readily available in any resuscitation room receiving children.

Notwithstanding the above, the ABCDE sequence of resuscitation that is followed in the child is the same as that in the adult: *a*irway with cervical spine control, *b*reathing with oxygen, *c*irculation with control of bleeding, *d*isability, *e*xposure.

Irrespective of the fluid chosen, it must be warmed to 37–38°C before infusion to prevent hypothermia and aggravating coagulation deficits. This is achieved with in-line warming devices that infuse the fluid at the required temperature, regardless of flow rate.

Intravenous fluid administration is initially dictated by the nature of the patient's injuries, an estimate of the current volume deficit, and the clinical and haemodynamic responses to treatment. Failure to respond to the first 1–2 litres of volume replacement suggests that the volume deficit is great (> 40% of circulating volume). It is, however, inappropriate to correct haemodynamic measurements in isolation, and there are situations where, in the presence of an uncontrolled bleeding site (for example, in the pelvis or peritoneum), increasing blood pressure will simply exacerbate blood losses.

Blood transfusion requirements depend upon the magnitude of blood loss and the physiological response. It is usual to replace losses with the aim of maintaining the patient's haematocrit at ~30%. Where there is immediately life-threatening haemorrhage, group O Rhesus-negative blood is given, but more usually fully cross-matched or type-specific blood can be supplied. Most transfusion services supply packed red cells. There is no evidence that 'fresh' whole blood is preferable. In situations of massive blood loss, where replacement of more than the equivalent of one circulating blood volume is needed, coagulation problems should be anticipated. Military experience has led to development of massive transfusion guidelines including early use of platelets and coagulation factors, often

EBM 7.3 **Antifibrinolytic treatment**

'Uncontrolled bleeding is an important cause of death in trauma victims. Antifibrinolytic treatment with tranexamic acid (TXA) reduces mortality in bleeding trauma patients without increasing the risk of adverse events although further trials are needed to determine its efficacy and safety in isolated traumatic brain injury.'

Roberts I, Shakur H, Ker K, Coats T, on behalf of the CRASH-2 Trial collaborators. Antifibrinolytic drugs for acute traumatic injury. Cochrane Database of Systematic Reviews 2011, Issue 1. Art. No.: CD004896. DOI: 10.1002/14651858.CD004896.pub3.

directed by 'near-patient' testing of coagulation. Recently, tranexamic acid (an antifibrinolytic agent) has been shown to improve morbidity and mortality in trauma patients at risk of major bleeding (EBM 7.3). Close liaison with the Blood Transfusion Service and haematology laboratories is essential for optimal management.

SUMMARY BOX 7.5

Initial blood samples in the trauma patient

- Blood grouping and cross-matching
- Full blood count and haematocrit
- Urea and electrolytes
- Plasma glucose
- Arterial blood gases
- Kleihauer–Betke analysis (in pregnant patients).

Measurement of urine output (> 1 ml/kg body weight/hr normally implies adequate renal perfusion), continuous intra-arterial blood pressure monitoring and serial lactate levels assist in monitoring the response to infusion. In this situation, intra-arterial blood pressure monitoring is significantly more accurate than standard cuff methods, and has the additional advantage that the in-dwelling cannula permits regular arterial blood sampling without additional patient discomfort. Continuous electrocardiogram (ECG) monitoring, oxygen saturation SpO_2 (by pulse oximetry), core temperature and serial blood pressure measurements are standard requirements and augment clinical judgement. A low or falling GCS may indicate cerebral hypoperfusion due to hypovolaemia or worsening intracranial injury. More sophisticated means of cardiovascular assessment can provide additional information and should be used at an early stage, but techniques such as central venous and pulmonary artery wedge pressure and cardiac output measurement are usually impractical in the immediate resuscitative phase. They will be used later, particularly if vasoactive agents such as vasopressors or inotropes are employed.

SUMMARY BOX 7.6

Monitoring the trauma patient

- Heart rate
- Blood pressure (cuff and intra-arterial) (in both arms if suspected aortic injury)
- Capillary refill
- Respiratory rate
- Glasgow Coma Scale
- Urine output
- ECG
- Pulse oximetry
- Core temperature.

Analgesia

A calm, gentle and reassuring approach does much to relieve anxiety and is the first step in pain relief. Adequate analgesia is often neglected – or worse, thought to be unnecessary or hazardous in trauma patients. Physiological responses to pain produce adverse effects – for example, by increasing intracranial and arterial pressure – and so analgesia is essential. Further, it must be given according to the patient's individual requirements, rather than as a rigid process.

In cooperative, fully conscious patients without respiratory problems, Entonox (50% nitrous oxide, 50% oxygen) is useful for short-duration procedures such as manipulation of dislocations and fractures. Its value is limited by the need for patient cooperation (the euphoric effect may be associated with confusion and disorientation), its short duration of action and its limited analgesic effect.

Opioid drugs such as morphine or diamorphine, given in small intravenous (intramuscular absorption may be poor and inconsistent) doses titrated to effect are unsurpassed for analgesia. Provided the drug is given like this, haemodynamic disturbance or respiratory depression is rare and the need for antiemetics e.g. cyclizine uncommon. The newer synthetic opioids have no advantages.

Head injury or suspected head injury is not an *absolute* contraindication to opioid administration, provided that the agent is given as above and that the patient's airway, ventilation and haemodynamic status are carefully monitored. If necessary, naloxone can be given, if there is doubt as to whether alterations in conscious level are due to the opioid or to the head injury and its effects.

Local anaesthetic techniques are generally of limited value in the early management of major trauma, but an exception is the use of a femoral nerve block for patients with femoral shaft fractures. Long-bone fractures need to be immobilized to reduce pain and blood loss from the fracture site, to facilitate the taking of X-rays, patient movement and transfer, and to reduce the chances of fat embolism syndrome. Inflatable or foam-cushioned splints are suitable for upper-limb or below-knee injuries; adjustable traction splints are best for femoral fractures.

The next phase

The above assessments and interventions represent only the immediately life-saving procedures and should occupy just the first 10 minutes after arrival in the emergency department. Then, provided the patient's condition permits, a more detailed history and examination is undertaken, with appropriate laboratory and imaging investigations to determine the full extent of the patient's injuries and the requirement for surgery or other care. This review, or secondary survey, should enable a definitive management plan to be formulated. Throughout, the continuing priorities of *A*irway, *B*reathing and *C*irculation must be constantly reviewed and managed as necessary.

The patient is examined from top to toe to ensure that no wound, bruise or swelling is missed. The back and spine are examined with the patient 'log-rolled', looking specifically for localized tenderness, swelling, bruising or a 'step'. The perineum is examined and a rectal examination performed (Table 7.3).

The neurological status of the patient is recorded regularly, including the GCS, pupil sizes and reactions, and any focal deficit). The ears, nose and mastoid areas are carefully examined for evidence of skull-base injury, such as blood/cerebrospinal fluid otorrhoea or rhinorrhoea, or bruising. Muscle power should be tested and recorded using the MRC

Table 7.3 Rectal examination in the trauma patient

- Anal sphincter tone
- Prostate: position, bogginess
- Blood in the rectum
- Pelvic fractures
- Perineal injury

Table 7.4 Assessing muscle power: the MRC scale

No flicker of movement	0
A flicker of contraction, but no movement	1
Movement, with gravity neutralized	2
Movement against gravity	3
Movement against added resistance	4
Normal power	5

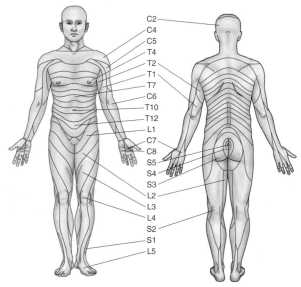

Fig. 7.13 Sensory dermatomes.

(Medical Research Council) scale (Table 7.4), and the tendon reflexes examined. It is vital to test sensation in a methodical fashion (Fig. 7.13). The perineal area must be included (this is most easily achieved at the time of rectal examination), as the lowest (sacral) dermatomes are in this area.

 SUMMARY BOX **7.7**

Causes of early neurological deterioration in the trauma patient

Intracranial

- Haematoma
- Cerebral oedema
- Fitting.

Extracranial

- Hypoxia
- Hypotension
- Hyper-/hypocarbia
- Hyper-/hypoglycaemia.

Drugs

Any decrease in the patient's conscious level (i.e. a numerical fall in GCS) must prompt an immediate search for, and correction of, a primary cause, such as intracranial haematoma, or secondary factors such as hypoxia, hypercarbia, hypotension or hypoglycaemia. Confounding factors may render the assessment of the GCS difficult, especially if the patient has taken alcohol or other drugs, but altered consciousness or other neurological deficit should never be assumed to be due solely to alcohol or other drugs alone until proven otherwise.

IMAGING AND OTHER DIAGNOSTIC AIDS

The radiological investigations needed in the initial phase of the management of a major trauma patient are limited but important. It is important to obtain the best-quality views, and fixed overhead X-ray facilities in the resuscitation room itself are invaluable, as transfer of the patient to a main X-ray department can be hazardous. A portable machine brought to the resuscitation room is preferable to transfer, although the images obtained will be of poorer quality.

There are three primary X-ray views in the blunt trauma patient, but these do have limitations:

- The *chest X-ray* may demonstrate thoracic injuries previously unrecognized on clinical examination, but even on a good-quality erect view over half of the rib fractures actually present will be missed (Fig. 7.14). The patient's condition often precludes an erect film, and on a supine view pneumothoraces and/or haemothoraces are difficult to detect; even in the absence of pathology, the mediastinal contours are displaced and widened.
- The *lateral view of the cervical spine* should be a cross-table film and must include *all* of the vertebrae from C1 to T1. This provides valuable information on acute bony injury (Fig. 7.15), but a 'normal' neck X-ray does not exclude significant injury to soft tissues, including the cervical cord.
- On *a plain antero-posterior view of the pelvis*, injuries to the posterior elements are difficult to see (especially around the sacroiliac regions, which may lead to significant occult haemorrhage).

The use of additional imaging techniques depends upon their availability and the clinical state of the patient. For head, spinal and pelvic injury, CT is unsurpassed and rapid. In contrast to the information provided by conventional skull

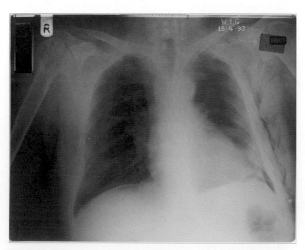

Fig. 7.14 Chest X-ray showing rib fractures and subcutaneous emphysema.

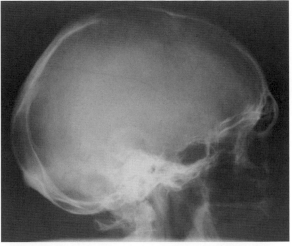

Fig. 7.16 Lateral X-ray of the skull, showing a fracture.

X-rays (Fig. 7.16), CT defines the nature and magnitude of the intracranial insult (Fig. 7.17). It is therefore invaluable in providing the information the physician needs to determine the requirement for neurosurgical intervention (EBM 7.4).

In experienced hands, ultrasound examination of the abdomen is a quick, non-invasive and accurate method of detecting free intraperitoneal fluid. It can be performed in the resuscitation room and has largely supplanted diagnostic peritoneal lavage, although this technique remains a simple and rapid method for establishing the presence of intraperitoneal bleeding if ultrasound is not available. Injury to some solid organs, the retroperitoneum and hollow viscera is less easily demonstrated on ultrasound, and CT – with contrast as necessary – is preferable, provided that the patient is stable and can be transferred safely to the CT suite.

AFTER THE RESUSCITATION ROOM

The immediate aim of the resuscitation team is to assess and treat life-threatening injuries. There is no absolute guide as to the length of time this process will take, but the procedures and referral must be performed expediently, without compromising patient care. The result should be a patient with a patent airway and adequate gas exchange, whose circulatory status is normal or in the process of being adequately corrected. Long-bone fractures should have been splinted appropriately and cervical spine control maintained throughout.

Continuing care then involves identifying the correct destination for the patient. The nature and extent of the injuries and the patient's physiological response to treatment dictate this. In some situations, it is impossible to 'stabilize' the patient without immediate surgical intervention. Examples include patients with exsanguinating intra-abdominal or intrathoracic haemorrhage, in whom immediate laparotomy or thoracotomy is mandated.

More commonly, the patient is, at least temporarily, stable so that further investigation can be undertaken beyond the resuscitation room prior to definitive surgical or intensive care unit admission. Senior anaesthetic and surgical staff must accompany the patient in these situations, so that, if sudden deterioration occurs, the patient can be transferred directly to theatre. Full monitoring and resuscitation equipment is mandatory for the transfer.

The subsequent destination of the patient then depends upon their overall condition and the findings of these investigations. Intensive care admission is required if ventilation is needed or anticipated, if there are multiple

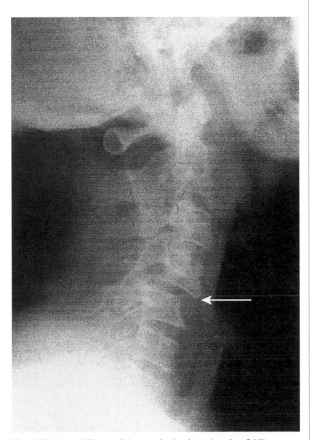

Fig. 7.15 Lateral X-ray of the cervical spine, showing C4/5 subluxation (arrowed).

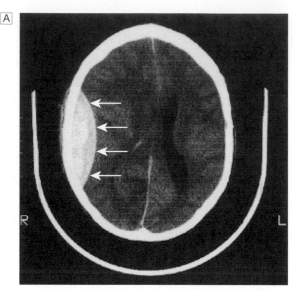

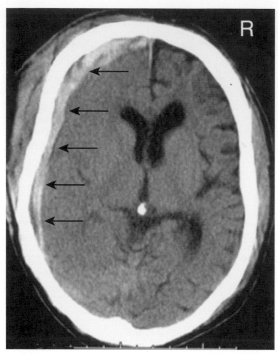

Fig. 7.17 Computed tomography in head injury. A Right-sided extradural haematoma (arrows) with midline shift towards the left. B Left-sided subdural haematoma (arrows).

injuries involving main systems, or if the patient needs invasive monitoring. Stable, self-ventilating patients with less severe injuries may be managed in a high-dependency unit, but the attending staff must be familiar with multiple trauma assessment and the relevant specialties must liaise closely to ensure a multidisciplinary approach. Previous or underlying medical conditions may play a crucial part in the subsequent course of the patient's course. The role of conditions such as coronary artery disease, diabetes etc. (and the medications required for these conditions) are well established. It is becoming increasingly recognized, however, that changes in immune function after injury may lead not only to local bacterial infections, but also to reactivation of diseases such as malaria which may compromise recovery.

It may be necessary to transfer the patient to another hospital for emergency investigation not available in the receiving hospital, or as part of definitive treatment by a specialist service. Inter- and intrahospital transfer is hazardous and must be performed by experienced anaesthetic and nursing staff with relevant monitoring and resuscitation equipment. The aspects of airway, ventilation and circulation control must be secured prior to transfer. The receiving unit must be informed of the relevant patient details, allowing it to prepare effectively for his or her arrival. The notes, details of investigations, X-rays, scans and observation charts must

accompany the patient. The type of transport used will depend upon the distance and geography of the journey involved, but may involve air transportation with all its attendant specific considerations. Regular updates should be supplied to the receiving specialist.

↻ SUMMARY BOX 7.9

Information required by the receiving unit or hospital

- Patient's name, age and sex
- Previous health status and medications (if known)
- Pulse, blood pressure and respiratory rate (at scene, on arrival and current)
- Glasgow Coma Scale (at scene, on arrival and at present)
- Summary of injuries, including signs of head injury and any lateralizing signs
- Summary of i.v. fluids (including blood), and the haemodynamic and urine output responses
- X-ray, CT or other imaging results
- Blood grouping/cross-matching, haematology and biochemistry results
- Tetanus status/cover provided, antibiotics and other drugs given (include doses and timing).

R.W. Parks

08

Practical procedures and patient investigation

INTRODUCTION

Every practical procedure performed on a conscious patient should be preceded by an explanation, which should include the reasons for the procedure and what it will entail. Appropriate reassurance should always be given. Many patients find comfort in continuing reassurance throughout the procedure, and most are helped by a description of sensations they are likely to experience before these occur. Where appropriate, informed written consent should be obtained. A record that the procedure was performed should be made in the case notes.

GENERAL PRECAUTIONS

It is important to be aware of the risk of infection or trauma to patient, operator and assistant during any practical procedure. These risks are minimized by following a few simple rules:

- Needles should not be resheathed and all disposable sharp instruments discarded by the operator should be placed in an appropriate container to minimize the risk of needle-stick injury
- Drapes and other soiled equipment should be placed in appropriate containers
- Gloves and gown should only be removed after all used instruments and disposable equipment have been placed in appropriate containers.

ASEPTIC TECHNIQUE

Transmission of infection is an ever-present problem, and the risk of spread should be minimized. As a minimum precaution, the skin should be cleansed with an antiseptic solution before all procedures, and sterile instruments used. For some procedures, such as central venous catheterization, bladder catheterization, insertion of chest drains and lumbar puncture, a full aseptic technique must be employed. The steps required are outlined in Table 8.1.

LOCAL ANAESTHESIA

Local anaesthetic agents inhibit membrane depolarization and hence block the transmission of nerve impulses. They may be used topically, i.e. painted or sprayed on mucous membranes and wound surfaces, so that they are absorbed locally to produce analgesia. Areas suitable for topical analgesia include the urethra, eye, nose, throat and bronchial tree. Local anaesthesia may also be administered by local infiltration, and this is used widely for minor surgical procedures. Local anaesthetic drugs are potentially toxic and care must be taken to avoid inadvertent intravascular injection. The first sign of toxicity is often numbness or tingling of the tongue or around the mouth, followed by lightheadedness and tinnitus. At higher blood levels, there is loss of consciousness, convulsions and apnoea.

Table 8.1 Aseptic technique

- An assistant is desirable to open non-sterile packs and 'drop' required instruments or solutions on to the sterile field
- Hand-washing for aseptic techniques ('scrubbing up') should last a full 3 minutes. The hands and forearms are wetted under a running tap and thoroughly washed with an antiseptic solution such as povidone-iodine (Betadine) or chlorhexidine (Hibiscrub)
- A sterile brush is then used to scrub the hands: in particular, the ulnar border, the interdigital clefts and the nails
- After the wash is completed, the hands are rinsed and held hands up/elbows down, so that water from the hands runs from the elbows into the sink
- The hands are dried on a sterile towel and the operator puts on a sterile gown and gloves. Thereafter, the operator must not touch anything other than sterile equipment or instruments
- The operative field is now cleansed with an antiseptic solution such as povidone-iodine or chlorhexidine, using sterile instruments and swabs. The area prepared should be much greater than the anticipated operative field, and cleansing should start from the centre and work outwards
- The operative field is then encircled with sterile drapes, which are secured so as to leave the operative field at the centre and provide the operator with as wide a sterile surrounding as possible

Cardiovascular collapse eventually occurs as a result of myocardial depression, vasodilatation and hypoxia. In general, efficacy is related to correct placement and toxicity to total dose. Where there is doubt about placement or a wide area of infiltration is anticipated, it is safer to calculate the maximum recommended dose and dilute it to the desired volume with 0.9% saline.

Lidocaine is the most widely used local anaesthetic agent and is available in 0.5–2% solutions. The maximum recommended dose is 3 mg/kg. Lidocaine is a short-acting anaesthetic (lasting up to 2 hours), whereas bupivacaine is longer-acting (up to 8 hours). A mixture of the two can be administered.

Solutions of local anaesthetic mixed with a 1:200 000 concentration of adrenaline (epinephrine) are also available. Adrenaline acts as a vasoconstrictor. It minimizes bleeding and reduces redistribution of the anaesthetic agent, thereby increasing its efficacy and duration of action. Local anaesthetic agents with adrenaline should not be used in anatomical areas supplied by an end-artery, such as the digits, because of the risk of vasoconstriction, ischaemia and gangrene.

SUTURING

The purpose of suturing is to approximate tissue in such a manner as to allow optimum primary healing to take place or to ligate bleeding vessels to arrest haemorrhage. Needles can be straight or curved. Straight needles are usually hand-held whereas curved needles are designed for use with a needle holder. The thread is 'swaged' inside the needle, which can be cutting or round-bodied. The latter push tissue aside and can be used to reduce the risk of needle-stick injuries e.g. for closing the linea alba in abdominal wound closure, or for bowel/vascular anastomosis. Cutting needles are more commonly used for skin closure.

Suture materials

Non-absorbable sutures

Non-absorbable sutures may be classified into three groups:

1. *Natural braided sutures* (e.g. silk, linen) have good handling qualities and knot easily and securely. Their disadvantage is increased tissue reaction and suture line sepsis, caused by the capillary action of the braided material drawing micro-organisms into the suture track. Such materials also lose tensile strength quickly with time, or when wet.
2. *Synthetic braided materials* (e.g. Nurolon, Ethibond, Mersilene) cause less tissue reaction than natural materials. They have good handling qualities and knot easily and securely.
3. *Synthetic monofilament materials* (e.g. nylon, polypropylene) have less drag through the tissues and cause little tissue reaction. They are free from the capillary effect of braided sutures and cause less suture track sepsis. However, they handle less well because of increased 'memory' (i.e. they retain the configuration in which they were packaged). Knots in monofilament sutures are less secure than those in braided or natural sutures, requiring multiple throws on each one.

Absorbable sutures

Absorbable sutures are generally made from synthetic materials. They cause relatively little tissue reaction, retain their tensile strength and are absorbed slowly. They can be multifilament, such as Dexon (polyglycolic acid) and Vicryl (polyglycolic plus polylactic acid), or monofilament, such as Maxon (polyglyconate) and PDS (polydioxonone). These synthetic sutures are commonly used for intra-abdominal procedures and subcuticular wound closure. Interrupted sutures with each knot buried are used for small wounds, whereas in longer wounds a continuous subcuticular suture is employed.

Suturing the skin

Skin wounds are sutured under as near-sterile conditions as possible, using a strict aseptic technique. A few basic principles underlie good wound care:

- Tissue should be handled gently. The wound should not be rubbed with swabs. Blood in a wound is removed by pressing a swab on to it
- Haemostasis should be meticulous to prevent wound haematoma
- All foreign material and devitalized tissues should be removed. Where this is prevented by heavy contamination, delayed primary suture or secondary suture should be considered
- Potential spaces (dead space) in the wound should be closed using absorbable suture material such as Vicryl. Where this is not possible, a suction drain is led from the potential space before more superficial layers are closed
- The tension on knots is critical. If they are tied too tightly, the suture line may become ischaemic, leading to delayed healing or non-healing and an increased risk of wound infection. Equally, insufficient tension on the suture may result in failure to appose the wound edges or inadequate haemostasis.

Table 8.2 **Times recommended for removal of sutures**	
• Face and neck	4 days
• Scalp	7 days
• Abdomen and chest	7–10 days
• Limbs	7 days
• Feet	10–14 days

Cutting needles are used to suture skin. Non-absorbable sutures are generally preferred, but require subsequent removal. Interrupted sutures have the advantage over a continuous suture in that the removal of one or two appropriately sited stitches may allow adequate drainage if the wound becomes infected. The sutures should be placed equidistant from one another, taking equal 'bites' on either side of the wound. A sufficient number should be inserted to maintain apposition without the skin edges gaping. The size of bite is determined by the amount of subcutaneous fat and by whether or not the fat has been separately sutured. For abdominal wounds, 5 mm bites are taken on either side of the wound, whereas on the face a 1–2 mm bite is preferred. The wound edge is picked up with toothed dissecting forceps, then the needle is introduced through the skin at an angle as close to vertical as possible and brought out on the other side at a similar angle.

Similar principles apply when using a continuous suture. A subcuticular continuous suture is preferred by some surgeons and avoids the small pinpoint scars at the site of entry and exit of interrupted sutures, or the ugly cross-hatching that results if sutures are tied too tightly or left in too long. Table 8.2 gives the suggested times for removal of sutures. Cosmetic results as good as those achieved by subcuticular suturing can be obtained by removing sutures in half the times listed in Table 8.2 and by replacing them with adhesive strips (e.g. Steristrip). Skin stapling is commonly used for closure of wounds at any site, as it can be undertaken rapidly. The staples are supplied in disposable cartridges for single patient use and are easily removed.

AIRWAY PROCEDURES

Maintaining the airway

The ability to maintain the airway is a basic skill that every doctor, nurse, paramedic and indeed member of the general public should have. Its simplicity belies its importance, but it is a life-saving skill, which must be learnt through practice.

In the unconscious patient, muscles that normally maintain a clear airway become lax. The tongue and soft tissue fall backwards, particularly in the supine patient, occluding the airway. Maintaining a clear airway allows the patient to breathe or allows the lungs to be ventilated.

Procedure

The simplest manoeuvre is to place the patient on their side with the neck extended in the so-called 'recovery position'. This allows the tongue and soft tissues to fall clear of the larynx and provide a patent airway. The mouth and pharynx should be checked and cleared of debris, such as dentures, vomit or food.

When the patient has to be kept supine, the neck should be extended. The mouth is opened slightly and the mandible pulled firmly forward by pressure applied behind both angles of the jaw. The mandible is held in this position by closing the mouth and using the teeth as a splint. Forward

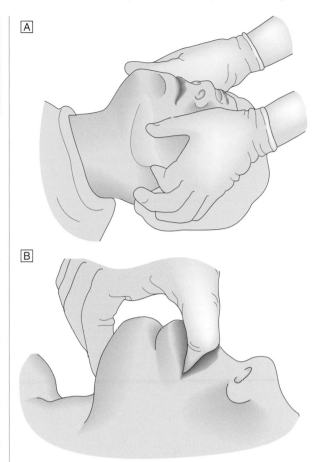

Fig. 8.1 Maintaining the airway. [A] The jaw-thrust manoeuvre. [B] The chin-lift manoeuvre.

pressure is maintained behind the angles of the jaw (*jaw-thrust* manoeuvre) or submentally (*chin-lift* manoeuvre), avoiding pressure on the soft tissues (Fig. 8.1). In some cases, particularly in edentulous patients, an oropharyngeal airway helps to maintain a patent airway.

Ventilation by mask

The lungs may be ventilated by mask and bag, using one of two systems. The first is a rebreathing bag with an adjustable valve and fresh gas supply (which should be present in each anaesthetic room, intensive therapy unit and resuscitation room). The second and more widespread is the self-reinflating type of bag, such as the 'Ambu' or 'Laerdal' bags, which do not rely on a gas supply but to which supplemental oxygen can be added. For the inexperienced, this technique is best performed with the help of an assistant.

Procedure

The airway is held patent with the patient supine, as described above. A mask is applied to the face and held in position using the thumb and index fingers of both hands. The little fingers of each hand are placed behind the angles of the jaw and used to lift the mandible forward. The ring and middle fingers are placed on the mandible to help maintain this position. The assistant squeezes the bag to ventilate the lungs. The adequacy of ventilation is assessed by observing appropriate chest movement.

With more experience, it is possible to maintain a patent airway and hold the mask on with one hand, and squeeze the bag with the other.

The laryngeal mask airway

This airway device is designed to be inserted into the pharynx, and has a cuff that, when inflated, forms a cup around the larynx. It is not a replacement for endotracheal intubation and does not protect the airway from aspiration. It does, however, provide a patent airway when positioned correctly, and allows effective ventilation of the lungs. As with other procedures, insertion should be learned under supervision.

Procedure

For men a size 4 is suitable, and for women a size 3, with smaller sizes being available for children. The cuff should be deflated and lubricated with gel. The patient's head is maintained in an extended position using the left hand, and the airway is held in the right hand and introduced into the mouth (Fig. 8.2). The airway is passed backwards over the tongue until resistance is felt. It should then be at the level of the larynx. The cuff is inflated and the airway should be seen to rise slightly out of the mouth. Position is confirmed by the ability to ventilate the lungs.

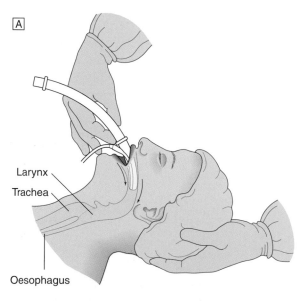

Larynx

Trachea

Oesophagus

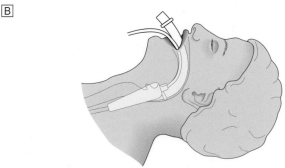

Fig. 8.2 Insertion of a laryngeal mask airway. A Gentle insertion of airway with head in extended position. B Advancement of airway.

Endotracheal intubation

Endotracheal intubation can be life-saving; it can maintain a patent airway, facilitate oxygenation and prevent aspiration. Every opportunity should be taken to acquire this skill in the elective situation in the anaesthetic room.

Procedure

The patient's neck is flexed and the head extended at the atlanto-occipital joint. Retaining a pillow under the head but leaving a space free from beneath the shoulders will usually help to attain this position. Failure to position the patient correctly is one of the most common causes of difficulty in intubation.

The laryngoscope is held in the left hand; its blade is inserted into the right side of the patient's mouth and passed backwards along the side of the tongue into the oropharynx. The blade is designed to push the tongue over to the left side of the mouth. Care is taken to avoid damage to the lips and teeth. The laryngoscope is *pulled* upwards and forwards, *not* used as a lever, to lift the tongue and jaw and reveal the epiglottis (Fig. 8.3). The blade is then advanced to the base of the epiglottis and the laryngoscope pulled further upwards and forwards to reveal the vocal cords.

For men, a 9 mm cuffed tube is usually appropriate, and for women an 8 mm tube is generally used. For children, a rough rule of thumb to gauge tube size is age divided by 4, + 4.5 mm. Normally, an uncuffed tube is used in children.

The endotracheal tube is passed through the vocal cords into the trachea and advanced until its cuff is about 1 cm through. Many endotracheal tubes have a mark to indicate this position. The laryngoscope blade is then withdrawn and the cuff inflated to provide an airtight seal in the trachea.

The most serious complication of endotracheal intubation is failure to recognize misplacement of the tube, particularly in the oesophagus or, to a lesser degree, in the right main bronchus. Misplacement is best avoided by direct visualization

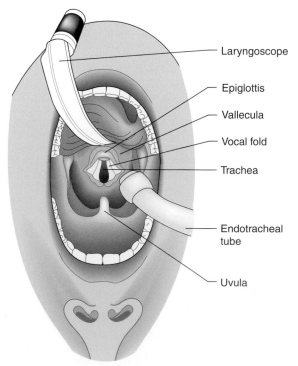

Laryngoscope

Epiglottis

Vallecula

Vocal fold

Trachea

Endotracheal tube

Uvula

Fig. 8.3 Oral endotracheal intubation.

of passage of the tube between the vocal cords, inspection of the chest wall for equal movement of both sides of the chest, and auscultation for breath sounds bilaterally in the mid-axillary line. Absence of breath sounds or the presence of only quiet ones in the epigastrium is a further reassuring sign. If there is any doubt about the position of the tube, it should be removed and ventilation instituted by mask.

Surgical airway

Inability to intubate the trachea is an indication for creating a surgical airway. In the emergency situation, such as in patients with severe facial trauma or pharyngeal oedema secondary to burns, the insertion of a large-calibre plastic cannula through the cricothyroid membrane (**needle cricothyroidotomy**) below the level of the obstruction can be life-saving. Intermittent jet insufflation of oxygen at 15 litres/min (1 sec inspiration and 4 secs to allow expiration) can provide oxygenation for a limited period (30–45 minutes) until a more definitive procedure can be undertaken.

Surgical cricothyroidotomy is performed by making an incision that extends through the cricothyroid membrane and inserting a tracheostomy tube.

In children, care must be taken to avoid damage to the cricoid cartilage, which is the only circumferential support to the upper trachea. Surgical cricothyroidotomy is therefore not recommended for children under 12 years of age.

Procedure

It is important to check all equipment and connections before starting. With the patient in the supine position and the neck in a neutral position, the thyroid cartilage (Adam's apple) and cricoid cartilage are palpated. The cricothyroid membrane lies between the lower border of the thyroid cartilage and the upper border of the cricoid cartilage. The skin is cleansed with antiseptic solution and local anaesthetic infiltrated into the skin, if the patient is conscious. The thyroid cartilage is stabilized with the left hand and a small transverse skin incision made over the cricothyroid membrane. The blade of the scalpel is inserted through the membrane and then rotated through 90° to open the airway. An artery clip or tracheal spreader may be inserted to enlarge the opening enough to admit a cuffed endotracheal or tracheostomy tube (Fig. 8.4). The central trocar of the tube is removed and the tube connected to a bag-valve or ventilator circuit. The cuff is then inflated and air entry to each side of the chest is checked. The tube is secured to prevent dislodgement.

Formal open tracheostomy may be performed as an emergency procedure, but is more commonly undertaken in critically ill patients requiring long-term ventilation. It is a procedure for an experienced clinician and involves making an inverted U-shaped opening through the second, third and fourth tracheal rings.

Changing a tracheostomy tube

It is common practice to change a tracheostomy tube every 7 days. Suction must be available.

Procedure

If a cuffed tube is to be inserted, the integrity of the cuff is checked and it is then fully deflated. Lubricant gel is applied to both the cuff and tube. The patient is placed semi-recumbent with the neck extended. If replacement is likely to be difficult, a suction catheter inserted into the old tracheostomy tube can be used as an introducer for the new tube.

The cuff of the old tube is deflated. Secretions often collect above the cuff and enter the trachea when it is deflated, causing the patient to cough; both patient and operator should be alert to this. Because the tube is curved, it should be removed with an 'arc-like' movement. The site is then cleansed and any secretions are removed. In the spontaneously breathing stable patient, there is no need for undue haste. The new tube is inserted with a similar movement to that employed for removal, and its cuff inflated.

Any signs of respiratory distress should raise suspicion of the possibility of misplacement or occlusion of the tube. The tube and trachea are immediately checked for patency by passing a suction catheter through the tube. If the catheter passes easily into the respiratory tract, usually signified by the patient coughing as the catheter touches the carina, other causes for respiratory distress should be sought.

When the tracheostomy is no longer needed, an airtight dressing is applied over the site after removing the tube. There is no need for formal surgical closure at this stage, as in most instances the wound will close and heal spontaneously. For the first few days, patients should be encouraged to press firmly on the dressing when they wish to cough, so as to avoid air leakage through the tracheostomy site.

THORACIC PROCEDURES

Intercostal tube drainage

Intercostal intubation is used to drain a large pneumothorax, haemothorax or pleural effusion. To drain a pneumothorax, a size 14–16 Fr catheter is inserted, using a lateral approach in the mid-axillary line of the sixth intercostal space. Drainage of an effusion or haemothorax requires a larger drain (20–26 Fr), which should be inserted in the seventh, eighth or ninth intercostal space in the posterior axillary line. A slightly higher insertion in the mid-axillary line may be technically easier in supine, acutely ill patients.

Procedure

If a low lateral approach is to be used, reference should be made to the chest X-ray to ensure that the drain will not be inserted subdiaphragmatically. A strict aseptic technique must be used. The skin, intercostal muscles and pleura are infiltrated with local anaesthetic. If a rib is encountered by the needle, the tip is 'walked' up the rib to enter the pleura above the rib edge. The depth at which the pleural space is entered is determined by aspiration with the syringe. A 3 cm horizontal incision is now made in the skin. A tract is developed by blunt dissection through the subcutaneous tissues and the intercostal muscles are separated just superior to the top of the rib to avoid damage to the neurovascular bundle. The parietal pleura is punctured with the tip of a pair of artery forceps and a gloved finger is inserted into the pleural cavity (Fig. 8.5). This ensures the incision is correctly placed, prevents injury to other organs, and permits any adhesions or clots to be cleared. The trocar is removed from the thoracostomy tube, the proximal end is clamped, and the tube is advanced into the pleural space to the desired length. The tube is sutured to the skin with a heavy suture to prevent accidental dislodgement. A 'Z' suture is placed around the incision, wrapped tightly around the drainage tube and tied, thus securing the tube. A sterile dressing and an adhesive bandage are applied to form an airtight seal and prevent aspiration of air around the tube. The drainage tube is attached to an underwater drainage system and a chest X-ray is then obtained. Low-pressure suction may be applied to the drainage bottle to assist drainage or re-expansion of the lung.

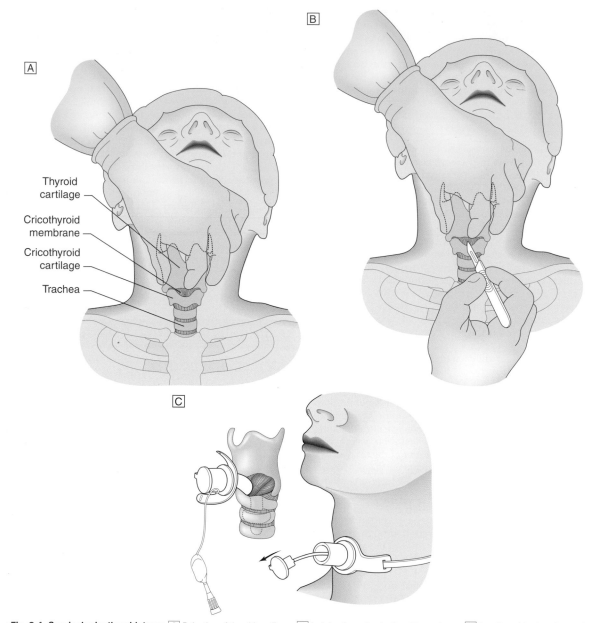

Fig. 8.4 Surgical cricothyroidotomy. [A] Palpation of thyroid cartilage. [B] Incision through cricothyroid membrane. [C] Insertion of tracheostomy tube.

Removal of an intercostal drainage tube

The drainage tube may be removed 12–24 hours after cessation of drainage. As a precaution in the case of pneumothorax, the tube is first clamped for several hours and a chest X-ray taken to ensure that there has been no recurrence.

Procedure

The 'Z' suture is freed from the tube and can be used to close the wound. Where this is not possible, the suture should be totally removed and a new one inserted around the wound. Patients are asked to hold their breath in expiration and the tube is withdrawn, after which the skin is firmly closed with the previously inserted suture. A sterile dressing is firmly applied over the wound and a chest X-ray repeated to confirm that there is no pneumothorax.

Pleural aspiration

Aspiration of fluid from the pleural cavity is performed for diagnostic or therapeutic purposes. Protein or amylase content, and cytological or bacteriological examination may be diagnostic. Complete aspiration of large effusions allows fuller expansion of the lungs and may improve ventilation.

Procedure

Where aspiration is to be undertaken for diagnostic purposes only, a 21-gauge needle and syringe are adequate. For therapeutic aspiration, a larger-bore needle, 50 ml syringe and three-way tap system should be used. The procedure is carried out using a strict aseptic technique.

The patient is positioned sitting up, resting the arms and elbows on a table. The position and size of the effusion

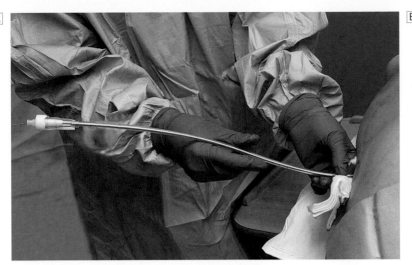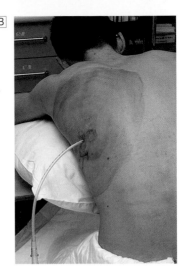

Fig. 8.5 Chest drain. A Insertion. B In situ.

should be outlined by percussion and chest X-ray. The lower border of the effusion is determined, particularly on the right to avoid puncturing the liver. In the case of small effusions, ultrasound guidance is helpful.

The skin, intercostal muscles and pleura are infiltrated with local anaesthetic in the seventh or eighth space, in line with the inferior angle of the scapula. The needle is advanced over the upper border of the rib to avoid damage to the neurovascular bundle. Continuous suction should be applied to the syringe and the needle advanced no further than is required to aspirate fluid freely, thereby avoiding damage to the underlying lung.

If the volume of fluid to be removed is greater than the volume of the syringe being used, a three-way tap greatly reduces the risk of air entry and allows the syringe to be emptied into a collection vessel (Fig. 8.6); this avoids having to disconnect the syringe each time it is filled. It is normally recommended that no more than 1–1.5 litres of fluid be removed at any one time. This reduces the risk of sudden mediastinal shift or the development of pulmonary oedema

associated with rapid re-expansion of a collapsed lung. Coughing or pain on aspiration is an indication that visceral pleura is in close contact with the end of the cannula, which should be repositioned or withdrawn.

At the end of the procedure, the needle is withdrawn and a sterile dressing applied. A chest X-ray is taken to assess the amount of residual fluid present and to exclude a pneumothorax.

ABDOMINAL PROCEDURES

Nasogastric tube insertion

A nasogastric tube is inserted to drain stomach contents in conditions such as intestinal obstruction, or to administer enteral nutrition. In most situations, a 14–16 Fr single-lumen radio-opaque nasogastric tube with multiple distal openings will suffice. Double-lumen tubes are occasionally used to allow continuous low-pressure suction and to prevent the lumen from becoming blocked by gastric mucosa.

Procedure

The nose is inspected for any deformity and the more patent nasal passage is chosen for insertion. The patient is placed in the sitting position and a local anaesthetic spray may be used to anaesthetize the nasal passage. The tube is well lubricated with gel and passed backwards along the floor of the nasal passage (Fig. 8.7). A slight resistance may be felt as the tube passes from the nasopharynx to the oropharynx, and the patient should be warned that a retching sensation may be experienced at this point.

The patient is now asked to swallow, and with each swallow the tube is advanced down the oesophagus. It is important not to push the tube rapidly and force its insertion in a patient who is retching; rather, slow and steady progress should be sought, with small advancements made during each act of swallowing. The oesophago-gastric junction is about 40 cm from the incisor teeth, and ideally, about 10–15 cm of the tube should be placed into the stomach. Most nasogastric tubes have markings to allow measurement of the length inserted. Correct placement of the tube is confirmed by free aspiration of gastric contents, and by auscultation in the epigastrium while 20 ml of air is insufflated. Once in place, the tube is fixed to the nose with adhesive tape.

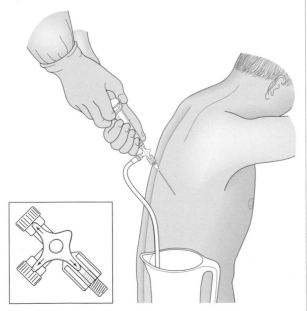

Fig. 8.6 Pleural aspiration.

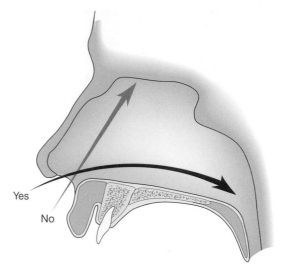

Yes

No

Fig. 8.7 Nasogastric intubation. Note the correct direction for inserting the tube.

In patients with head injuries, the nasal route is avoided because of the risk of introducing infection – or even the nasogastric tube itself – into the central nervous system through an open fracture of the skull base. The oral route is also considered in patients with serious coagulopathy, as passage of the tube through the nose may result in significant haemorrhage. Finally, blind passage of a tube in the early period following oesophagectomy should never be attempted, as this may disrupt the anastomosis.

Fine-bore nasogastric tubes

Elemental diets tend to have an unpleasant taste and are poorly tolerated when swallowed normally. Such diets are therefore best given by infusion through a fine-bore nasogastric tube, which is more comfortable and less likely to cause oesophageal erosions than a standard nasogastric tube. It does, however, require great care in insertion, as it can easily pass into the respiratory tract. A chest X-ray should be obtained to confirm placement in the stomach and not the lung before feeding commences.

Procedure

Fine-bore nasogastric tubes have a wire stylet to facilitate passage. The tube is passed in the same way as a standard nasogastric tube. Again, it is important not to force the tube but to advance it slowly and steadily with each swallowing action made by the patient. The position of the tube is confirmed by X-ray, and only then is the stylet removed. Once removed, it must never be reintroduced while the tube remains in place, as there is a significant risk of perforating both the tube and the oesophagus. The tube tends to collapse if aspirated, so that aspiration cannot be used to check its position.

It is often advantageous to position the fine-bore feeding tube in the jejunum. This can be achieved using a radiological imaging technique or by the use of an enteral feeding tube with a mercury-filled tip that 'self-propels' into the jejunum.

Gastric lavage

The most common indication for gastric lavage is the removal of ingested poisons or drugs. Much less frequently, it is used to lower or raise the core body temperature.

Aspiration of gastric contents is a serious risk. If there is any doubt about the patient's ability to maintain the airway, expert assistance must be sought and endotracheal intubation considered prior to the procedure. The patient's level of consciousness, the presence of a gag reflex and the ability to cough are the most useful guides to the need for endotracheal intubation.

Procedure

After the need for endotracheal intubation is assessed, the patient is placed on the left side in the recovery position, with a 15° head-down tilt of the trolley. A large-bore gastric tube is introduced into the mouth. A mouth gag is useful to prevent the patient from biting the tube. As the tube is passed into the oropharynx and upper oesophagus, the patient is likely to gag and even to vomit. The tube is advanced into the stomach and its correct position confirmed by the free flow of gastric contents. If there is doubt, auscultation of the epigastrium during injection of air down the tube will confirm correct placement. About 100–200 ml of warm water is passed down the tube into the stomach. The end of the tube is then lowered below the level of the stomach into a collecting bucket, and gastric contents are allowed to syphon out. The manoeuvre is repeated until the returned water becomes clear. It is important to avoid over-distension of the stomach. Activated charcoal can be instilled into the stomach to act as an absorbent, if this is appropriate. On completion of lavage, the tube is removed.

Oesophageal tamponade

The Sengstaken tube is a gastric aspiration tube with inflatable gastric and oesophageal balloons, which may be used for emergency treatment of bleeding oesophageal varices. A modification, the Sengstaken–Blakemore or Minnesota tube (see Fig. 14.9), has an additional channel to allow the aspiration of saliva from the oesophagus above the level of the oesophageal balloon.

The use of a Sengstaken–Blakemore tube is generally a temporary measure to control haemorrhage prior to definitive treatment, or to allow transfer of the patient to a specialist centre. It is advisable to deflate the oesophageal balloon for 5 minutes every 6 hours to avoid the risk of ischaemic necrosis and ulceration of the oesophageal mucosa. The tube is not normally kept in place for more than 24 hours.

Procedure

The Sengstaken–Blakemore tube should be stored in a refrigerator, as this renders it less pliable and thus facilitates insertion. The oesophageal and gastric balloons are checked for leaks and then completely deflated using an aspiration syringe prior to insertion. The tube is inserted in the same way as a normal nasogastric tube. However, it is much more uncomfortable and local anaesthesia is recommended for nasal passage. A patient with bleeding varices is unlikely to cooperate fully and the tube may have to be passed with the patient on his or her side. If there is difficulty inserting the tube via the nasal route, the oral route may be used.

The tube is advanced approximately 60 cm and the gastric balloon inflated with 150–200 ml of air or water. The tube is then drawn back until this lower balloon impacts at the cardia. An assistant holds the tube in this position under slight tension, and the oesophageal balloon is inflated with air to a pressure of approximately 40 mmHg, checked by attaching a sphygmomanometer. The tube is secured in position with tape, but no additional traction is necessary.

The stomach is aspirated regularly through the main lumen of the tube to check for further bleeding. This lumen may also be used for the administration of medication, such as lactulose and neomycin. A fourth lumen allows aspiration of the upper oesophagus and pharynx and reduces the risk of bronchial aspiration. In patients who are stuporose or comatose, the airway should be protected by an endotracheal tube.

Abdominal paracentesis

Abdominal paracentesis is performed to relieve the discomfort caused by distension with ascitic fluid, or to obtain fluid for cytological examination. The bladder must be emptied, if necessary by preliminary catheterization. A 'Trocath' peritoneal dialysis catheter with multiple side perforations over a length of 8 cm is inserted under sterile conditions.

Procedure

The operator scrubs up and wears a gown and gloves. A site is chosen for insertion of the catheter. This can be either in the midline (one-third of the way from the umbilicus to the pubic symphysis), or in the right or left iliac fossa (at the junction of the outer and middle thirds of a line drawn from the umbilicus to the anterior superior iliac spine). The vicinity of scars should be avoided, as adhesions increase the risk of bowel perforation. Local anaesthetic is infiltrated through all layers of the abdominal wall. The depth at which the peritoneum is entered is determined by aspiration with the syringe.

A 3 mm stab incision is made in the skin with a scalpel. The trocar is introduced into the catheter and the shaft of the catheter is held firmly between left thumb and index finger some 4–5 cm higher than the estimated depth of the peritoneum. This prevents 'overshoot' as the right hand inserts the trocar and catheter through the abdominal wall into the peritoneum (Fig. 8.8).

The catheter is then advanced further with the left hand while the trocar is withdrawn with the right. If any resistance is encountered, the catheter is withdrawn 2–3 cm, rotated 180° and then advanced again. The minimum final length of catheter within the peritoneal cavity must be 10 cm. If this position is not obtained, the side perforations of the catheter may lie within the abdominal wall and allow troublesome extravasation of ascitic fluid into the subcutaneous tissues. The catheter is secured to the skin and attached via a connection tube with a flow-control clamp to a sterile drainage bag (Fig. 8.9).

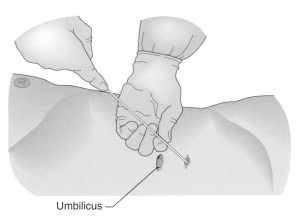

Umbilicus

Fig. 8.8 Insertion of a peritoneal dialysis catheter.

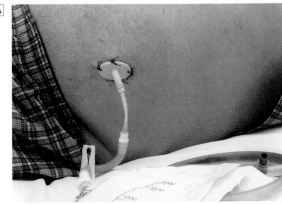

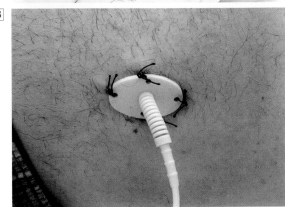

Fig. 8.9 Abdominal paracentesis catheter in situ. [A] Catheter inserted in left iliac fossa. [B] Flange of catheter secured with sutures.

Drainage of large volumes of ascitic fluid must be accompanied by intravenous infusion of albumin in order to avoid precipitating a marked shift of fluid from the intravascular compartment into the peritoneal cavity. This prevents significant haemodynamic changes and reduces the risk of developing cardiovascular instability, renal impairment or hepatic encephalopathy.

Diagnostic peritoneal lavage

This procedure may be undertaken to look for the presence of blood or intestinal contents following blunt abdominal trauma. If the patient is stable, a CT scan of the abdomen is the investigation of choice; however, diagnostic peritoneal lavage (DPL) is indicated in unconscious trauma patients, in patients with multiple injuries and unexplained shock, or in patients with equivocal physical signs. The patient should have a nasogastric tube and a urethral or suprapubic catheter inserted prior to DPL, to reduce the risk of injury to the stomach or bladder.

Procedure

This procedure can be performed using a closed or open technique, the latter being favoured to minimize the risk of intra-abdominal injury. Under sterile conditions and following the instillation of local anaesthesia, a 5 cm vertical subumbilical incision is made and dissection continued through the subcutaneous tissue and linea alba. The peritoneum is opened and a cannula inserted into the peritoneal cavity and advanced into the pelvis. A syringe is connected to the dialysis catheter, and if frank blood is immediately aspirated, this is a positive DPL result. If gross blood is not obtained, 1 litre of warm sterile isotonic saline is infused and

8

allowed to distribute evenly throughout the peritoneal cavity. The fluid is then retrieved by placing the infusion bag on the floor and allowing the effluent to drain from the abdomen by gravity. An unequivocal test will reveal gross evidence of blood, bile or faeces. If necessary, fluid can be sent to the laboratory for analysis. A positive result is obtained if the red cell count is $> 100 \times 10^9$, the white cell count is $> 0.5 \times 10^9$ or the amylase is $> 175\,U/ml$.

VASCULAR PROCEDURES

Venepuncture

The antecubital fossa is the most convenient site, as the median cubital vein, median vein of the forearm and the cephalic vein are all easily accessible (Fig. 8.10). Care must be taken to avoid the brachial artery. Sampling from smaller veins on the forearm or the back of the hand may at first sight appear more attractive, but these veins collapse easily on aspiration and adequate samples are difficult to obtain. In cases of extreme difficulty, the femoral vein should be considered. This vessel lies medial to the femoral artery, which is used as a landmark. In adults, a 21-gauge needle is used; in children, a 23- or 25-gauge will suffice.

Procedure

A venous tourniquet is applied to the upper arm and the patient is encouraged to clench the fist several times to increase venous filling. The position of the vein is identified and the skin cleansed. The needle is advanced through the skin and into the vein, with the needle bevel facing upwards. This manoeuvre is carried out in a 'two-step' fashion, first through the skin and then through the vein wall. Entry through the skin with a decisive action causes much less discomfort than a slow hesitant movement. The needle is advanced 2–3 mm into the vein and the position of the needle and syringe stabilized with one hand. The

plunger of the syringe is slowly withdrawn with the other hand until the required amount of blood is obtained. The tourniquet is then released, the needle withdrawn and pressure immediately applied over the site of entry into the vein to prevent haematoma formation, which is painful for the patient and makes subsequent sampling more difficult.

The blood is placed into the appropriate sample tubes after removal of the needle from the syringe. With pre-vacuumed sample tubes, the needle should be left on the syringe in order to fill the tubes. Haemolysis invalidates some results – for example, potassium and phosphate levels – and is more likely to occur when smaller needles are used. It can be minimized by slow withdrawal of blood into the syringe.

Safety measures

Used needles and syringes should be placed in specially reinforced carriers – 'cin-bins' – to avoid the risk of needle-stick injury or blood contamination to portering or other staff. To further reduce the risk of blood spillage or contamination to medical and laboratory staff, systems have now been introduced in which the sample tubes themselves are modified so that they may be used as syringes, and sent to the laboratory without the need to transfer blood from syringe to tube.

Venepuncture for blood culture

This procedure is carried out for microbiological culture and identification of organisms that may be present in the blood. The procedure is similar to venepuncture but particular care must be taken to avoid contamination. The skin must be thoroughly cleansed and a strict 'no-touch' technique used.

Procedure

A venous tourniquet is applied, as before. The patient's skin is thoroughly cleansed with an appropriate solution, using a sterile swab or cotton wool ball. Venepuncture is performed without the operator touching the skin around the site of entry of the needle. After withdrawal, the needle is removed from the syringe and a second sterile needle substituted. This is then used to introduce the appropriate aliquot of blood into both aerobic and anaerobic culture bottles. Exact volumes of blood required and the number of bottles filled will depend on local laboratory policies. All blood culture bottles should be sent immediately to the laboratory or, if this is not possible, placed in an incubator at 37°C until transport is available.

Peripheral venous cannulation

Most intravenous infusions are given into the forearm. The veins of the leg are generally avoided because of the greater risk of thrombosis. Intravenous cannulae should not be sited over joints, if possible, as this necessitates splinting and reduces the free use of the arm by the patient. Even with splinting, cannulae are subject to more movement in these positions and are prone to more complications.

A wide range of cannulae are commercially available but all consist essentially of an outer flexible sheath and an inner metal needle. A 16- or 18-gauge cannula will suffice for most purposes in adults. Where rapid infusions of large quantities of fluid are required, a larger cannula should be used.

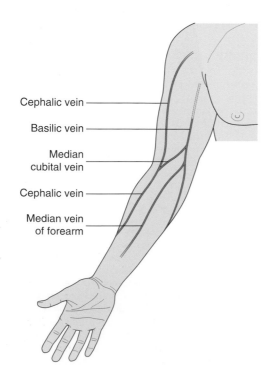

Cephalic vein
Basilic vein
Median cubital vein
Cephalic vein
Median vein of forearm

Fig. 8.10 Venepuncture sites.

Procedure

A venous tourniquet is applied, the site of insertion chosen and the skin is cleansed. Venepuncture is made in the 'two-step' fashion described above and confirmed by a 'flashback' of blood into the cannula. The cannula is initially advanced 2–3 mm into the vein, and then the cannula sheath is advanced into the vein with one hand while the metal needle is partially withdrawn with the other.

Once the cannula sheath is fully inserted into the vein, the tourniquet is released and gentle pressure applied over the vein at the tip of the cannula. The metal needle is then fully withdrawn from the cannula and the giving set, previously primed with normal saline, is connected. The cannula and distal 10–15 cm of the giving set are securely fixed to the skin with adhesive tape.

Cannulation sites should be inspected regularly for signs of swelling, erythema or tenderness, which may indicate extravasation, thrombophlebitis or infection. If any of these is present or the patient complains of pain at the site, the infusion must be stopped and the cannula resited. Extravasation may cause tissue necrosis. Thrombophlebitis occurs more readily when small veins are used, or when the pH of the infusate differs significantly from blood pH. The chances of infection increase the longer a cannula is left in situ, and infusion sites must be changed regularly.

Bolus injections through an intravenous cannula should not be made without first ensuring that the cannula is patent and that there is no extravasation.

Venous cutdown

Venous cutdown for fluid replacement is rarely required, except in seriously hypovolaemic patients, usually following trauma and should only be regarded as a temporary measure for resuscitation. The most common site is the long saphenous vein at the ankle (Fig. 8.11) or at the saphenofemoral junction

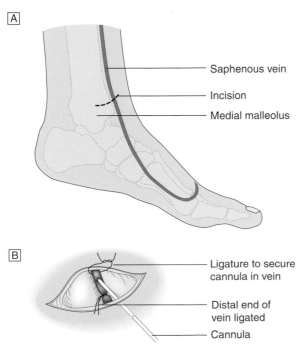

in the groin. Other sites include the basilic vein in the antecubital fossa or the cephalic vein at the wrist.

Procedure

Venous cutdown is performed with an aseptic technique. A transverse incision is made in the skin over the vein, which is then identified by blunt dissection. At the ankle, the site of cutdown is 2–3 cm anterior to the medial malleolus. The vein should be cleared for a distance of 1–2 cm. The distal end of the vein is ligated with an absorbable ligature. A second absorbable ligature is placed under the proximal end of the exposed vein and is elevated to prevent backflow of blood. A transverse incision is then made in the vein. A large-bore cannula is passed through the skin 2 cm below the skin incision and guided into the vein. The cannula is advanced beyond the proximal ligature, which is then tied securely.

The intravenous infusion is then commenced to ensure it flows freely, and the wound is closed with non-absorbable sutures. The cannula is sutured to the skin to prevent accidental displacement and a sterile dressing is applied.

Central venous catheter insertion

Placement of a central venous catheter is indicated for monitoring of the central venous pressure (CVP) and for prolonged drug administration or parenteral nutrition. It is recommended that all central lines are placed under ultrasound guidance to reduce complications arising for collateral damage to surrounding structures

Strict aseptic technique is needed, as infection is one of the most common complications of this procedure. If the catheter is to be used for drug therapy or parenteral nutrition, the procedure should be carried out in the operating theatre. The common sites of insertion of catheters into the superior vena cava are from the internal jugular vein in the neck, from the subclavian vein, or occasionally from a peripheral vein in the antecubital fossa.

Internal jugular vein cannulation

A high approach at the level of the thyroid cartilage carries the least risk. The right internal jugular vein is preferred, as this provides a straighter route into the superior vena cava and avoids the risk of damaging the thoracic duct on the left. In general, the Seldinger technique is used; several commercial kits are available containing the necessary equipment.

Procedure

The patient is placed in a supine position, with at least 15° head-down tilt to distend the neck veins and reduce the risk of air embolism. The patient's head is turned to the left, unless there is potential for a cervical spine injury following trauma. A wide area on the right side of the neck is cleansed and draped.

The carotid artery is identified at the level of the thyroid cartilage, using the index and middle fingers of the left hand. The internal jugular vein lies just lateral and parallel to it. A bleb of local anaesthetic can be infiltrated into the skin at the proposed puncture site.

Using ultrasound guidance an 18-gauge needle on a 10 ml syringe held in the right hand, the needle is advanced through the skin just lateral to the carotid pulsation, at an angle of 60° to the skin and in the line of the vein (Fig. 8.12). Free aspiration of blood confirms the position of the vein. This manoeuvre is repeated to place a larger (16-gauge) needle in the vein. The flexible 'J' end of the guidewire is now passed through this needle into the vein, and the needle

Fig. 8.11 Saphenous venous cutdown. **A** Incision made anterior to the medial malleolus. **B** Cannula inserted in a proximal direction after ligation of the distal vein.

Labels for figure: Saphenous vein · Incision · Medial malleolus · Ligature to secure cannula in vein · Distal end of vein ligated · Cannula

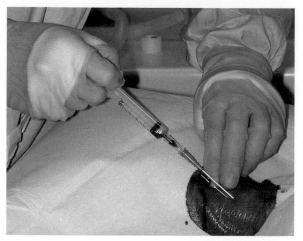

Fig. 8.12 Cannulation of the internal jugular vein. Note the triangle between the sternal and clavicular heads of the sternocleidomastoid muscle.

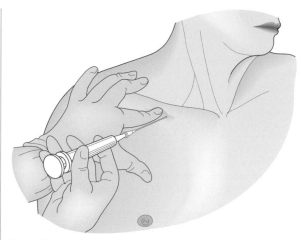

Fig. 8.13 Cannulation of the subclavian vein.

removed over it. This leaves the guidewire in the internal jugular vein. A dilator is now passed over the wire into the vein and then withdrawn. The catheter is advanced over the wire and then the wire is removed, leaving the catheter in situ. In most adults, no more than 15 cm of catheter need be advanced into the vein to ensure correct placement. Blood is then aspirated from the catheter to confirm its position in the major vein. Heparinized saline (5 ml) is injected and the catheter is sutured to the skin to fix it in position. A chest X-ray is taken to check the position of the catheter and to exclude the presence of a pneumothorax, which is a recognized complication.

Subclavian vein cannulation

Subclavian vein cannulation carries a significant risk of causing a pneumothorax or puncturing the subclavian artery and should only be attempted by an experienced operator.

Procedure

The Seldinger technique is generally used to insert a subclavian catheter. The patient should be placed in a supine position, with head-down tilt of at least 15°. A small pad is placed between the shoulder blades to allow the shoulders to drop backwards. Local anaesthetic is infiltrated into the skin and subcutaneous tissue. Under aseptic conditions, a large-calibre needle attached to a 10 ml syringe is introduced 1 cm below the junction of the middle and medial thirds of the clavicle. The needle is directed medially, slightly cephalad and posteriorly behind the clavicle towards the tip of a finger placed in the suprasternal notch (Fig. 8.13). Applying suction, the needle is advanced until blood is withdrawn into the syringe. The syringe is then disconnected, a flexible guidewire inserted through the needle and the needle removed. The catheter is subsequently passed over the guidewire and the latter is withdrawn. The catheter is flushed with heparinized saline and fixed in position. A chest X-ray is taken to check the position and exclude a pneumothorax. An occlusive dressing covers the skin entry point.

Peripheral venous catheterization

In theory, this is the safest approach, as it avoids the risk of pneumothorax. Haemorrhage from accidental arterial puncture or as a result of a coagulopathy can be controlled by pressure. Thrombosis and thrombophlebitis are, however, more frequent compared to the internal jugular or subclavian route.

 SUMMARY BOX **8.1**

Central venous cannulation

- Air embolism is always a risk, even in the head-down position
- When using a guidewire, always hold it at some point along its length while it remains in the patient
- Blood should be easily aspirated from the catheter, if it is correctly positioned
- A chest X-ray should always be taken to confirm the absence of a pneumothorax and correct positioning. A rough guide to position is that the tip of the catheter should lie at the level of the carina on X-ray
- Cannulae inserted for intravenous nutrition are tunnelled in the subcutaneous tissue to emerge on the chest wall at a distance from the site of entry into the vein (Fig. 8.14). This minimizes the risk of sepsis spreading down the tract into the vein.

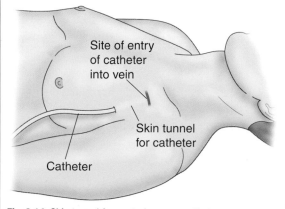

Fig. 8.14 Skin tunnel for central venous catheter.

Procedure

A venous tourniquet is applied to the arm, and a suitable vein selected in the antecubital fossa through which the catheter can be passed. The area is prepared using an aseptic technique and local anaesthetic is infiltrated into the skin at an appropriate site. A large cannula is inserted into the vein, as for normal intravenous cannulation, and the needle withdrawn. The long catheter is passed through the cannula into the vein and the venous tourniquet is then released.

The catheter is advanced up the basilic vein and into the superior vena cava. A guide is often provided to gauge the length of catheter inserted. Difficulty is frequently experienced in advancing the catheter past the axilla, and extension and abduction of the arm may help overcome this. The insertion cannula is then withdrawn from the vein, leaving the long catheter in place. A chest X-ray is taken to confirm placement.

Arterial blood sampling

Arterial blood sampling is undertaken to measure arterial PO_2, PCO_2, $[H^+]$ and standard $[HCO_3^-]$. The radial artery at the wrist is the site of choice. The femoral artery or brachial artery at the elbow may also be used.

A heparinized sample is required to prevent blockage in the blood gas analyzer as a result of coagulation of the sample. There are several commercially available prepeparinized syringes, but an ordinary 2 ml syringe that has been preheparinized as described below will suffice.

Procedure

If the syringe is not preheparinized, up to 0.5 ml of 1000 U/ml heparin is drawn into the syringe. The plunger is then fully withdrawn, following which the air and excess heparin are expelled from the syringe. The residual heparin will be sufficient to anticoagulate the sample. A 23-gauge needle is suitable for arterial puncture.

The course of the artery is defined by palpating the pulse between the index and middle fingers held 2 cm apart. The skin is cleansed and the needle, with its bevel upwards, introduced through the skin at an angle of about 60°. The needle is then advanced into the artery. Correct positioning is confirmed by blood pulsating into the syringe under pressure; 1–1.5 ml is normally sufficient.

The needle is withdrawn and firm pressure applied over the puncture site for 3 minutes to avoid haematoma formation. The needle is removed from the syringe and any air bubbles expelled before capping the syringe. The syringe is gently inverted several times to ensure mixing of the heparin. The sample is sent immediately for analysis. Where delay is anticipated, it should be transported in ice.

Needle pericardiocentesis

Cardiac tamponade may result from penetrating or blunt trauma to the chest. Cardiac function may be significantly impaired by a minimal amount of blood within the fixed, fibrous pericardium. The classic signs are elevated CVP, hypotension and muffled heart sounds (Beck's triad). Immediate pericardiocentesis may be life-saving.

Procedure

The patient should be monitored throughout this procedure, with particular reference to the vital signs, CVP and electrocardiogram (ECG). An aseptic technique is used and the skin in the subxiphoid region is infiltrated with local anaesthetic. The skin is punctured 1–2 cm inferior to the left xiphochondral junction, using a wide-bore plastic-sheathed needle (at least 15 cm in length) with a syringe attached. The needle is angled at 45° and aimed towards the tip of the left scapula (Fig. 8.15). The syringe is aspirated as the needle is advanced, until it easily fills with blood. ECG changes suggest the needle has been advanced too far. Positive pericardiocentesis must be followed by surgical exploration.

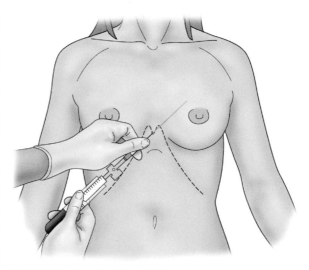

Fig. 8.15 Needle pericardiocentesis.

URINARY PROCEDURES

Urethral catheterization

This procedure may be carried out to relieve urinary retention or to determine urine output when it needs to be closely monitored. Occasionally, catheterization is necessary to facilitate nursing the incontinent patient. Anatomical obstruction may often be the cause of urinary retention in the male. It is particularly important to avoid forcing the passage of the catheter in this procedure, and if difficulty is experienced, assistance should be sought. A full aseptic technique is required for both male and female catheterization.

Procedure in the male

The shaft of the penis is held with a sterile swab, the foreskin if present is retracted and the urethral orifice cleansed with a non-alcoholic, non-iodine-containing solution. The shaft of the penis is held erect with a sterile swab in the left hand and traction applied to elongate the urethra. Lidocaine gel is instilled into the urethra slowly and carefully, with light but steady pressure. It is important to leave the local anaesthetic agent for a sufficient length of time before proceeding with catheterization, as difficulty in male catheterization is often caused by poor analgesia.

The urinary catheter is introduced into the urethra with a 'no-touch' technique and advanced fully to ensure the balloon on the catheter is within the bladder (Fig. 8.16). Correct placement is confirmed by the passage of urine down the catheter. If this does not occur, suprapubic pressure may help. Alternatively, a bladder syringe can be attached to the catheter and aspiration used. With the passage of urine, the balloon on the catheter is inflated with the recommended volume of sterile water (generally, 10–30 ml). The catheter is gently withdrawn until the balloon engages the bladder neck, and it is then connected to the drainage tubing. It is very important that the foreskin, where present, should be replaced over the glans to prevent paraphimosis.

Procedure in the female

A 16–18 Fr catheter is suitable for this procedure. The labia minora are separated with the thumb and fingers of the left hand to expose the urethral meatus on the anterior vaginal wall. The pudenda are now swabbed with antiseptic

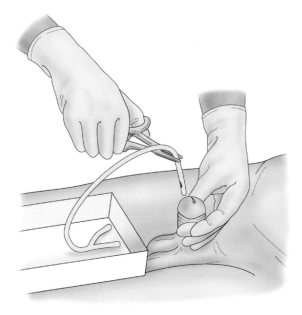

Fig. 8.16 Male catheterization.

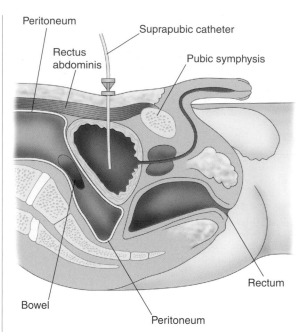

Fig. 8.17 Suprapubic catheterization.

solution. Two swabs are used, each being swept once across the pudenda from anterior to posterior and then discarded.

In general, the catheter need only be inserted for half its length before the passage of urine confirms correct placement. The balloon is inflated and the catheter withdrawn until the balloon impacts in the bladder neck.

Suprapubic catheterization

This procedure is only appropriate when the bladder is distended and urethral catheterization has failed or is contraindicated. It is carried out with a full aseptic technique.

Procedure

The position of the bladder is determined by percussion. Where available, ultrasound guidance is helpful. Generally, the point of insertion lies two finger-breadths above the pubic symphysis in the midline.

The area is cleansed and draped. Local anaesthetic is then infiltrated through all layers of the anterior abdominal wall, using an 18-gauge needle. The depth and position of the bladder can be gauged by the free aspiration of urine through this needle. The needle is withdrawn and a stab incision made in the skin. The trocar and catheter are advanced through the incision, into the bladder (Fig. 8.17). Entry into the bladder is confirmed by the loss of resistance, at which point the catheter is advanced as the trocar is withdrawn. Free passage of urine confirms correct placement. The catheter must be advanced far enough into the bladder so that the balloon, when inflated, is well within the bladder. The balloon is then filled with 10 ml of water and a sterile dressing is applied.

CENTRAL NERVOUS SYSTEM PROCEDURES

Lumbar puncture

Lumbar puncture is carried out to obtain a sample of cerebrospinal fluid (CSF) for diagnostic purposes, to measure the CSF pressure or to introduce materials into the CSF.

It is important to examine the patient beforehand for evidence of raised intracranial pressure, examining the fundi in particular for evidence of papilloedema. Lumbar puncture is contraindicated if there is any suggestion of raised intracranial pressure, as it may result in 'coning' in such patients. The advent of computed tomography (CT) has provided a non-invasive aid to the detection of raised intracranial pressure, and in some conditions, such as subarachnoid haemorrhage, has removed the need for lumbar puncture.

Procedure

Lumbar puncture is carried out using a strict aseptic technique. Patients are placed on one side (usually the left), with their back at the edge of the bed or trolley. They are then asked to curl up as much as possible, to flex the lumbar spine and open up the interspinous spaces (see Fig. 5.4).

The skin is thoroughly cleansed and drapes are applied. The space between the spinous processes of the third and fourth lumbar vertebrae is identified by the point at which a vertical line dropped from the highest point of the iliac crest crosses the spine. Local anaesthetic is infiltrated into the skin and subcutaneous tissues to a depth of about 2 cm. A small stab incision is made in the midline, midway between the two spinous processes.

For most purposes, a 22-gauge spinal needle is adequate. The needle is inserted through the stab incision and advanced in the midline in a slightly headward direction. Entry into the subarachnoid space is felt with a distinct loss of resistance, and will occur in most adults at a depth of 4–6 cm from the skin.

The stylet is withdrawn from the needle and the position confirmed by the free flow of CSF. If the subarachnoid space is not entered or bone is encountered, the position of the needle in the midline should be checked. This is best done by observing (from the side) the angle of the needle in relation to the patient's back. If the needle is in the midline, it should be withdrawn and reinserted in a slightly more headward direction. If the patient experiences pain, a nerve has been touched. The needle should be immediately withdrawn and repositioned.

Once the procedure is complete, the needle is withdrawn and a sterile dressing applied. The patient is usually advised to remain supine for at least 12 hours to minimize the risk of developing a 'spinal' headache. Persistent headache may be a result of continued CSF leakage through the puncture in the dura. In these circumstances, an anaesthetist should be asked to advise on an epidural 'blood patch'. With modern needles, the risk of CSF leakage is lessened and the advice to remain supine for 12–24 hours may be unnecessary.

EXCISION OF LUMPS AND SWELLINGS (E.G. SEBACEOUS CYST, LIPOMA, DERMOID, LYMPH NODE)

The area is cleansed and draped. Local anaesthetic with adrenaline (7 mg/kg) is used to provide a field block. The skin and subcutaneous tissue is incised overlying the swelling and a plane is developed around the swelling using a haemostat. Small blood vessels may be cauterized or ligated. Usually a clean plane of loose areolar tissue is present around these swellings which can be developed by sharp dissection using scissors. Feeding vessels should be deliberately looked for and ligated or cauterized. Special care is required in the case of a sebaceous cyst where skin incision should encircle the punctum to avoid opening the cyst. After excision is completed, haemostasis is ensured and the subcutaneous tissue approximated using absorbable suture. The skin may be closed using subcuticular or interrupted sutures or Steristrips.

IMAGING

Radiological imaging has a central role in the management of surgical patients and may guide various therapeutic procedures. A number of imaging techniques are now available that provide information on the structure and function of systems and organs. The principal imaging techniques include radiography (including plain X-rays, contrast studies and CT), ultrasound, magnetic resonance imaging (MRI) and isotope scanning.

Plain radiography

Radiographs account for the highest proportion of all imaging examinations. X-rays penetrate the body and cast an image either on film or on a fluorescent screen. The image is formed by the differences in attenuation of the various tissues through which the X-rays pass, producing a two-dimensional impression of a three-dimensional structure. On a plain radiograph, bone absorbs most X-rays and appears radio-opaque (white), whereas gas and fat absorb few X-rays and appear radiolucent (dark). If X-ray power (kilovoltage) and exposure time are altered, tissues of varying densities can be visualized. Other calcified tissues, such as most urinary tract stones, old tuberculous lymph nodes and calcified atheromatous plaques, are radio-opaque. Foreign materials, such as metal or glass, are also radio-opaque, but wood and plastic are radiolucent and invisible to X-rays.

Ionizing radiation is potentially harmful. Therefore, unnecessary investigations should be avoided and radiation exposure of patients and staff should be minimized. As the inverse square law determines radiation fall-off with distance, workers should maintain a good distance from the X-ray source during exposure. Radiation received by staff should be monitored by the wearing of X-ray-sensitive film badges, and protective lead aprons should be worn when staff are in exposed situations.

Contrast studies

Radio-opaque contrast media may be used to demonstrate the gastrointestinal, biliary, vascular and urinary tracts. They can either be used to outline anatomical structures directly, or else be concentrated physiologically in an organ (indirect imaging). Barium sulphate is insoluble and is used extensively to investigate the gastrointestinal tract. Gastrografin is a water-soluble contrast medium used if leakage from the gastrointestinal tract into the peritoneal cavity is likely. A barium swallow is used to assess the oesophagus and a barium meal to investigate the stomach and duodenum. Progress of contrast can be observed by fluoroscopic screening, using a technique known as image intensification. The large bowel is studied by giving contrast material rectally (barium enema). A single-contrast enema may be used to determine whether there is a complete mechanical obstruction in the emergency setting; however, improved mucosal detail will be obtained by using a double-contrast technique with barium and gas. Buscopan may be given at the same time to abolish spasm. In the biliary, vascular and urinary tracts, iodine-containing agents are used. The risk of life-threatening anaphylactic reactions with the newer, low-osmolar, non-ionic agents is minimal but these are still recognized complications of intravascular administration. Intravenous contrast is also potentially nephrotoxic in patients with impaired renal function.

Computed tomography (CT)

CT involves use of a series of X-rays directed at a narrow transverse section of the body and detected by multiple receptors. More modern machines spiral around the patient (spiral CT), resulting in more rapid image capture and higher resolution of images. Each element of the beam is attenuated according to the density of the tissue it traverses, and is converted into a grey-scale image that is displayed on a screen as a two-dimensional image. Further information can be gained after administration of oral, rectal or intravenous contrast. Three-dimensional reconstruction can be performed to assess relationships between structures and aid in the discrimination of abnormalities.

Ultrasonography

This is a safe, non-invasive, painless technique that allows the visualization of solid internal organs. Using 1–15 MHz mechanical vibrations (above the range of human hearing), generated and detected by a transducer, an image is obtained because of differences in the reflection of the transmitted sound at the interface of tissues with different impedance. For transcutaneous ultrasonography, the probe must be 'coupled' to the skin with conduction gel to exclude an air interface. Calcified tissue, such as stones, causes an abrupt and marked change in acoustic impedance, resulting in virtually complete reflection of ultrasound and a posterior acoustic shadow. For biliary ultrasound, the patient should be fasted to minimize bowel gas shadows and to reduce gallbladder contraction. Ultrasonography of the pelvis is aided by a full bladder, as this provides a fluid-filled, non-reflective window to scan the pelvic organs.

8

Special probes have now been developed for insertion into various body orifices, such as rectum, vagina and oesophagus, and also through laparoscopic and endoscopic equipment. These probes can be placed closer to the target organ, allowing the use of higher-frequency sound that has lower penetration but greater resolution. Ultrasound can be employed to study blood flow using the Doppler principle. Ultrasound is reflected from the red blood cells, the movement of which causes a frequency shift related to the velocity. This is used to generate an audible signal that can be used to assess whether flow is normal or abnormal. The term duplex ultrasonography is used when the grey scale conventional ultrasound is combined with the Doppler ultrasound to study the vascularity of a limb.

Magnetic resonance imaging (MRI)

MRI, formerly known as nuclear magnetic resonance, involves the application of a powerful magnetic field to the body; this causes the protons of all hydrogen nuclei to behave like magnets. They are initially aligned and then excited by pulses of radio waves at a frequency that causes them to resonate and emit radio signals. These are recorded electronically and, using sophisticated computer technology, images can be displayed in any anatomical plane. T1 and T2 refer to the relaxation times for the hydrogen ions. On a T2 weighted scan, all fluid containing tissues and water are seen as bright images (mimicking contrast) whereas the fat containing tissues remain dark. The reverse of this holds good for T1 weighted scans. Intravenous administration of gadolinium may be used for delineating vascular structures. MRI does not use ionizing radiation, is harmless and provides very good images of soft tissues. It has the disadvantages that it is expensive, time-consuming and unsuitable for patients with pacemakers or metallic implants. An exciting new application of MRI is the study of blood flow and cardiac function. Magnetic resonance angiography (MRA) avoids intravascular injections and is replacing some conventional techniques. Magnetic resonance cholangiopancreatography (MRCP), a type of T2 weighted scan, has now replaced endoscopic retrograde cholangiopancreatography (ERCP) for diagnostic imaging of the biliary tract, as it avoids the potential complications of pancreatitis and bleeding, although ERCP remains a valuable therapeutic tool.

Radioisotope imaging

Radioisotope imaging provides more information about function than structure. Suitable tracer agents combine a substance taken up by the target tissue and a radioactive label. Radioisotopes in common usage include ^{99m}Tc (technetium), ^{123}I and ^{131}I (iodine), ^{111}In (indium), ^{133}Xe (xenon), ^{67}Ga (gallium) and ^{201}Th (thallium). Distribution of radioisotopes is visualized using a gamma camera. The investigation is based upon the localization of the radioactive tracer in the target tissue with the help of the substance specific to the organ (e.g. bi-phosphonates labelled with ^{99m}Tc for bone scan) or the tracer uptake directly (e.g. ^{131}I itself for thyroid). Investigations employing radioisotope techniques include bone scanning, lung scanning to detect pulmonary emboli, renal scanning for detecting cortical scarring (DMSA) or renal function (DTPA), RBC scan for detection of obscure gastrointestinal bleeding, leucocyte scanning for inflammation and infection, and thyroid scanning.

Positron emission tomography (PET)

PET is a new, more expensive radioisotope technique that is proving useful in the imaging of physiological brain metabolism, tumour detection and functional cardiac imaging. It involves detection of positron emitting radionuclide tracer by a gamma camera. The tracer used is radioactive 2-fluorodeoxy-D-glucose (2FDG), which being an analogue of glucose is metabolized in metabolically active tissue. It is thus a measure of metabolically active tissue rather than the metastasis itself and needs clinical correlation. PET scan can be combined with CT for better anatomical delineation of the area.

9

Postoperative care and complications

INTRODUCTION

Following an operation, there are three phases of patient care. After a short period of immediate postoperative care in a recovery room to ensure the full return of consciousness, the patient is returned to surgical ward care, unless there are indications for transfer to a high-dependency unit or intensive therapy unit. On discharge from ward care, patients may still require rehabilitation and convalescence before they are ready to resume domestic or other activities. This chapter discusses the first two phases, during which attention focuses on the regulation of homeostasis and the prevention, detection and management of complications.

The major life-threatening complications that may arise in the recovery room are airway obstruction, myocardial infarction, cardiac arrest, haemorrhage and respiratory failure. These complications can also arise during ward care, but except for haemorrhage and cardiopulmonary catastrophe, many of the problems arising in this phase do not threaten life and are often specific to the operation performed.

A timeline showing typical times for the development of postoperative complications is given in Figure 9.1.

IMMEDIATE POSTOPERATIVE CARE

Patients who have received a general anaesthetic should be observed in the recovery room until they are conscious and their vital signs are stable. Acute pulmonary, cardiovascular and fluid derangements are the major causes of life-threatening complications in the early postoperative period, and the recovery room provides specially trained personnel and equipment for the observation and treatment of these problems.

In general, the anaesthetist exercises primary responsibility for the patient's cardiopulmonary function, and the surgeon is responsible for the operative site, the wound and any surgically placed drains. Clinical notes should accompany the patient. These include an operation note describing the procedure performed, an anaesthetic record of the patient's progress during surgery, a postoperative instruction sheet with regard to the administration of drugs and intravenous fluids, and a fluid balance sheet.

Monitoring of airway, breathing and circulation is the main priority in the immediate postoperative period (EBM 9.1). The nature of the surgery and the patient's premorbid medical condition will determine the intensity of postoperative monitoring required; however, the patient's colour, pulse, blood pressure, respiratory rate, oxygen saturation and level of consciousness will be routinely observed. The nature and volume of drainage into collecting bags or wound dressings, and urinary output are also monitored, if appropriate. Continuous electrocardiogram (ECG) monitoring is undertaken and oxygenation is assessed by the use of a pulse oximeter. Monitoring of central venous pressure (CVP) may be indicated if the patient is hypotensive, has borderline cardiac or respiratory function, or requires large amounts of intravenous fluids.

EBM 9.1 Optimal postoperative care

'Optimal postoperative care requires clinical assessment and monitoring; respiratory management; cardiovascular management; fluid, electrolyte and renal management; control of sepsis; and nutrition.'

SIGN guideline 77 Postoperative management in adults; 2004.

The patient may initially remain intubated, but following extubation should receive supplemental oxygen by face mask or nasal prongs and should be encouraged to take frequent deep breaths. The patient must breathe adequately and maintain a good colour. Shallow breathing may mean that the patient is still partially paralyzed. A dose of neostigmine can reverse the residual effects of curariform

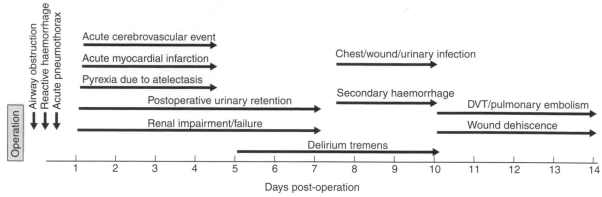

Fig. 9.1 Timeline showing typical times for development of postoperative complications.

agents. Cyanosis is an ominous sign indicating hypoxaemia due to inadequate oxygenation, and may be due to airway obstruction or impaired ventilation. Respiratory depression later on in the postoperative period is usually caused by over-sedation with opioid analgesic agents.

SUMMARY BOX 9.1

Immediate postoperative monitoring

- Airway: attention to maintenance of airway
- Breathing: ensure adequate ventilation
- Circulation: monitor for evidence of blood loss
- Assess the patient's
  - Colour
  - Pulse
  - Blood pressure
  - Respiratory rate
  - Oxygen saturation
  - Level of consciousness.

Airway obstruction

The main causes of airway obstruction are as follows:

- *Obstruction by the tongue* may occur with a depressed level of consciousness. Loss of muscle tone causes the tongue to fall back against the posterior pharyngeal wall, and may be aggravated by masseter spasm during emergence from anaesthesia. Bleeding into the tongue or soft tissues of the mouth or pharynx may be a complicating factor after operations involving these areas.
- *Obstruction by foreign bodies,* such as dentures, crowns and loose teeth. Dentures must be removed before operation and precautions taken to guard against displacement of crowns or teeth.
- *Laryngeal spasm* can occur at light levels of unconsciousness and is aggravated by stimulation.
- *Laryngeal oedema* may occur in small children after traumatic attempts at intubation, or when there is infection (epiglottitis).
- *Tracheal compression* may follow operations in the neck, and compression by haemorrhage is a particular anxiety after thyroidectomy.
- *Bronchospasm or bronchial obstruction* may follow inhalation of a foreign body or the aspiration of irritant material, such as gastric contents. It may also occur as an idiosyncratic reaction to drugs and as a complication of asthma.

Attention is directed at defining and rectifying the cause of airway obstruction as a matter of extreme urgency. Airway maintenance techniques include the chin-lift or jaw-thrust manoeuvres, which lift the mandible anteriorly and displace the tongue forward (see Chapter 8). The pharynx is then sucked out, an oropharyngeal airway is inserted to maintain the airway, and supplemental oxygen is administered. If cyanosis does not improve or if stridor persists, reintubation may be necessary.

Haemorrhage

Significant blood loss via a surgical drain, particularly if associated with hypovolaemic shock, is an indication for immediate transfer of the patient from the recovery room back to the operating theatre for re-exploration and control of the bleeding source. Reactive bleeding is usually caused by a slipped ligature or dislodgement of a diathermy coagulum as the blood pressure recovers from the operation. Superficial bleeding into the surgical wound rarely requires immediate action; however, patients who have undergone neck surgery must be observed for the accumulation of blood in the wound. If necessary, the wound can be reopened in the recovery room to prevent airway compression and asphyxia.

Late secondary haemorrhage typically occurs 7–10 days after an operation and is due to infection eroding a blood vessel. Rigid drain tubes may also occasionally erode a large vessel and cause dramatic late postoperative bleeding. Secondary haemorrhage associated with infection is often difficult to control. Interventional radiological techniques may achieve temporary control, but surgical re-exploration is usually indicated.

SURGICAL WARD CARE

General care

Monitoring of vital signs, including temperature, continues on return to the ward. In addition, output from the urinary catheter, nasogastric tube and surgical drains is monitored. The frequency of recordings or measurements can be reduced as the patient stabilizes.

Patients are normally visited morning and evening by the medical staff to ensure that there is steady progress. Anxiety, disorientation and minor changes in personality, behaviour or appearance are often the earliest manifestation of complications. The general circulatory state and adequacy of oxygenation are noted, and vital signs recorded on the nursing chart are checked. Temperature readings provide vital information regarding progress and may give early indication of potentially serious postoperative complications.

The chest is examined and all sputum inspected. Full chest expansion and coughing are encouraged. Following abdominal surgery, the abdomen is examined for evidence of excessive distension or tenderness. The return of bowel sounds and the free passage of flatus reflect recovery of gut peristalsis. The legs are checked for swelling, discoloration or calf tenderness.

Tubes, drains and catheters

If a nasogastric tube is in place, it is kept open at all times to serve as a vent for swallowed air. Free drainage of gastric contents may be supplemented by intermittent manual aspiration. Nasogastric tubes are removed once the volume of aspirate diminishes. It is not necessary to wait until bowel sounds have returned or flatus has been passed. Nasogastric tubes are uncomfortable and may prevent coughing with expectoration, and so they should not be retained for longer than necessary. Surgical drains are generally removed when the volume of effluent diminishes. If a urinary catheter has been placed, it should be removed once the patient is mobile.

Fluid balance

Fluid balance is reviewed regularly. The standard intravenous fluid requirement for an adult is 3 litres/day, of which 1 litre should ordinarily be normal (isotonic) saline and 2 litres should be 5% dextrose. In the first 24 hours after surgery, normal saline can be omitted and replaced by 5% dextrose due to sodium conservation as a result of metabolic response. However, this should be judged according to the patient's general circulatory status, the observed fluid losses, and the daily measurement of serum urea and electrolyte levels. Similarly, it is not necessary to replace potassium within the first 24–48 hours after surgery, as potassium is released from injured cells and tissues at the surgical site in sufficient quantity. Potassium supplements (60–80 mmol daily) can subsequently be added to intravenous fluids, provided urinary output is adequate. Intravenous fluid therapy is discontinued once oral fluid intake has been established.

Blood transfusion

Haemoglobin measurement will be a guide to the need for postoperative blood transfusion. A full blood count should be undertaken within 24 hours of surgery and, as a general rule, blood is administered if the Hb is less than 80 g/l. Above this level, patients can be prescribed oral iron, unless they have cardiovascular instability or are symptomatic from their anaemia. If a blood transfusion is given, pulse, blood pressure and temperature should be monitored to detect a transfusion reaction. Major ABO incompatibility can result in an anaphylactic hypersensitivity reaction, with severe bronchospasm and hypotension, whereas incompatibility of minor factors may result in tachycardia, pyrexia and rash. Other potential complications of blood transfusion are hypothermia (if the blood has not been adequately warmed), hyperkalaemia (due to leakage of potassium from the red blood cells), acidosis (if the blood has been stored for a long period) and coagulation abnormalities (as stored blood is deficient in clotting factors).

Nutrition

Nutrition in postoperative patients is frequently poorly managed. A few days of starvation may cause little harm, but enteral or parenteral nutrition is essential if starvation is prolonged. Enteral nutrition is preferred, as it is associated with fewer complications and is believed to augment gut barrier function. If a prolonged period of starvation is anticipated in the postoperative period, a feeding jejunostomy tube can be inserted at the time of abdominal surgery. Alternatively, a fine-bore nasogastric or nasojejunal feeding tube can be passed (see Chapter 8). If the enteral route cannot be used, total parenteral nutrition can be prescribed. Dietary intake should be monitored in all patients in the postoperative period, and oral high-calorie supplements given if appropriate.

COMPLICATIONS OF ANAESTHESIA AND SURGERY

General complications

Nausea and vomiting can be caused by surgery and/or anaesthesia, and an antiemetic can prove useful. If nausea has been associated with previous anaesthetics, antiemetic drugs should be administered prophylactically. Transient hiccups in the first few postoperative days are usually no more than a nuisance. Persistent hiccups can be a serious complication, exhausting the patient and interfering with sleep, and may be due to diaphragmatic irritation, gastric distension or metabolic causes, such as renal failure. If no precipitating cause can be found, small doses of chlorpromazine may be helpful.

Spinal anaesthesia may cause headache as a result of leakage of cerebrospinal fluid, and patients should remain recumbent for 12 hours after this form of anaesthesia. If headache persists, it may be necessary to seal the injection site in the dura-arachnoid with a 'blood patch' (i.e. an extradural injection of the patient's blood, which clots and so seals the leak). Myalgia affecting the chest, abdomen and neck is a specific complication of suxamethonium administration, and may last for up to a week.

Intravenous administration of irritant drugs or solutions can cause bruising, haematoma, phlebitis and venous thrombosis. Intravenous cannulae, particularly those placed in large veins, should be securely sealed to guard against air embolism. Sites of cannula insertion should be checked regularly for signs of infection, and the cannula replaced if necessary. Arterial cannulae and needle punctures are the most common cause of arterial injury, and may rarely lead to arterial occlusion and gangrene.

Pulmonary complications

Respiratory complications remain the largest single cause of postoperative morbidity and the second most common cause of postoperative death in patients over 60 years of age. Pulmonary complications are more common after emergency operations. Special hazards are posed by pre-existing chronic obstructive pulmonary disease (COPD). Once a patient has fully recovered from anaesthesia, the main respiratory problems are pulmonary collapse and pulmonary infection. Pleural effusion and pneumothorax occur less commonly. Pulmonary embolism is a major complication of deep venous thrombosis, which is considered later.

9

Pulmonary collapse

Inability to breathe deeply and cough up bronchial secretions is the primary cause of pulmonary collapse after surgery. Contributory factors include paralysis of cilia by anaesthetic agents, impairment of diaphragmatic movement, over-sedation, abdominal distension and wound pain. When there is complete obstruction of a bronchus or bronchiole, air in the lung distal to the obstruction is absorbed, the alveolar spaces close (atelectasis), and the affected portion of the lung contracts and becomes solid. Small bronchioles (1 mm or less) are prone to close when lung volume reaches a critical point (closing volume). The closing volume is higher in older patients and in smokers, owing to the loss of elastic recoil of the lung, which increases the risk of atelectasis. The extent of collapse varies from closure of a small segment to collapse of a lobe or, when a main bronchus is obstructed, the entire lung. Atelectasis is a very common complication of surgery and usually occurs within 24 hours. It is of clinical relevance because it leads to increased work of breathing and impaired gas exchange; if untreated, secondary bacterial infection will supervene, causing lobar or bronchopneumonia.

The clinical signs of pulmonary collapse include rapid respiration, tachycardia and mild pyrexia, with diminished breath sounds and dullness to percussion over the affected segment. Arterial P_aO_2 is low and the chest X-ray shows areas of increased opacification.

Preoperative measures to reduce the risk of pulmonary collapse following surgery include stopping smoking before the operation, physiotherapy for patients with COPD, and deferring elective surgery for at least 2 weeks in patients with a chest infection. Practising with an incentive spirometer preoperatively will help.

Postoperatively, pulmonary collapse is prevented by encouraging the patient to breathe deeply, cough and mobilize. Adequate analgesia and regular chest physiotherapy are of great importance in the postoperative period. Placement of an epidural catheter in patients undergoing major abdominal surgery may help alleviate postoperative wound pain. Hypoxia is treated by giving oxygen by mask or nasal prongs, and bronchospasm is relieved by inhalation of salbutamol.

When hypoxia is severe, endotracheal intubation, assisted ventilation and repeated bronchial aspiration may be needed. Posture is important and the patient should initially be placed on the unaffected side to aid expansion of the collapsed lung. Bronchoscopy may be needed to suck out a plug of inspissated secretion.

Pulmonary infection

Pulmonary infection commonly follows pulmonary collapse or the aspiration of gastric secretions. Pyrexia, tachypnoea and green sputum are typical. The chest signs are those of collapse with absent or diminished breath sounds, often in association with bronchial breathing and coarse crepitations from surrounding areas of partial bronchial occlusion. Chest X-ray usually demonstrates patchy fluffy opacities.

The patient is encouraged to cough, and antibiotics are prescribed after sputum is sent for bacteriological examination. Most pulmonary infections are caused by the respiratory commensals, *Streptococcus pneumoniae* and *Haemophilus influenzae,* but many postoperative pulmonary infections are caused by Gram-negative bacilli acquired by aspiration of oropharyngeal secretions. Antibiotics provide the mainstay of treatment. Oxygen is given if there is hypoxia, and more intensive measures, including bronchoscopy and assisted ventilation, are instituted if respiratory function continues to deteriorate.

Respiratory failure

Respiratory failure is defined as an inability to maintain normal partial pressures of oxygen and carbon dioxide (P_aO_2 and P_aCO_2) in arterial blood. Blood gas determinations are the key to its early recognition and should be repeated frequently in patients with previous respiratory problems. The normal P_aO_2 is > 13 kPa at the age of 20 years, falling to around 11.6 kPa at 60 years; respiratory failure is denoted by a value of less than 6.7 kPa. Severe hypoxaemia may result in visible central cyanosis. In type 1 respiratory failure there is hypoxia and in type 2 there is hypercarbia with hypoxia.

Acute respiratory distress syndrome (ARDS)

ARDS is characterized by impaired oxygenation, diffuse lung opacification on chest X-ray and an increasing 'stiffness' of the lungs (decreased compliance). It may result from pulmonary or systemic sepsis, following massive blood transfusion, or as a consequence of aspiration of gastric contents. The syndrome displays a wide spectrum of severity. Many minor and transient cases recover spontaneously, whereas in a proportion of cases, progressive respiratory insufficiency occurs. Tachypnoea with increasing ventilatory effort, restlessness and confusion develop. Hypoxia initially responds to an increase in the oxygen content of inspired air, but progressively increasing concentrations are required to prevent the P_aO_2 from falling. The pathophysiology is unclear, but endotoxin-activated leucocytes are thought to be deposited in the pulmonary capillaries, releasing oxygen-derived free radicals, cytokines and other chemical mediators. Damage to the vascular endothelium results in increased capillary permeability and leakage of fluid, causing widespread interstitial and alveolar oedema. This is seen as bilateral diffuse fluffy opacities on chest X-ray (Fig. 9.2). The lungs become increasingly stiff and difficult to ventilate.

Management includes supportive measures in the form of ventilation with positive end-expiratory pressure (PEEP) and treatment of the underlying condition, i.e. control of infection by antibiotics, drainage of any source of pus and correction of hypovolaemia. The mortality rate of severe ARDS is approximately 50%.

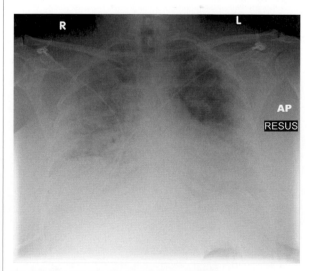

Fig. 9.2 Chest X-rays showing features of ARDS.

Pleural effusion

Small pleural effusions (Fig. 9.3) are not uncommon following upper abdominal surgery, but are usually of no clinical significance. They may be secondary to other pulmonary pathology, such as collapse/consolidation, pulmonary infarction or secondary tumour deposits. The appearance of a pleural effusion 2–3 weeks after an abdominal operation may suggest the presence of a subphrenic abscess. Small effusions may be left alone to reabsorb if they do not interfere with respiration. Alternatively, pleural aspiration is performed and the fluid sent for bacteriological culture.

Pneumothorax

The most common cause of postoperative pneumothorax is the insertion of a central venous line, and a chest X-ray is necessary after this procedure to exclude this potential complication. There is also an enhanced risk of pneumothorax in patients on positive-pressure ventilation, presumably owing to rupture of pre-existing bullae. The insertion of an underwater seal drain is usually followed by rapid expansion of the lung.

Cardiac complications

The risks of anaesthesia and surgery are increased in patients suffering from cardiovascular disease. Whenever possible, arrhythmias, unstable angina, heart failure or hypertension should be corrected before surgery. Valvular disease, especially aortic stenosis, impairs the ability of the heart to respond to the increased demand of the postoperative period. The administration of fluids to patients with severe aortic or mitral valve disease should be carefully monitored.

Myocardial ischaemia/infarction

Although in most cases there is a history of preceding cardiac disease, myocardial ischaemia or cardiac arrest can occur in an otherwise fit patient. Patients with ischaemia may complain of gripping chest pain, but this is not invariable (particularly in the elderly diabetic patient or in the early postoperative period) and hypotension may be the only sign. The absence of symptoms after operation is thought to be due to the residual effects of anaesthesia and to the administration of postoperative analgesia. If ischaemia is suspected, an ECG is performed urgently and arrangements are made for cardiac monitoring. A sample of blood is withdrawn to estimate concentrations of cardiac enzymes. One-third of postoperative myocardial infarctions are fatal.

Cardiac failure

Although acute cardiac failure occurs most often in the immediate postoperative period, patients with ischaemic or valvular heart disease, arrhythmias or major surgical insult can also go into failure in the subsequent recovery period. Clinical manifestations are progressive dyspnoea, hypoxaemia and diffuse congestion on chest X-ray. Excessive administration of fluid in the early postoperative period in patients with limited myocardial reserve is a common cause, which can be avoided by monitoring CVP. Treatment consists of avoiding further fluid overload, and the administration of diuretics and cardiac inotropes.

Arrhythmias

Sinus tachycardia is common and may be a physiological response to hypovolaemia or hypotension. It is also caused by pain, fever, shivering or restlessness. Tachycardia increases myocardial oxygen consumption and may decrease coronary artery perfusion. Sinus bradycardia may be due to vagal stimulation by neostigmine, pharyngeal irritation during suction, or the residual effects of anaesthetic agents. Atrial fibrillation is the most common postoperative arrhythmia. Fast atrial fibrillation may result in haemodynamic disturbances and may require pharmacological intervention. Refractory cases may require cardioversion.

Postoperative shock

Shock is defined as a failure to maintain adequate tissue perfusion. The three main types are hypovolaemic, cardiogenic and septic shock. Hypovolaemic shock may be caused by inadequate replacement of pre- or perioperative fluid losses or postoperative haemorrhage, whereas cardiogenic shock is usually secondary to acute myocardial ischaemia/infarction or an arrhythmia. Hypovolaemic and cardiogenic shock are characterized by tachycardia, hypotension, sweating, pallor and vasoconstriction. Septic shock is characterized in the early stages by a hyperdynamic circulation with fever, rigors, a warm vasodilated periphery and a bounding pulse. Later features include hypotension and peripheral vasoconstriction. Without appropriate management, shock will result in oliguria and the development of multisystem organ failure, and may lead to death.

Urinary complications

Postoperative urinary retention

Inability to void postoperatively is common, especially after groin, pelvic or perineal operations, or operations under spinal/epidural anaesthesia (Fig. 9.4). Postoperative pain, the effects of anaesthesia and drugs, and difficulties in initiating micturition while lying or sitting in bed may all contribute. Males tend to be more commonly affected than females. When its normal capacity of approximately 500 ml is exceeded, the bladder may be unable to contract and empty itself. Frequent dribbling or the passage of small volumes of urine may indicate overflow incontinence, and examination may reveal a distended bladder. The management of acute urinary retention is catheterization of the bladder, with removal of the catheter after 2–3 days (see Chapter 8).

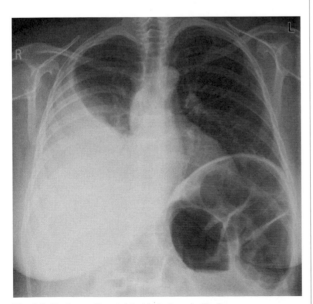

Fig. 9.3 Postoperative right-sided pleural effusion.

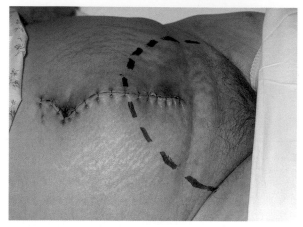

Fig. 9.4 Postoperative urinary retention.

Urinary tract infection

Urinary tract infections are most common after urological or gynaecological operations. Pre-existing contamination of the urinary tract, urinary retention and instrumentation are the principal factors contributing to postoperative urinary infection. Cystitis is manifested by frequency, dysuria and mild fever, and pyelonephritis by high fever and flank tenderness. Treatment involves adequate hydration, proper drainage of the bladder and appropriate antibiotics.

Renal failure

Acute renal failure after surgery results from protracted inadequate perfusion of the kidneys. The most common cause of postoperative oliguria is pre-renal vascular insufficiency from hypovolaemia, water depletion or extracellular fluid depletion. Hypoperfusion of the kidney may be aggravated by hypoxia, sepsis and nephrotoxic drugs. Patients with pre-existing renal disease and jaundice are particularly susceptible to hypoperfusion, and are more likely to develop acute renal failure.

The complication can largely be prevented by adequate fluid replacement before, during and after surgery, so that urine output is maintained at 0.5 ml/kg/hr or more. The importance of monitoring hourly urine output means that bladder catheterization is needed in all patients undergoing major surgery, and in those at risk of renal failure. Early recognition and treatment of bacterial and fungal infections is also important in the prevention of renal failure.

Urine output below 700 ml in 24 hours (or less than 0.5 ml/kg/hr for several hours on catheter drainage) should be considered pathological oliguria. Management involves the restoration of an adequate circulating intravascular compartment by the administration of intravenous fluids. A CVP line is usually required to measure circulating blood volume. Diuretics may be administered only if the patient is well hydrated; however, they should not be continually prescribed if the patient remains oliguric.

Acute postoperative renal failure occurs when the reversible stage of acute renal insufficiency progresses to acute tubular necrosis. Volume loading becomes potentially dangerous with established renal failure, and the mainstays of treatment at this stage are the replacement of observed fluid loss, plus an allowance of approximately 500 ml/day for insensible loss, and restriction of dietary protein intake to less than 20 g/day. Biochemical status is checked by frequent estimations of serum urea and electrolytes. Hyperkalaemia can be treated by intravenous administration of insulin and glucose, or cation exchange resins. Haemofiltration or haemodialysis may be indicated if conservative measures fail to prevent rapid rises in serum concentrations of urea and potassium. Recovery from acute tubular necrosis can be anticipated in survivors after 2–4 weeks. The patient will then enter a polyuric phase, in which fluid and electrolyte balance requires careful monitoring. The mortality rate in patients who develop postoperative renal failure is 50%.

Cerebral complications

Cerebrovascular accidents (CVA)

These are usually precipitated by sudden hypotension during or after surgery in elderly hypertensive patients with severe atherosclerosis. They are a specific complication of carotid endarterectomy, occurring in 1–3% of cases, but may also complicate cardiac surgery.

Neuropsychiatric disturbances

These occur frequently and cover a wide spectrum of disorders. The most common is mental confusion with agitation, restlessness and disorientation, and is known as delirium. It usually occurs in the elderly and may arise on a background of dementia due to cerebral atrophy, but is often precipitated by the use of sedative or hypnotic drugs. Acute toxic confusion state is a well-recognized acute psychiatric disorder that occurs in some patients during a serious illness or after a major surgical intervention. Many factors can contribute, and it is important to look for a treatable cause, such as hypoxia, sepsis, or a metabolic disturbance such as uraemia or electrolyte imbalance. Sleep deprivation, particularly in intensive care units, can also cause severe mental disturbance.

Delirium tremens (acute alcohol withdrawal syndrome)

Delirium tremens occurs in alcoholics who stop drinking suddenly. In most instances, this can be predicted from a detailed history. Prodromal symptoms include personality changes, anxiety and tremors. The fully developed condition is characterized by extreme agitation, visual hallucinations, restlessness, confusion and, rarely, convulsions and hyperthermia. If symptoms are mild, treatment involves the prescription of oral diazepam and vitamin B (thiamine). Control of extreme agitation may require intravenous administration of diazepam, or haloperidol.

Venous thrombosis and pulmonary embolism

These complications are discussed in detail in Chapter 21, but the essential details are summarized here for convenience.

Deep venous thrombosis (DVT)

The pathogenesis of venous thrombosis involves stasis, increased blood coagulability and damage to the blood vessel wall (Virchow's triad). The incidence of DVT varies with the type of operation and the associated risk factors, which include increasing age, obesity, prolonged operations, pelvic and hip surgery, malignant disease, previous DVT or pulmonary embolism (PE), varicose veins, pregnancy, and use of the oral contraceptive pill.

Measures to prevent DVT include taking care to avoid prolonged compression of the leg veins during and after the operation; the use of graded compression support stockings (TED stockings); mechanical or electrical compression of the calf muscles during surgery; and low molecular weight heparin (LMWH).

DVT is frequently asymptomatic, but may present with a painful, tender swollen calf. It may be the cause of a postoperative fever. Duplex ultrasonography is now the investigation of choice for diagnosing DVT.

Nowadays, most DVTs are treated with LMWH injected subcutaneously once daily rather than by means of an unfractionated heparin infusion. Heparin therapy is stopped once the patient is fully anticoagulated with warfarin, which is then normally continued for 3–6 months. The dose of warfarin is adjusted to maintain an international normalized ratio (INR) at 2–3 times normal.

Pulmonary embolism

Massive pulmonary embolus with severe chest pain, pallor and shock demands immediate cardiopulmonary resuscitation, heparinization and urgent CT pulmonary angiography. Fibrinolytic agents, such as streptokinase or urokinase, can be infused intravenously to encourage clot lysis if it is at least 6 days after surgical intervention, or in extreme cases the clot can be removed at open pulmonary embolectomy under cardiopulmonary bypass.

If a PE is suspected in a patient complaining of chest pain, sometimes in association with tachypnoea, haemoptysis and a pleural rub and effusion, a chest X-ray and ECG should be undertaken, mainly to rule out alternative causes of the symptoms. If these are negative, a CT pulmonary angiogram should then be performed and if this reveals lobar or segmental perfusion defects, the patient is heparinized and monitored carefully (Fig. 9.5). In such cases, it is also important to search for the source of the embolus; warfarin therapy is recommended in all patients who have sustained a pulmonary embolus, and therapy is normally continued for 6 months. If the patient cannot be anticoagulated, or sustains further PE despite anticoagulation then consideration can be given to placing an inferior vena caval (IVC) filter.

Wound complications

Infection

Infection (Fig. 9.6) is the most common complication in surgery. The incidence varies from less than 1% in clean operations to 20–30% in dirty cases. Subcutaneous haematoma is a common prelude to a wound infection, and large haematomas may require evacuation. The onset is usually within 7 days of operation. Symptoms include malaise, anorexia, and pain or discomfort at the operation site. Signs include local erythema, tenderness, swelling, cellulitis, wound discharge or frank abscess formation, as well as an elevated temperature and pulse rate. If a wound becomes infected, it may be necessary to remove one or more sutures or staples prematurely to allow the egress of infected material. The wound is then allowed to heal by secondary intention. Antibiotics are only required if there is evidence of associated cellulitis or septicaemia. If the wound infection is chronic, the presence of a suture sinus or an enterocutaneous fistula must be excluded.

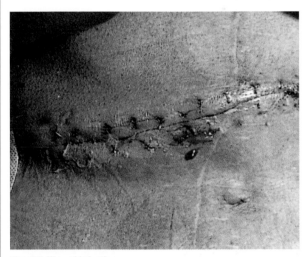

Fig. 9.6 Wound infection.

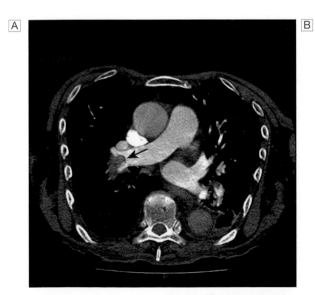 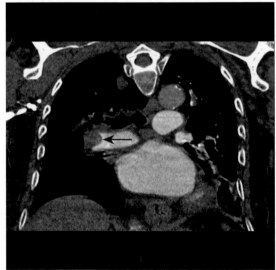

Fig. 9.5 CT pulmonary angiograms showing pulmonary embolus.

Dehiscence

The incidence of abdominal wound dehiscence should be less than 1%. Wound dehiscence (Fig. 9.7) may be partial (deep layers only) or complete (all layers, including skin). A serosanguinous discharge is characteristic of partial wound dehiscence. The extrusion of abdominal viscera through a complete abdominal wound dehiscence is known as evisceration. This rare complication usually occurs within the first 2 weeks after operation. Risk factors include obesity, smoking, respiratory disease, obstructive jaundice, nutritional deficiencies, renal failure, malignancy, diabetes and steroid therapy; however, the most important causes are poor surgical technique, persistently increased intra-abdominal pressure, and local tissue necrosis due to infection. The wound should be resutured under general anaesthesia. Incisional herniation complicates approximately 25% of cases.

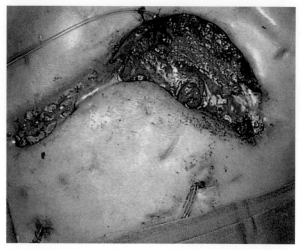

Fig. 9.7 Wound dehiscence.

 SUMMARY BOX **9.2**

Complications of anaesthesia and surgery

General complications
- Nausea and vomiting
- Hiccups
- Headache

Pulmonary complications
- Pulmonary collapse
- Pulmonary infection
- Respiratory failure
- Acute respiratory distress syndrome (ARDS)
- Pleural effusion
- Pneumothorax

Cardiac complications
- Myocardial ischaemia/infarction
- Cardiac failure
- Arrhythmias
- Postoperative shock

Urinary complications
- Urinary retention
- Urinary tract infection
- Renal failure

Cerebral complications
- Cerebrovascular accidents (CVA)
- Neuropsychiatric disturbances
- Delirium tremens

Venous thromboembolism
- Deep venous thrombosis
- Pulmonary embolism

Wound complications
- Wound infection
- Wound dehiscence.

Postoperative fever

Fever in a patient who has had surgery can be due to a variety of causes related to the primary disease or complications related to the surgical intervention or general anaesthesia. The common conditions that cause fever are listed in Box 9.3. The cause must be diligently identified and treated appropriately.

 SUMMARY BOX **9.3**

Causes of a fever in a postoperative patient

Days 0–2
- Physiological as response to tissue injury – low grade
- Pulmonary collapse / atelectasis
- Blood transfusions
- Thrombophlebitis

Days 3–5
- Sepsis – wound infection
- Biliary or urinary sepsis
- Intra-abdominal collection
- Pneumonia

Day 5–7
- Deep vein thrombosis (DVT)
- Enteric anastomotic leak

> 7 Days
- Intra-abdominal collection
- DVT
- Septicaemia.

D. McWhinnie

10

Day surgery

INTRODUCTION

Ambulatory surgery is the generic term for surgical procedures performed on a day-case basis or with a short hospital stay. Terminology is often confusing as in North America, 'day surgery' often refers to a 23-hour overnight stay, while in the UK and Europe, day surgery refers to the admission and discharge of the patient on the same day as surgery.

Day surgery is a process, not a procedure and its benefits relate to a well-defined and streamlined pathway. A hospital admission of only a few hours minimizes the risk of hospital acquired infection and early mobilization reduces the risk of venous thromboembolism (VTE). Patients like day surgery and prefer to recover from their procedure in the comfort of their own home. The economic benefit of shortening the postoperative length of stay in surgery relates to the closure of inpatient beds. A move from inpatient surgery to day surgery was incorporated in the United Kingdom government's health policy in 2000 and has resulted in the closure of many inpatient beds throughout the country.

 SUMMARY BOX **10.1**

Clinical effectiveness of day surgery

- The surgical outcomes of a procedure performed on a day case basis or as an inpatient should, in theory, be identical, as it is the patient pathway and not the surgery that is different
- In practice, surgical outcomes from patients undergoing day surgery rather than inpatient surgery are often better as day surgery patients are a preselected cohort of healthier patients with fewer comorbidities.

FACILITIES FOR DAY SURGERY

Day surgery facilities can be configured in a number of ways but all require a day ward, operating theatres and a recovery area. Most day units have abandoned beds in favour of trolleys and chairs and many now utilize specialized day surgery trolleys which can provide all the functions of a bed, trolley and operating table together. These trolleys accompany the day surgery patient throughout the entire patient journey, before transfer to a chair to complete second-stage recovery. Considerable time savings can be made in the theatre pathway by avoiding trolley transfers.

Free-standing units

Free-standing day units can be built within the community they serve. Patient travelling distances and times are minimized but a lack of overnight facilities constrains both patient eligibility and case mix. Only the fittest patients are accepted and surgery is of a minor or intermediate nature. Nevertheless, these units offer the most efficient use of resources, maximizing throughput of selected procedures and minimizing the cost per patient.

Any patient unable to be safely discharged when the free-standing unit closes in the evening requires ambulance transfer to the main hospital, often some distance away. Free-standing units are popular in the USA and in the last 5 years many have been built in the United Kingdom as 'Treatment Centres' or 'Ambulatory Care and Diagnostic Centres' (ACADs).

Hospital integrated units

Most hospitals now have dedicated day ward facilities. Performing day surgery through the in-patient ward offers inappropriate care to both the day patient and the in-patient. In-patients require more intensive nursing and medical care and the day patient is often neglected. The result is often an unplanned overnight admission or discharge without comprehensive discharge information requiring an unnecessary GP visit or hospital readmission. Day surgery theatres can either be separate or part of the existing theatre complex. Separate theatres can require duplication of specialized equipment but list cancellation is less likely from emergency or urgent elective cases.

10

Cost effectiveness of day surgery

- Same-day admission and discharge avoids the costs of an overnight inpatient bed
- Criteria based pre-assessment reduce unnecessary investigations
- Dedicated day or ambulatory theatre lists maximize surgical throughput
- Protocol-based discharge with comprehensive patient information reduces unplanned hospital readmissions.

THE PATIENT PATHWAY

First patient contact

An efficient and effective ambulatory pathway (Fig. 10.1) requires the patient to arrive at the day unit on the day of surgery fully prepared for their procedure both physically and mentally. Preparation for possible day surgery starts at first patient contact with their General Practitioner. Patients will often raise the topic of day surgery themselves as their preferred management option at their initial consultation. A brief 'health screen' with the GP referral letter detailing the patient's blood pressure, body mass index, medication and past medical history allows the surgeon at outpatients to consider appropriate pre-assessment required for the patient. If no diagnostic or other investigations are required, the patient can be listed for their surgical procedure and referred immediately for pre-assessment, avoiding a follow-up out-patient clinic appointment.

Exclusion criteria for ambulatory surgery

Day surgery remains an efficient and safe surgical process as long as only specified patients are accepted for operation. The basic criteria for acceptance for day surgery were evaluated in the 1990s and although the detail has changed, the principles remain the same i.e. body mass index (BMI) and the American Society of Anaesthesiologists' Physical Status Classification System (ASA status). Each hospital has its own set of admission criteria dependent on the day unit facilities available and the surgical case mix to be undertaken. Stand-alone units require more strictly defined criteria than hospital integrated units to minimize unplanned overnight admissions requiring transfer to another hospital.

BMI

Body mass index is calculated by the equation: BMI = Weight (kg)/Height (m²). Obesity is defined as a BMI of greater than 30 kg/m². The prevalence of obesity is rising and it has been estimated that 35% of the adult population, 14% of children aged 6 to 11 years and 12% of children aged 12 to 17 years are now officially categorized as obese. The practical risks of obesity in ambulatory surgery include the serious morbidities of diabetes and obstructive sleep apnoea. There is, however little evidence to support the view that obese patients suffer clinically relevant increased morbidity after day surgery leading to a higher overnight admission rate and the Department of Health suggests that most patients with a BMI of less than 40 are suitable for day surgery. However, clinical judgment must be exercised on a case-by-case basis in the context of the surgery required.

ASA status

This is used to assess the physical state of the patient prior to surgery and has been adopted worldwide (Table 10.1). Most day units accept ASA I and II patients. More advanced units and those that can deal safely with unplanned overnight admissions may accept some patients with ASA III status such as insulin-dependent diabetics.

Pre-assessment

Pre-assessment is the evaluation of a patient's fitness for elective surgery and is best performed by a specialized pre-assessment team of nursing staff. The team should be supported by consultant anaesthetic sessions where more

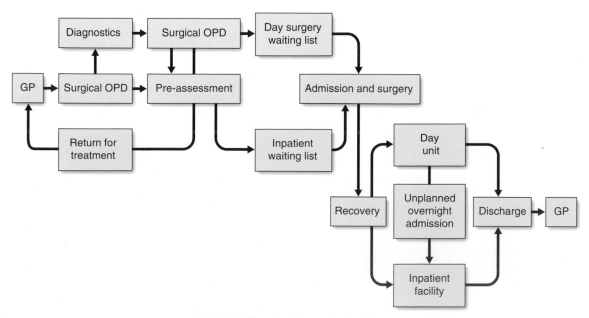

Fig. 10.1 The ambulatory patient pathway.

Table 10.1 American Society of Anaesthesiologists classification of physical status

ASA I	Normal healthy patients. Little or no risk for surgery.
ASA II	Patients with mild systemic disease. Minimal risk during treatment. Examples include well-controlled non-insulin dependent diabetes, mild hypertension, epilepsy or asthma.
ASA III	Patients with severe systemic disease that limits activity but is not incapacitating. These patients need medical input before surgery. Examples include insulin-dependent diabetes or a history of myocardial infarction, congestive heart failure or cerebrovascular accident in the preceding six months.
ASA IV	Patients with severe systemic disease limiting activity and is a constant threat to life. Elective surgery is contradicted and emergency surgery requires urgent medical input. Examples include unstable diabetes, hypertension and epilepsy or a recent myocardial infarction.
ASA V	Patients who are moribund and not expected to survive more than 24 hours without an operation

complex patients are evaluated and where a final decision can be made regarding patients suitability for day surgery. The role of the pre-assessment team is to safely and accurately allocate patients for day, 23-hour or in-patient surgery as well as ensuring they have adequate social support. Pre-assessment provides an opportunity to answer patient questions and allay fears, and has been shown to reduce the rates of cancellation and non-attendance for surgery.

All elective surgical patients should initially be regarded as day cases until proved otherwise. The final decision as to the appropriate management pathway should lie with the pre-assessment team except when the surgeon for clinical reasons specifies that the patient should remain in hospital overnight. The pre-assessment process consists of a consultation, appropriate investigations if required and written information regarding admission, operation and discharge. The consultation should occur as early as possible in the pathway to enable problems to be addressed and to allow time for optimization prior to the scheduled operating date. Many hospitals require some of the optimization to be performed in primary care (e.g. blood pressure control) before accepting the patient for clinic referral. Pre-assessment performed shortly before the date of surgery may result in late postponement if unexpected medical problems are discovered. Ideally no patient should be listed for surgery until they have been deemed fit and have received sufficient information for them to give informed consent.

Pre-assessment is offered to the patient in a number of options:

1. At source in the GP surgery. This model is used in surgical outreach clinics when the pre-assessment nurse accompanies the surgeon to the clinic. It is more cost effective however to train a practice nurse to perform the routine pre-assessments and refer more complex patients for hospital pre-assessment.
2. At the pre-assessment clinic. Formal pre-assessment consultations can be programmed in advance for 30–60 minute interviews depending on the complexity of the patient.
3. At the surgical outpatient clinic. Where a number of surgical clinics are running concurrently, it is cost

effective to offer patients a 'one-stop' pre-assessment service. Patients requiring more complex pre-assessment can be deferred to a planned pre-assessment clinic at a later date.

4. By telephone, postal questionnaire or internet (e-mail or on-line). This model is suitable for fit patients undergoing straightforward procedures especially if they have already had a basic health screen performed at the GP surgery.

Regardless of the mode of pre-assessment, it is essential patients feel relaxed and unhurried. Adequate time is required for patient questions and clarification of detail. Patients often remember little of their consultation with the surgeon due to anxiety and pressure of time. The pre-assessment consultation offers the patient a reprise of their intended procedure and reinforcement of salient points. Relatives or the patient's carer are encouraged to attend as they may remember important information forgotten by the patient. Written information regarding admission, discharge and the procedure itself is an essential component of the day surgery process.

The admission proforma should be standardized for all subspecialties and best practice suggests it should consist of a generic section addressing the basic health screen, current and past medication, past medical history, social factors and a supplementary section pertinent to the surgical subspecialty such as ophthalmology, orthopaedics, urology or gynaecology.

Basic health screen

This consists of the patient's demography, BMI, blood pressure, medication and past medical history and allows ASA status to be evaluated.

Medication

A full list of current medications including dosages and indications for each drug should be obtained. Significant numbers of patients, particularly older patients, take anticoagulants or anti-platelet agents but not all patients undergoing surgery require complete cessation of this therapy beforehand. The decision is based on the consequences of stopping therapy versus the risks of bleeding during or after surgery. Many surgeons would consider performing superficial surgery such as inguinal hernia repair or excision of a large lipoma with an INR of <1.8. In contrast, any surgery within the abdominal cavity at this INR would be contraindicated due to latent bleeding.

Warfarin

When considering cessation of warfarin, the original indication for the drug dictates the management plan.

- Atrial fibrillation (AF): Anticoagulation with warfarin reduces the annual embolic stroke rate from 4% to 2%. Stopping warfarin one week prior to surgery to normalize coagulation poses little risk of stroke.
- VTE: After DVT or PE patients are usually anticoagulated for 3–6 months. Ideally, surgery should be deferred until the course of anticoagulation has ceased. If this is not possible then conversion to heparin therapy preoperatively is advocated.
- Prosthetic heart valves: Mitral valves are intolerant of normal coagulation and conversion to heparin therapy is required, thereby excluding such patients from day surgery. Aortic valves are less susceptible to embolization due to high blood flows and closing pressures and warfarin can be safely stopped 3 days before surgery and restarted immediately after operation.

Anti-platelet agents

The most common indication for long-term therapy is arterial disease and short-term cessation of therapy carries little risk. Patients taking anti-platelet therapy for transient ischaemic attacks or for a xenograft heart valve should not have their therapy stopped and are unsuitable for day surgery. Following arterial stenting, patients usually continue therapy for one year and non-essential surgery should be suitably delayed. Aspirin or dipyridamole should be stopped 4 days before surgery and clopidogrel 7 days before surgery to ensure normal platelet function.

Past medical history

The most common problems encountered by the pre-assessment team are those of heart disease and diabetes.

Heart disease

Patients with high blood pressure can be referred back to the GP for therapy: more extensive heart disease may require a cardiology referral for optimization. The risk of myocardial ischaemia during anaesthesia is increased in the hypertensive patient and elevated blood pressure remains the most common reason for 'on the day' cancellations. However, the specific blood pressure where patient safety becomes compromised is unknown but admission systolic and diastolic pressures of less than 180 and 110 mmHg respectively do not increase perioperative complications and there is no need to routinely cancel patients with an elevated blood pressure below these parameters.

Diabetes

Patients with diabetes can be day cases but the resource implications for pre-assessment and their admission are considerable. Strict protocols are required. Type I diabetic patients are more difficult to manage in the perioperative period than Type II patients and are more liable to unplanned overnight admission. Random blood glucose estimation is of no value in assessing suitability for day surgery and should only be performed on the day of surgery to help guide perioperative management. Stability of the disease in the months before surgery is essential in dictating the success of the admission, especially in the Type I patient. The stability of the diabetic patient can be assessed by the patient's self-monitored blood glucose profiles in the preceding few months and by estimation of their glycosylated haemoglobin (HbA1c). This measurement is a reflection of the integrated blood glucose control over the preceding 2–3 months with extra weighting for the one month preceding the sample. The normal range for HbA1c is about 4–6% in the non-diabetic patient. An HbA1c of less then 8% suggests that the patient will be suitable for day surgery. Values above 8% indicate unsuitability for day surgery as results above this level are associated with higher fasting blood glucose, making perioperative blood glucose control more difficult to manage. An HbA1c of over 9% indicates that a review of their diabetic management should be undertaken before any elective surgery is undertaken.

All the other usual criteria for day surgery should be met and there should be no history of repeated hypoglycaemic attacks nor of recent hospital admissions due to the complications of diabetes.

Most minor and intermediate surgical procedures can be safely undertaken in adult diabetic patients with the possible exception of laparoscopic cholecystectomy due to the high risk of postoperative nausea and vomiting. Wherever possible, the patient should be managed with local anaesthesia as this may remove the need for the patient to starve preoperatively.

The three key principles in managing the diabetic patient as a day case are:
- Diabetic medication should be omitted on the morning of surgery
- The procedure should be scheduled as early as possible on the operating list
- Return the patient as soon as possible postoperatively to their usual diet and medication.

Type II patients treated with oral hypoglycaemic drugs with a fasting blood glucose <10 mmol/l can be monitored safely but patients with higher fasting glucose should be managed either with a GKI (glucose/potassium/insulin) infusion or separate glucose drip and insulin infusion.

Type I patients will all require an infusion until they are ready for a meal after surgery and are likely to require significant anaesthetic assistance. After discharge, the patient and carer should be able to monitor and measure blood sugar at home and they should be aware of the possibilities of hyperglycaemia and delayed hypoglycaemia, especially if hypoglycaemic medication was taken significantly later on the day of surgery.

Social factors

The population of the United Kingdom has never been more mobile. Large numbers of young people are in higher education and living away from home. There are more single households than ever before and with the concept of the extended family in decline it is often difficult to identify a carer for the day case patient. Nevertheless if no other exclusion criteria are apparent, the pre-assessment nurse can explore all possibilities with the patient to ensure a responsible adult is at home the night of the procedure in case of problems. Patients' home conditions should be appropriate for a safe and comfortable recovery with a readily accessible toilet available and access to a telephone in case of emergency. The day surgery patient should live within about 90 minutes travel to the hospital but if the patient has undergone a procedure where postoperative haemorrhage is a risk, then local protocols may dictate a shorter journey time. It is difficult for patients living in remote areas to fulfil these requirements and there may have to be an acceptance that they might have to stay overnight. However, as postoperative medical facilities are not required, they can be lodged, with their carer in local hotel accommodation overnight. Indeed, the concept of the 'hospital hotel' may be an option for hospitals serving rural and remote communities whereby their day surgery is performed in the hospital's day unit but they are discharged to 'hotel' facilities, without medical or nursing supervision, but within the hospital campus, at a lower cost than an in-patient hospital bed.

Investigations

Many preoperative assessment clinics take blood and record 12-lead electrocardiograms for their patients but this is not evidence-based. NICE (National Institute for Clinical Evidence) conducted an extensive systematic review of routine preoperative tests and concluded that the evidence for investigations did not exist. The NICE guidelines are therefore based on the consensus opinion of healthcare professionals and relate to the grade of surgery being performed (Table 10.2), the patient's age (Table 10.3), and the severity of any underlying disease, whether cardiovascular, respiratory or renal (Table 10.4).

A pregnancy test should be conducted if the patient says she may be pregnant although many units now perform pregnancy tests routinely.

Table 10.2 Grade of surgery related to NICE preoperative investigations	
Grade 1	Diagnostic laparoscopy or endoscopy, breast biopsy
Grade 2	Inguinal hernia, varicose veins, knee arthroscopy, tonsillectomy
Grade 3	Thyroidectomy, abdominal hysterectomy, TURP
Grade 4	Colonic resection, joint replacement, artery reconstruction

A sickle cell test is required for:
- patients of African or Afro-Caribbean descent
- patients with a family history of homozygous sickle cell disease or heterozygous trait
- patients from the Eastern Mediterranean, Middle East and Asia.

Hospitals should develop their own protocols for pre-assessment based on the NICE guidelines. The more variation in the process, the more likely an unintentional adverse outcome can occur.

SUMMARY BOX 10.3

Pre-assessment

- All elective surgical patients should be pre-assessed
- All patients undergoing a procedure suitable for day surgery should initially be defaulted to day surgery, and only if not clinically fit should they be allocated to an overnight stay
- The pre-assessment team should be empowered to allocate the appropriate length of stay to each individual patient
- Pre-assessment should be performed early in the patient pathway to avoid late cancellation for surgery. This can occur if the patient is found to be unfit for day surgery, with insufficient time to optimize their health.

The surgical waiting list

Before leaving the pre-assessment clinic, the patient should have an idea of when their operation is likely to be scheduled. Dates when the patient is unavailable due to

10

Table 10.3 Investigations depending on patient's age and grade of surgery.

Grade of Surgery	Age	CXR	ECG	FBC	INR/ APTT	U+E+ Creat	Glucose Random	Urine
Grade 1	< 16	No	No	No	No	No	No	No
Grade 1	16–60	No	No	No	No	No	No	No
Grade 1	61–80	No	No	No	No	No	No	No
Grade 1	> 80	No	Yes	No	No	No	No	No
Grade 2	< 16	No	No	No	No	No	No	No
Grade 2	16–60	No	No	No	No	No	No	No
Grade 2	61–80	No	No	Yes	No	No	No	No
Grade 2	> 80	No	Yes	Yes	No	No	No	No
Grade 3	< 16	No	No	No	No	No	No	No
Grade 3	16–60	No	No	Yes	No	No	No	No
Grade 3	61–80	No	Yes	Yes	No	Yes	No	No
Grade 3	> 80	No	Yes	Yes	No	Yes	No	No
Grade 4	< 16	No	No	No	No	No	No	No
Grade 4	16–60	No	No	Yes	No	Yes	No	No
Grade 4	61–80	No	Yes	Yes	No	Yes	No	No
Grade 4	> 80	No	Yes	Yes	No	Yes	No	No

Table 10.4 Investigations depending on patient's disease type and severity.

Disease	Severity	CXR	ECG	FBC	INR/ APTT	U+E+ Creat	Blood gases	Lung function
Cardiovascular	Mild	No	Yes	No	No	No	No	No
Cardiovascular	Severe	No	Yes	No	No	Yes	No	No
Respiratory	Mild	No	No	No	No	No	No	No
Respiratory	Severe	No	No	No	No	No	No	No
Renal	Mild	No	No	No	No	Yes	No	No
Renal	Severe	No	Yes	Yes	No	Yes	No	No

holidays or work commitments should be noted. Contact telephone numbers are recorded and the patient should be asked if they would consider a short notice cancellation date for their operation. As waiting times for different surgeons for day surgery can be variable, many hospitals have adopted a policy of 'pooling' the more common day procedures such as hernia, laparoscopic cholecystectomy and varicose vein surgery. This ensures surgical waiting times for day surgery are equitable between surgeons.

Admission for surgery

An efficient and effective ambulatory pathway requires the patient to arrive at the day unit on the day of surgery fully prepared for their procedure both physically and mentally (Fig. 10.2). Admission administration is minimal. Patients can sign their consent form to confirm they wish to proceed with their operation at any appropriate point before their procedure. If the patient signs the form in advance, a health professional involved in their care on the day should also sign it to confirm the patient still wishes to proceed. The diagnosis and planned surgery should be confirmed as still appropriate and the operation site marked. Although consent remains valid indefinitely unless withdrawn by the patient, many hospitals time-limit consent forms to 3 months after dating on safety grounds.

Scheduling for theatre

Day surgery patients should have their operation as early as possible on the operating list to ensure safe and comfortable discharge before the end of the day. With dedicated day lists, patients requiring the longest recovery time either because of the length of operation or the nature of the surgery, should be prioritized. Afternoon day lists may require scheduling of local anaesthetic cases towards the end of the list to ensure all patients can be successfully discharged. Adding day cases to major surgery lists has advantages and disadvantages. Where there is more than one anaesthetist allocated to a list, it is possible to start with a minor or intermediate day case while the major case is being prepared for anaesthesia in the anaesthetic room. Delays can inevitably occur and many surgeons prefer to commence the list with a major procedure so that if complications do occur they are often manifest in the afternoon rather than late in the evening. Mixed ambulatory lists, where available, offer the

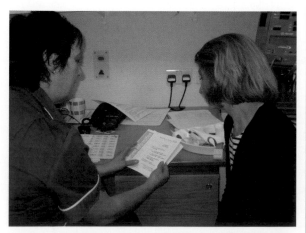

Fig. 10.2 Successful day surgery depends on careful explanation to the patient in advance of the surgical appointment.

optimal use of the operating theatre with the true day cases early in the day and those patients scheduled for a 23-hour stay receiving their surgery later.

Anaesthesia and analgesia

Day surgery may be performed under general, local or regional anaesthesia. General anaesthesia remains the most popular mode of anaesthesia in this country but local and regional techniques are gaining popularity with both patients and professionals alike due to the absence of postoperative cerebral upset. While there is no 'ideal' day case general anaesthetic, the aim is to provide rapid and safe recovery with minimal pain or postoperative nausea or vomiting. Modern anaesthetic agents such as desflurane or sevoflurane are ideally suited to day surgery as is total intravenous anaesthesia (TIVA) with Propofol. The use of the laryngeal mask rather than endotracheal intubation has changed anaesthetic practice in day surgery since its introduction in 1988, allowing a more rapid turnaround of patients.

Prior to the procedure, non-steroidal anti-inflammatory drugs should be given where there are no contraindications. It is not necessary to provide the drug intravenously or by the PR route as oral administration one hour before surgery produces better and longer-lasting pain relief. Paracetamol may also be given preoperatively to reduce the need for more potent opioids and their unwanted side effects. It is more effective when given intravenously with analgesic effects similar to those of NSAIDs.

Local anaesthesia has always been useful in day surgery for the removal of 'lumps and bumps' but increasingly, it provides an excellent and safe technique for the repair of inguinal herniae and other abdominal wall herniae, especially in patients with major comorbidities. Furthermore, patients can usefully be scheduled late on the day list late ensuring maximal utilization of theatres.

Recovery

The recovery of patients after day surgery starts at the end of anaesthesia and finishes with the return to normal activities. Recovery consists of three phases.

- First stage – until the patient is awake after anaesthesia
- Second stage – until the patient is discharged from hospital
- Late – until the patient has returned to normal activities.

The two most common problems encountered in first and second stage recovery are postoperative pain and nausea (PONV).

The management of pain in recovery is best managed using a pain score protocol. For moderate pain, oral analgesia can be given as soon as the patient is awake and able to swallow safely.

Suitable drugs include paracetamol, paracetamol/codeine compounds and NSAIDs if not already administered pre- or perioperatively. Severe pain is best treated with a rapid onset, short-acting opiate such as intravenous fentanyl.

The management of PONV can be divided into general measures given to all patients and specific medication given to those at higher risk (Table 10.5). General measures include the use of short-acting anaesthetics, pre-emptive non-opioid analgesia and a reduction in the fluid deficit by minimizing the preoperative fast and giving IV fluids peroperatively. Patients at risk for PONV may require the routine administration of a 5HT3 antagonist such as ondansetron or granisetron; if at very high risk, dexamethasone 4–8 mg may be given in addition.

Table 10.5 Risk factors for PONV

Key risk factors	Additional surgical risk factors
Female gender	Oral or ENT surgery
Non-smoker	Squint surgery
Previous history of PONV	Laparoscopic surgery
Suffers motion sickness	
Perioperative use of opioids	

Discharge criteria

The decision as to when a patient is fit for discharge from the day unit should be taken by trained nursing staff using agreed discharge criteria protocols (Table 10.6). A postoperative visit by the surgeon and anaesthetist is encouraged at the end of the operating list, but awaiting a member of the busy surgical team to discharge the patient usually results in delay.

The criterion of being able to take oral fluids before discharge has now been abandoned as encouragement to drink postoperatively increases the incidence of PONV. Oral intake remains necessary in selected patients such as diabetics. Voiding before discharge in patients with a low risk of urinary retention is also considered unnecessary.

When the discharge criteria are met, the patient and their carer should be offered both generic and procedure-specific written discharge information to encompass:

- medication
- wound care dressing renewal and suture removal (if required)
- bathing or showering
- return to normal activities including work, sexual activities and exercise
- signs and symptoms which may indicate a problem
- contact emergency telephone number and follow-up arrangements
- travel after day surgery.

Patients may return to driving a minimum of 48 hours after general anaesthesia due to impaired reaction times. The procedure undertaken and its surgical site will also determine resumption of driving which can only occur when the patient can safely perform an emergency stop. It is unclear after what time period patients can safely fly after surgery and it will vary with the complexity and extent of the procedure. Air travel where trapped gas or air may still remain within a body cavity as in laparoscopic or middle ear procedures requires extra caution as retained gas expands in flight due to the lower atmospheric pressure. The immobility associated with continuous travel of more than 3 hours within 4 weeks of surgery raises the risk of venous thromboembolism.

Table 10.6 Discharge criteria for day surgery

- Vital signs stable and comparable to those recorded on admission
- Orientation to time, place and person
- Pain controlled and oral analgesics supplied
- Understands the use of medications issued and written information supplied
- Ability to dress and walk (if appropriate)
- Minimal nausea or vomiting
- Minimal wound bleeding
- Has a responsible adult to take them home
- Has a carer at home for the next 24 hours

SUMMARY BOX 10.4

Principles of day surgery care

- Patient information
- Patient counselling
- Exclusion criteria
- Pre-assessment
- Optimization of health
- Day of surgery admission
- Theatre scheduling
- Minimally invasive surgery
- Pre-emptive analgesia
- Regular analgesia
- Avoid opiate analgesia if possible
- Minimize postoperative nausea and vomiting
- Fluid therapy
- Early mobilization
- Discharge criteria
- Discharge information
- Nurse-led discharge.

DAY SURGERY PROCEDURES

The rapid expansion of minimal access techniques in surgery over the last 20 years has offered many possibilities for converting a surgical procedure from an in-patient to a day case. Anaesthesia and analgesia have markedly improved and procedures up to 2 hours long can even be performed on a day case basis provided they are scheduled early in the day. For many years the Audit Commission 'Basket of 25' surgical procedures provided a template for day surgery (Table 10.7). However, as most of these procedures are minor or intermediate in nature (accounting for only about 25% of all day surgery) and several others are now obsolete, the

Table 10.7 Audit Commission 'basket of 25 procedures'

1. Orchidopexy
2. Circumcision
3. Inguinal hernia repair
4. Excision breast lump
5. Anal fissure dilatation or excision
6. Haemorrhoidectomy
7. Laparoscopic cholecystectomy
8. Varicose vein stripping or ligation
9. Transurethral resection of bladder tumour
10. Excision of Dupuytren's contracture
11. Carpal tunnel decompression
12. Excision of ganglion
13. Arthroscopy
14. Bunion operations
15. Removal of metal ware
16. Extraction of cataract
17. Correction of squint
18. Myringotomy
19. Tonsillectomy
20. Sub mucous resection
21. Reduction of nasal fracture
22. Operation for bat ears
23. D & C / hysteroscopy
24. Laparoscopy
25. Termination of pregnancy

Table 10.8 **BADS directory of procedures – aspirational percentages for selected surgical operations.**

Subspecialty	Operation	Day case	23-hour stay	< 72-hour stay
Breast	Wide local excision	15	75	10
	Sentinel node resection	80	20	–
	Simple mastectomy	15	75	–
ENT	Submucous resection	60	35	–
	Tonsillectomy	80	20	–
General	Haemorrhoidectomy	65	30	5
	Lap cholecystectomy	60	30	10
	Lap fundoplication	40	40	20
	Lap gastric banding	10	45	45
	Primary inguinal hernia	95	5	–
	Recurrent inguinal hernia	70	30	–
Gynaecology	Therapeutic laparoscopy	70	20	10
	Cone biopsy of cervix	95	5	–
Head and neck	Branchial cyst excision	10	70	20
	Partial thyroidectomy	10	50	40
Orthopaedics	Knee arthroscopy	95	5	–
	Bunion operations	85	15	–
	Subacromial decompression	80	15	5
Urology	Laser prostatectomy	90	10	–
	Lap pyeloplasty	10	80	10
Vascular	Varicose vein surgery	75	25	–

'Basket' is now of limited value. There is also a realization that reducing the length of stay of the short stay surgical pathway for each patient by one day provides a similar reduction in overnight bed days as converting a patient from a 23-hour stay to a day case. The British Association of Day Surgery (BADS) directory of procedures offers information on over 200 day and short stay surgical procedures indicating the percentage of a particular procedure which could be performed as a day case, as an overnight 23-hour stay or a short stay admission up to 72 hours given ideal theatre and organizational conditions. A selection of these aspirational percentages for common day and short stay surgical procedures is shown in Table 10.8.

Many surgeons and anaesthetists are concerned about patient safety after discharge and often cite risk of postoperative haemorrhage at home as a reason for keeping the patient in hospital overnight. Primary (reactionary) haemorrhage occurs within the first 4–6 hours after surgery and although uncommon can be addressed within the working day. Secondary haemorrhage occurs 2–4 days after surgery and even if the patient had an in-patient procedure, they would still have returned home by the time this event occurred.

23-HOUR SURGERY

In 23-hour surgery, the patient is admitted early in the morning for a morning list or late morning for an afternoon list and remains in hospital overnight. The following morning transfer to a discharge lounge for breakfast occurs before admission of the next day's patients. Twenty-three hour surgery provides a resource for patients with significant comorbidities but requiring a day case procedure, or for patients undergoing more major surgery where the length of stay has been significantly reduced by enhanced recovery techniques such as in laparoscopic colorectal procedures. The 23-hour unit is a useful intermediate management option for evaluating procedures new to day surgery in a safe environment before scheduling them through the day unit.

SECTION 2

Gastrointestinal surgery

A.C. de Beaux

11

The abdominal wall and hernia

UMBILICUS

Developmental abnormalities

Persistent vitello-intestinal duct

The vitello-intestinal duct runs in intrauterine life from the apex of the midgut loop to the yolk sac. It is normally obliterated long before birth, but part of it may persist as a Meckel's diverticulum on the antimesenteric border of the ileum. Rarer abnormalities include persistence of a band attaching the umbilicus to a Meckel's diverticulum or a loop of ileum; a patent communication (fistula) between the ileum and umbilicus; an encysted portion of the duct that does not connect with the ileum (enterocystoma); an umbilical sinus; and a persistent umbilical portion of the duct, which forms a polypoidal raspberry-like tumour of the umbilicus (enteroteratoma) (Fig. 11.1). Symptomatic remnants may have to be excised, although a broad-based Meckel's diverticulum is usually left alone if found incidentally at laparotomy. Persisting bands can cause intestinal obstruction.

Urachus

The urachus runs from the apex of the bladder to the umbilicus. It is normally obliterated at birth but may give rise to cysts, a urinary fistula, or a discharging umbilical sinus if parts of it remain patent. Symptomatic remnants require excision.

Umbilical sepsis

Umbilical sepsis in neonates may give rise to portal thrombophlebitis, liver abscess formation, jaundice and portal vein thrombosis, which may result in portal hypertension. Tetanus can follow the application of cow dung to the umbilicus, as was once practised in some underdeveloped societies.

In adults, sepsis can result from retention of inspissated sebum within the folds of the umbilicus, and from infection of a pilonidal sinus of the umbilicus. Infection is usually mixed staphylococcal and streptococcal, characterized by erythema, tenderness and swelling. Treatment involves drainage of any pus and the prescription of systemic antibiotics.

Umbilical tumours

The umbilicus may rarely be involved by primary neoplasms (e.g. squamous carcinoma or melanoma), or by secondary tumour that has tracked along the ligamentum teres from the liver or lymph nodes in the porta hepatis. Neoplasia is an occasional unexpected finding in an umbilicus that has been excised because of persistent discharge.

DISORDERS OF THE RECTUS MUSCLE

Haematoma of the rectus sheath

Spontaneous or traumatic rupture of a branch of the inferior epigastric artery can result in a painful swelling within the rectus sheath in association with rigidity of the affected side of the abdominal wall. This condition is rare, but may represent an unusual presentation of acute abdominal pain in the elderly patient, especially if they are on anticoagulation therapy. A history of excessive physical exertion may precede the onset of symptoms. Ultrasonography can be used to confirm the diagnosis. Spontaneous resolution is typical but rarely evacuation of clot may be indicated for symptom control.

Desmoid tumour

This rare tumour is thought to arise from fibrous intramuscular septa in the lower rectus abdominis muscle. It is more common in women of child-bearing age and can be associated with intestinal polyposis in Gardner's syndrome. The lesion must be excised widely, as it is prone to recur and can become malignant (fibrosarcoma).

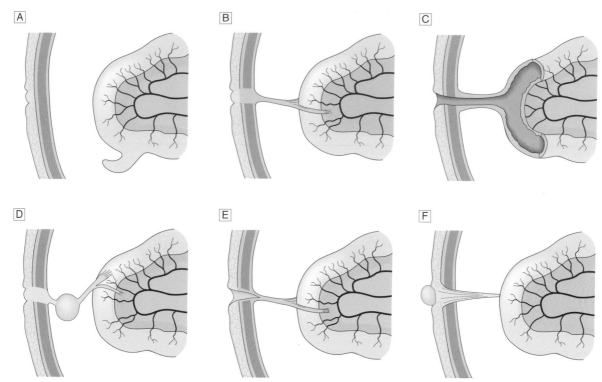

Fig. 11.1 Persistence of the vitello-intestinal duct, giving rise to developmental abnormalities. **A** A Meckel's diverticulum. **B** A fibrous cord to the ileum. **C** An umbilical intestinal fistula. **D** An enterocystoma. **E** An umbilical sinus. **F** An enteroteratoma.

ABDOMINAL HERNIA

A hernia is an abnormal protrusion of a cavity's contents, through a weakness in the wall of the cavity, taking with it all the linings of the cavity, although these may be markedly attenuated (Fig. 11.2). Hernias of the abdominal wall are common. Multiple factors contribute to the development of hernias. In essence, hernias can be considered design faults, either anatomical or through inherited collagen disorders, although these two factors work together in the majority of patients. Hernias may exploit natural openings such as the inguinal and femoral canals, umbilicus, obturator canal or oesophageal hiatus, or protrude through areas weakened by stretching (e.g. epigastric hernia) or surgical incision. In addition to these 'weak' anatomical areas, the collagen make up of the tissues, especially the Type I to III collagen ratio is also important. Type I imparts the strength to the tendon or fascia, Type III provides elastic recoil to the tissue. The Type I/III collagen ratio varies between individuals but is constant in all the fascia of a particular individual. Hernias can be considered as a disease of collagen metabolism.

The hernia is immediately invested by a peritoneal sac drawn from the lining of the abdominal wall (Fig. 11.2). The sac is covered in turn by those tissues that are stretched in front of it as the hernia enlarges (i.e. the coverings). The neck of the sac is the constriction formed by the orifice in the abdominal wall through which the hernia passes. A hernia may contain any intra-abdominal structure but most commonly contains omentum and/or small bowel. A hernia may involve only part of the circumference of the bowel (Richter's hernia), a Meckel's diverticulum (Littré's hernia) or an incarcerated appendix (Amyand's hernia). A sliding inguinal hernia is defined as one in which a viscus forms a portion of the wall of the hernia sac. Most commonly, the viscus involved is caecum, sigmoid colon or urinary bladder. In the early stages of a hernia, sometimes the hernial contents are pre-peritoneal fat only, such as a lipoma of the cord which can mimic an inguinal hernia.

 SUMMARY BOX 11.1

Hernia

- A hernia is an abnormal protrusion of a cavity's contents through a weakness in the wall of the cavity, but takes with it all the linings of the cavity
- Hernias of the abdominal wall are common and may exploit natural openings or weak areas caused by stretching or surgical incisions in association with a defect in collagen metabolism
- Abdominal hernias have a peritoneal sac, the neck of which is often unyielding and constitutes a potential source of compression of the hernial contents
- Hernia may be classified as reducible or irreducible, and the contents (e.g. bowel) may become obstructed or strangulated
- Strangulation denotes compromise of the blood supply of the contents and its development significantly increases morbidity and mortality. The low-pressure venous drainage is occluded first and then the arterial supply becomes occluded, with the development of gangrene.

Inguinal hernia

Groin hernias account for three-quarters of all abdominal wall hernias, and inguinal herniorrhaphy is one of the most frequently performed general surgical procedures. The most common types of groin hernia are indirect inguinal (60%),

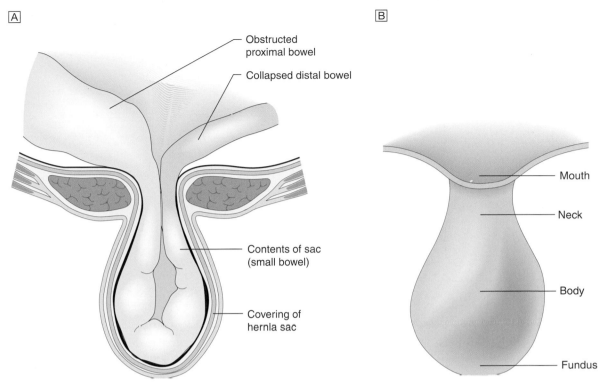

Fig. 11.2 Hernia. **A** Anatomical structure. **B** Parts of the hernial sac.

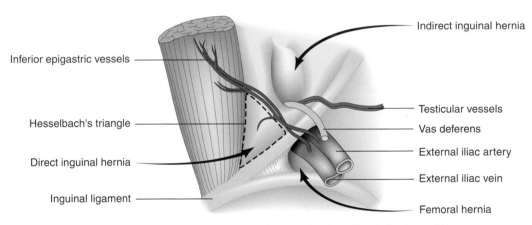

Fig. 11.3 Anatomy of the internal inguinal ring, showing sites of herniation from within.

direct inguinal (25%) and femoral (15%) (Fig. 11.3). Most (85%) groin hernias occur in males. Inguinal hernias occur in 1–3% of all newborn males. The incidence in premature infants is 30 times that seen at term. In early life, an indirect inguinal hernia is by far the most common variety. After middle age, weakness of the abdominal musculature leads to an increasing incidence of direct inguinal hernias. Femoral hernias are relatively more common in females (possibly because of stretching of ligaments and widening of the femoral ring in pregnancy), but an indirect inguinal hernia is still the most common type of groin hernia in women.

Surgical anatomy

The inguinal canal is an oblique passage in the lower anterior abdominal wall, through which the spermatic cord passes to the testis in the male, or the round ligament to the labium majus in the female. The processus vaginalis traversing the canal is normally obliterated at birth, but persistence in whole or in part presents an anatomical predisposition to an indirect inguinal hernia (Fig. 11.4). The openings of the canal are formed by the internal and external rings. The internal (deep) inguinal ring is an opening in the transversalis fascia, which lies approximately 1 cm above the mid-inguinal point (midway between the pubic tubercle and the anterior superior iliac spine). The internal inguinal ring is bounded medially by the inferior epigastric artery (Fig. 11.3). The inguinal canal ends at the external (superficial) inguinal ring, which is an opening in the aponeurosis of the external oblique muscle just above and medial to the pubic tubercle. At birth, the internal and external rings lie on top of each other, so that the inguinal canal is short and straight; with growth, the two rings move apart so that the canal becomes longer and oblique.

The testis and spermatic cord receive a covering from each of the layers as they pass through the abdominal wall.

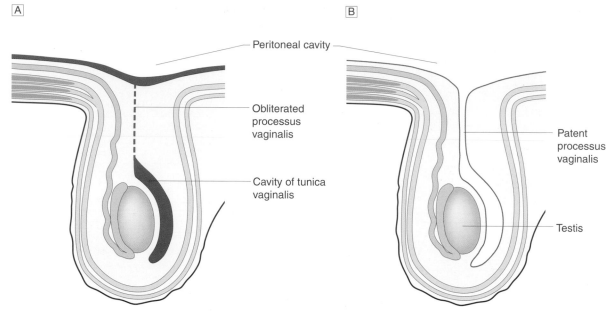

Fig. 11.4 **Processus vaginalis testis.** A Normal obliteration of processus vaginalis. B Persistence of patent processus.

The innermost layer is derived from the transversalis fascia (the internal spermatic fascia), the middle layer from the internal oblique muscle (the cremasteric muscle and fascia), and the outer layer from the external oblique aponeurosis (the external spermatic fascia). Within the inguinal canal, the spermatic cord is covered only by the cremasteric and internal spermatic fasciae. The spermatic cord consists of the vas deferens, the artery of the vas (branch of the inferior vesical artery), the testicular artery (branch of the aorta on the right and renal artery on the left), the cremasteric artery (branch of the inferior epigastric artery), the pampiniform plexus of veins, the ilio-inguinal nerve, the genital branch of the genitofemoral nerve and lymphatics.

Indirect inguinal hernia

An indirect inguinal hernia enters the internal (deep) inguinal ring and descends within the coverings of the spermatic cord so that it can pass on down into the scrotum, the so-called inguino-scrotal hernia. Very occasionally, it enlarges between the muscle layers of the abdominal wall to form an interstitial hernia.

Clinical features

Inguinal hernias typically develop over months to years. While such hernia may cause no symptoms, there may be a dragging discomfort in the groin, particularly during lifting or straining, or at the end of the day. Following a period of rest, such symptoms may improve until further strenuous activity. It is not unusual for a patient to present with a lump in the groin rather than because of painful symptoms.

The hernia forms a swelling in the inguinal canal, which may extend into the scrotum. It is often readily visible when the patient stands or is asked to cough. However, as the population becomes fatter, and patients tend to present earlier with symptoms or a small swelling, the diagnosis may not be so obvious on inspection of the groin. However, look for signs of asymmetry between the two groins. While bilateral inguinal hernias are not unusual, it is unusual for both hernias to be of similar size (Fig. 11.5). An inguinal hernia, which passes into the scrotum, passes above and medial to the pubic tubercle, in contrast to a femoral hernia, which bulges below and lateral to the tubercle (Fig. 11.6). Again, in

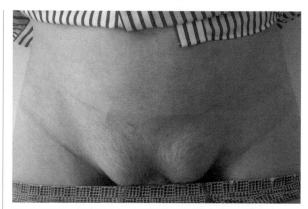

Fig. 11.5 **Clinical photograph of bilateral inguinal hernia.**

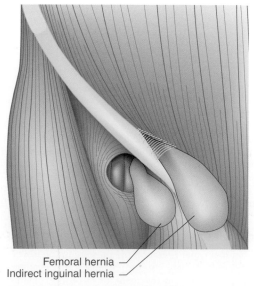

Femoral hernia
Indirect inguinal hernia

Fig. 11.6 **Exit of femoral and inguinal hernias.**

more obese patients, such landmarks can be difficult to palpate with confidence. A cough impulse is normally palpable, and bowel sounds can often be heard within the hernia on auscultation. If there is no visible swelling, a cough impulse is sought with the patient standing.

The hernia often reduces spontaneously when the patient lies down, or it may be reduced by gentle pressure applied in an upward and lateral direction. It may be possible to control the hernia, once reduced, by placing a finger over the internal (deep) inguinal ring.

Direct inguinal hernia

Direct hernias are due to weakness of the abdominal wall and may be precipitated by increases in intra-abdominal pressure (e.g. obstructive airways disease, prostatism or chronic constipation). The hernia protrudes through the transversalis fascia in the posterior wall of the inguinal canal. The defect is bounded above by the conjoint tendon, below by the inguinal ligament, and laterally by the inferior epigastric vessels (Fig. 11.3). These boundaries mark the area known as Hesselbach's triangle. The hernia occasionally bulges through the external (superficial) inguinal ring, but the transversalis fascia cannot stretch sufficiently to allow it to descend down into the scrotum. The sac has a wide neck, so that the hernia seldom becomes irreducible, obstructs or strangulates. As shown in Figure 11.3, the neck of the sac of a direct inguinal hernia lies medial to the inferior epigastric vessels, whereas that of an indirect hernia lies lateral to them. A combined indirect and direct hernia may occur on the same side (pantaloon or saddle-bag hernia), with sacs straddling the inferior epigastric vessels.

Clinical features

The hernia forms a diffuse bulge in the region of the medial part of the inguinal canal. It is usually readily reduced by backward pressure, and the edges of the defect may then be palpable. Clinically, it is frequently impossible to determine whether a hernia confined to the inguinal canal is of the direct or the indirect variety.

Management of uncomplicated inguinal hernia

The identification of an inguinal hernia in any child is *nearly always* an indication to operate. Elective surgery is usually undertaken on a day-case basis, with liberal use of local anaesthetic blocks for postoperative pain relief.

Adults with a symptomatic inguinal hernia should be offered surgery. Open mesh repair or laparoscopic mesh repair aims to reduce postoperative pain to a minimum, enabling most procedures to be undertaken as day cases EBM 11.1. Inguinal hernias can be controlled by a truss, but this is uncomfortable and is now seldom indicated, as repair using local or regional anaesthestic techniques can be employed in higher-risk patients.

EBM 11.1 Laparoscopic inguinal hernia repair

'Laparoscopic inguinal hernia repair is associated with less acute and chronic pain, less nerve injuries such as numbness, quicker return to normal activity and work, and significantly fewer postoperative complications such as infection and haematoma formation than open inguinal hernia repair. Hospital costs are higher for laparoscopic repair and it requires the use of general anaesthetic.'

www.nice.org.uk/TA083guidance,2010

Indirect inguinal hernia

The first step in the open approach is to open the inguinal canal, free the hernial sac from the spermatic cord (Fig. 11.7) and excise it after transfixing and ligating its neck. Simple excision of the sac (herniotomy) is all that is needed in young children. In older children and adults, the internal ring is usually stretched and widened, and therefore after herniotomy it is necessary to tighten the deep ring and/or strengthen the posterior wall with a mesh (herniorrhaphy or hernioplasty). Suture repair alone is rare in developed countries in adults, but still has a place in the repair of groin hernias in adolescents (a rare age for presentation of groin hernias).

Direct hernia

In a direct hernia, the sac, following mobilization from the spermatic cord, is not normally excised and it is simply invaginated by sutures placed in the transversalis fascia. Insertion of a synthetic mesh is currently used to reinforce the posterior wall of the inguinal canal EBM 11.2.

EBM 11.2 Use of mesh in hernia repair

'Mesh reduces the risk of hernia recurrence.'

Flum et al, Ann Surg 2003;237:129.

In all hernia repairs, it is important to avoid constricting the spermatic cord by making the deep inguinal ring too tight. This may compromise the blood supply to the testis, particularly in large or recurrent hernias. In older patients, removal of the testis may be considered so that the inguinal canal can be completely obliterated in recurrent hernias.

The most common surgical procedure now performed is the Lichtenstein open tension-free repair, which involves the insertion of a synthetic mesh underneath the spermatic cord (Fig. 11.8). The mesh is secured to the aponeurotic tissue overlying the pubic bone medially, the inguinal ligament inferiorly, and the internal oblique aponeurosis and conjoint tendon superiorly. Laterally, the mesh is divided and its two sides wrapped around the spermatic cord and sutured in place.

Laparoscopic hernia repair, using a transperitoneal or pre-peritoneal approach, is increasing in popularity. The technique involves reducing the hernial sac and inserting

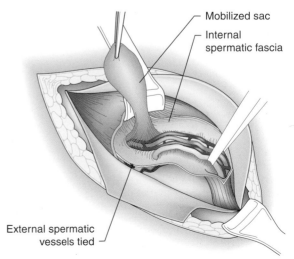

Mobilized sac

Internal spermatic fascia

External spermatic vessels tied

Fig. 11.7 Principle of dissection in the repair of a right inguinal hernia.

11

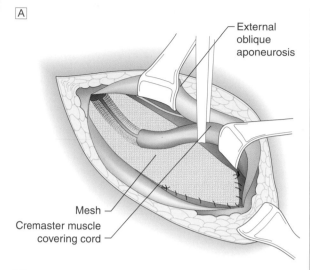

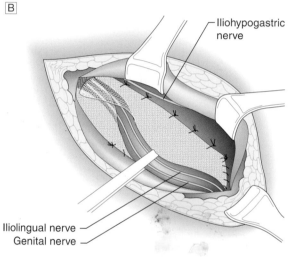

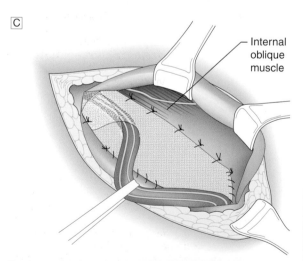

Fig. 11.8 Lichtenstein open mesh repair – right sided hernia. **A** The lower border of the mesh is secured in place with a continuous suture to the inguinal ligament. **B** Interrupted sutures are placed between the upper edge of the mesh and the underlying aponeurosis. **C** A suture is placed laterally to close the two tails around the internal ring.

a mesh. Proponents of these techniques emphasize minimal pain, both acute and chronic, a more rapid return to normal activities and work, improved cosmesis and fewer infective complications; however, critics emphasize the necessity for a general anaesthetic, the violation of the peritoneal cavity (with the transperitoneal approach), increased hospital costs and the technical difficulty of the surgery. An additional benefit of laparoscopic surgery is that the mesh is larger than that used at open surgery, and covers the direct, indirect and femoral hernial orifices. It is generally accepted that the laparoscopic approach is particularly useful for patients with recurrent inguinal hernias or bilateral inguinal hernias, or exploration of the groin when a symptomatic hernia is suspected from the history but is not obvious on clinical examination.

The asymptomatic inguinal hernia does not always require repair. However, the majority of such hernias become symptomatic within several years, at which time they can be repaired.

Approximately 5% of hernias will recur. Early recurrence within 2 years is usually a result of an inadequate primary operation, whereas late recurrence reflects progression of the underlying muscular weakness. Recurrent hernias can be difficult to repair and the laparoscopic approach may be of particular benefit to these patients.

Sportsman's hernia

Groin injury leading to chronic groin pain is often referred to as the sportsman's hernia. However, the definition, investigation and treatment of this condition remain controversial. The differential diagnosis includes musculotendinous injuries, osteitis pubis, nerve entrapment, urological pathology or bone and joint disease. In many cases, clinical signs are lacking, despite the patient's symptoms. Herniography studies have demonstrated a significant incidence of symptomatic impalpable hernia in patients presenting with obscure groin pain. Dynamic ultrasound (ultrasound examination of the groin with the patient at rest and when straining) is replacing herniography as it is non-invasive. MRI scanning is also used, more to exclude other pathology that might be causing the groin pain rather than to diagnose a sportsman's hernia.

A deficiency of the posterior inguinal wall is the most common operative finding in patients with chronic groin pain. Some authors have described a tear in the conjoint tendon as the cause of the pain, whereas in Gilmore's description, a tear in the external oblique aponeurosis, causing dilatation of the external (superficial) inguinal ring, was implicated. Surgical intervention is recommended only when conservative management has failed. Appropriate repair of the posterior wall of the inguinal canal has proved to be of therapeutic benefit in selected patients.

Femoral hernia

A femoral hernia projects through the femoral ring and passes down the femoral canal. The ring is bounded laterally by the femoral vein, superiorly by the inguinal ligament, medially by the lacunar ligament, and inferiorly by the superior ramus of the pubis and the reflected part of the inguinal ligament (pectineal ligament of Astley Cooper) (Fig. 11.9). As the hernia enlarges, it passes through the saphenous opening in the deep fascia of the thigh (the site of penetration of the long saphenous vein to join the femoral vein) and then turns upwards to lie in front of the inguinal ligament. The hernia has many coverings and may be deceptively small, sometimes escaping detection. It frequently contains omentum or small bowel, but the urinary bladder can 'slide' into the medial wall of the sac.

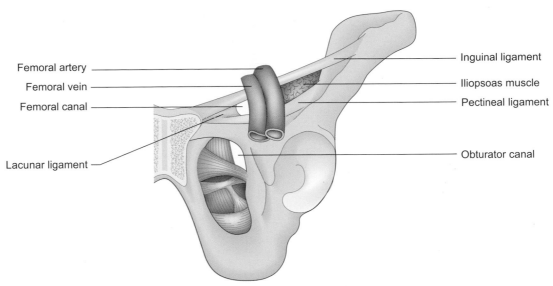

Fig. 11.9 Anatomy of the femoral ring.

Femoral artery

Femoral vein

Femoral canal

Lacunar ligament

Inguinal ligament

Iliopsoas muscle

Pectineal ligament

Obturator canal

Clinical features

The hernia forms a bulge in the upper inner aspect of the thigh. While a lump or swelling may be the presenting symptom, groin pain related to exercise is also a common presentation. It can sometimes be difficult to differentiate between an inguinal and a femoral hernia, but as indicated earlier, the former passes above and medial to the pubic tubercle as it enters the groin, whereas the latter passes below and lateral to it. Tracing the tendon of adductor longus upwards to its insertion can be a useful guide to the position of the pubic tubercle.

A femoral hernia is frequently difficult or impossible to reduce because of its J-shaped course and the tight neck of the sac. As well as needing to be differentiated from inguinal hernia, it can be confused with an inguinal lymph node (no cough impulse, irreducible), saphenous varix (positive cough impulse or 'saphenous thrill', which is prominent on standing but disappears on elevating the leg), ectopic testis, psoas abscess, hydrocoele of the spermatic cord or a lipoma.

Surgical repair of femoral hernia

A femoral hernia is particularly likely to obstruct and strangulate (indeed 40% of such hernias present this way), and therefore surgical intervention is indicated EBM 11.3. As with inguinal hernia, repair can be carried out under local or general anaesthesia.

EBM 11.3 Emergency hernia surgery

'Infarcted bowel is the main risk factor for death in hernia surgery.'

Derici et al, Hernia 2007;11:341.

The aim of operation is to reduce the sac and obliterate the femoral ring by suturing the inguinal ligament to the pectineal ligament. The femoral canal can be approached from below the inguinal ligament, through the inguinal canal, or from above by entering the rectus sheath and displacing the rectus abdominis medially. The approach from above (McEvedy approach) gives the best access, and is particularly useful if the hernia contains strangulated bowel and intestinal resection is required. The laparoscopic approach is an alternative 'high' approach.

SUMMARY BOX 11.2

Groin hernias

- Indirect inguinal hernias comprise 60% of all groin hernias and commence at the deep inguinal ring, lateral to the inferior epigastric vessels
- Direct inguinal hernias account for 25% of all groin hernias and bulge through a weakness in the back wall of the inguinal canal, medial to the inferior epigastric vessels. They rarely obstruct or strangulate
- Indirect inguinal hernias may pass down within the coverings of the spermatic cord to the scrotum; direct hernias do not descend into the scrotum
- Asymptomatic inguinal hernias do not have to be repaired, especially in the elderly
- Femoral hernias account for 15% of all groin hernias and pass through the femoral canal, emerging below and lateral to the pubic tubercle (in contrast to inguinal hernias, which pass medially to the tubercle and may descend to the scrotum)
- Femoral hernias are often small and easy to miss on clinical examination, but are prone to obstruct and strangulate.

Ventral hernia

Ventral hernias occur through areas of weakness in the anterior abdominal wall (Fig. 11.10): namely, the linea alba (epigastric hernia), the umbilicus (umbilical and paraumbilical hernia), the lateral border of the rectus sheath (Spigelian hernia), and the scar tissue of surgical incisions (incisional hernia). Such incisions include scars from laparoscopic surgery, the so-called port-site hernia.

Epigastric hernia

Epigastric hernias protrude through the linea alba above the level of the umbilicus. The herniation may consist of extraperitoneal fat or may be a protrusion of peritoneum containing omentum. The hernia is common in thin individuals and can cause local discomfort. Unless large, epigastric hernias

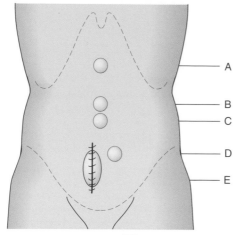

Fig. 11.10 Types of ventral hernia. [A] Epigastric: through the linea alba. [B] Umbilical: through an umbilical scar. [C] Para-umbilical: above or below the umbilicus. [D] Spigelian: lateral edge of rectus muscle. [E] Incisional: anywhere.

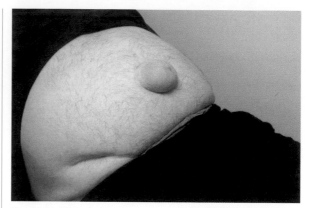

Fig. 11.11 Clinical photograph of a para-umbilical hernia – note the appendicectomy scar.

are rarely visible on inspection, but are palpable as a firm midline lump. It is repaired by closing the defect with non-absorbable sutures, or by inserting a small mesh, or by laparoscopic intraperitoneal mesh repair.

Umbilical hernia

True umbilical hernias occur in infants. The small sac protrudes through the umbilicus, particularly as the child cries, but is easily reduced. Over 95% of these hernias close spontaneously in the first 3 years of life. Persistence after the third birthday is an indication for elective repair. Surgery involves excision of the hernial sac and closure of the defect in the fascia of the abdominal wall.

Para-umbilical hernia

This hernia is caused by gradual weakening of the tissues around the umbilicus (Fig. 11.11). It most often affects obese multiparous women, and passes through the attenuated linea alba just above or below the umbilicus. The peritoneal sac is often preceded by the extrusion of a small knuckle of extraperitoneal fat through the linea alba. The hernia gradually enlarges, the covering tissues become stretched and thin, and eventually loops of bowel may become visible under parchment-like skin. The sac is often multilocular and may be irreducible because of adhesions that form between omentum and loops of bowel. The skin may become reddened, excoriated and ulcerated, and rarely an intestinal fistula may even develop.

Operation is advised because of the risk of obstruction and strangulation. Unless there is a large protrusion of the umbilicus itself, most surgical repairs can be performed preserving the umbilicus. Through a transverse subumbilical incision, the anterior layer of the rectus sheath is exposed. The sac is opened and the contents are reduced. The classic Mayo repair involves the development of a flap of rectus sheath and linea alba above and below the hernial defect. The defect is closed by overlapping the layers, using mattress sutures of non-absorbable material in a 'double-breasted' fashion. Alternatively, the defect can be closed using non-absorbable transverse sutures or the insertion of a mesh. Like epigastric hernias, there is increasing use of laparoscopic mesh repair, especially for a large hernia or a small hernia in a fat patient.

Incisional hernia

Incisional hernias occur after 5% of all abdominal operations. Over half of incisional hernias occur in the first 5 years after the original surgery. Midline vertical incisions are most often affected, and poor surgical technique, wound infection, obesity and chest infection are important predisposing factors, in addition to the collagen metabolism status of the patient. The diffuse bulge in the wound is best seen when the patient coughs or raises the head and shoulders from a pillow, thereby contracting the abdominal muscles (Fig. 11.12). Strangulation is rare, but surgical repair is usually advised.

Again, open or laparoscopic mesh repair is possible. At open surgery, the mesh can be inserted as an onlay, inlay, sublay or intraperitoneal position (Fig. 11.13). The sublay operation is associated with the lowest incidence of wound complications and recurrence of the hernia. Many incisional hernia wounds are cosmetically poor, so laparoscopic surgery for cosmesis is not so clear cut. However, laparoscopic surgery is associated with less pain, shorter hospital stay and more rapid return to activities. However, it is difficult to restore the normal anatomy by bringing the muscles together again at laparoscopic surgery, and thus such an approach is mainly used for smaller incisional hernias.

Parastomal hernia

These occur after the formation of an abdominal wall stoma. The majority of patients with a stoma will develop a parastomal hernia with time. The best way to treat such a hernia includes reversing the stoma, if possible. Otherwise, the

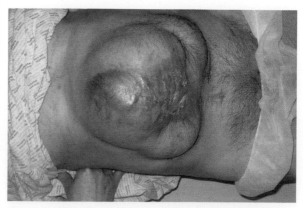

Fig. 11.12 Clinical photograph of a midline incisional hernia.

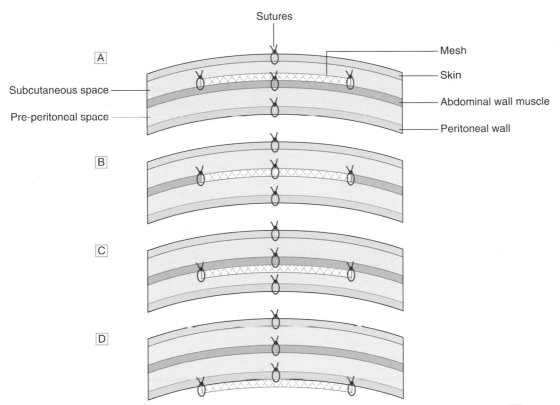

Fig. 11.13 Position of mesh at open incisional hernia repair. **A** Onlay – mesh anterior to the muscles in the subcutaneous space. **B** Inlay – mesh bridges the gap in the muscles. **C** Sublay – mesh within the muscle layers and/or the pre-peritoneal space. **D** Intra-peritoneal onlay mesh (IPOM).

techniques for incisional hernia are relevant here including repositioning of the stoma. There is evidence to support the use of mesh reinforcement at the time of creation of the stoma to minimize the risk of parastomal hernia development. Such prophylactic use of mesh is also considered in other high risk groups, such as midline incisions in the obese.

Rare external hernia

- A *Spigelian hernia* occurs through the linea semilunaris at the outer border of the rectus abdominis muscle. Treatment is surgical, as the hernia is liable to strangulate
- A *lumbar hernia* forms a diffuse bulge above the iliac crest between the posterior borders of the external oblique and latissimus dorsi muscles. It seldom requires treatment
- An *obturator hernia* is a rare hernia that is more common in women and passes through the obturator canal. Patients may present with knee pain owing to pressure on the obturator nerve; however, the diagnosis is frequently made only when the hernia has strangulated and is discovered at laparotomy.

Internal hernia

Herniation of the stomach through the oesophageal hiatus in the diaphragm (hiatus hernia) is a common cause of internal herniation and is considered in Chapter 13. A variety of cul-de-sacs and peritoneal defects resulting from rotation

of the bowel and other abnormalities of development may be responsible for the entrapment of bowel and acute intestinal obstruction. For example, herniation may occur through the foramen of Winslow (opening of the lesser sac) and through various openings in the diaphragm, including the oesophageal hiatus (Fig. 11.14). In addition, bowel operations, such as the development of a Roux loop can lead to 'iatrogenic' sites for internal hernia formation.

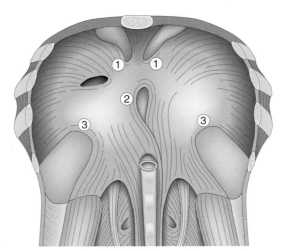

Fig. 11.14 Sites of diaphragmatic herniation. **1** Parasternal, between the sternal and costal slips of the diaphragm (foramen of Morgagni). **2** Oesophageal hiatus. **3** Pleuroperitoneal canal (foramen of Bochdalek).

11

Complications of hernia

Irreducibility

An irreducible hernia is one in which the contents cannot be manipulated back into the abdominal cavity. This may be due to narrowing of the neck of the sac by fibrosis, distension of the contained bowel, or adhesions to the walls of the sac.

Obstruction

An irreducible hernia may progress to intestinal obstruction. Abdominal pain, vomiting and distension signal the need for urgent operation *before* strangulation supervenes.

Strangulation

The vessels supplying the bowel within a hernia may be compressed by the neck of the sac or by the constricting ring through which the hernia passes. The contents initially become swollen as a result of venous congestion, and there is exudation of a blood-stained fluid. The arterial supply is subsequently compromised and gangrene follows. Bacteria and toxins pass out through the bowel wall, causing local peritonitis.

The patient complains of pain in the hernia and usually has features of intestinal obstruction (vomiting, abdominal distension). The skin overlying the hernia is red, warm to touch and tender, the cough impulse is lost, and there may be increasing evidence of circulatory collapse and sepsis. In a Richter's hernia, only part of the circumference of the bowel is strangulated, and there may be no evidence of intestinal obstruction. Strangulation is the main risk factor for death in such cases EBM 11.3.

Management of complicated hernia

If there is no evidence of strangulation, an attempt can be made to reduce an apparently irreducible hernia by giving analgesia, putting the patient to bed with the foot of the bed elevated, and applying gentle pressure. Undue force must never be used for fear of rupturing the bowel or returning the entire hernia to the abdomen with the bowel still trapped within it (reduction en masse). If the hernia does not reduce readily, emergency same day surgery is advised to avoid further complications. Femoral hernias are the least likely hernia (of the common hernias) to be reduced in this way. Following successful reduction of a hernia, the patient can be discharged from the Accident and Emergency department with a plan to repair the hernia within a month.

In infants and children, the majority of 'irreducible' inguinal hernias can, in fact, be safely reduced by a suitably trained clinician. Small doses of intravenous opiate analgesia administered in the presence of suitably trained paediatric nursing staff can relax the child and assist with the reduction process. The hernia can then be repaired within 72 hours on the next available operating list. The child should be detained in hospital pending repair to allow early detection of further episodes of incarceration. Failure to reduce a hernia in this manner necessitates emergency surgery which is often more difficult than when the hernia has been reduced prior to surgery.

Urgent operation is indicated for all obstructed hernias, as one can never be certain that strangulation is not present. Occasionally, a CT scan is indicated in such cases, especially if an underlying malignancy is suspected, such as anaemia, significant weight loss or palpable mass away from the hernia. At surgery, the hernial sac is opened and the contents are inspected carefully. If they are viable, they can be returned to the abdominal cavity and the hernia repaired. If there is doubt about the viability of a loop of bowel or omentum, the devitalized tissue must be resected before proceeding to repair. The use of mesh in potentially infected fields remains controversial. Sometimes bowel resection and simple suture repair is indicated, with planned mesh repair reserved for later recurrence of the hernia.

Mesh, like any prosthesis, can become infected. Often this requires removal of the mesh, with increased risk of recurrence of the hernia.

S. Paterson-Brown

12

The acute abdomen and intestinal obstruction

INTRODUCTION

The 'acute abdomen' is a term used to encompass a spectrum of surgical, medical and gynaecological conditions, ranging from the trivial to the life-threatening, which require hospital admission, investigation and treatment. The primary symptom of the condition is abdominal pain. For the purposes of multicentre studies looking at acute abdominal pain, the definition is taken as 'abdominal pain of less than 1 week's duration requiring admission to hospital, which has not been previously investigated or treated'. Acute abdominal pain following trauma is usually considered separately.

The acute abdomen is a very common clinical entity. It has been estimated that at least 50% of general surgical admissions are emergencies and, of these, 50% present with acute abdominal pain. The acute abdomen therefore represents a significant part of the general surgical workload. Furthermore, patients with acute abdominal pain have significant morbidity and mortality. Studies have shown a 30-day mortality of 4% among patients admitted with acute abdominal pain, rising to 8% in those who undergo operative treatment. Not surprisingly, the mortality rate varies with age, being the highest at the extremes of age. The highest mortality rates are associated with laparotomy for unresectable cancer, ruptured abdominal aortic aneurysm and perforated bowel.

Individual conditions presenting with acute abdominal pain will not be dealt with in depth in this chapter, but will be covered elsewhere.

AETIOLOGY

The causes of the acute abdomen may be subdivided into surgical, medical and gynaecological disorders. Surgical causes may be classified according to the organ involved, as well as the underlying pathological process (Table 12.1). The most common causes in any population will vary according to age, sex and race, as well as genetic and environmental factors (Tables 12.2 & 12.3).

The remainder of this chapter will be concerned principally with surgical conditions, although it should be borne in mind that medical and gynaecological conditions may present with acute abdominal pain.

PATHOPHYSIOLOGY OF ABDOMINAL PAIN

To be able to make an accurate clinical assessment of the patient presenting with acute abdominal pain, it is necessary to understand the pathophysiology. Abdominal pain can be divided into somatic and visceral types.

Somatic pain

The parietal peritoneum covers the anterior and posterior abdominal walls, the undersurface of the diaphragm and the pelvic cavity. It develops from the somato-pleural layer of the lateral plate mesoderm and its nerve supply

Table 12.1 Possible causes of acute abdominal pain

Surgical Inflammation • Inflammatory bowel disease • Acute appendicitis • Acute diverticulitis • Acute pancreatitis • Acute cholecystitis • Acute cholangitis • Meckel's diverticulitis	Abdominal wall conditions • Rectus sheath haematoma
Obstruction • Intestinal obstruction • Biliary colic • Ureteric colic • Acute retention of urine	Genitourinary • Urinary tract infection • Pyelonephritis
	Neurological • Tabes dorsalis
Ischaemia • Mesenteric ischaemia • Torsion of a viscus	Haematological • Sickle cell disease • Malaria • Hereditary spherocytosis
Perforation • Perforated peptic ulcer disease • Perforated diverticular disease • Perforated appendix • Toxic megacolon with perforation • Acute cholecystitis and perforation • Perforated oesophagus • Perforated bladder • Perforation of a length of strangulated bowel • Ruptured abdominal aortic aneurysm	Endocrine • Diabetes mellitus • Thyrotoxicosis • Addison's disease
	Metabolic • Uraemia • Hypercalcaemia • Porphyria
	Infective • Herpes zoster

Medical
Cardiovascular
• Myocardial ischaemia
• Myocardial infarction (inferior)
	Gynaecological
	• Ectopic pregnancy
	• Ovarian cyst
	    Torsion
	    Rupture
	    Haemorrhage
	    Infarction
	    Infection
	• Pelvic inflammatory disease
	• Fibroid degeneration
	• Salpingitis
	• Mittelschmerz
	• Endometriosis

Gastrointestinal • Gastritis • Gastroenteritis • Mesenteric adenitis • Hepatitis • Hepatic abscess • Curtis–FitzHugh syndrome • Primary peritonitis	

is therefore derived from somatic nerves supplying the abdominal wall musculature and the skin (T5–L2). The exception to this is the diaphragmatic portion, which is supplied centrally by afferent nerves in the phrenic nerve (C3–C5), and peripherally in the lower six intercostal and subcostal nerves.

The parietal peritoneum is sensitive to mechanical, thermal or chemical stimulation, and cannot be handled, cut or cauterized painlessly. As a result of its innervation, when the parietal peritoneum is irritated, there is reflex contraction of the corresponding segmental area of muscle, causing rigidity of the abdominal wall (guarding) and hyperaesthesia of the overlying skin.

When the diaphragmatic portion of the parietal peritoneum is irritated peripherally, there will be pain, tenderness and rigidity in the distribution of the lower spinal nerves, but when it is irritated centrally, pain is referred to the cutaneous distribution of C3, 4 and 5 (i.e. the shoulder area, Fig. 12.1). Somatic pain is classically described as sharp or knife-like in nature, and is usually well localized to the affected area.

Visceral pain

The visceral peritoneum forms a partial or complete investment of the intra-abdominal viscera. It is derived from the splanchno-pleural layer of the lateral plate mesoderm, and shares its nerve supply with the viscera (i.e. the autonomic nerves). Visceral pain is mediated through the sympathetic branches of the autonomic nervous system, with afferent nerves joining the pre-sacral and splanchnic nerves, which eventually join thoracic (T6–T12) and lumbar (L1–L2) segments of the spinal cord. The visceral peritoneum and the viscera are insensitive to mechanical, thermal or chemical stimulation, and can therefore be handled, cut or cauterized painlessly. However, they are sensitive to tension, whether due to overdistension or traction on mesenteries, visceral muscle spasm and ischaemia.

Visceral pain is typically described as dull and deep-seated. It is usually localized vaguely to the area occupied by the viscus during development, and is referred to the

Table 12.2 Common causes of acute abdominal pain in UK adults requiring admission to hospital

Condition	Approximate incidence (%)
Non-specific abdominal pain	35
Acute appendicitis	30
Acute cholecystitis and biliary colic	10
Peptic ulcer disease	5
Small bowel obstruction	5
Gynaecological disorders	5
Acute pancreatitis	2
Renal and ureteric colic	2
Malignant disease	2
Acute diverticulitis	2
Dyspepsia	1
Miscellaneous	1

Table 12.3 Common causes of acute abdominal pain in UK children

- Acute appendicitis
- Urinary tract infection
- Mesenteric adenitis
- Gastroenteritis

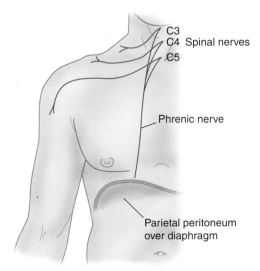

Fig. 12.1 The shared sensory innervation of the shoulder and diaphragm.

overlying skin of the abdominal wall according to the dermatome level with the sympathetic supply, as mentioned above. Therefore, pain arising from the intestine and its outgrowths (the liver, biliary system and pancreas) is usually felt in the midline. Irritation of foregut structures (the lower oesophagus to the second part of the duodenum) is usually felt in the epigastric area. Pain from midgut structures (the second part of the duodenum to the splenic flexure) is felt around the umbilicus. Pain from hindgut

structures (the splenic flexure to the rectum) is felt in the hypogastrium.

Although the division of abdominal pain into visceral and somatic pain is useful, it is important to realize that some pathological conditions will result in a mixed picture. For example, acute appendicitis classically presents with acute abdominal pain that is initially felt in the umbilical area resulting from appendicular obstruction, which gradually localizes to the right iliac fossa and becomes sharper in nature as the overlying parietal peritoneum becomes inflamed.

 SUMMARY BOX 12.1

Abdominal pain

- Visceral abdominal pain is mediated by the sympathetic nervous system and is typically deep-seated and ill localized to the area originally occupied by the viscus during intrauterine life
- Colic is a form of visceral pain that arises from a hollow viscus with muscle in its walls (e.g. gut, gallbladder, ureter), and results from excessive muscle contraction, often against an obstructing agent
- Patients experiencing colic are usually unable to remain still during the bout of pain but are pain-free between attacks. 'Biliary colic' is an exception (and the term colic may be a misnomer), in that pain often waxes and wanes on a plateau and there are no pain-free intervals
- Parietal pain, such as that caused by parietal peritonitis, is mediated by somatic nerves and is localized to the area of inflammation
- Reflex guarding and rigidity of the overlying muscles is usually present, and the patient is reluctant to move for fear of exacerbating the pain
- Some areas of the peritoneum (e.g. the pelvis, posterior abdominal wall) are 'non-demonstrative' in that parietal peritonitis may be present without tenderness or guarding of overlying muscles.

PATHOGENESIS

As one can see from the list of surgical conditions that may present with acute abdominal pain (Table 12.1), there are two main underlying pathological processes involved: inflammation and obstruction. These processes may be triggered by a variety of underlying abnormalities. It is important to realize that in any one patient a combination of abnormalities and processes may be involved.

Inflammation

Acute inflammation of an intra-abdominal organ or the peritoneum may occur as a result of a variety of irritants. These may be broadly classified into infective or non-infective in nature (Table 12.4).

No matter what the trigger of the inflammation, the subsequent pathological process is the same. There is reactive hyperaemia of the injured tissue as a result of capillary and arteriolar dilatation; exudation of fluid into the tissues as a result of an increase in the permeability of the vascular endothelium; and an increase in filtration pressure. Finally, there is migration of leucocytes from the vessels into the inflamed tissues.

12

Table 12.4 Injurious agents causing inflammation

Infective
- Bacterial
- Viral
- Fungal
- Parasitic

Non-infective
- Chemical
- Ischaemic
- Physical trauma
  heat
  cold
  radiation
  immune mechanisms

Table 12.5 Classification of peritonitis

Generalized peritonitis

Primary: infection of the peritoneal fluid without intra-abdominal disease
- Haematogenous spread
- Lymphatic spread
- Direct spread: usually associated with continuous ambulatory peritoneal dialysis (CAPD) catheters
- Ascending infection: from the female genital tract

Secondary: inflammation of the peritoneum arising from an intra-abdominal source
- Infectious
- Non-infectious
  Blood
  Ischaemia
  Bile
  Chemical
  Foreign body
- Perforation

Localized peritonitis
- Usually due to spreading inflammation across the wall of an intra-abdominal viscus

The clinical consequences of the inflammatory process depend upon a multitude of factors, the most important being the underlying condition, its severity and duration, the organ involved, the patient's age and comorbidity. In general, the patient will complain of abdominal pain and tenderness, which occurs as a result of tissue stretching and distortion and is due to the release of inflammatory mediators, some of which also mediate pain. On general examination, the patient may be pyrexial and have a tachycardia; investigations may reveal a raised white cell count. Examination of the abdomen will reveal tenderness in the affected area, with guarding and rigidity if the parietal peritoneum is involved.

Peritonitis

Inflammation of the peritoneum (peritonitis) may be classified according to extent (either localized or generalized) and aetiology (Table 12.5). In a surgical setting, the most common cause of generalized peritonitis is perforation of an intra-abdominal viscus. Inflammation of the peritoneum results in an increase in its blood supply and local oedema formation. There is transudation of fluid into the peritoneal cavity, followed by the accumulation of a protein-rich fibrinous exudate. In the normal state, the greater omentum constantly alters its position within the abdominal cavity as a result of intestinal peristalsis and abdominal muscle contraction. In the presence of inflammation, the greater omentum will adhere to and surround the abnormal organ. The fibrinous exudate effectively glues the omentum to the inflamed viscus, walling it off and preventing the further spread of inflammation. In addition, the exudate inhibits intestinal peristalsis, resulting in a paralytic ileus which also limits the spread of the inflammation and infection. As a result of the ileus, fluid accumulates within the lumen of the intestine and, along with the formation of large volumes of intra-peritoneal transudate and exudate, this will lead to a decrease in the intravascular volume, producing the clinical features of hypovolaemia.

Clinical features

The clinical features of peritonitis will again vary according to a wide variety of factors. The most common symptom is abdominal pain, which is constant and often described as sharp. The pain is usually well localized if it is secondary to inflammation of an intra-abdominal viscus, but may spread to involve the whole peritoneal cavity. Primary peritonitis can present rather more subtly, and as many as 30% of affected individuals may be asymptomatic.

The term 'peritonitis' or 'peritonism detected on clinical examination' is used to describe the collection of signs associated with inflammation of the parietal peritoneum, and includes 'guarding' and 'rebound' tenderness. Evidence of inflammation of the parietal peritoneum in association with inflammation of an intra-abdominal viscus is often a strong indication that the patient requires some form of surgical intervention.

Infarction

An infarct is an area of ischaemic necrosis caused either by an occlusion of the arterial supply or the venous drainage in a particular tissue, or by a generalized hypoperfusion in the context of shock (Table 12.6). The typical histological feature of infarction is ischaemic coagulative necrosis. An inflammatory response begins to develop along the margins of an infarct within a few hours, stimulated by the presence of the necrotic tissue.

Table 12.6 Aetiology of infarction

Occlusive
Arterial
- Embolism
- Thrombosis
- Extrinsic compression

Venous
- Thrombosis
- Extrinsic compression

Non-occlusive
Shock
- Hypovolaemia
- Cardiogenic
- Sepsis

Vasoconstrictor drugs

The consequences of decreased perfusion of a tissue depend on several factors: the availability of an alternative vascular supply, the rate of development of the hypoperfusion, the vulnerability of the tissue to hypoxia, and the blood oxygen content. In the context of acute abdominal pain, intestinal infarction is the most common cause. Other organs that may infarct include the ovaries, kidneys, testes, liver, spleen and pancreas.

Clinical features

In general, the patient will complain of severe abdominal pain and the onset will depend on the nature of the underlying process. Embolization will result in a sudden onset of pain, whereas the onset in thrombosis is likely to be more gradual. Infarction and ischaemia are potent triggers of inflammation of the affected structure, and the clinical features reflect this.

Perforation

Spontaneous perforation of an intra-abdominal viscus may be the result of a range of pathological processes. Weakening of the wall of the viscus, which might follow degeneration, inflammation, infection or ischaemia, will predispose to perforation. An increase in the intraluminal pressure of a viscus, such as occurs in a closed-loop obstruction (Fig. 12.2), will predispose to perforation, as will peptic ulceration, acute appendicitis and acute diverticulitis. Other less common causes are carcinoma of the colon, inflammatory bowel disease and acute cholecystitis.

Perforation can also be iatrogenic, and may occur during the insertion of a Verres needle at laparoscopy, because of a careless cut or suture placement during surgery, and during the course of an endoscopic procedure.

Clinical features

Spontaneous perforation of a viscus usually results in the sudden onset of severe abdominal pain, which is usually well localized to the affected area. The resultant clinical picture depends on the nature of the perforated viscus and the relative sterility and toxicity of the material that is spilt into the abdominal cavity, in addition to the speed with which the perforation is surrounded and sealed (if at all) by the adjacent structures and omentum. The inevitable peritoneal contamination will lead to either localized or generalized peritonitis, and the associated symptoms and signs, as already discussed. Intestinal content, blood and bile are all irritant to the peritoneum.

Obstruction

The term 'obstruction' refers to impedance of the normal flow of material through a hollow viscus. It may be caused by the presence of a lesion within the lumen of the viscus, an abnormality in its wall, or a lesion outside the viscus causing extrinsic compression.

The smooth muscle in the wall of the obstructed viscus will contract reflexly in an effort to overcome the impedance. This reflex contraction produces 'colicky abdominal pain'. The exception to this rule is 'biliary colic'. The gallbladder and biliary system has little smooth muscle in its wall and attempts at contraction tend to be more continuous than 'colicky'.

If the obstruction is not overcome, there will be an increase in intraluminal pressure and proximal dilatation. The end result depends on the anatomical location of the obstruction, whether it is partial or complete, and whether the blood supply to the organ is compromised. For example, a urinary bladder calculus causing partial urinary outflow obstruction may result in a dilatation of the ureter and renal pelvis, and subsequent 'post-renal' renal failure. An obstructed inguinal hernia, on the other hand, will not only produce proximal dilatation of the intestine (usually associated with vomiting) but may also result in ischaemia of the bowel wall, leading to infarction and perforation.

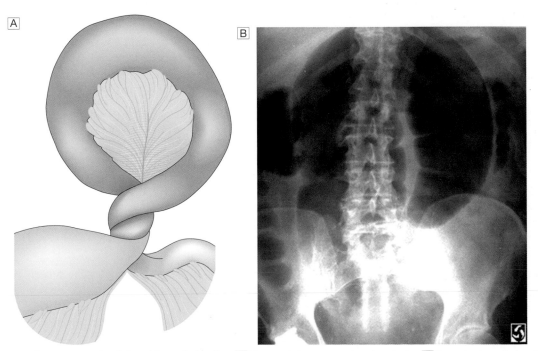

Fig. 12.2 Volvulus: an example of closed-loop obstruction. A Diagrammatic representation of a volvulus. B X-ray showing volvulus of sigmoid colon.

12

CLINICAL ASSESSMENT

The ability to make an accurate assessment by taking a good history and performing an appropriate examination is a vital skill in the management of the patient with acute abdominal pain. Although an exact diagnosis is often impossible to make after the initial assessment and often relies on further investigations, it is the formulation of an appropriate, safe and effective management plan that is the most important issue. In most cases, it is possible to take a full history and perform a thorough examination, but this is not always so, and occasionally a rapid evaluation followed by immediate resuscitation is required.

History

The main presenting complaint of patients with an acute abdomen is pain. The characteristics of the pain (Table 12.7) give important clues to the likely underlying diagnosis, and these should be explored in depth. However, the importance of a full history cannot be overemphasized and is essential in all patients.

Site of pain

The site of abdominal pain is perhaps the most valuable pointer to the underlying diagnosis. In order to describe the site of pain, the abdomen is traditionally divided into either quarters or ninths (Figs 12.3 and 12.4).

Table 12.7 Characteristics of abdominal pain

- Site
- Nature
- Radiation
- Time and mode of onset
- Severity
- Progression
- Duration
- Exacerbating/relieving factors

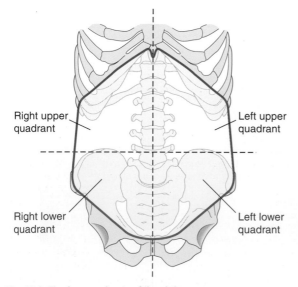

Fig. 12.3 The four quadrants of the abdomen.

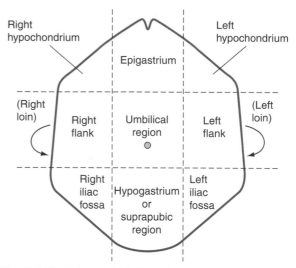

Fig. 12.4 The abdomen divided into ninths.

Nature of pain

As discussed above, there are two main pathological mechanisms in the development of abdominal pain: obstruction and inflammation.

Inflammation produces a constant pain made worse by local or general disturbance, and pain which is made worse by movement or coughing suggests inflammation of the parietal peritoneum. In this situation, the patient will often be seen to lie very still in order not to exacerbate the pain.

Obstruction of a muscular viscus produces a colicky pain which comes and goes in 'spasms', often only lasting a few minutes at a time but returning at frequent intervals. It may be described as 'gripping' in nature, and between spasms the patient is usually pain-free. The pain itself is severe and may be helped by moving around or drawing the knees up towards the chest. Underlying inflammation must be suspected when a colicky pain does not disappear between spasms, or becomes continuous. In the case of intestinal obstruction, this might mean strangulation, for which urgent surgery is required.

Radiation of pain

Radiation is the process whereby pain extends directly from one place to another, while usually remaining present at the site of onset. When a pain radiates, it signifies that other structures are becoming involved. For example, pain from a duodenal ulcer may radiate through to the back, indicating that inflammation has occurred through the wall of the duodenum to involve structures of the posterior abdominal wall, such as the pancreas. Ureteric pain radiates to the tip of the penis in men and to the labium majoris in women.

Onset of pain

The onset of pain can be sudden or gradual. Typically, pain from a perforation is sudden and that from inflammation is gradual. Patients with the former can usually remember exactly what they were doing at the time of onset, whereas in the latter localization in time is more difficult. The various characteristics of abdominal pain, as shown in Figure 12.5, are essential in helping the clinician formulate a differential diagnosis.

Severity of pain

A patient's description of the severity of pain is very subjective. Every individual has a different reaction to pain, and

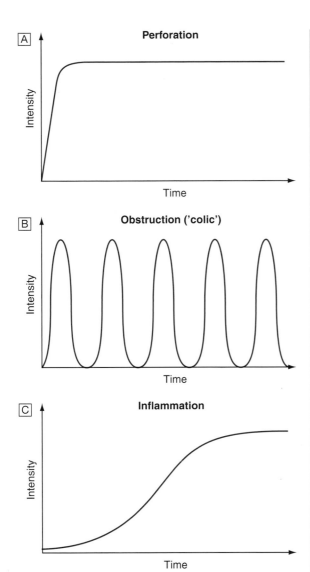

Fig. 12.5 Time vs intensity graphs for acute abdominal pain.

12

this is often more reflective of the patient's personality than of the underlying pathology. A better indication is to assess the effect of the pain on the patients' lives. For example, did they call their GP? Were they unable to attend work? Did the pain interfere with their sleep? Furthermore, it is often useful to ask the patient to rate pain severity using a score on a numerical or pictorial scale.

Progression of pain

Once a pain has occurred, it may remain exactly the same, may gradually improve or worsen, or may fluctuate.

Movement of pain

It is also useful to note whether the pain moves. Acute appendicitis is a classic example of pain that moves, starting as a vague central 'referred' pain and then moving to the right iliac fossa as the adjacent parietal peritoneum becomes inflamed.

Examination

During the course of taking a history it is possible to form a general impression of the state of the patient. The unwell patient with acute abdominal pain may look pale and sweaty, lie flat on the bed, be cerebrally obtunded, and be unable to move without experiencing pain. Others, however, may look surprisingly well, have a good colour, sit up in bed, talk normally and be able to move freely. All these observations should be noted and recorded, along with the temperature, pulse, blood pressure and respiratory rate.

Other important features to look for on general examination include clinical evidence of anaemia, jaundice, cyanosis and dehydration. It is important to bear in mind that physical signs are often less obvious than might be expected in the elderly, the obese, the generally unwell and those taking steroids. As in every emergency patient, a full examination, including the cardiovascular, respiratory and neurological systems, in addition to the abdomen and pelvis, must be carried out and the results documented. Specific details relating to the abdominal examination are described below and in Table 12.8.

In small children with abdominal pain, it is useful to ask the child to 'blow out' and 'suck in' their abdomen and to cough. These three movements will usually elicit pain in the presence of peritonism without laying a hand on the child's abdomen. Rebound tenderness should *never* be elicited in children. Gentle tapping with the percussing finger will elicit the same information (tap tenderness) in a much less cruel way. The history of pain on moving or coughing is also a good indicative as to the presence of rebound tenderness.

Inspection of the abdomen

In order to examine the abdomen, the patient must be adequately exposed and positioned. The full extent of the abdomen should be visible, and by convention the patient should be exposed from 'nipples to knees'. This prevents the common mistake of not examining the breasts, groins and external genitalia. Patient dignity should be maintained and the breasts and genitalia covered once assessed. Patients should be positioned supine on the bed or trolley with a single pillow behind the head and shoulders and with the arms resting by their side.

Inspection of the abdomen may reveal a wealth of information. Abdominal swellings due to abnormal enlargement of the liver, kidneys or spleen, and tumours of the bowel, ovaries or other intra-abdominal or retroperitoneal structures may be visible. Scars from previous abdominal or pelvic surgery may be observed, and are of importance in the presence of bowel obstruction, which may be secondary to adhesions. All scars should be tested for the presence of herniation. Distended veins on the abdominal wall may be secondary to portal hypertension or occlusion of the inferior vena cava. The abdomen may be generally distended by intra-abdominal blood or fluid, or as a result of intestinal obstruction. In cases of obstruction, intestinal peristalsis may be visible, if the patient is thin.

Palpation

Palpation of the abdomen should be carried out in a systematic manner, beginning with gentle superficial examination of the whole abdomen looking for tenderness. This should start away from the site of maximum pain and move towards the tender site, encompassing all areas, as shown in Figures 12.3 and 12.4. Palpation over an area of tenderness will cause pain, which in turn will stimulate the patient to contract the overlying muscles (voluntary guarding). If the pain is due to inflammation, the approximation of the parietal peritoneum on to the inflammatory area will result in a reflex contraction of the overlying muscles (involuntary guarding). If the whole peritoneal cavity is inflamed, then there will be generalized peritonitis and the abdominal wall will be rigid (board-like rigidity). When the palpating

Table 12.8 Checklist for examination of the acute abdomen

Method	Question	Significance
Inspection	What is the abdominal contour?	Distension: intestinal obstruction or ascites
	Does the abdomen move with respiration?	Rigid abdomen: peritonitis
	Can the patient blow out/suck in the abdomen?	Rigid abdomen: peritonitis
	Does the patient lie still or writhe about?	Fear of movement: peritonitis
		Writhes about: colic
	Are there visible abnormalities?	Scars: relevant previous illness, adhesions
		Hernia: intestinal obstruction
		Visible peristalsis: intestinal obstruction
		Visible masses: relevant pathology
Gentle palpation	Is there tenderness, guarding or rigidity?	Tenderness/guarding: inflamed parietal peritoneum
		Rigidity: peritonitis
Deep palpation	Are there abnormal masses/palpable organs?	Palpable organs/masses: relevant pathology
	Is there rebound tenderness?	Rebound tenderness: peritonitis
Percussion	Is the percussion note abnormal?	Resonance: intestinal obstruction
		Loss of liver dullness: gastrointestinal perforation
		Dullness: free fluid, full bladder
		Shifting dullness: free fluid
Auscultation	Are bowel sounds present/abnormal?	Absent sounds: paralytic ileus
		Hyperactive sounds: mechanical obstruction, gastroenteritis
	Is there a bruit?	Bruit: vascular disease

Do not forget to:

Examine the groin

Consider a digital rectal examination

Consider a vaginal examination when appropriate

Examine the chest

hand, which has been pushing the parietal peritoneum against the inflamed viscus, is suddenly released, the viscus will bounce back and hit the parietal peritoneum, causing an additional sharp pain (rebound tenderness). This is an excellent indication of underlying peritoneal inflammation (peritonism) but is very painful and is better tested by light percussion. As already mentioned earlier, history of pain on coughing or moving is also a good indication of peritoneal inflammation.

If light palpation of the whole abdomen elicits no pain, the process is repeated pressing more firmly to detect deep tenderness. This will allow for the detection of organomegaly and the presence of any masses.

In the past, opiate analgesia was traditionally withheld from patients with acute abdominal pain on the assumption that it might mask important clinical signs, particularly of localized tenderness. This has now been shown not to be the case, and analgesia should never be withheld from a patient pending formal examination. Indeed, the administration of analgesia relaxes the patient and may often help the examination. However, repeated administration of opiate analgesia to a patient with abdominal pain in whom a definite diagnosis has not been made cannot be supported without regular reassessment, as this suggests progression of the disease process and that surgical intervention may be indicated.

During the general examination, particular attention should be paid to the supraclavicular fossae, axillae and cervical regions for the presence of lymphadenopathy. The hernial orifices must also be specifically examined, as must the male external genitalia, looking for tenderness and masses within the scrotum.

Percussion

Percussion is useful in the localization and assessment of tenderness, particularly in the assessment of rebound tenderness, in addition to determining the presence of fluid within the peritoneal cavity. The normal abdomen is universally resonant because of the presence of gas-containing bowel lying in front of the solid retroperitoneal structures, and because the normal pelvic viscera lie entirely within the bony pelvis.

The liver gives a dull note to percussion anteriorly from the level of the right fifth rib to the right costal margin, and loss of liver dullness to percussion may represent free intra-peritoneal gas. The presence of suprapubic dullness may indicate a full bladder due to urinary retention. If there is free intra-peritoneal fluid, the percussion note will be dull in the flanks. The site of the dullness moves as the patient rolls on to his or her side (shifting dullness). One litre or more of fluid is required before this sign can be elicited.

Auscultation

Bowel will only produce gurgling noises if it contains a mixture of fluid and gas. Normal bowel sounds are low-pitched and occur every few seconds. Their absence over a 30-second period suggests that peristalsis has ceased, a condition termed ileus. This may be due to generalized peritonitis or atony of the bowel smooth muscle, such as might follow a prolonged period of obstruction. Increased peristalsis produces a higher volume, pitch and frequency of the bowel sounds and can be heard in mechanical obstruction (often described as 'tinkling'), in addition to conditions such as gastroenteritis. In general, bowel sounds should be described as present and normal, present and abnormal, or absent.

Auscultation should continue over the course of the aorta and the iliac arteries, listening for the presence of bruits, which are indicative of turbulent flow.

If gastric outlet obstruction is clinically suspected, the patient's abdomen may be shaken from side to side in an attempt to elicit a 'succussion splash'.

Rectal examination

Finally, a rectal examination is performed to assess the pelvis and, if a gynaecological disorder is suspected, a vaginal examination is indicated. Although examination of the rectum is considered 'routine' it may be omitted, particularly in young patients, when a diagnosis and management plan have already been made and are unlikely to be influenced by any information obtained. Useful information that might be obtained from a rectal examination includes the presence of masses, tenderness and blood.

Specific clinical signs in acute abdominal pain

Murphy's sign

In acute cholecystitis, a deep breath taken by the patient elicits acute pain when the examiner presses downwards into the right upper quadrant. This is caused by the movement of the inflamed gallbladder striking the examining hand.

Boas's sign

In acute cholecystitis, pain radiates to the tip of the scapula and there is a tender area of skin just below the scapula, which is hyperaesthetic.

Grey Turner's and Cullen's signs

In patients with severe acute pancreatitis, bruising and discoloration may be seen around the umbilicus (Cullen's sign) and in the left flank (Grey Turner's sign). Cullen's sign was actually first described in relation to ruptured ectopic pregnancy, but is now often also associated with acute pancreatitis.

Rovsing's sign

In acute appendicitis, palpation in the left iliac fossa produces pain in the right iliac fossa.

Investigations

Following initial clinical assessment, and during assessment in the critically ill, measures should be taken to resuscitate the patient. During this period, further investigations can be organized to help in the diagnostic process. It is important to remember that in all patients a working list of differential diagnoses must be made after clinical assessment so that only appropriate investigations are instituted. There is no point in organizing investigations the results of which will not influence the clinical management.

The most common investigations carried out on the patient with acute abdominal pain include full blood count (FBC), urea and electrolytes (U&Es), amylase, C-reactive protein, liver function tests, plain radiology (erect chest and supine abdominal X-rays) and an ultrasound scan.

Blood tests

Blood tests can be very useful in confirming a diagnosis (amylase for acute pancreatitis), identifying an underlying inflammatory cause for the pain (raised C-reactive protein and leucocytosis) and biliary disorders (liver function tests).

It is also very useful to have baseline results for FBC and U&Es for future reference.

FBC, C-reactive protein and U&Es

A single reading of a raised white cell count taken on its own is fairly non-discriminatory, but a persistent elevation or a rise suggests underlying inflammation and/or infection; similarly for C-reactive protein levels. In the assessment of patients with possible appendicitis, recent studies have demonstrated that, in the presence of a normal C-reactive protein *and* white cell count, acute appendicitis is very unlikely. Obviously U&Es are essential in patients who might be hypovolaemic in order to monitor fluid replacement, particularly if surgery is being considered. Similarly, an abnormal haemoglobin level may be significant and require correction.

Serum amylase

A serum amylase greater than three times the upper limit of normal is highly suggestive of acute pancreatitis. Lesser values are non-specific and can be the result of a wide range of conditions. However, as many as 20% of patients with acute pancreatitis may have normal amylase levels on admission. Other causes of a raised amylase are shown in Table 12.9. In patients with acute pancreatitis who present more than 48 hours after the onset of pain, the serum amylase may have returned to normal. In these patients, measurement of the urinary amylase may be of value.

Liver function tests

Liver function tests are increasingly becoming available on an emergency rather than a routine basis in many hospitals, as clinicians have recognized their value in the assessment and subsequent management of acute hepatobiliary and pancreatic disorders (see chapter 14). The measurement of gamma glutamyl transferase (GGT) is a particularly sensitive test for possible stones in the common bile duct (choledocholithiasis).

Blood gas analysis

Arterial blood sampling is often used to monitor the acid-base status and the efficacy of gas exchange in the seriously ill patient. Patients with sepsis and intestinal ischaemia are likely to demonstrate a metabolic acidosis with an elevated lactate level.

Table 12.9 Causes of hyperamylasaemia

Pancreatic conditions
- Acute pancreatitis
- Pancreatic cancer
- Pancreatic trauma

Other intra-abdominal pathology
- Perforated peptic ulcer
- Acute appendicitis
- Ectopic pregnancy
- Intestinal infarction
- Acute cholecystitis

Decreased clearance of amylase
- Renal failure
- Macroamylaseaemia

Miscellaneous
- Head injury
- Diabetic ketoacidosis
- Drugs (e.g. opiates)

Serum calcium

Patients with hypercalcaemia may complain of abdominal pain as a result of abnormal gastrointestinal motility, nephrolithiasis, peptic ulcer disease, pancreatitis or malignancy. A low calcium level is one of the poor prognostic factors in patients with severe acute pancreatitis.

Sickle tests

Sickle cell crises are a rare cause of acute abdominal pain. Blood should be sent for testing on all at-risk patients.

Blood glucose

Measurement of blood glucose is important, as diabetic ketoacidosis may present with acute abdominal pain, and also because any serious illness can result in poor glycaemic control, particularly in diabetic patients.

Urinalysis

Dipstick testing

Haematuria may result from a wide range of conditions but in the context of acute abdominal pain may indicate a urinary tract tumour, infection or nephrolithiasis. Glucose or ketones in the urine indicate recent starvation or possible diabetic ketoacidosis. Protein, bilirubin or casts in the urine suggest renal or liver disease. In patients with an inflamed retrocaecal appendix, urine testing may demonstrate the presence of protein, and urgent microscopy (which will confirm or refute the presence of bacteria) should be arranged to determine whether there is an underlying urinary tract infection or whether another condition, such as appendicitis, might be the cause.

Bacteriology

If the clinical picture is suggestive of a urinary tract infection and the urine dipstick demonstrates blood, protein or nitrites, urgent microscopy and culture should be requested. Specimens from any other potential sites of infection should also be submitted for bacteriological analysis (stool, blood, pus etc.).

Pregnancy test

A pregnancy test should be performed in all women of child-bearing age who present with acute abdominal pain and in whom the chance of pregnancy cannot be excluded. Not only is this important if X-rays are to be taken, but it will also reveal the possibility of an ectopic pregnancy if positive.

Urinary porphobilinogen

Quantitative assay of urinary porphobilinogen is the most important diagnostic test for porphyria, which is a rare condition that may present with acute abdominal pain and should be considered in difficult cases.

Radiological investigations

Plain X-rays

The role of plain radiography in the investigation of the patient with acute abdominal pain has been well studied. The erect chest X-ray (CXR) is the most appropriate investigation for the detection of free intra-peritoneal gas (Fig. 12.6) and should be carried out in any patient who might have a perforation. If the condition of the patient prevents an erect film being taken, then a left lateral abdominal decubitus film might be helpful. Although a visceral perforation is the most common cause of free intra-peritoneal gas, other causes exist and should be considered where appropriate (Table 12.10). An erect CXR is also useful in identifying a respiratory condition which may present with upper abdominal pain.

The role of plain abdominal radiographs remains controversial despite many studies that have demonstrated that,

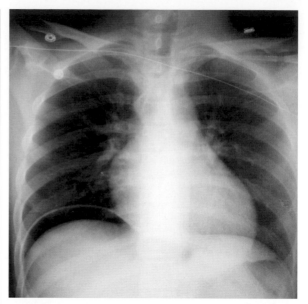

Fig. 12.6 Gas under the diaphragm seen on the erect chest X-ray in a patient with a perforated peptic ulcer.

Table 12.10 Causes of free subdiaphragmatic gas on abdominal X-ray

- Perforation of an intra-abdominal viscus
- Gas-forming infection
- Pleuroperitoneal fistula
- Iatrogenic: laparoscopy, laparotomy
- Gas introduced per vaginam: post-partum
- Interposition of bowel between liver and diaphragm

---

with the exception of suspected intestinal obstruction (Fig. 12.7), they rarely help in the diagnosis and have even less role in altering the clinical decision (EBM 12.1). However, the supine abdominal X-ray (AXR) can be of use in patients whose diagnosis is unclear and in whom the presence of calcification (e.g. ureteric colic) and abnormal gas shadows (e.g. possible intestinal ischaemia) may be helpful. They should however *not* be performed routinely, and have no role in the investigation of patients with suspected appendicitis.

An erect AXR is only of value in patients with intestinal obstruction, although it is well known that even then the information obtained over and above that from the supine film is small. In patients with suspected obstruction whose supine film does not show significant bowel dilatation, an erect film might reveal fluid levels.

EBM 12.1 Abdominal radiography

'Plain abdominal radiography has a limited role in the assessment of the acute abdomen, particularly when the diagnosis is likely to be peptic ulcer disease, acute biliary disease or acute appendicitis. It is valuable when the diagnosis is uncertain and in patients with other suspected acute gastrointestinal conditions such as obstruction.'

Paterson-Brown S. In: Paterson-Brown S, ed. A companion to specialist surgical practice: core topics in general and emergency surgery, 4th edn. London: Elsevier; 2009: 81-95.

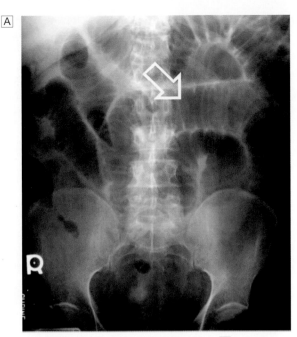

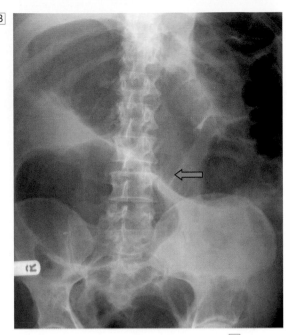

Fig. 12.7 Abdominal X-rays in bowel obstruction. [A] Supine film in a patient with small bowel obstruction showing valvulae comitantes. [B] X-ray demonstrating large bowel obstruction with arrow at a haustration.

Contrast radiology

Contrast may be administered orally, down a nasogastric or nasojejunal tube, or per rectum to examine the bowel in patients with acute abdominal pain. In the emergency setting, the contrast used is usually water-soluble, as free egress of barium into the peritoneal cavity can make subsequent surgery more difficult and will remain for a very long time making subsequent X-ray examinations more difficult to interpret. As water-soluble contrast does not adhere well to the bowel mucosa, the information obtained is less specific and detailed than with barium, but in the patient with acute abdominal pain, the main issue that requires the use of contrast X-rays is determining the presence or absence of obstruction or perforation.

In up to 50% of patients with a perforated peptic ulcer, no free gas can be identified on plain radiography. If the diagnosis remains uncertain based on clinical assessment, a water-soluble contrast meal might be diagnostic (Fig. 12.8). In patients with small bowel obstruction, a water-soluble small bowel follow-up can help not only in confirming or refuting obstruction, but also in predicting which patient is likely to require surgery. Failure of contrast to reach the caecum by 4 hours suggests obstruction and these patients will not usually settle with non-operative management (Fig. 12.9).

A water-soluble contrast enema used to be considered essential in the assessment of patients with large bowel obstruction in order to differentiate between pseudo-obstruction and an obstruction caused by a mechanical problem (Fig. 12.10). However computed tomography (CT) with rectal contrast is now more commonly performed (see Ch. 16). Carrying out an unnecessary operation on a patient with pseudo-obstruction is associated with a high morbidity and mortality and cannot be defended.

Intravenous pyelography confirms the diagnosis of renal obstruction by calculi and may be helpful in the diagnosis of other types of renal pain. Again CT is now more commonly used to detect renal tract calculi.

Ultrasonography

Ultrasound is the most common investigation used in patients with acute abdominal pain. As a general investigation it might reveal small amounts of intra-peritoneal fluid in conditions such as perforation and infection, whereas in specific

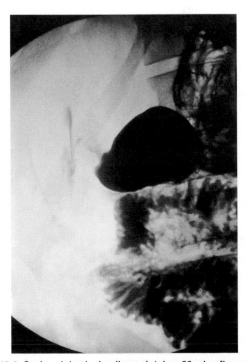

Fig. 12.8 Supine abdominal radiograph taken 20 min after oral administration of 50 ml of water-soluble contrast in a patient with suspected perforated peptic ulcer, in whom the erect chest radiograph was normal. Note the small trickle of contrast through the perforation. These findings were confirmed at laparotomy (from Ellis BW, Paterson-Brown S (eds) 2000 Hamilton Bailey's Emergency Surgery, 13th edn. Hodder Arnold, with permission).

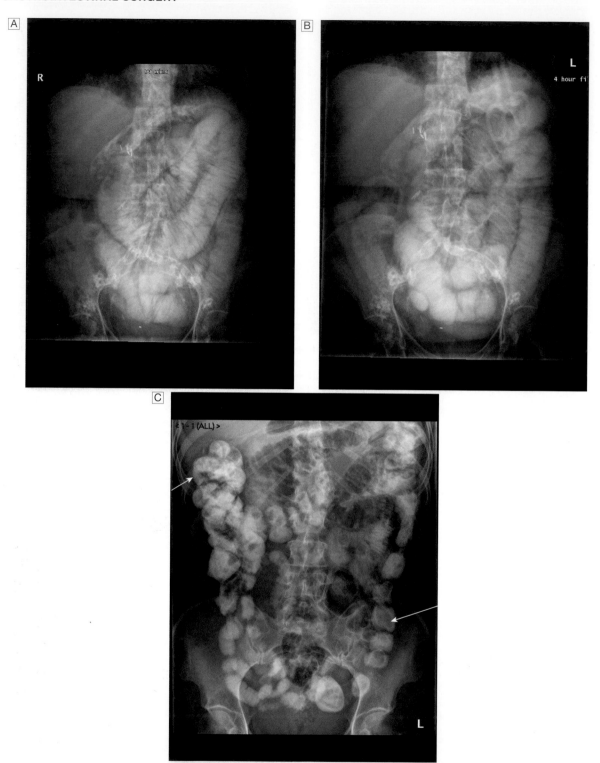

Fig. 12.9 Supine abdominal radiographs taken after oral administration of 50 ml of water-soluble contrast material. **A** 90 minutes after administration. **B** 4 hours after. Note failure of contrast to reach the caecum and the obvious small bowel obstruction. Laparotomy confirmed small bowel obstruction due to adhesions. **C** 90 minutes after administration of contrast in another patient showing contrast in the large bowel (arrows) excluding small bowel obstruction.

conditions such as acute cholecystitis, biliary obstruction, aortic aneurysms and ovarian cysts it can be diagnostic. Although some studies have reported high levels of sensitivity and specificity in the diagnosis of acute appendicitis, ultrasonography in these cases is highly operator-dependent and a negative result cannot be relied upon, particularly if the clinical picture suggests otherwise.

Computed tomography (CT)

The current multi-slice CT scanners have such good organ definition that they are increasingly being used early in the investigation of the acute abdomen where they can reliably identify free intra-abdominal gas, ischaemic bowel, acute inflammation such as appendicitis and diverticulitis. In general, because of the radiation used, the use of CT should

12

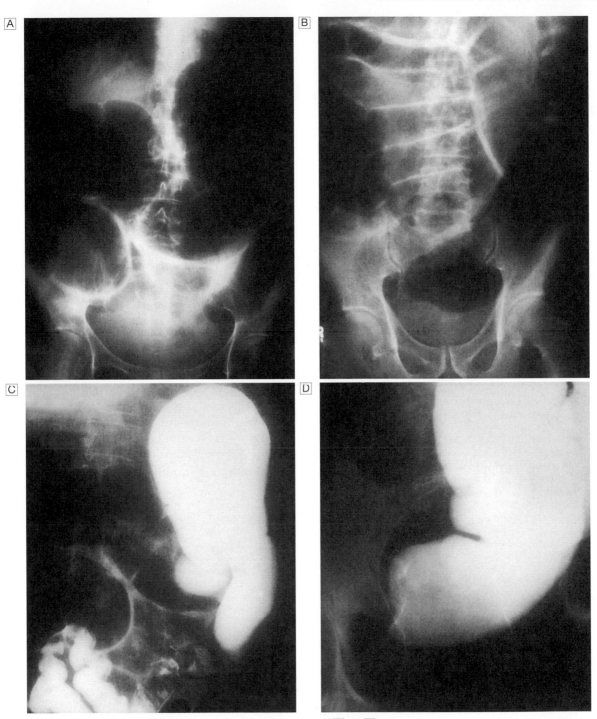

Fig. 12.10 Contrast radiology in the diagnosis of large bowel obstruction. A and B Supine abdominal X-rays in patients with large bowel obstruction. C Contrast enema in patient A shows no mechanical cause, i.e. pseudo-obstruction. D An obstructing carcinoma of the sigmoid colon in patient B.

be limited to cases of diagnostic difficulty and to evaluate traumatic injuries and intra-abdominal sepsis in patients who may have an intra-abdominal collection or abscess, in addition to suspected leaking abdominal aortic aneurysms. Contrast-enhanced CT is also used routinely to detect pancreatic necrosis in patients with severe acute pancreatitis. CT should not be used routinely in young patients with suspected appendicitis.

Angiography

Mesenteric angiography used to be the investigation of choice in suspected mesenteric ischaemia, but has now been superseded by CT angiography, which can also reliably

differentiate arterial from venous causes, and distinguish occlusive from non-occlusive disease. CT angiography can also be used in the diagnosis and management of lower gastrointestinal haemorrhage, although this rarely presents with acute abdominal pain. Obviously, if embolization is required, formal angiography is necessary.

Endoscopic investigations

Flexible sigmoidoscopy is commonly performed on patients who present with an acute abdomen associated with rectal bleeding and in those patients with large bowel obstruction to evaluate the anorectum. Additional information can be obtained from a colonoscopy. Furthermore, a sigmoid volvulus can often be deflated by careful sigmoidoscopy (see chapter 16). Upper gastrointestinal endoscopy is used to investigate patients with acute upper abdominal pain in whom a perforated peptic ulcer has been excluded, as discussed above.

Peritoneal investigations

Peritoneal lavage

Peritoneal lavage was used for many years as a first-line investigation in patients suspected of having intra-abdominal injury from trauma. However its use has now been taken over by CT. Many Emergency Departments are now using FAST (Focussed Abdominal Scans for Trauma); ultrasound scans in the immediate assessment of patients with abdominal trauma in order to identify free fluid (i.e. blood or bowel contents). In patients where free fluid is seen, CT scans can then be organized if required, or alternatively, depending on the state of the patients, immediate surgery can be planned. Occasionally some patients on the intensive care unit requiring large amounts of cardiac support are too unstable to be transferred to the CT scanner. In these patients peritoneal lavage can be helpful in confirming or excluding a surgical cause of a patient's condition. It is carried out by inserting a dialysis catheter into the peritoneal cavity under local anaesthetic and infusing 1 litre of normal saline. The effluent is removed and examined for white cell count, amylase, bacteria and bile.

Laparoscopy

Many studies have demonstrated that laparoscopy (Fig. 12.11) can significantly improve surgical decision-making in patients with acute abdominal pain. It is particularly useful in patients for whom the decision to operate is in doubt, and in the elderly when findings from the history and examination can be misleading. Young women probably benefit the most from laparoscopy, as it is so difficult in this group to accurately differentiate acute appendicitis from acute gynaecological conditions, many of which do not require surgery. As laparoscopic appendicectomy increases in use, more patients will undergo diagnostic laparoscopy first.

MANAGEMENT

All patients admitted with acute abdominal pain require resuscitation and close monitoring, with regular re-evaluation. It is a good clinical rule that initial treatment should be based around the ABC principle (airway, breathing and circulation). Except in the management of overwhelming haemorrhage (e.g. ruptured abdominal aortic aneurysm and ruptured ectopic pregnancy) when resuscitation takes place on the way to the operating theatre, all patients with acute abdominal pain, including those requiring urgent surgery, benefit from adequate resuscitation. This will usually involve the administration of several litres of normal saline and/or a colloid solution, intravenous antibiotics and oxygen by face mask (see chapters 1 and 5). Monitoring by means of temperature, pulse, blood pressure, urine output and central venous pressure will depend on the clinical circumstances and will not be detailed further here. Suffice to say that good preoperative assessment, resuscitation, monitoring and regular reviewing of the patient with acute abdominal pain (initially every 30 minutes to 2 hours, depending on the state of the patient) is a prerequisite for a satisfactory clinical outcome. Indeed, following the first assessment, close observation and regular reassessment should be carried out on *all* patients without a definitive diagnosis, as their condition may well change and the underlying cause or the correct management may become more obvious. Until this time, it is common practice to keep the patient fasted; if there are signs or symptoms of obstruction, a nasogastric tube is inserted. Appropriate analgesia should be administered early to keep the patient as comfortable as possible. Deep venous thrombosis prophylaxis should also be commenced as a routine.

The management of most conditions presenting as an acute abdomen will be covered in detail in the relevant chapters. The remainder of this chapter will cover the principles that underpin the management of peritonitis, acute appendicitis, non-specific abdominal pain and gynaecological causes of the acute abdomen.

PERITONITIS

As discussed above, inflammation of the peritoneum is a common feature of the acute abdomen. It can be classified as acute or chronic, septic or aseptic, and primary or secondary. Acute suppurative peritonitis secondary to visceral disease is the most common form of peritonitis in surgical practice and primary peritonitis is rare. Chronic peritonitis due to tuberculosis is now rare, and is more commonly found in patients undergoing peritoneal dialysis. It results in abdominal pain, ascites or obstruction due to matting of the bowel by dense adhesions. Treatment is by removal of the catheter and drainage of any loculated collections, usually under ultrasound guidance, but occasionally laparotomy is required. Aseptic peritonitis is generally due to chemical (e.g. urine, bile, gastric contents, blood, meconium)

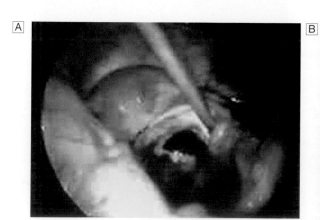
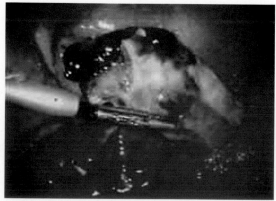

Fig. 12.11 Diagnostic laparoscopy. [A] Bleeding ovarian cyst. [B] Acute appendicitis.

or foreign-body irritants (e.g. starch, talc, cellulose), and is frequently followed by secondary bacterial peritonitis.

The primary objective is to deal promptly and effectively with the underlying cause. For example, perforation of a viscus must be repaired, infarcted bowel must be resected, and infective foci should be removed or drained. Operation is undertaken with minimal delay. The only time that should be spent before operation is that needed to resuscitate an ill patient. It is imperative that extracellular fluid volume is replaced adequately, and central venous pressure monitoring is essential in critically ill and elderly patients. A nasogastric tube should be inserted to empty the stomach and prevent further vomiting, and a urinary catheter should also be placed to monitor urinary output. Antibiotic cover is indicated early in all patients with established secondary peritonitis and is directed against gut flora in the first instance (e.g. piperacillin-tazobactam or gentamicin and metronidazole). Thorough peritoneal lavage is an essential adjunct to operation, and many surgeons employ an antibiotic-containing solution.

Primary peritonitis

Primary peritonitis is uncommon, although in childhood it can account for up to 15% of acute abdominal emergencies. The condition used to be common in young girls following the ascent of pneumococcal or streptococcal infection from the genital tract.

Escherichia coli is now the predominant causal organism and probably gains access through the gut wall, or rarely by bloodborne spread from a distant focus. In adults, spontaneous bacterial peritonitis (SBP) may occur in patients with the nephrotic syndrome, but is more frequently seen in those with liver cirrhosis or chronic renal failure (particularly in patients on peritoneal dialysis). The mortality rate for patients with primary bacterial peritonitis varies from 20% to 80%.

Classically, diffuse peritonitis with generalized abdominal tenderness and rigidity develops within 24 hours. Fever and leucocytosis occur early. Abdominal rigidity is relatively uncommon. A sample of peritoneal fluid, which is usually turbid, is sent for Gram staining and bacterial culture. Antibiotic therapy is the mainstay of treatment, but either laparoscopy or laparotomy may be needed to rule out a surgical cause, if this is suggested by the culture of enteric organisms.

Postoperative peritonitis

Peritonitis after abdominal surgery may be a residual effect of the original disease or a direct complication of its operative management (e.g. anastomotic leakage). Diagnosis is difficult, as:

- the patient is usually receiving analgesia and/or sedation, and may not complain of pain
- any pain and tenderness may be attributed to the wound
- there is often a 24–48-hour period after abdominal surgery when bowel sounds are absent and the abdomen is distended.

Persisting abdominal distension or the development of vomiting and distension after an initial return to normality should raise the suspicion of peritoneal infection. Suspicion is heightened if the patient looks unwell and has fever, tachycardia and an altered mental state. Plain abdominal films may merely show dilatation of the intestine and ultrasonography can be used to detect collections. However contrast enhanced CT with oral contrast/rectal contrast is the best investigation and will identify anastomotic leakage and any associated collections.

Fluid and electrolyte replacement, nasogastric suction and broad-spectrum antibiotic therapy are instituted, and the need for reoperation is considered. Patients with a small anastomotic leak which is well drained (by drains left at the time of the original surgery) may be managed non-operatively and intra-peritoneal collections can be drained by percutaneous drainage under radiological guidance. Patients with more widespread peritonitis require repeat laparotomy. There is an increasing role for re-look laparotomy in patients with severe sepsis identified at the time of the first operation in order to further washout the peritoneal cavity, if after the first few days they are still exhibiting signs of severe sepsis. This is usually preceded by CT to help identify any collections which may have occurred.

Intra-abdominal abscess

An intra-abdominal abscess may develop in conjunction with an underlying inflammatory process or be a complication of peritonitis or intra-abdominal surgery. The abscess gives rise to pyrexia, tachycardia and clinical signs of toxicity. Leucocytosis and raised C-reactive protein are usual. Common sites for abscess formation are the subphrenic and subhepatic spaces, the pelvis, and between loops of bowel. Complications include rupture with generalized peritonitis, the erosion of blood vessels with potentially catastrophic bleeding, and septicaemia. Occasionally, subphrenic abscesses rupture into the pleural cavity, and pelvic abscesses sometimes discharge spontaneously through the rectum.

The site of the abscess may be suspected from the history and clinical examination, but localizing signs can be surprisingly few, particularly with subphrenic abscess, hence the expression 'pus somewhere, pus nowhere else, pus under the diaphragm'. Unexplained fever after peritoneal infection or operation should always raise the suspicion of abscess formation. Tachycardia is usual. Pain and tenderness over the ribcage, shoulder-tip pain and a 'sympathetic' pleural effusion strengthen the suspicion of subphrenic abscess, whereas urgency of defaecation, diarrhoea and a boggy swelling in the pouch of Douglas on rectal examination are features of a pelvic abscess (Fig. 12.12).

12

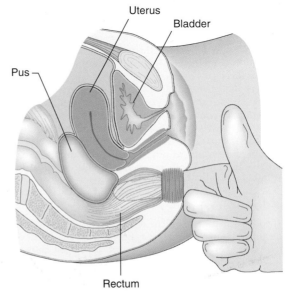

Fig. 12.12 Rectal examination for pelvic abscess.

Uterus

Bladder

Pus

Rectum

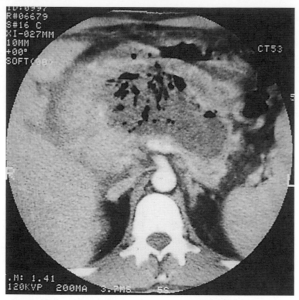

Fig. 12.13 CT scan of upper abdomen showing pancreatic abscess containing streaks of gas.

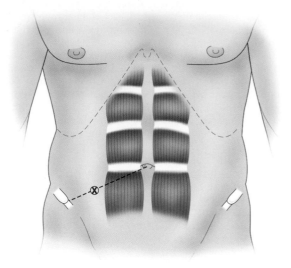

Fig. 12.14 McBurney's point.

Ultrasound and/or CT are of immense value in diagnosis (Fig. 12.13), aspiration to obtain material for bacteriological culture and subsequent drainage. However, surgical drainage may still be needed to ensure effective drainage, particularly if the collection is loculated. Pelvic abscesses frequently rupture spontaneously into the rectum, but may require incision and drainage through the anterior rectal wall. Antibiotic therapy is used in conjunction with drainage of the abscess. Signs usually resolve rapidly following effective drainage.

ACUTE APPENDICITIS

Anatomy

The appendix is a worm-shaped blind-ending tube that arises from the posteromedial wall of the caecum 2 cm below the ileocaecal valve. It varies in length from 2 to 25 cm, but is most commonly 6–9 cm long. On the external surface of the bowel, the base of the appendix is found at the point of convergence of the three taeniae coli of the caecum. On the surface of the abdomen, this point lies one-third of the way along a line drawn between the right anterior superior iliac spine and the umbilicus (McBurney's point; Fig. 12.14). The appendix has its own mesentery, the mesoappendix, and its blood supply comes from the appendicular artery, a branch of the ileocolic artery. The position of the appendix is variable, depending on its length and mobility. In cadaveric dissections the most common site is retrocaecal, but data from diagnostic laparoscopy indicate that the pelvic position is probably more common (Fig. 12.15). In children, there are abundant lymphoid follicles in the submucosa, but these atrophy with age.

Epidemiology

In the UK, appendicitis is the most common cause of acute abdominal pain requiring surgery, and it has been estimated that 16% of the population of developed countries will undergo appendicectomy for presumed appendicitis during their lifetime. There has been a decline in the incidence of appendicitis over the last 20 years, but the reason for this is unknown. There is an equal incidence in males

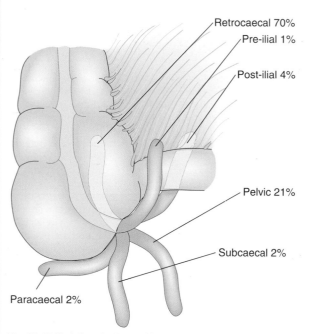

Fig. 12.15 Variations in the position of the appendix.

and females. Appendicitis is uncommon in patients below the age of 2 and above the age of 65, and is most common in the under-40s, with a peak incidence between 8 and 14 years. There is a geographical variation in the incidence, being rare in Asia and Central Africa, which is thought to be due to environmental factors. In Western countries, it is seen more frequently in cities than in rural areas.

Aetiology

Despite its prevalence, the aetiology of acute appendicitis remains unclear. Several different mechanisms have been proposed, one of the more popular causes being a diet lacking in fibre and a consequent slow transit time and alteration in bacterial flora. However, this theory is challenged by a decline in incidence of appendicitis over recent years that has not been matched by an increase in dietary fibre intake. Others have suggested that viral infection may be an aetiological agent, as there is an association between appendicitis and concurrent viral illness and because there is a seasonal variation in the incidence of appendicitis.

Pathogenesis

Obstruction of the lumen of the appendix is thought to play the main role in the initiation of inflammation. Faecoliths, lymphoid hyperplasia, foreign bodies, carcinoid tumours and strictures may all cause luminal obstruction and subsequently lead to acute appendicitis. Following obstruction, the wall of the appendix becomes inflamed, commencing in the mucosa and spreading to involve the submucosal, muscular and serosal layers. A fibrinopurulent exudate forms on the serosal surface and extends to any adjacent peritoneal surface. Inflammation of the wall of the appendix causes venous congestion, which may compromise arterial inflow, leading to ischaemia and infarction. Organisms from the lumen of the appendix enter the submucosa through an ischaemic ulcer, causing liquefaction of the wall and ultimately perforation.

As a result of the transmural inflammation, small bowel and omentum adhere to the appendix, creating a localized area of sepsis. If left untreated, this may progress to form an appendix mass or even an abscess. If perforation occurs early in the clinical course, the inflamed area will not have had time to be walled off, and generalized peritonitis follows.

Clinical features

History

Classically, the onset of acute appendicitis is associated with the gradual onset of poorly localized central abdominal pain. After a variable amount of time, the pain moves to the right iliac fossa and changes in character, to become sharper, constant and well localized. It is aggravated by movement and coughing. As described earlier, this change in the nature of the pain occurs when the parietal peritoneum overlying the appendix becomes involved in the inflammatory process. In general, most patients present within 24 hours of the onset of the central abdominal pain. Many patients also admit to anorexia and occasional vomiting.

In children, the classic history and physical findings of appendicitis are often not seen. Non-specific symptoms (anorexia, nausea, vomiting, diarrhoea) and signs (fever, fetor, pallor, abdominal distension) can confuse the inexperienced clinician. The finding of tenderness and guarding in the right iliac fossa usually makes the diagnosis without the need for other investigations.

Examination

The patient with established acute appendicitis looks unwell, is flushed and has a dry furred tongue with a fetor. The temperature is usually only mildly elevated (37.3–38.5°C) and there is often a tachycardia. Classically, the area of maximal tenderness is over McBurney's point, with guarding and rebound (percussion) tenderness. Palpation in the left iliac fossa may reproduce the pain in the right iliac fossa (Rovsing's sign) and the patient may find it painful to extend the right hip owing to irritation of the psoas muscle (psoas stretch sign). Although rectal and vaginal examinations are frequently normal, they can be useful when the abdominal signs are vague, particularly if the acutely inflamed appendix lies within the pelvis, when tenderness may be elicited with the examining finger. In young women, either rectal or vaginal examination is extremely useful in helping to differentiate acute appendicitis from acute gynaecological disorders.

Variations in clinical features

The symptoms and signs of acute appendicitis are influenced by a variety of factors, which include age, sex, personality and the position of the appendix. Only 50% of patients with acute appendicitis give a typical history. An inflamed retrocaecal appendix may produce poorly localized abdominal pain, and an inflamed pelvic appendix lying close to the bladder may produce symptoms of frequency and dysuria. In this scenario, as with a retrocaecal appendix that overlies the ureter, it may be quite difficult to differentiate between urinary infection and acute appendicitis. Dipstick examination of the urine may reveal microscopic haematuria and proteinuria in both cases. However, urgent microscopy and Gram stain of the urine will demonstrate bacteria in urinary tract infection. An inflamed pelvic appendix lying near the rectum causes irritation and diarrhoea, and is commonly mistaken for gastroenteritis. However, gastroenteritis is a dangerous diagnosis to make in the acute abdomen as it almost never causes abdominal tenderness (compared to abdominal pain). A very long appendix extending up to the right upper quadrant might even mimic acute cholecystitis.

Acute appendicitis is most dangerous in the very young, the very old and pregnant women. As it is uncommon under the age of 2 years, when it does occur, it is often incorrectly diagnosed as gastroenteritis. The symptoms and signs are atypical and generalized peritonitis quickly develops. In contrast, in elderly patients, the onset is more insidious. The inflamed area tends to wall off, with the development of a mass, and symptoms and signs of obstruction may be present. In the pregnant patient, the appendix is displaced upwards by the enlarged uterus, and the site of the pain and tenderness is high in the abdomen. Appendicitis in pregnancy carries a high rate of morbidity and mortality for both mother and fetus.

A list of conditions that should be considered in the differential diagnosis of acute appendicitis is given in Table 12.11.

Complications

Gangrenous appendicitis and perforation tend to occur after a significantly more prolonged period of pain than uncomplicated appendicitis. Generalized peritonitis results if the inflamed area is not walled off by omentum and loops of bowel. If walling off does occur, either an appendix mass or an abscess will develop. A perforated pelvic appendix will lead to a pelvic abscess, and on examination there may be very little in the way of abdominal signs.

12

Table 12.11 Differential diagnosis of acute appendicitis
• Mesenteric adenitis
• Meckel's diverticulitis
• Regional ileitis (Crohn's disease)
• Carcinoma of the caecum
Gynaecological disorders
• Ruptured ovarian follicle (Mittelschmerz)
• Acute salpingitis
• Ruptured ectopic pregnancy
• Torsion of an ovarian cyst
Genitourinary
• Pyelonephritis
• Ureteric colic
• Urinary tract infection
• Right-sided testicular torsion

Investigations

The various investigations used in patients with suspected appendicitis have already been discussed earlier in the chapter. However, the diagnosis of acute appendicitis is based on clinical assessment and there are no specific diagnostic tests. Ultrasonography in skilled hands might demonstrate a swollen non-compressible appendix, free fluid or even a mass in the right iliac fossa. If, after clinical assessment, the diagnosis remains in doubt, the clinician must proceed along one of two lines: either to carry out laparoscopy and undertake appendicectomy if indicated, or to institute a short policy of close and repeated observation with reassessment every hour. On occasions when there is diagnostic difficulty, and particularly in the elderly, abdominal CT can be helpful in making the diagnosis in addition to excluding other conditions (Fig. 12.16).

Management

The treatment of appendicitis is almost always surgical; increasingly, laparoscopic appendicectomy is being carried out, especially if a diagnostic laparoscopy has been performed first to establish the diagnosis (EBM 12.2). Although the laparoscopic approach is undoubtedly associated with less postoperative pain, most studies have so far failed to show significant advantages in shortening hospital stay or returning to normal activities. This is probably because of the underlying sepsis, which slows recovery. It is also possible to treat patients who do not have overt peritonitis non-operatively with antibiotics, and this is often done in areas of the world where ready access to surgery is impossible. In these conditions, there is a high incidence of recurrent problems and as such this practice is not favoured. If, by the time the patient presents, a mass can be felt, non-operative management with intravenous fluids and antibiotics is the treatment of choice, provided there are no signs of peritonitis (when an operation should be carried out). In these patients, an ultrasound scan should be arranged to look for an underlying abscess; if one is present, it should be drained either under radiological guidance or surgically.

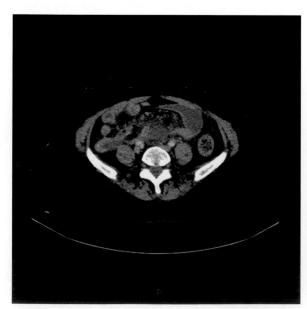

Fig. 12.16 CT scan demonstrating perforated appendicitis.
The thickened and inflamed appendix can be seen extending from the caecum medially associated with some flecks of gas near the tip.

Following successful non-operative treatment of an appendix mass, it used to be traditional practice to carry out an interval appendicectomy 3–6 months later. This prevents further attacks, and in the elderly makes sure that there is no underlying carcinoma of the caecum. However, several studies have now confirmed that after the successful non-operative treatment of either an appendix mass or an abscess, only a few patients develop recurrent problems, and most of them do so within the first few months. It is therefore reasonable not to carry out an interval appendicectomy unless the patient experiences further symptoms or complications (EBM 12.3). It is still important, especially in older patients, to exclude a carcinoma of the caecum by either double-contrast barium enema or colonoscopy. An interval appendicectomy should be undertaken if this course is not pursued.

Prognosis

The overall mortality of appendicitis is less than 1%, rising to 5% if perforation occurs and increasing with age. The postoperative morbidity is mainly related to wound infection and late-onset intestinal obstruction from adhesions. The former can be kept to a minimum by perioperative prophylactic antibiotics (metronidazole), and the latter by careful surgery and perhaps the increasing use of laparoscopic appendicectomy. It used to be thought that fertility in female patients was adversely affected by acute appendicitis, but this no longer seems to be the case. Even in cases of perforated appendicitis, there appears to be no increased risk of infertility.

NON-SPECIFIC ABDOMINAL PAIN (NSAP)

This term is often applied to patients in whom no cause can be found for their abdominal pain. In studies, its incidence has been found to be around 40% for all patients admitted with acute abdominal pain, dropping to around 25%

Appendicitis

- Incidence has declined, but appendicitis is still the most common acute abdominal condition in childhood, adolescence and early adulthood
- The typical history of periumbilical colic (visceral midgut pain), followed within several hours by right iliac fossa pain (somatic pain from parietal peritonitis), is not always present
- Tenderness and muscle guarding in the right iliac fossa are the most reliable signs of acute appendicitis. Leucocytosis, high temperature and radiological signs are manifestations that may denote gangrene and perforation
- The diagnosis should be made and appendicectomy undertaken before gangrene and perforation supervene
- Gangrene and perforation are common and/or particularly dangerous in infants, during pregnancy and in the elderly.

if investigations such as laparoscopy are used to improve diagnostic accuracy. The major concern in reaching a diagnosis of NSAP is that a serious underlying condition has been missed. It has been reported that 10% of patients over 50 years of age who are discharged with NSAP from hospital after an acute admission with abdominal pain have an underlying malignancy, of which half are colonic. Another group of patients who tend to be diagnosed with NSAP are young females who may have a gynaecological condition, such as pelvic inflammatory disease or ovarian cyst pathology. With the more widespread use of laparoscopy in the investigation of patients with acute abdominal pain, the incidence of NSAP will continue to fall.

GYNAECOLOGICAL CAUSES OF THE ACUTE ABDOMEN

Gynaecological conditions commonly present to the on-call surgical team as 'lower abdominal/pelvic pain', mimicking acute surgical conditions such as acute appendicitis and acute diverticulitis. A detailed gynaecological and sexual history is essential to help differentiate these conditions, in addition to obtaining urine for microscopy and a pregnancy test. Where gynaecological conditions are suspected or confirmed, discussion and referral to the on-call gynaecological team is indicated. However a general knowledge of the common gynaecological conditions which often present to the on-call surgical team and their treatment is required.

Mittelschmerz and ruptured corpus luteum

The Graafian follicle normally ruptures 14 days after the start of the last menstrual period, and release of the ovum may be complicated by bleeding. The follicle normally becomes a corpus luteum, which degenerates before the start of the next period unless conception occurs. Bleeding from the corpus luteum is an occasional cause of pain in the late stages of the menstrual cycle.

Patients with these causes of pain are usually between 15 and 25 years of age, and experience sudden pain in one or other iliac fossa. Tenderness and guarding in the right iliac fossa can simulate acute appendicitis, and a few patients bleed sufficiently to suggest rupture of an ectopic pregnancy.

Rectal or vaginal examination may reveal tenderness in the rectovaginal pouch. Ultrasonography may demonstrate free fluid in the pelvis.

The patient is treated non-operatively, unless appendicitis or ruptured ectopic pregnancy cannot be excluded when laparoscopy should be performed.

Ruptured ectopic pregnancy

A fertilized ovum implants at an abnormal site in 1 in 200 pregnancies; the fallopian tube is by far the most common site. The erosive trophoblast may penetrate the wall of the tube, and often ruptures after about 6 weeks. Alternatively, the conceptus may be extruded from the fimbrial end of the tube.

Bouts of cramping iliac fossa pain may be associated with fainting and vaginal bleeding. Rupture produces sudden severe pain, bleeding and circulatory collapse, with the abdominal pain often becoming generalized. Immediate surgery is required. A missed period is reported by most patients and a raised beta human chorionic gonadotrophin (β-HCG) level in the presence of abdominal pain should always raise the suspicion of an ectopic pregnancy.

Complications of an ovarian cyst

Benign ovarian cysts are a common cause of torsion, rupture and bleeding. Dermoid cysts often have a long pedicle and account for 50% of torsions in young women. Pain from rupture/bleeding can be sudden and severe and may mimic other causes of lower abdominal peritonitis, particularly acute appendicitis.

Pain from a torted ovarian cyst is often severe and cramp-like and sometimes associated with a smooth round mobile mass that lies higher in the abdomen than might be expected. Tenderness and guarding may be present. Torsion of a fibroid may produce a similar picture.

At laparoscopy the twisted pedicle is transfixed and ligated and the cyst is removed. Care must be taken to avoid rupture in case the cyst is malignant. Further radical surgery may be needed if histological examination reveals malignancy. In many cases the cyst has actually resulted in torsion of the whole ovary and by the time of surgery this is usually dead and requires removal, although if caught early untwisting may result in salvage of the ovary. Obviously in all such cases the gynaecology team should be involved in management.

Acute salpingitis

Acute salpingitis is most commonly caused by chlamydial infection, but streptococcal, gonococcal or even tuberculous infection can also be responsible. Both tubes are often involved and adhesions may seal the fimbriated end, producing a pyosalpinx, and subsequent infertility.

Bilateral pain is felt just above the pubis and inguinal ligaments. There may be urinary frequency, irregular menstruation, pyrexia, leucocytosis and raised C-reactive protein. Vaginal examination reveals unusual warmth, a tender cervix and a vaginal discharge. The cervix appears red and inflamed, and a swab reveals the causative organism. Vaginal findings may be less marked when there is a closed pyosalpinx.

Treatment consists of antibiotic therapy. Laparoscopy is used increasingly to avoid unnecessary laparotomy if acute appendicitis cannot be ruled out. The tubes appear inflamed and oedematous, and 'milking' them gently produces a purulent discharge from which a bacteriological swab can be taken.

SUMMARY BOX **12.3**

Gynaecological causes of pain and the acute abdomen

- Non-specific abdominal pain (i.e. pain for which no cause is defined) is particularly common in female adolescents and young women, and often mimics acute appendicitis. Laparoscopy may prove increasingly valuable when the diagnosis is in doubt and the need for surgery cannot be excluded
- Minor intraperitoneal bleeding at the time of rupture of the Graafian follicle may cause mid-cycle pain (Mittelschmerz) in the iliac fossa in young girls
- Rupture of an ectopic pregnancy causes intraperitoneal bleeding and more severe abdominal pain, with circulatory collapse. Signs of pregnancy are seldom present and pregnancy testing may be unhelpful. Elevation of the foot of the bed may produce shoulder-tip pain and underline the need for laparotomy
- Torsion of an ovarian cyst often causes cramping lower abdominal pain. Ovarian cysts can become very large and produce visible abdominal swellings which lie higher than might be expected. Some cysts prove to be malignant and care must be taken to avoid rupture at operation
- Acute salpingitis is often due to gonococcal infection and produces bilateral suprapubic pain which is often associated with urinary frequency, a tender cervix and vaginal discharge.

R.H. Hardwick

13

The oesophagus, stomach and duodenum

SURGICAL ANATOMY

Oesophagus

The oesophagus extends from the cricoid cartilage (at the level of vertebra C6) to the gastric cardia and is 25 cm long. It has cervical, thoracic and abdominal portions. The oesophagus passes through the diaphragm at the level of the 10th thoracic vertebra and the final 2–4 cm lie within the peritoneal cavity. The relationships are shown in Figure 13.1.

The oesophagus has an upper sphincter, the cricopharyngeus, and a lower sphincter that cannot be defined anatomically but is a 3–5 cm high-pressure area located in the region of the oesophageal hiatus of the diaphragm. The oesophagus is held loosely in the hiatus by a thickening of fascia, the phreno-oesophageal ligament. The healthy oesophagus is lined by squamous epithelium and its wall can be divided into two principle layers, muscular and mucosal. The muscular layer has two components with longitudinal fibres outside and circular fibres inside; the upper third of the oesophagus is striated muscle and the remainder is smooth muscle. Between the muscle and the mucosa is the submucosa where numerous mucous glands and lymphatics are found.

The oesophagus receives its blood supply from the inferior thyroid artery in the cervical region, the bronchial arteries and branches from the thoracic aorta in the thorax, and the inferior phrenic and left gastric arteries in the abdomen.

Venous drainage is to the inferior thyroid veins in the neck, the hemi-azygous and azygous veins (systemic circulation) in the thorax, and the left gastric (portal circulation) in the abdomen. The connection between these veins is important in the development of varices in patients with portal hypertension.

Sympathetic nerve supply is derived from pre-ganglionic fibres from spinal cord segments T5 and T6, and post-ganglionic fibres from the cervical vertebral and coeliac ganglia. Parasympathetic supply comes from the glossopharyngeal, recurrent laryngeal and vagus nerves.

The lymphatics run in the submucosa and drain to the regional lymph nodes, and subsequently to the posterior mediastinal, supraclavicular and coeliac lymph nodes.

Stomach and duodenum

The stomach is an easily distensible viscus partly covered by the left costal margin. The diaphragm and left lobe of the liver lie on its anterior surface. Posteriorly, the stomach bed is formed by the diaphragm, spleen, left adrenal, upper part of the left kidney, splenic artery and pancreas. The greater and lesser curvatures correspond to the long and short borders of the stomach respectively, and the organ can be further divided anatomically into four distinct areas based on the microscopic mucosal appearance: namely, the

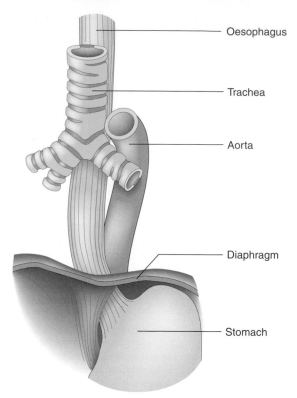

Fig. 13.1 Anatomical relationships of the oesophagus.

cardia, fundus, body and antrum. The stomach is limited at its proximal end by the oesophagogastric junction situated just below the lower oesophageal sphincter, a physiological sphincter that prevents stomach contents from regurgitating into the oesophagus. Distally, the stomach is limited by the pylorus, a true anatomical sphincter. It is composed of greatly thickened inner circular muscle that helps to regulate the emptying of stomach contents into the duodenum.

The duodenum is divided into four parts, which are closely applied to the head of the pancreas. The first part is approximately 5 cm in length; its importance lies in the fact that it is the most common site for peptic ulceration to occur. The second part has on its medial wall the ampulla of Vater, where the conjoined pancreatic duct and common bile duct deliver their contents to the gastrointestinal tract. The third and fourth parts pass behind the transverse mesocolon into the infracolic compartment.

The stomach has an extensive blood supply (Fig. 13.2) derived from the coeliac axis. When the stomach is used as a conduit in the chest, as in an oesophagectomy, the left gastric, left gastroepiploic and short gastric vessels are divided, and the stomach then relies on the right gastric and right gastroepiploic vessels for viability. Ischaemia does not usually result because of the free communication between the vessels supplying the stomach. The blood supply to the duodenum is derived from both the coeliac axis (via the gastroduodenal artery) and branches from the superior mesenteric artery. The veins from the stomach and the duodenum accompany the arteries and drain into the portal venous system.

The lymphatics from the stomach accompany the arteries and drainage is to nodes around these vessels. Thereafter, drainage is to other groups around the aorta, liver, splenic hilum and pancreas, and then to the coeliac nodes. The lymphatics of the duodenum drain into the nodes located at the coeliac axis and superior mesenteric vessels.

The parasympathetic nerve supply to the stomach is derived from the anterior and posterior vagal trunks. These pass through the diaphragm with the oesophagus. The anterior trunk gives off branches to the liver and gallbladder and descends along the lesser curvature. The posterior trunk gives off a coeliac branch and descends along the lesser curvature of the stomach, going on to supply the pancreas, small intestine and large intestine as far as the distal transverse colon. The parasympathetic system supplies motor fibres to the stomach wall, inhibitory fibres to the pyloric sphincter (thus effecting relaxation of the sphincter), and secretomotor fibres to the glands of the stomach. Sympathetic

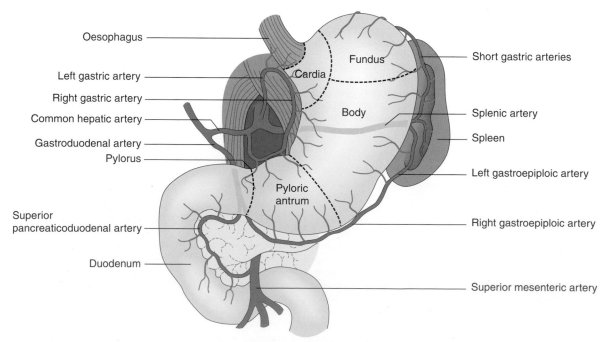

Fig. 13.2 Blood supply and anatomical relationships of the stomach and duodenum.

fibres accompany the gastric arteries to reach the stomach from the coeliac ganglion. These provide motor fibres to the pyloric sphincter. The duodenum receives a sympathetic and parasympathetic supply from the coeliac and superior mesenteric plexuses

SURGICAL PHYSIOLOGY

Oesophagus

Oesophageal peristalsis is initiated by swallowing (primary) or luminal distension (secondary) and progresses distally at around 2–4cm/s requiring the coordinated contraction and relaxation of oesophageal muscle. The lower sphincter relaxes momentarily 2–3 seconds before the peristaltic wave arrives and pressures of about 80mmHg are usually generated in the oesophageal body. Disruption of any part of this process can result in difficulties with swallowing and/or pain.

Between the outer longitudinal muscle layer and the inner circular layer is a nerve plexus (Auerbach's or myenteric plexus) receiving parasympathetic motor innervation to smooth muscle cells from vagal nuclei in the dorsal motor nucleus of the brain stem. Between the inner muscular layer and the submucosa is another nerve plexus (Meissner's or submucosal plexus), which relays signals from the numerous free nerve endings in the mucosa and submucosa to vagal afferent fibres. This sensory information is sent back to the brain via the vagus nerve trunks. Sympathetic innervation arrives via pre-ganglionic sympathetic fibres from the spinal cord that synapse with post-ganglionic nerve cells in sympathetic ganglia before passing with the blood vessels to the oesophagus. Together, the myenteric and submucosal plexuses constitute part of the enteric nervous system of the gut and can be influenced by both neural and hormonal stimuli.

Around one litre of alkaline saliva is produced each day by the salivary glands which helps lubricate the food bolus and neutralizes refluxed gastric acid.

Stomach

Food is passed from the oesophagus into the stomach, where it is stored, ground and partially digested. As food enters the stomach, the muscles in the stomach walls relax and intragastric pressure rises only slightly. This effect is known as receptive relaxation, and is mediated by the vagus nerve. It is followed by muscular contractions that increase in amplitude and frequency, starting in the fundus and moving down towards the body and antrum. In the antrum, the main role is the grinding of food and propulsion of small amounts (now called chyme) into the duodenum when the pyloric sphincter relaxes.

Gastric emptying is controlled by two mechanisms: hormonal feedback and a neural reflex called the enterogastric reflex. In the former, fat in the chyme is the main stimulus for the production of a number of hormones, the most powerful being cholecystokinin, which exerts a negative feedback effect on the stomach, decreasing its motility. The enterogastric reflex is initiated in the duodenal wall, and this further slows stomach emptying and secretion.

Gastric secretions

Classically, gastric secretion has been divided into three phases:

- *Cephalic (neural) phase.* Signals arise in the central cortex or appetite centres, triggered by the sight, smell, taste and thought of food, and travel down the vagus nerves to the stomach
- *Gastric phase.* Food (in particular protein digestion products) causes the release of acid, this release controlled by a negative feedback mechanism dependent upon the pH of the stomach. The gastric phase accounts for the greatest part of daily secretion, approximately 1.5 litres
- *Intestinal phase.* The presence of food in the duodenum triggers the release of a number of hormones, including duodenal gastrin. These exert a positive feedback effect on the stomach, causing a small increase in gastric secretion.

Mucus is produced by all regions of the stomach. It is composed mainly of glycoproteins, water and electrolytes, and serves two important functions. It acts as a lubricant, and it protects the surface of the stomach against the powerful digestive properties of acid and pepsin. Bicarbonate ions are secreted into the mucus gel layer and this creates a protective buffer zone against the effects of the low pH secretions. Alkaline mucus is produced in the duodenum and small intestine, where it has a similar function of mucosal protection.

The parietal cells in the stomach are responsible for the production of acid. Acid secretion by these cells is stimulated by two main factors: acetylcholine, released by the vagus nerve, and gastrin from the antrum. Acetylcholine and gastrin act on neuroendocrine cells located close to the parietal cells. On stimulation, these cells release histamine, which has a paracrine action on the parietal cell, stimulating acid production and secretion. Parietal cells secrete acid via an active transport mechanism, the proton pump. Somatostatin, gastric inhibitory peptide and vasoactive intestinal peptide inhibit acid secretion.

Pepsin is a proteolytic enzyme produced in its precursor form, pepsinogen, by the peptic cells found in the body and fundus of the stomach. Pepsinogen production is stimulated by acetylcholine from the vagus nerve. The precursor is then converted to its active form, pepsin, by the acid contents of the stomach.

Intrinsic factor is also produced by the parietal cells. It is a glycoprotein that binds to vitamin B_{12} present in the diet and carries it to the terminal ileum. Here specific receptors for intrinsic factor exist and the complex is taken up by the mucosa. Intrinsic factor is broken down and vitamin B_{12} is then absorbed into the bloodstream.

HISTORY AND SYMPTOMS

Dysphagia

Dysphagia is defined as difficulty in swallowing. It is a serious symptom and requires proper investigation regardless of clinical diagnosis. Certain points in the history, however, are often helpful in making a differential diagnosis:

- *Onset.* Sudden onset suggests a foreign body. In carcinoma, the dysphagia occurs over a period of weeks, whereas in achalasia and benign strictures, symptoms tend to develop over a number of years
- *Site.* The actual site of obstruction correlates poorly in general to where the patient feels the discomfort, although some patients who feel the obstruction to be high may have a pharyngeal pouch
- *Progression.* Dysphagia due to an oesophageal stricture (benign or malignant) tends to be progressive whereas patients with motility disorders will often have intermittent symptoms.

13

Table 13.1 **Causes of dysphagia**

Intraluminal	Intramural	Extrinsic
Pharynx/upper oesophagus		
Foreign body	Pharyngitis/tonsillitis	Thyroid enlargement
	Moniliasis	Pharyngeal pouch
	Sideropenic web	
	Corrosives	
	Carcinoma	
	Myasthenia gravis	
	Bulbar palsy	
Body of oesophagus		
Foreign body	Corrosives	Mediastinal lymph nodes
	Peptic oesophagitis	Aortic aneurysm
	Carcinoma	
Lower oesophagus		
Foreign body	Corrosives	Para-oesophageal hernia
	Peptic oesophagitis	
	Carcinoma	
	Diffuse oesophageal spasm	
	Systemic sclerosis	
	Achalasia	
	Post-vagotomy	

- *Severity.* Difficulty in swallowing solids is initially typical of carcinoma, whereas achalasia and other motility disorders tends to be associated with dysphagia to liquids as well
- *Causes.* A list of the common causes of dysphagia is shown in Table 13.1.

Odynophagia

This symptom is defined as pain on swallowing. It may occur in patients with oesophagitis or due to oesophageal spasm. The latter may be due to a mechanical obstruction (benign or malignant) or due to intrinsic dysmotility of the oesophageal musculature.

Heartburn

Retrosternal pain is a very common symptom and most people will have experienced it at some time. It is usually associated with gastro-oesophageal reflux and may be brought on by eating a heavy meal, alcohol or bending over. General practitioners will see many patients in their clinical practice who complain of heartburn and will treat them effectively with acid suppressing medication such as proton pump inhibitors.

Dyspepsia

Dyspepsia is something of a 'catch all' term used to describe the symptoms of indigestion. Patients may have some or all of the following; epigastric pain, belching, heartburn, nausea, early satiety or reduced appetite. These symptoms are very common in the general population. Current guidance from the National Institute for Clinical Excellence (NICE) in the UK, recommends lifestyle advice, medication review and empirical treatment for the majority of patients with dyspepsia but without so-called alarm symptoms

(weight loss, progressive dysphagia, iron deficiency anaemia, epigastric mass and persistent vomiting) (EBM 13.1). Unfortunately, the symptoms of early upper GI malignancy are very similar to dyspepsia and only advanced malignancies tend to cause alarm symptoms. Patients with advanced upper GI malignancy have a poor prognosis despite aggressive therapy, which creates a dilemma; which patients with dyspepsia should be referred for endoscopy? NICE guidance on dyspepsia should be applied with caution and doctors should have a low threshold for endoscopy in any patient who does not improve quickly with simple treatment. It is also imperative that a careful history is taken and anaemia excluded.

EBM 13.1 **NICE guidance on dyspepsia**

'Urgent specialist referral for endoscopic investigation is indicated in patients of any age with dyspepsia when presenting with any of chronic GI bleeding, progressive unintentional weight loss, progressive difficulty swallowing, persistent vomiting, iron deficiency anaemia, epigastric mass or suspicious barium meal.'

North of England Dyspepsia Guideline Development Group 2004 Dyspepsia: Managing dyspepsia in adults in primary care. Centre for Health Services Report No. 112. University of Newcastle upon Tyne. Crown Copyright. http://guidance.nice.org.uk/CG17/Guidance/pdf/English.

Regurgitation and Vomiting

Regurgitation is an effortless process whereby food is regurgitated into the mouth and is associated with achalasia, hiatus hernia and pharyngeal pouches. In severe cases regurgitation can lead to aspiration with coughing/choking, asthma and aspiration pneumonia. Vomiting is an active process whereby the stomach contents are forcefully expelled by powerful contractions of the abdominal musculature at the same time as relaxation of the lower oesophageal sphincter. Potential causes of vomiting are multiple and include infection, inflammation, endocrine disorders, drugs and medication, gastrointestinal obstruction, and physiological such as morning sickness in pregnancy.

Abdominal pain

Epigastric pain is a common upper gastrointestinal symptom. Pain relieved by eating traditionally suggests a duodenal ulcer whereas gastric ulcer pain is aggravated by food. However, the differential diagnosis for epigastric pain is extensive and includes conditions such as liver metastasis, pancreatic pathology, abdominal aortic aneurysm, gall stones, irritable bowel and even myocardial infarction.

EXAMINATION

Physical examination might reveal signs that will aid in the diagnosis of upper GI disorders. A smooth tongue, pallor and koilonychia are signs of iron deficiency anaemia, which can be present in oesophageal carcinoma, oesophagitis and Plummer–Vinson syndrome (see p. 176).

Lymphadenopathy, particularly in the supraclavicular region, hepatomegaly, abdominal mass, ascites and evidence of weight loss are associated with malignancy. A mass felt in the upper abdomen is usually a bad sign suggesting incurable malignancy. Crepitus in the neck of a patient who has been vomiting is a sign of surgical emphysema and suggests an oesophageal perforation. A succussion splash heard over the epigastrium when the patient is gently shaken suggests gastric outlet obstruction.

INVESTIGATIONS

Blood tests

A full blood count may reveal evidence of anaemia or infection. Serum urea and electrolytes tests may show dehydration, renal failure, hypokalaemia and hyponatraemia secondary to dysphagia or vomiting. Liver function tests might show low plasma proteins, abnormal clotting and elevated enzymes in the presence of metastatic disease, and portal hypertension.

Helicobacter pylori tests

Patients with dyspepsia should normally be tested for infection with *Helicobacter pylori*, the commonest cause of peptic ulceration and gastric adenocarcinoma world wide. *H. pylori* can be detected in the following ways:

- Blood tests to detect evidence of an immune response to *H. pylori*
- Stool tests looking for *H. pylori* antigens
- Urea breath tests
- CLO tests on endoscopic biopsies
- Histology of endoscopic biopsies.

Chest X-ray

A simple chest X-ray may show any of the following signs: pulmonary consolidation and fibrosis following aspiration in patients with oesophageal motility disorders and oesophageal carcinoma, an air-fluid level behind the heart shadow from a large hiatus hernia with intrathoracic stomach (Fig. 13.3), a mediastinal mass of lymph nodes and pulmonary metastases in oesophagogastric cancer, air in the mediastinum and neck after perforation of the oesophagus (Fig. 13.4) or under the diaphragm from a perforated peptic ulcer (Fig.13.5).

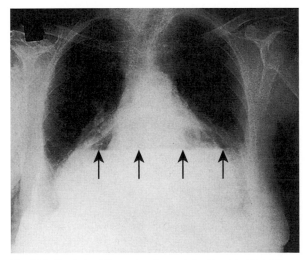

Fig. 13.3 Erect chest X-ray showing an intra-thoracic stomach secondary to a giant hiatus hernia. Note the air-fluid level.

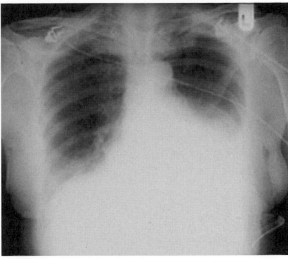

Fig. 13.4 Erect chest X-ray showing left hydro-pneumothorax in a patient with Boerhaave's syndrome.

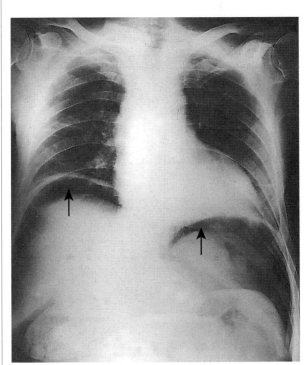

Fig. 13.5 Erect chest X-ray showing free air under both hemidiaphragms secondary to a perforated duodenal ulcer.

Contrast swallow/meal

A contrast swallow/meal using barium liquid or water soluble contrast may be useful:

- As a primary investigation when access to endoscopy is limited (Fig. 13.6)
- In a very frail patient with dysphagia or vomiting who might not be deemed fit enough for endoscopy (rare)
- To exclude a pharyngeal pouch prior to endoscopy
- To complement endoscopy and provide additional anatomical information (i.e. for patients with a large hiatus hernia) (Fig. 13.7)
- To diagnose a suspected upper GI perforation.

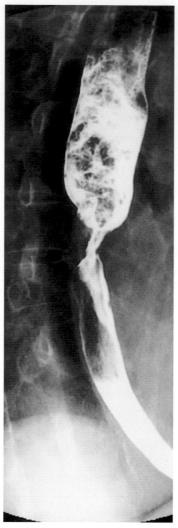

Fig. 13.6 Barium swallow showing a malignant looking stricture of the mid-oesophagus.

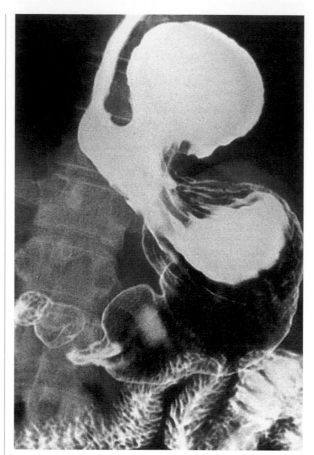

Fig. 13.7 Barium meal showing a large para-oesophageal hiatus hernia.

Endoscopy

Flexible oesophagogastroduodenoscopy (OGD) is now the first-line investigation for almost all upper GI symptoms. Flexible OGD is carried out either under light intravenous sedation or a local anaesthetic throat spray. The patient should be fasted for 4 hours before the procedure. It is important to monitor pulse and oxygen saturation throughout the procedure to identify and rectify any possible respiratory depression that might follow sedation. Therapeutic procedures can also be done at the time of OGD including dilatation of strictures, insertion of stents, thermal ablation of tumours, removal of foreign bodies and control of bleeding.

Computed tomography (CT)

CT is used most commonly to investigate and stage malignancy but may also be helpful when investigating patients with benign conditions such as large hiatus hernias, a suspected gastric volvulus or upper GI perforation. Staging upper GI CT scans are often done after the patient has drunk

water to distend the oesophagus and stomach. Emergency scans looking for evidence of gut perforation will use oral water soluble contrast.

Gastric emptying studies

These nuclear medicine scans require the patient to swallow radio-labelled liquid and solids (a two-phase study). The speed that the stomach empties can then be monitored using a gamma ray detector. Patients whose major complaint is nausea and vomiting but appear to have no structural abnormality of their upper GI tract should undergo a two-phase gastric emptying study to look for gastroparesis, a common condition in diabetics secondary to autonomic neuropathy.

Endoluminal ultrasound

Endoscopic ultrasonography (EUS) uses a variety of endoscopes containing high frequency ultrasound probes at their tips to investigate patients with upper GI disorders. By placing the probe within the GI lumen great detail of the underlying structures can be obtained. EUS is mostly used for staging the 'T' and 'N' component of TNM staging for oesophagogastric cancer (Fig. 13.8). In addition, EUS is increasingly being used to allow fine needle biopsy of suspicious lymph nodes, especially when the status (positive or negative for cancer) will have profound implications for

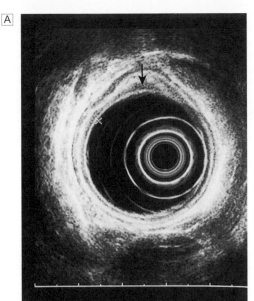

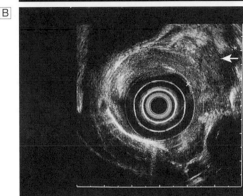

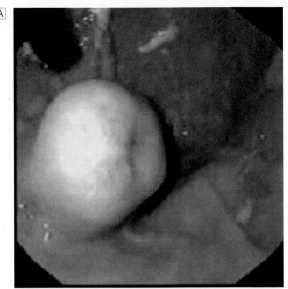

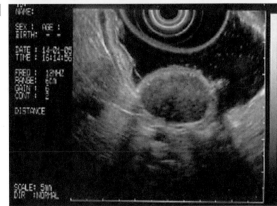

Fig. 13.8 Endoscopic ultrasound (EUS). **A** The normal layers of the oesophagus and a small T1 cancer confined to the mucosa marked with an arrow. **B** A full-thickness T3 tumour of the oesophagus. Note the complete destruction of the normal oesophageal layers.

Fig. 13.9 **A** Endoscopic view of a 2-cm diameter polypoid submucosal gastric lesion. **B** EUS confirms the lesion is arising from the muscularis propria and likely to be a GIST.

the intention of a patient's treatment (curative or palliative). EUS is also useful for investigating submucosal lesions of the stomach such as gastrointestinal stromal tumours (GISTs) (Fig. 13.9) (see p. 176).

Manometry and pH studies

Measurements of lower oesophageal pH can be made over a 24-hour period using an intraluminal electrode placed 5 cm proximal to the lower oesophageal sphincter attached to a catheter passed through the nose and pharynx. Alternatively, oesophageal pH can be measured over three days using a Bravo capsule® which is clipped to the oesophageal mucosa and is wireless (Fig. 13.10). Patients can indicate symptom events during the recording and these can be correlated with the pH trace. A composite scoring system (the DeMeester score) is then used to diagnose pathological GORD. Oesophageal pressure and peristalsis can also be analysed during a series of swallows (station manometry) or over a longer period (ambulatory manometry) (Fig. 13.11). To diagnose gastro-oesophageal bile reflux in patients with duodenogastric reflux a Bilitec probe® is used.

DIAGNOSIS AND MANAGEMENT – OESOPHAGUS

Gastro-oesophageal reflux disease (GORD) and Barrett's oesophagus

Patients typically complain of heartburn, regurgitation of acid into the back of their throat, nausea, waterbrash (hypersalivation), epigastric pain and occasionally vomiting. Reflux symptoms are very common affecting up to 30% of the population. The lower oesophageal sphincter usually prevents reflux by the following mechanisms:

- a physiological high-pressure zone (not a true sphincter) in the lower end of the oesophagus
- the mucosal rosette at the cardia, which acts like a plug
- the angle at which the oesophagus joins the stomach between the left border of the oesophagus and the fundus (angle of His)
- the diaphragmatic sling (crura), which acts like a pinchcock at the lower end of the oesophagus
- the high-pressure area at the lower end of the oesophagus, caused by the positive intra-abdominal pressure.

13

173

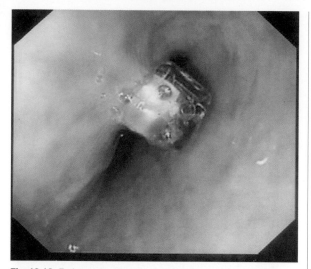

Fig. 13.10 Endoscopic view of a wireless Bravo capsule clipped to the oesophageal mucosa 5cm proximal to the gastro-oesophageal junction. These record for up to 72 hours before falling off and passing harmlessly through the gut.

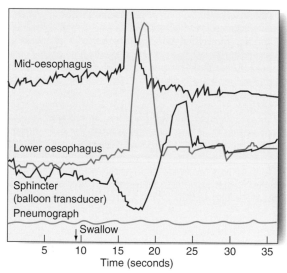

Fig. 13.11 Recording of the intraluminal pressure of the oesophagus.

Diagnosis and management

GORD is diagnosed by taking a good history, performing an endoscopy and sometimes a 24-hour oesophageal pH study. In young patients and those without alarm symptoms, empirical treatment may be appropriate without doing any investigations. Patients should be advised about lifestyle changes including weight loss if obese, stopping smoking, eating less fatty and spicy food, and drinking less caffeine and alcohol. Many patients will already have tried over-the-counter remedies such as antacids, alginates or low dose H2 antagonists. Definitive treatment, however, is provided by a course of proton pump inhibitors. Prokinetic agents such as metoclopramide may also help patients by improving the lower oesophageal muscle tone, promoting gastric emptying and reducing nausea.

Barrett's oesophagus is a histological diagnosis made after endoscopic biopsies. GORD can cause oesophagitis and in some patients this leads to a metaplastic change

in the mucosa from squamous to columnar type. Barrett's oesophagus is of interest as it can become dysplastic which in turn can lead to oesophageal adenocarcinoma. This disease is increasing in incidence and Barrett's patients offer a target group for surveillance to detect early neoplastic disease (EBM 13.2).

EBM 13.2 **Barrett's oesophagus guidelines**

'It is vitally important for accurate diagnosis that the precise sites of biopsies taken are recorded by the endoscopist in terms of distance from the incisor teeth and relation to the oesophagogastric junction (Recommendation grade C).'

British Society of Gastroenterology guidelines on surveillance of patients with Barrett's oesophagus. http://www.bsg.org.uk/clinical-guidelines/ oesophageal/guidelines-for-the-diagnosis-and-management-of-barrett-s-columnar-lined-oesophagus.html.

Anti-reflux surgery

Although surgical treatment of patients with severe anti-reflux disease has always been associated with good long-term outcomes, it has taken the introduction and refinements of laparoscopic techniques to bring the surgical option to more patients. The indications for surgery include those whose symptoms cannot be controlled by medical therapy, those with recurrent strictures despite treatment, and young patients who do not wish to continue taking acid suppression therapy for several decades. Symptoms that fail to be brought under control with acid suppression therapy are usually due to high-volume alkaline reflux, and surgery is an extremely effective cure (EBM 13.3). The presence of Barrett's metaplasia alone is not considered a suitable indication for anti-reflux surgery.

EBM 13.3 **Surgery for gastro-oesophageal reflux disease**

'It has been shown that, following anti-reflux surgery, quality of life is improved and costs are reduced significantly compared with medical treatment. Anti-reflux surgery should be offered to patients with proven symptomatic reflux that cannot be controlled symptomatically with medical therapy.'

For further information: www.acg.gi.org/physicians/guidelines/ GERDTreatment.pdf.

Surgery involves reduction of the hiatus hernia if present, approximation of the crura around the lower oesophagus, and some form of fundoplication. This takes the form of mobilizing the fundus of the stomach from its attachments to the undersurface of the left hemidiaphragm and the left crus, and then wrapping it around the oesophagus, either anteriorly or posteriorly. The most common procedure currently performed is the Nissen fundoplication, in which the fundus is taken posteriorly around the lower oesophagus and sutured to the left anterior surface of the left side of the proximal stomach as a 360° wrap (Fig. 13.12). Other procedures involving a partial (incomplete) fundoplication include the Toupet (posterior 270° wrap) and the Watson (anterior 180° wrap) repairs. Current data do not demonstrate much difference between the various approaches although early postoperative dysphagia is commoner with 360° wraps compared to the partial wraps. All procedures have a success rate in curing the symptoms of reflux of around 90% at a year and 70–80% at 10 years. Unwanted complications after surgery include gas bloat

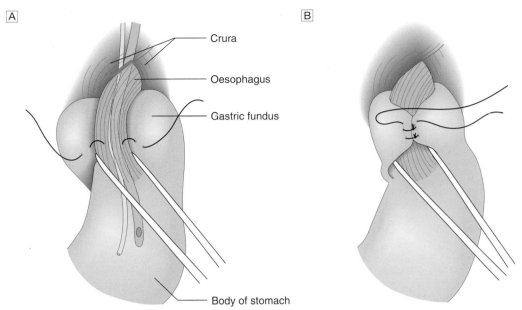

Fig. 13.12 Fundoplication for GORD. **A** Gastric fundus wrapped around the lower oesophagus. **B** Fundal wrap sutured in position.

(inability to belch), dysphagia, early satiety and increased flatus. These operations are now carried out laparoscopically, with excellent results in skilled hands.

SUMMARY BOX 13.1

Gastro-oesophageal reflux disease

- Reflux type symptoms are very common
- 'Life style' advice to patients is important (i.e. smoking, dieting etc)
- Proton pump inhibitors are generally effective treatment
- GORD for > 10 years (especially men) is a risk factor for Barrett's oesophagus
- Screening and surveillance for Barrett's patients increasingly relevant
- Laparoscopic anti-reflux surgery is clinically effective and cost efficient.

Hiatus hernia

A hiatus hernia is an abnormal protrusion of the stomach through the oesophageal diaphragmatic hiatus into the thorax. There are two types, sliding (90%) and rolling (10%) (Fig. 13.13). A sliding hernia occurs when the stomach slides through the diaphragmatic hiatus, so that the gastro-oesophageal junction lies within the chest cavity. It is covered anteriorly by peritoneum, and posteriorly is extraperitoneal. A rolling or para-oesophageal hernia is formed when the stomach rolls up anteriorly through the hiatus; the cardia remains in its normal position and therefore the cardio-oesophageal sphincter remains intact.

Rolling and sliding hernias are caused by weakness of the muscles around the hiatus. They tend to occur in middle-aged and elderly patients. Women are affected more frequently than men and there is a higher incidence in the obese.

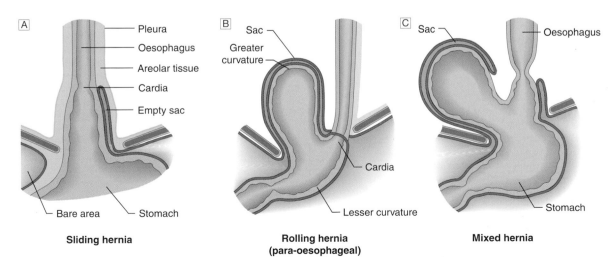

Fig. 13.13 Types of hiatus hernia. **A** Sliding hernia. **B** Rolling hernia (para-oesophageal). **C** Mixed hernia.

Clinical features

Hiatus hernias are often asymptomatic, but can produce some of or all the following symptoms:

- *Heartburn and regurgitation* owing to an incompetent lower oesophageal sphincter, which is aggravated by stooping and lying flat at night, and can be relieved by antacids.
- *Oesophagitis* resulting from persistent acid reflux, which leads to ulceration, bleeding with anaemia, fibrosis and stricture formation.
- *Epigastric and lower chest pain,* especially in para-oesophageal hernias, as the herniated part of the stomach (usually the fundus) becomes trapped in the hiatus. This can be a surgical emergency owing to the obstruction and strangulation of the stomach.
- *Palpitations and hiccups,* symptoms caused by the mass effect of the hernia in the thoracic cavity irritating the pericardium and the diaphragm. In patients with a large rolling hiatus hernia, displacement of the whole stomach may result in a volvulus into the chest, producing symptoms of vomiting from gastric outflow obstruction.

Management

Treatment is as for gastro-oesophageal reflux disease although patients with obstructive symptoms such as vomiting and regurgitation or breathlessness due to reduced lung capacity should be considered for surgical repair. Patients who present as an emergency with an obstructed hiatus hernia should have it decompressed with a nasogastric tube or endoscopically to prevent strangulation. Emergency surgery is occasionally necessary except if conservative therapy fails or gastric necrosis is suspected. Even large hiatus hernias can be repaired laparoscopically although the risk of conversion to open surgery is higher.

Achalasia

This disorder affects the whole oesophagus. The main feature is failure of relaxation of the lower oesophageal sphincter; as the disease progresses, the obstructed lower oesophagus dilates and peristalsis becomes uncoordinated.

Achalasia is thought to be due to a partial or complete degeneration of the myenteric plexus of Auerbach, and in the later stages of the disease loss of the dorsal vagal nuclei within the brain stem can be demonstrated. Infestation with the protozoon, *Trypanosoma cruzi,* which occurs in South America (Chagas' disease), also causes degeneration of the myenteric plexus, leading to a motor disorder of the oesophagus that is indistinguishable from achalasia.

Clinical features

The disease affects 1 in 100 000 of the population of developed countries. The patient is typically aged between 30 and 40 years, and females are affected more often than males (3:2). There is progressive dysphagia over several years, often for both solids and liquids. Gravity rather than peristalsis is responsible for food leaving the oesophagus and the patient finds it easier to eat when standing. There may also be retrosternal pain, which gradually decreases in severity as the oesophagus loses peristaltic activity. Other common symptoms include weight loss, halitosis and regurgitation of undigested food, which can lead to aspiration pneumonia, particularly at night, resulting in bouts of coughing and recurrent chest infections. In the longer term, achalasia can predispose to squamous cell carcinoma of the oesophagus.

Management

Treatment involves either balloon dilatation of the lower oesophageal sphincter or surgical myotomy (division of the muscles over the lower oesophagus and proximal stomach). Endoscopic injection of the lower oesophageal sphincter with botulinum toxin can give temporary symptom relief but the effects wear off quite quickly. Balloon dilatation of the gastro-oesophageal junction disrupts the lower oesophageal sphincter and improves symptoms in 80–90% of patients, but carries with it the risk of oesophageal perforation.

Operative treatment involves a laparoscopic Heller's myotomy. Via an abdominal approach the lower oesophageal sphincter is divided down to the mucosa for 5 cm above the oesophago-gastric junction and 3 cm down the stomach. Early complications include perforation and late complications include reflux oesophagitis, and recurrent dysphagia from an inadequate myotomy. In order to reduce the incidence of GORD after myotomy, surgeons carry out an anterior partial fundoplication at the same time.

Diffuse oesophageal spasm

This disorder tends to occur in middle-aged to elderly patients. Complaints are of intermittent dysphagia and retrosternal pain, which can mimic angina. The symptoms are caused by repetitive irregular peristalsis of the oesophageal body and oesophageal manometry is required to make the diagnosis. Diffuse oesophageal spasm can be precipitated by GORD and this should be excluded by 24-hour pH studies.

Management

Medical treatment includes calcium channel blockers, sublingual GTN and proton pump inhibitors. Surgical treatment involves a long myotomy but the results are unpredictable and most patients will be treated medically.

Nutcracker oesophagus

In this uncommon disorder, the symptoms are caused by repetitive forceful peristalsis. Manometry demonstrates normal peristalsis but with excessive amplitudes and pressures exceeding 150 mmHg. Medical treatment is similar to that of diffuse oesophageal spasm, but the results are disappointing. Dilatation and surgical myotomy also have poor results.

Plummer–Vinson syndrome

This syndrome, first described by Paterson and Brown Kelly, is characterized by a post-cricoid web that results in dysphagia. The web is related to iron deficiency anaemia, but may be congenital or traumatic in origin. The squamous epithelium becomes hyperplastic and there is hyperkeratosis and desquamation, which leads to web formation.

Clinical features

Patients are commonly middle-aged women. Dysphagia is the main presenting complaint, but there may also be symptoms and signs of anaemia, including koilonychia, smooth tongue and angular stomatitis.

Investigations

A full blood count will show hypochromic microcytic anaemia and serum ferritin levels will be low. Barium swallow demonstrates a narrowing of the upper oesophagus with a web in the anterior wall; this is confirmed by endoscopy, during which a friable web can be seen across the lumen of the oesophagus.

Management

The web is dilated endoscopically and biopsies should also be taken, as there is an association with post-cricoid carcinoma. The iron deficiency status is corrected by oral iron therapy.

Pouches

Pouches are protrusions of mucosa through a weak area in the muscle wall. The best-known type of pouch lies in the pharynx and is associated with raised cricopharyngeal pressure, with the pouch developing through Killian's dehiscence, between the thyropharyngeus and cricopharyngeus muscles. Incoordination of swallowing and failure of relaxation of the cricopharyngeus muscle cause the herniation. The pharyngeal pouch usually develops posteriorly and is then forced by the vertebral column to deviate to the side, usually the left. Oesophageal pouches can occur around the tracheobronchial tree in relation to pressure from adjacent lymph nodes, if enlarged, and also just above the gastro-oesophageal junction in patients with raised lower oesophageal sphincter pressure.

Clinical features

Most patients are elderly and males are more commonly affected. Symptoms include regurgitation of food, halitosis, dysphagia, gurgling in the throat, aspiration and a lump in the neck (pharyngeal pouch); alternatively, the patient may be asymptomatic.

Investigations

Barium swallow demonstrates the pouch and the uncoordinated swallowing. Endoscopy also confirms the diagnosis but must be performed with care to avoid accidental perforation of the pouch.

Management

Surgical myotomy of the cricopharyngeus and resection of the pouch used to be the surgical treatment of choice, but endoscopic stapling has now superseded this. A special linear stapling device is placed perorally under direct vision with one limb of the device in the oesophageal lumen and the other in the pouch before the stapler is closed and fired. This creates a common lumen between pouch and oesophagus and divides the cricopharyngeal sphincter at the same time.

Perforation

Aetiology

Intraluminal

This is caused by a swallowed foreign body or by removal of a foreign body during instrumentation, with rigid endoscopy carrying a much greater risk than flexible. The most common sites of perforation tend to coincide with the sites of anatomical narrowing. The commonest causes are iatrogenic, occurring during diagnostic endoscopy (rare) or therapeutic procedures such as dilatation (commoner).

Outside the wall

These are caused by penetrating injuries such as knife wounds to the neck but are rare.

Spontaneous

This follows episodes of violent vomiting (Boerhaave's syndrome). The perforation is frequently on the left posterolateral aspect of the lower oesophagus. A tear to the oesophageal mucosa only, following vomiting, is known as a Mallory–Weiss tear and tends to cause haematemesis and pain.

Clinical features

The clinical symptoms depend to some extent on the site and size of the perforation. If the perforation is in the cervical region, the patient complains of pain in the neck and local tenderness, and surgical emphysema is present. Perforation of the thoracic oesophagus causes retrosternal chest pain and dysphagia. Clinically, the patient may be shocked, short of breath and cyanosed owing to a pneumothorax or pleural effusion, if the pleural space is involved. Perforation in this area can lead to mediastinitis and septic shock. Perforation of the abdominal oesophagus can lead to peritonitis and a rigid abdomen.

Investigations

The most important factor in diagnosing oesophageal perforation early on is the examining doctor including it in his or her differential diagnosis of any patient who collapses with chest pain, shortness of breath or vomiting.

Erect chest X-ray

In addition to excluding a perforated duodenal ulcer (air under the diaphragm), an erect chest X-ray may show surgical emphysema with gas in the soft tissues of the mediastinum, often extending up to the neck. The mediastinum may also be widened, and if the pleural cavity has also been ruptured, there will be a hydropneumothorax.

CT scan and contrast swallow

The diagnosis is confirmed by a chest CT scan or water-soluble contrast swallow, which will also demonstrate whether the perforation is localized to the mediastinum or open to the pleural or peritoneal cavities (Fig. 13.14). If oesophageal perforation cannot be excluded after radiological imaging and clinical suspicion remains high an experienced

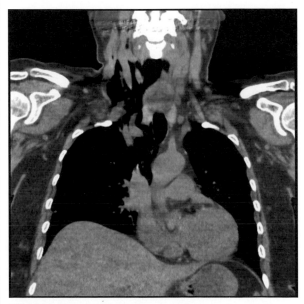

Fig. 13.14 Coronal CT image showing iatrogenic pharyngeal perforation with massive surgical emphysema.

endoscopist should perform an OGD. One potential catch is spontaneous pneumomediastinum which can occur in young adults and teenagers after violent vomiting or coughing and is thought to be due to the rupture of a pulmonary bullous. There is no oesophageal injury and the treatment is conservative.

Management

Following diagnosis of oesophageal perforation, patients should be discussed with and usually transferred to a regional oesophagogastric centre as soon as possible. Perforation of the cervical oesophagus can be treated non-operatively with intravenous fluids, withdrawal of oral fluid and diet, and the administration of antibiotics and antifungals. If an abscess develops in the superior mediastinum, this will require surgical drainage.

Perforation of the thoracic oesophagus has a much higher morbidity and mortality. Localized and small perforations that do not communicate with either pleural cavity can be treated non-operatively, as outlined above. If the perforation follows the dilatation of a carcinoma in a patient suitable for resection, emergency oesophagogastrectomy may be indicated although longer term survival in this situation is very rare and many specialists would now recommend placing a stent in the this situation. As a general rule, small perforations with minimal mediastinal contamination can often be managed conservatively whereas large defects will require surgery. If the perforation is detected early a primary repair of the defect may be possible. Late presentation with heavy contamination is best treated by repairing the defect over a T-tube to create a controlled oesophagocutaneous fistula; prolonged mediastinal drainage, antibiotics, antifungals and enteral feeding via a jejunostomy are also required in this life threatening situation.

TUMOURS OF THE OESOPHAGUS

Benign tumours

These account for less than 1% of oesophageal neoplasms. The most common is the benign leiomyoma which is often asymptomatic but may cause bleeding or dysphagia. It is best treated by local enucleation, with good results.

Carcinoma of the oesophagus

The incidence of carcinoma of the oesophagus has risen in populations of developed countries over the last two decades to a figure of around 15/100 000 in parts of the UK, due primarily to an increase in adenocarcinoma. The male to female ratio is 3:1 and adenocarcinoma is predominantly a disease of Western white males. In the Far East and other parts of the world, particularly among some black males, there is a greater incidence of squamous cell carcinoma.

The most important risk factors for adenocarcinoma of the oesophagus are reflux and obesity, with a slightly increased risk of cardia tumours with smoking. Risk factors for squamous cell carcinoma include alcohol, smoking, leucoplakia, achalasia, the consumption of salted fish or pickled vegetables, and chewing tobacco and betel nuts.

Clinical features

Progressive dysphagia to solids is the most common presentation. The average duration of symptoms at the time of presentation is between 3 and 9 months, and as a result, around 70% of patients are not operable at the time of diagnosis.

Occasionally, patients may present with metastatic disease, including enlarged cervical lymph nodes, jaundice, hepatomegaly, hoarseness from recurrent laryngeal nerve involvement, and chest pain from mediastinal invasion. Other general features of malignancy include weight loss, anorexia, anaemia and lassitude.

Investigations

Even if the diagnosis is made initially by barium swallow, it must always be confirmed by endoscopy and biopsy. For this reason, endoscopy is the best first-line investigation for anyone with dysphagia. Thereafter, investigations are aimed at accurate staging of the disease so as to assess resectability, determine a prognosis and identify patients who might benefit from neoadjuvant therapy. Local T (tumour) stage and N (nodal) spread are best assessed by endoscopic ultrasonography. M (metastases) stage is best assessed by CT and PET scans (lung, liver and bone metastases, distant lymphadenopathy), and laparoscopy (peritoneal metastases). Routine blood tests may reveal anaemia, liver disease and malnutrition, all of which require full assessment if surgery is to be considered. In those patients with proximal and middle-third tumours adjacent to the tracheobronchial tree, bronchoscopy can be a valuable investigation to assess airway invasion. If enlarged distant lymph nodes are detected, these should be aspirated for cytology, as surgical resection is contraindicated if they are positive for malignancy.

Management

The aim of treatment is to offer radical treatment to those with potentially curable disease and improve the quality of life for the remainder. The overall 5-year survival rate remains very low (<10%), although in patients who are suitable for resection, 5-year survival figures of 20–30% are possible. Multi-modal therapy involving perioperative chemotherapy and surgery is now the standard of care for oesophageal cancer when the treatment intent is curative.

Surgical resection

Patients with disease confined to the oesophagus and who are fit for surgery should be considered for resection in a high volume cancer centre. Oesophagectomy with palliative intent is no longer appropriate as few patients recover enough to gain any benefit before they die of their disease.

There are several methods currently used to resect the oesophagus:

- *Ivor Lewis two-phase oesophagectomy.* This involves a laparotomy during which the stomach is fully mobilized on its vascular pedicles, along with the lower oesophagus. A right thoracotomy is then carried out to resect the oesophagus, and the mobilized stomach is brought up into the chest and anastomosed to the proximal oesophagus. This is the preferred choice for middle and lower-third tumours (Fig. 13.15)
- *Left thoracolaparotomy.* This is a good approach for tumours around the oesophagogastric junction, particularly when the tumour extends down into the proximal stomach and a more extensive gastric resection is required
- *Transhiatal oesophagectomy.* This approach involves mobilization of the stomach via an abdominal incision, the oesophagus (some of it by blunt dissection) through the hiatus, and the cervical oesophagus via a left sided neck incision. Once the oesophagus is removed, the stomach is brought up into the neck and anastomosed to the cervical oesophagus. This technique is best

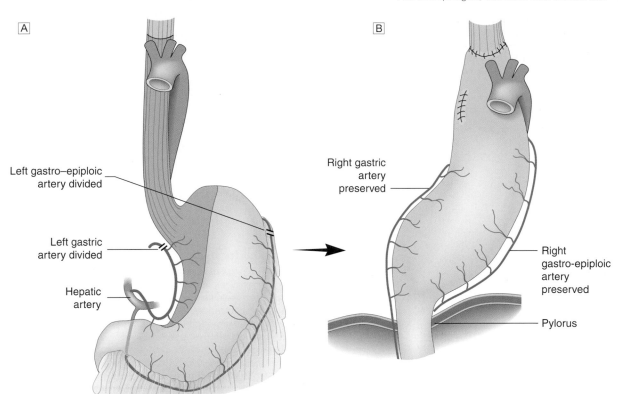

Fig. 13.15 Reconstruction after Ivor–Lewis oesophagectomy.

suited for very early tumours not requiring a radical lymphadenectomy but is rapidly being replaced by minimally invasive surgery

• *Minimally invasive oesophagectomy*. Increasingly surgeons are using laparoscopic and thoracoscopic techniques to mobilize the oesophagus. The commonest technique is to mobilize the stomach laparoscopically and then perform a thoracotomy to resect the oesophagus and perform an anastomosis, a so called 'hybrid technique'. Alternatively both the abdominal and chest phase of the surgery can be done using minimally invasive techniques.

Postoperative care

Uncomplicated recovery after oesophagectomy hinges on good surgical technique, good pain relief (often by epidural analgesia), the avoidance of excess intravenous fluid, early mobilization and effective chest physiotherapy. Many surgeons place a feeding jejunostomy at the time of oesophagectomy to allow early enteral feeding. The early recognition of postoperative complications and their aggressive management has done much to reduce the perioperative mortality of this major operation to around 5% (EBM 13.4).

EBM 13.4 **Oesophagogastric cancer report**

'The 30-day postoperative mortality rate for oesophagectomy and gastrectomy was 3.8 per cent (95 per cent CI 3.1 to 4.7) and 4.5 per cent (95 per cent CI 3.4 to 5.7), respectively. National oesophagogastric cancer audit report for England & Wales 2010. http://www.ic.nhs.uk/webfiles/Services/NCASP/audits%20and%20 reports/NHS%20IC%20OGC%20Audit%202010%20interactive.pdf

---

Radiotherapy and chemotherapy

All patients with locally advanced tumours should be considered for perioperative chemotherapy. Randomized clinical trials are in progress to discover the most effective combination of agents. Chemo-radiotherapy can also be used preoperatively, particularly for squamous carcinoma of the oesophagus although postoperative complications for these patients may be higher. Up to a third of patients will have a complete pathological response (no residual tumour when resected) and this has prompted trials of chemo-radiotherapy as definitive treatment.

Palliation

The majority of patients who present with oesophageal cancer (about 70%) will have palliative rather than curative treatment. It is therefore essential that a full range of palliative treatments are easily available and that an experienced hospital clinician with good specialist nurse support co-ordinates the care, working closely with community services.

Best supportive care: Some patients are too frail for any interventional treatment and require a holistic approach to their symptoms involving medication to counter nausea, vomiting and pain. Emotional and dietary support are also important.

Endoscopic stent: Patients with significant dysphagia who are not candidates for radical therapy should be considered for a palliative stent as this is a safe and effective method of relieving the distress of not being able to swallow (Fig. 13.16). They are inserted under intravenous sedation endoscopically but can also be screened into position by interventional radiologists. Chest pain for the first few days after insertion is common and patients should be started on a proton pump inhibitor to reduce reflux symptoms. Complications include perforation during insertion, migration of the stent,

13

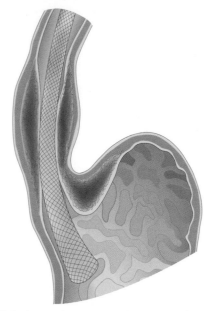

Fig. 13.16 Self-expanding metal stent inserted to relieve dysphagia from an incurable oesophageal tumour.

blockage and tumour ingrowth. The latter can be rectified by laser ablation or placement of a second stent. Stents cannot be used for very proximal tumours involving the cervical oesophagus.

Palliative chemotherapy: This has been shown in a number of randomized clinical trials to improve patients' symptoms (i.e. dysphagia) and double life expectancy for those with advanced oesophagogastric cancer.

Palliative radiotherapy and brachytherapy: Intraluminal radiotherapy (brachytherapy) has been shown to provide a better quality of life for patients with incurable oesophageal cancer than a stent. However, availability of this treatment in the UK is still limited. External beam radiotherapy can provide good palliative care for squamous oesophageal carcinoma but requires more visits by the patient to hospital.

 SUMMARY BOX **13.2**

Oesophageal cancer

- Always investigate dysphagia
- GORD, Barrett's and oesophageal adenocarcinoma are linked
- Early diagnosis can allow curative endoscopic or surgical therapy
- Late diagnosis (the norm) results in poor prognosis
- Curative treatment now usually multimodal
- Surgical outcomes better in high volume centres.

DIAGNOSIS AND MANAGEMENT – GASTRODUODENAL

Peptic ulceration

Peptic ulceration affects areas of mucosa exposed to acidic gastric contents. The main pathology is an imbalance between the acid-pepsin system and the mucosal ability to resist digestion. Duodenal ulcers occur four times more commonly than gastric ulcers.

Pathology

Duodenal ulcers usually occur in the first part of the duodenum and 50% occur on the anterior wall. The majority of gastric ulcers develop on the lesser curvature in the distal half of the stomach. They may co-exist with duodenal ulcers in 10% of patients. Duodenal ulcers may be acute (Fig. 13.17) or chronic. Ulcers with a history of less than 3 months' duration and with no evidence of fibrosis are considered to be acute. Gastric ulcers generally run a chronic course.

Gastric ulcers may be benign or malignant. Malignancy was once thought to be a complicating factor of benign gastric ulceration. It is now realized that malignant change in a benign ulcer is rare, and that such ulcers are in fact probably malignant from the outset. Duodenal ulcers are very rarely malignant.

Aetiology

Helicobacter pylori

H. pylori is present in around 50% of the world's population, its prevalence increasing with age. It is more prevalent in developing countries, where poor and crowded living conditions are commonplace, and here the infection is probably acquired in early life via the faecal–oral or oral–oral route. Once an individual is infected, the *H. pylori* persists; in the majority of patients, there are no symptoms.

H. pylori is detected in 95% of patients with duodenal ulceration. It infects the mucosa of the antrum of the stomach, where it causes an inflammatory response. This gastritis stimulates the gastrin-producing (G) cells of the antrum to increase gastrin production. The subsequent hypersecretion of acid provides an ideal environment for gastric metaplasia of the duodenal mucosa to occur. The colonization of the metaplastic areas by *H. pylori* further damages the mucosa, and ultimately duodenal ulceration occurs.

H. pylori is found in approximately 75% of cases of gastric ulcers, although its role here is less well defined. It may be that the gastritis facilitates the access of acid and pepsin to the stomach mucosa. It seems that the key factor is decreased mucosal resistance, with excess acid having less of a role. Indeed, most patients with gastric ulceration have a normal or decreased secretory capacity.

Nonsteroidal anti-inflammatory drugs (NSAIDs)

This group of drugs includes aspirin, ibuprofen and diclofenac. Their role as anti-inflammatory agents centres on their inhibition of prostaglandin synthesis by inhibiting the action of cyclo-oxygenase. In the stomach, prostaglandins are responsible for the production of mucus

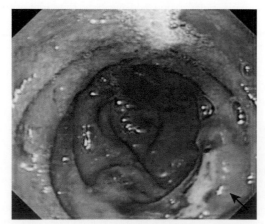

Fig. 13.17 Endoscopic view of an acute duodenal ulcer.

and bicarbonate. These both help to protect the stomach mucosa from acid by maintaining an alkaline buffer zone. By inhibiting prostaglandin synthesis, NSAIDs damage the gastric mucosa and are implicated in 30% of gastric ulcers. They may also be responsible for the small number of *H. pylori*-negative duodenal ulcers.

Smoking

This is an aetiological factor in both duodenal and gastric ulceration, but is more important in gastric ulceration. Smoking also delays ulcer healing, and there is an increased likelihood of complications (e.g. bleeding or perforation) developing in smokers.

Genetic factors

First-degree relatives of patients with a duodenal ulcer are at increased risk of developing a duodenal ulcer themselves. This risk is further increased if ulcers develop in patients under 20 years of age. First-degree relatives of patients with gastric ulcers are also at increased risk of developing gastric ulcers.

Zollinger–Ellison syndrome

This is a rare syndrome caused by a gastrin-secreting tumour (gastrinoma), which is normally found in the pancreas but may occasionally be found in the duodenum or stomach. Approximately 30% of patients have features consistent with multiple endocrine neoplasia syndrome (MEN I). Hypergastrinaemia results in a greatly increased risk of peptic ulceration. Diarrhoea may be a prominent feature, owing to large volumes of acid being secreted into the small intestine. Inactivation of the pancreatic lipase causes steatorrhoea. Complications of ulceration (pain, bleeding and stenosis) are common.

The diagnosis of Zollinger–Ellison is problematic, but ulceration in unusual sites, at an early age, or ulcers persisting despite medical treatment should be reviewed with a high index of suspicion and serum gastrin measured. Computed tomography (CT) or magnetic resonance imaging (MRI) and selective angiography may be used to localize the tumour.

Cure is effected by removal of the tumour wherever possible, although this may be made more difficult by the presence of metastatic disease, a very small tumour or multifocal disease. Removal is often supplemented with control of acid secretion using proton pump inhibitors.

Other factors

Other patients at risk of peptic ulceration include those with blood group O and those with hyperparathyroidism. Hyperparathyroidism causes elevated calcium levels, thus stimulating acid secretion. With treatment of the underlying condition, spontaneous ulcer healing usually occurs.

Clinical features

Recurrent well-localized epigastric pain is typical of peptic ulcer disease. Classically, the pain of a gastric ulcer occurs during eating and is relieved by vomiting. Patients with duodenal ulceration characteristically describe pain when they are hungry. This pain is relieved by food, antacids, milk and vomiting. Often, however, these well-defined features are not present, and it is usually impossible to differentiate between the pain of gastric ulceration and that of duodenal ulceration. Other symptoms associated with peptic ulcer disease include heartburn, anorexia, waterbrash (a sudden flow of saliva into the mouth) and intolerance of certain foods. Intermittent vomiting may occur. Where persistent vomiting is troublesome, the possibility of gastric outlet obstruction should be considered. Such vomiting tends to be projectile and may contain recognizable food eaten many hours previously.

Diagnosis

As already described, endoscopy and biopsy is essential in the diagnosis of peptic ulceration. In addition *H. pylori* can be diagnosed using the CLO test; a biopsy specimen taken from the antrum is placed in a gel containing urea. Ammonia released by the action of the *H. pylori*-derived urease is detected and causes a colour change – in most kits, from yellow to pink/red. Biopsy of gastric ulcers is particularly important, as malignancy needs to be excluded.

Special forms of ulceration

Stress ulceration refers to erosions or ulceration of the stomach or duodenum occurring in certain circumstances. These include severe illness, trauma, prolonged mechanical ventilation, multiple organ failure, sepsis and major surgery. The aetiology is not fully defined, although acid and mucosal ischaemia appear to be key elements. Medical prophylaxis using proton pump inhibitors may be useful in such circumstances.

Cushing's and Curling's ulcers are special forms of stress ulceration that occur following central nervous injury and burns, respectively. Hypersecretion of acid is not always essential for stress ulceration to occur, but does appear to be important in both of these conditions. In neurosurgical injury, raised intracranial pressure may be responsible for an increase in vagal activity and hence the increase in gastric secretion. The ulcers resulting from hypersecretion are usually single and, in common with other forms of peptic ulceration, may be complicated by perforation and bleeding.

MANAGEMENT OF UNCOMPLICATED PEPTIC ULCER DISEASE

Medical management

General measures helpful in the management of peptic ulcers include the avoidance of NSAIDs, smoking and excessive alcohol. If NSAIDs cannot be avoided in patients with a history of peptic ulceration PPIs should be prescribed (e.g. omeprazole or lansoprazole). These agents act by irreversibly inhibiting H^+/K^+ ATPase and thus are powerful inhibitors of acid secretion.

Eradication of *H. pylori*

Duodenal ulcers

Eradication of the *H. pylori* has become the mainstay of management in patients with a duodenal ulcer (EBM 13.5). Eradication therapies comprise an antisecretory agent, typically a PPI, together with one or more antibiotics. This 'triple therapy' is usually given for 7 days followed by a healing dose of PPI for 4–6 weeks. Eradication rates of greater than 90% occur with good compliance, although reinfection following successful eradication is possible. Without eradication therapy, approximately 80% of ulcers will recur within 1 year. Complete resolution of symptoms is a good indicator of successful eradication. However, where symptoms persist, it is advisable to recheck the *H. pylori* status.

13

EBM 13.5 The role of *H. pylori* eradication in the treatment of peptic ulceration

'RCTs have found that Helicobacter eradication is superior to acid-lowering drugs in duodenal ulcer healing, and both are superior to no treatment. In preventing duodenal ulcer recurrence, eradication therapy was similar to maintenance acid-lowering drugs, but eradication therapy was superior to no treatment. In gastric ulcer healing, eradication therapy was similar to acid-lowering drugs. In preventing gastric ulcer recurrence, eradication therapy was superior to no treatment.'

Ford A, et al. Cochrane Database of Systematic Reviews 2004; CD003840.

Gastric ulcers

Malignancy should be excluded by endoscopic biopsy before a diagnosis of benign gastric ulcer is made. Where a patient is found to be *H. pylori*-positive at endoscopy, eradication therapy should be instituted. Without eradication, the relapse rate is in the region of 50%, but this falls to less than 10% with successful eradication therapy. Endoscopic surveillance of a treated ulcer should continue until healing is complete. Failure to heal warrants further biopsies.

Surgical management

Duodenal ulceration

Surgery for uncomplicated duodenal ulceration is now extremely rare. Operations such as a truncal vagotomy, highly selective vagotomy, or gastric resectional surgery have had little role since the introduction of eradication therapy.

Gastric ulceration

Failure of conservative therapy to heal a gastric ulcer is an indication for surgical intervention. Where malignancy cannot be excluded or is suspected, resection of the ulcer is the treatment of choice. The extent and type of resection will be determined by the position of the ulcer within the stomach and its suspected malignant potential. Benign distal ulcers may be treated by a Billroth I gastrectomy, whereby the distal part of the stomach is removed and the proximal stump anastomosed to the duodenum. More proximal ulcers usually necessitate a Polya-type reconstruction involving anastomosis of the gastric remnant to the jejunum (Fig. 13.18).

Many patients who had surgery for ulcer disease in the 1960s and 70s are still alive today and suffer long-term side effects similar to those experienced by patients having a gastrectomy for cancer.

Dumping

This arises in up to 20% of patients following gastric resection and encompasses a range of vasomotor symptoms, including light-headedness, tachycardia, flushing, sweats and palpitations. Occasionally, these are accompanied by diarrhoea and vomiting.

Early dumping (or dumping syndrome proper) occurs 15–30 minutes after eating. The rapid emptying of hyperosmolar (mainly carbohydrate) gastric contents into the small intestine leads to the influx of fluid down an osmotic gradient into the bowel lumen. The symptoms associated with the syndrome are due to both the sudden contraction of the extracellular fluid compartment and intestinal distension causing increased peristalsis. The patient often needs to lie down until the symptoms pass. In the majority of patients, symptoms improve spontaneously with conservative measures, which include taking smaller, dry and frequent meals, avoiding excessive carbohydrate intake, and avoiding liquids at mealtimes.

Late dumping is much less common than early dumping. It is a reactive hypoglycaemia caused by more rapid absorption of glucose from the upper small intestine. This causes hyperglycaemia, which in turn leads to increased insulin production and rebound hypoglycaemia. The symptoms are of a similar nature to those of the dumping syndrome proper (or early dumping), but may include hunger and confusion and occur 1–3 hours after eating. Late dumping is symptomatically controlled with carbohydrate.

Diarrhoea

Rapid influx of gastric contents into the small intestine and an interruption of vagal fibres to abdominal viscera are thought to be responsible. The diarrhoea may be associated with mild steatorrhoea. Codeine-related compounds or loperamide may be used to treat the diarrhoea, although they are not always helpful. Eating small, dry meals lacking in refined carbohydrates can help.

Weight loss

Weight loss following gastric surgery is common. Reduced oral intake is the main cause; this may be due to early satiety, nausea, vomiting, abdominal pain or simply a poor

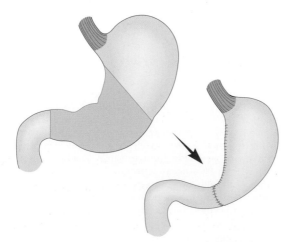
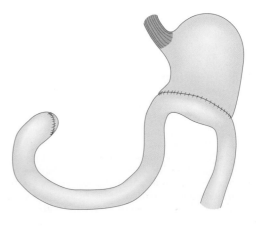

Fig. 13.18 Gastrectomy for peptic ulceration.

appetite. Malabsorption may also play a role in weight loss due to accelerated emptying of gastric contents into the small intestine or bacterial overgrowth.

Anaemia

This may occur after any form of gastric surgery and is particularly common following complete gastrectomy. The picture may be one of iron, B_{12} or folate deficiency, or a mixture of the three. Iron deficiency is the most common and may be part of a generalized poor intake, as described above. It may also result from depressed acid-dependent reduction of iron salts, this process being necessary for the body's utilization of iron. B_{12} deficiency occurs when insufficient intrinsic factor is available for its absorption. This usually only arises after extensive gastric resection, as the stomach generally produces far more intrinsic factor than is actually needed for B_{12} absorption. Folate deficiency may result from poor oral intake.

Osteoporosis and osteomalacia

These conditions are associated with partial gastrectomy owing to decreased absorption of calcium and vitamin D. Such bone disease may manifest itself many years postoperatively as pathological fractures. Vitamin D and calcium supplementation is indicated on a long-term basis, especially in women.

Carcinoma

Patients who have had peptic ulcer surgery are at increased risk of developing gastric adenocarcinoma. The reason is thought to be due to reflux of carcinogenic bile salts into the gastric remnant. Consequently, such patients should be offered long term endoscopic surveillance.

COMPLICATIONS OF PEPTIC ULCERATION REQUIRING OPERATIVE INTERVENTION

Perforation

Duodenal ulcers

Up to 50% of patients will have had no previous ulcer symptoms. The incidence of duodenal ulcer perforation is decreasing, probably due in part to improvements in the medical management of duodenal ulcers. Perforation usually occurs in acute ulcers on the anterior wall of the duodenum.

Gastric ulcers

Gastric ulcer perforation is less common than duodenal ulcer perforation. It has a peak incidence in the elderly, and consequently the associated morbidity and mortality are higher. Gastric perforation has a strong association with NSAID use.

Clinical features

The acute onset of severe unremitting epigastric pain is strongly suggestive of the possibility of perforation. Thereafter, the range of symptoms depends on the intra-abdominal course. The patient may be pale, shocked and peripherally shut down secondary to generalized peritonitis. Irritant stomach contents in the peritoneal cavity may give rise to shoulder-tip pain, resulting from irritation of the diaphragm. Vomiting may occur. The abdomen does not move freely with respiration, and marked tenderness, guarding, fear of movement and board-like rigidity may be found on examination. Respiration is shallow and bowel sounds are usually absent.

Generalized peritonitis does not occur in some patients because the perforation seals over with omentum. In others, the fluid tracks down the right paracolic gutter, simulating acute appendicitis. Silent perforations may also occur, and are only found incidentally on a chest X-ray.

Diagnosis

In 60% of cases of perforation, an erect chest X-ray will demonstrate free air under the diaphragm, although the absence of free air does not exclude a perforation (see Fig. 13.5). A lateral decubitus film can be useful where an erect chest X-ray is not feasible, e.g. because of shock or disability.

A moderate hyperamylasaemia may be found with a perforated duodenal ulcer. High amylase levels are more suggestive of pancreatitis. Where there is still doubt over the diagnosis, an emergency water-soluble contrast meal or an abdominal CT scan may be indicated.

Management

The initial management, as for other causes of peritonitis, consists of resuscitation, oxygen therapy, intravenous fluids and broad spectrum antibiotics, and the passage of a naso-gastric tube. Intravenous opiate analgesia and PPIs should be given as necessary. A urinary catheter enables close monitoring of urine output.

Operative management is usually indicated although patients who do not have generalized peritoneal signs or systemic sepsis may be successfully managed conservatively so long as frequent reassessment shows no deterioration in their condition. Surgeons are increasingly using a laparoscopic approach to treatment but open surgery should not be considered inferior.

Duodenal ulcers

Surgery usually involves simple closure, whereby the ulcer is under-run with sutures or plugged using an omental patch (Fig. 13.19), coupled with a thorough peritoneal lavage. All patients should receive 72 hours of intravenous PPI therapy and then *H. pylori* eradication therapy and a healing course of oral PPIs.

Gastric ulcers

Approximately 15% of perforated gastric ulcers prove ultimately to be malignant. However, current practice suggests biopsy of the ulcer wall, followed by simple closure or local excision of the ulcer, is best. If the ulcer turns out to be malignant, a minority will progress to gastric resection following tumour staging (see below).

SUMMARY BOX **13.3**

Peptic ulcer disease

- *Helicobacter pylori* is the most important cause – eradicate it
- NSAID medication next commonest cause
- Surgery now only for complications (bleeding and perforation)
- Always biopsy a gastric ulcer – some will be malignant
- If an ulcer fails to heal with medical therapy look for rare causes (i.e. ZE).

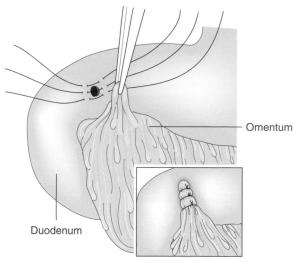

Omentum

Duodenum

Fig. 13.19 Closure of perforated duodenal ulcer.

Acute haemorrhage

The differential diagnosis of upper gastrointestinal bleeding is summarized in Table 13.2. Upper gastrointestinal bleeding presents with haematemesis (vomiting blood) and/or melaena (the passage of black tarry stool that has a very characteristic smell). Melaena results from the digestion of blood by enzymes and bacteria. Less commonly, melaena may be the result of a bleed from the right colon. Very rarely, if bleeding is very brisk, upper gastrointestinal bleeding may present as fresh rectal bleeding, in which case signs of cardiovascular instability are present. Slow chronic blood loss may be asymptomatic and detected on rectal examination by a positive faecal occult blood test.

Diagnosis

History and examination

A full history and examination are essential in determining the cause of the bleeding. Pointers to the diagnosis include the past medical history (peptic ulcer disease, previous bleeding, liver disease, previous surgery, coagulopathies), drug history (most importantly, NSAIDs and anticoagulants) and social history (alcohol abuse).

Specific features to be looked for include those suggestive of acute substantial blood loss and shock (hypotension, tachycardia, tachypnoea and pallor), and signs of liver

disease and portal hypertension (spider naevi, portosystemic shunting and bruising). The latter are particularly important, as variceal haemorrhage necessitates specific treatment.

Blood tests

The full blood count may be normal immediately after an acute bleed but will fall once haemodilution has occurred. The test may show anaemia, suggestive of more chronic blood loss. Urea is often high following a gastrointestinal bleed, due to the absorption of blood and its subsequent metabolism by the liver. Coagulation derangement occurs in the presence of significant liver disease.

Management

Resuscitation

Bleeding is now the most common cause of death from peptic ulcer disease and resuscitation is vital. Following the administration of high-flow oxygen, intravenous access is obtained and blood taken for the investigations noted above. A sample is also taken for blood cross-matching and intravenous fluids started.

A nasogastric tube is passed to monitor the bleeding and prevent aspiration. A urinary catheter is inserted. A central or arterial line may aid resuscitation. Volume replacement is gauged against pulse, blood pressure, urine output and central venous pressure. Over-transfusion or rapid transfusion in those with compromised cardiac function can lead to pulmonary oedema.

Detection and endoscopic treatment

The aims of management of bleeding peptic ulcers are to identify the bleeding point, arrest the bleeding (bleeding ceases spontaneously in 90% of patients) and prevent recurrence. Once resuscitation has occurred, endoscopy is used to detect the site of bleeding (Fig. 13.20), doing so in 80–90% of cases. The endoscopist should also have the necessary experience and training to attempt control of the bleeding using techniques such as adrenaline (epinephrine) 1:10 000 injection and application of heater probes and clips. Bleeding from the ulcer base, the presence of a visible vessel and adherent clot overlying the ulcer are features associated with a significantly increased risk of further bleeding.

In patients in whom endoscopy does not identify the bleeding point, angiography may be used, but the limitation of this investigation is that it can only detect active bleeding of greater than 1 ml/min. In these patients, selective embolization can be used to stop the bleeding and thus avoid the need for surgery.

Table 13.2 **Causes of upper gastrointestinal bleeding.**	
• Peptic ulceration	50%
• Mucosal lesions including gastritis, duodenitis and erosions	30%
• Mallory-Weiss tear	5–10%
• Varices	5–10%
• Reflux oesophagitis	5%
• Angiodysplasia	2%
• Carcinoma	Uncommon
• Aortoduodenal fistula	Uncommon
• Dieulafoy syndrome (rupture of a large tortuous submucosal artery normally found in the body of the stomach)	Rare
• Coagulopathies	Uncommon

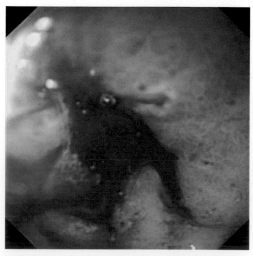

Fig. 13.20 Endoscopic view of bleeding duodenal ulcer.

Surgical management

Emergency surgery may be indicated if endoscopy reveals bleeding from a major artery and where attempted injection sclerotherapy is unable to control the bleeding directly; 50% of patients with active arterial bleeding and 30% with a visible vessel at the ulcer base are ultimately likely to require surgery. When bleeding recurs after therapeutic endoscopy, a further endoscopy may be able to control the bleeding. Recurrent bleeding is associated with significant morbidity and mortality, particularly in the elderly. Continuing bleeding is particularly common in those with a chronic ulcer and is more common in gastric ulceration. The type of operation used depends on the site of the bleeding ulcer and the co-morbidity of the patient:

- *Duodenal ulcers.* A bleeding duodenal ulcer may simply be under-run with sutures, through a duodenotomy (opening of the anterior wall of the duodenum) to gain access to the ulcer. Once tolerating oral fluids, the patient should be started on *H. pylori* eradication therapy empirically.
- *Gastric ulcers.* With a bleeding gastric ulcer, the possibility of malignancy must be considered. The ulcer must be biopsied in all cases to determine its nature. In young fit patients, the ulcer should be excised completely by taking a small wedge resection. In elderly patients or those with significant co-morbidity, under-running of the ulcer may be preferable, at least in the first instance. If the pathology result confirms malignancy, then the patient should have accurate staging and further treatment as indicated. If the ulcer proves to be benign, *H. pylori* eradication is indicated. NSAIDs should be avoided.

GASTRIC NEOPLASIA

Benign gastric neoplasms

Benign tumours of the stomach may arise from epithelial or mesenchymal tissue. Adenomatous polyps may be single or multiple and are the most common benign epithelial neoplasm. Gastrointestinal stromal tumours (GISTs) arise from the pacemaker cells in the gastric wall and have a variable natural history. Diagnosis is usually by endoscopy and EUS; biopsies are rarely helpful as the lesions are submucosal. Small asymptomatic GISTs (up to 2cm diameter) can safely be left alone but larger ones should be either kept under surveillance (2–5cm) or resected (>5cm). Symptomatic gastric GISTs (bleeding, pain, obstruction) should usually be resected (Fig. 13.21) and laparoscopic techniques are often possible.

Malignant gastric neoplasms

Gastric carcinoma
Epidemiology

Adenocarcinoma is the most common malignancy affecting the stomach. It accounts for 90% of malignant tumours found within the stomach; lymphomas, carcinoids and gastrointestinal stromal tumours make up the rest. The incidence of gastric cancer has decreased substantially in the last 50 years. Gastric cancer principally affects those in the 60–80-year age group, but is not infrequently seen in younger patients. Where once the tumour was more commonly noted in the gastric antrum, its incidence in this region has diminished and a corresponding increase in incidence in the proximal stomach has occurred. The male:female ratio is 2:1. Gastric cancer has the fifth poorest 5-year survival rate after cancer of the pancreas, liver, oesophagus and lung.

Aetiology

- *Diet.* Gastric cancer is noted more commonly where malnutrition is prevalent. It has also been associated with the use of certain preservatives in food; nitrates, nitrites and nitrosamines have been implicated. Where soils are rich in nitrates or dietary intake is high, gastric carcinoma is more common. A high vitamin intake is thought to be protective against the development of cancer of the stomach. Diets rich in carotene and vitamins C and E have been shown to reduce the incidence of intestinal metaplasia in the stomach, a condition thought to be associated with malignant change.
- *H. pylori infection.* Recent epidemiological studies have suggested that *H. pylori* may be associated with an increased incidence of malignant change within the stomach (EBM 13.6). At the present time, it is thought that its ability to produce ammonia as well as other mutagenic chemicals may play a part in neoplastic transformation of the gastric mucosa. Such changes are thought to be enhanced by lack of vitamin C.
- *Gastric polyps.* Hyperplastic and adenomatous polyps are the most frequently found, but only the latter have significant malignant potential. Studies have shown that over one-quarter of adenomatous polyps may show malignant changes within them. Furthermore, gastric carcinoma is frequently encountered in stomachs affected by polyps. This suggests that conditions necessary for the development of polyps may also enhance the development of malignancy.

13

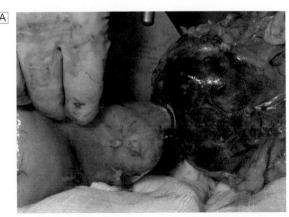 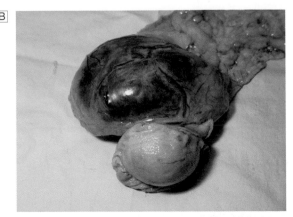

Fig. 13.21 **A** Large dumb-bell shaped gastric GIST lesion in situ. **B** Lesion resected showing intact gastric mucosa over its luminal aspect.

EBM **13.6** The role of *H. pylori* eradication in the prevention of gastric cancer

'RCTs have found that Helicobacter eradication reduces the risk of developing gastric cancer as long as premalignant lesions do not pre-exist at the time of eradication.'

Ley C, et al. Cancer Epidemiol Biomarkers Prev 2004;13:4–10.
Wong BC, et al. JAMA 2004; 291:187–194.

- *Gastroenterostomy.* Where there has been a previous gastric resection or duodenal bypass for benign disease and the remaining stomach has been anastomosed to the bile-containing upper gastrointestinal tract, the stomach remnant is more vulnerable to malignant change than the intact stomach. The risk of malignant change increases with the time elapsed since surgery. Patients who have had gastric resections with gastroenterostomy may be 4–5 times more liable to develop gastric carcinoma in the stomach remnant than the normal population.
- *Chronic atrophic gastritis.* This condition is associated with a loss of the gastric glands from the stomach mucosa. It has been noted to be more frequent in patients at increased risk of developing stomach cancer. Chronic atrophic gastritis is associated with pernicious anaemia, which is linked to an increased risk of gastric cancer. Such patients have a four-fold increased risk compared to the normal population.
- *Intestinal metaplasia.* This condition arises when the gastric mucosa is replaced by mucosa containing glands that have features more in common with those found in the small intestine. Such changes are usually found in the distal part of the stomach and are associated with an increased risk of development of gastric carcinoma.
- *Gastric dysplasia.* When the gastric mucosal cells become less uniform in size, shape and organization, dysplastic changes may result and may be low- or high-grade. Patients with high-grade dysplasia often have associated malignant change.
- *Hereditary diffuse gastric cancer*: Inherited mutations of the E-cadherin gene can result in an aggressive form of signet ring gastric adenocarcinoma affecting young patients. Once symptomatic these patients are rarely curable. Consequently, patients with a strong family history of gastric cancer should be referred for genetic counselling and, if appropriate, offered endoscopic surveillance and/or a prophylactic total gastrectomy (EBM 13.7).

EBM **13.7** Hereditary diffuse gastric cancer – gastrectomy

'...a multidisciplinary approach to preoperative counselling involving a gastroenterologist, surgeon, dietician, genetic counsellor and specialist nurse is absolutely necessary.'

Fitzgerald RC, Hardwick RH, Huntsman D et al. 2010 Updated consensus guidelines for the clinical management and directions for future research. J Med Genet 47: 436-444. http://jmg.bmj.com/content/47/7/436.full.html#related-urls

Early gastric cancer

Early gastric cancer results when neoplastic cells are limited to the mucosa or submucosal layers of the stomach wall. By definition, this type of cancer is confined to the most super-ficial layers of the stomach wall but it can be associated in a small minority of patients with lymph node metastases. Such tumours, if adequately treated surgically, are associated with 5-year survival rates in excess of 90%. The survival rate will depend upon the depth of invasion of the tumour and the presence or absence of lymph node metastases at the time of surgical excision. Early gastric cancer in the UK accounts for approximately 10% of all resected cases of gastric adenocarcinoma whereas in Japan (a high incidence country for gastric cancer) it makes up well over 50%. The explanation for this is multifactorial but includes the Japanese public's awareness of the symptoms of gastric cancer and a national screening programme to detect early disease.

Advanced gastric cancer

The vast majority of malignant gastric tumours found in Western countries are locally advanced gastric adenocarcinomas. These tumours have invaded into the muscularis propria and sometimes through to the serosa. The risk of peritoneal metastases and lympho-vascular invasion is much higher than for early tumours. Advanced gastric tumours often invade the adjacent gastric wall via submucosal lymphatics creating a diffusely thickened and rigid stomach (linitis plastica) (Fig. 13.22). Invasion into adjacent structures such as the pancreas can also occur (Fig. 13.23).

Factors affecting survival in advanced gastric cancer

The survival of patients with advanced gastric cancer depends upon the stage of the tumour at presentation and on the general fitness of the patient. Treatment with curative intent implies surgical resection, increasingly combined with perioperative chemotherapy. For surgery to be curative, excision of the primary tumour must be adequate, with margins clear of the tumour and with satisfactory en bloc resection of all possible involved lymph nodes (EBM 13.8).

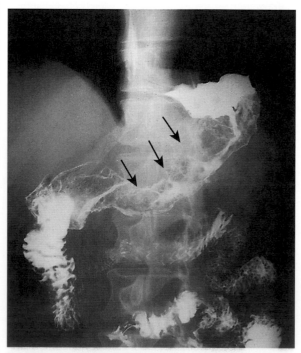

Fig. 13.22 Barium meal showing extensive gastric carcinoma with narrowing of the lumen (arrowed).

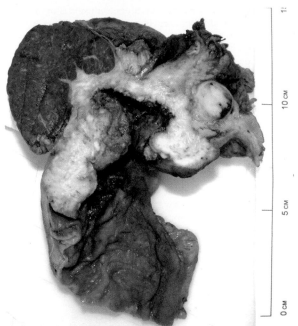

Fig. 13.23 Resection specimen showing invasion of a gastric cancer into the tail of the pancreas. The spleen has been removed en bloc with the stomach and distal pancreas.

EBM	13.8 D1 versus D2 (radical) lymph node dissection in gastric cancer

'Subgroup analysis suggests a survival benefit for T_3 and T_4 tumours with more radical surgery. Learning curves of surgeons and centres performing low-volume cancer surgery may confound any benefit of more radical surgery.'

McCulloch P, et al. Cochrane Database of Systemic Reviews 2004; CD001964.

Poor survival has been correlated with depth of tumour invasion through the stomach wall, involvement of tumour resection margins and the presence of lymph node metastases. Transgression of the tumour through the stomach wall is associated with poor survival, as the tumour is able to spread transperitoneally and therefore seed the peritoneum with malignant cells, making complete surgical excision impossible.

A comprehensive pathological classification of tumours has enabled the prognosis of a particular stage of cancer to be estimated. Such staging is usually classified according to the tumour size (T), the node status (N), and the presence or absence of distant metastases (M) (Table 13.3).

Clinical features of gastric malignancy

The symptomatology of gastric carcinoma may be subtle, and mild symptoms of indigestion, flatulence or dyspepsia may be the early signs of malignancy. Such symptoms should not be overlooked and should not be treated without further investigation, particularly in patients in a vulnerable age group (> 40 years).

The severity of symptoms is not invariably associated with the stage of disease. More advanced gastric cancer tends to be associated with weight loss, anaemia, dysphagia, vomiting, epigastric or back pain, or the presence of an epigastric mass. The patient may also manifest signs of more widespread distant metastases, such as jaundice (liver secondaries or compression of the biliary tree by enlarged

Table 13.3 TNM classification of gastric carcinoma*

T (Tumour)	
T_1	Tumour invades lamina propria or submucosa
T_2	Tumour invades muscularis propria or subserosa
T_3	Tumour invades serosa
T_4	Tumour invades adjacent structures
N (Node)	
N_0	No lymph node involvement
N_1	Fewer than 7 lymph nodes involved by tumour
N_2	7–15 lymph nodes involved by tumour
N_3	More than 15 lymph nodes involved by tumour
M (Metastases)	
M_0	No metastases
M_1	Metastases present

*Greene FL, Page DL, Fleming ID, et al, eds. AJCC cancer staging manual. 6th edn. Springer-Verlag: New York; 2002.

lymph nodes), ascites, spurious diarrhoea (secondary to pelvic infiltration), and signs and symptoms of intestinal obstruction secondary to malignant deposits on the bowel.

Diagnosis

Diagnosis is made on the basis of a thorough medical history, clinical examination and an upper gastrointestinal endoscopy and biopsy. Following histological diagnosis the patient should meet with an experienced clinician to be told their diagnosis in an appropriate environment preferably with the support of a family member and a specialist upper GI nurse. Patients deemed potentially fit enough for radical therapy should have a series of staging investigations.

Staging of gastric carcinoma

- *CT:* Any patient with a histological diagnosis of gastric cancer should undergo a CT scan of their chest, abdomen and pelvis unless they are very frail. This should provide information about the M-stage (liver, lung, peritoneum and distant nodes) and can help exclude T4 involvement of adjacent structures such as the pancreas.
- *EUS:* EUS is excellent at determining T-stage. High frequency probes (10 MHz or more) can accurately differentiate between T1–4 disease and add information of local nodal status (N-Stage).
- *Staging laparoscopy:* This procedure is essential in patients with locally advanced tumours to detect small volume peritoneal and liver metastases that cannot be detected by CT (Fig. 13.24). Peritoneal washings are also helpful as patients with positive peritoneal cytology for malignancy have a very poor prognosis and rarely benefit from surgery.
- *PET-CT:* Gastric adenocarcinomas are not always PET-avid. This limits PET's application as a routine staging procedure looking for metastatic disease.

Treatment with curative intent

All patients should have their case discussed by a multidisciplinary Upper GI team. Those with potentially curable disease who are deemed fit enough for radical therapy have the following options:

- *Surgery alone:* Patient with early gastric cancer should undergo a distal (subtotal) or total D_2 gastrectomy (depending upon the site of the tumour) done by an experienced surgeon working in a high volume cancer

13

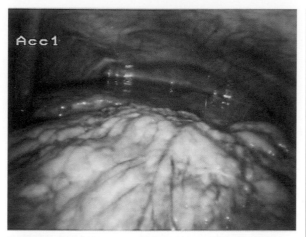

Fig. 13.24 Staging laparoscopy showing omental metastases and ascites secondary to advanced gastric cancer.

centre. The 'D$_2$' description refers to the excision of both the first tier of perigastric lymph nodes and the second tier of nodes along the gastric arteries (Fig. 13.25). Reconstruction of the gastrointestinal tract is usually by Roux en-Y to prevent bile reflux (Fig. 13.26). When oncologically safe to do so, a distal gastrectomy is preferable to a total gastrectomy as it gives a better quality of life

- *Combined therapy*: Randomized clinical trials in the UK have shown improved survival for patients who have perioperative chemotherapy and surgery compared to those who have surgery alone. The effect seems most pronounced for advanced tumours; the neo-adjuvant or preoperative component of the chemotherapy seems to have the biggest impact on survival (EBM 13.9). Further trials continue to discover if newer agents such as Bevacizumab can improve survival further. The surgery is the same regardless of whether chemotherapy is given or not.

EBM	**13.9 Combination surgery and chemotherapy in gastric cancer**

'*In patients with operable gastric or lower esophageal adenocarcinomas, a perioperative regimen of ECF decreased tumor size and stage and significantly improved progression-free and overall survival.*'

Cunningham D, Allum WH, Stenning SP, Thompson JN, Van de Velde CJ, Nicolson M, et al. Perioperative chemotherapy versus surgery alone for resectable gastroesophageal cancer. N Engl J Med 2006; 355(1):11-20.

Palliation

- *Best supportive care*: Some patients are too frail for any anticancer therapy and all focus should be on relieving their symptoms and supporting them and their families through their terminal illness. Nausea and vomiting is treated with antiemetics such as cyclizine or ondansetron. Poor appetite may respond to steroids such as dexamethasone. Pain often requires opiate analgesia. Eating can be particularly difficult for patients with advanced gastric cancer and dietetic

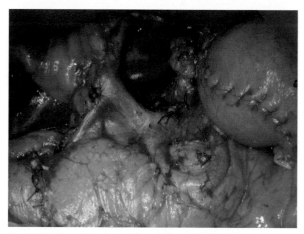

Fig. 13.25 Operative view of the coeliac axis after D2 nodal dissection and removal of all lymph nodes.

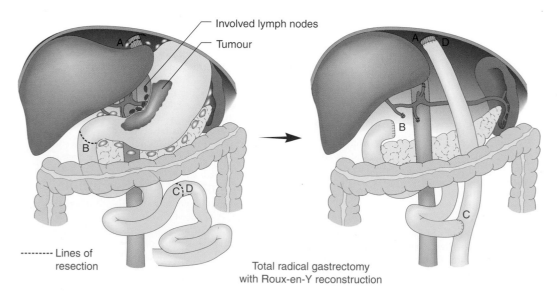

Involved lymph nodes

Tumour

-------- Lines of resection

Total radical gastrectomy with Roux-en-Y reconstruction

Fig. 13.26 Total gastrectomy with curative intent.

support is essential. Towards the end of a patient's life they may need medication via a subcutaneous infusion from a portable syringe driver.

- *Palliative chemotherapy*: For patients who are fit enough, valuable improvements in quality of life can be achieved with palliative chemotherapy using combinations of drugs such as epirubicin, cisplatin and 5-fluorouracil. In addition, life expectancy can be extended if the tumour is chemosensitive (EBM 13.10).

EBM 13.10 The role of palliative chemotherapy in gastric cancer

'Systematic reviews show a modest survival benefit for palliative chemotherapy in gastric cancer, with ECF (epirubicin, cisplatin and 5-fluorouracil) regimens currently amongst the more effective. Newer combinations with irinotecan- or taxane-based regimens show promising results.'

Wohrer SS, et al. Ann Oncol 2004; 15:1585–1595.

- *Palliative radiotherapy*: Bleeding from advanced gastric tumours can be troublesome and can be greatly reduced by a short course of external beam radiation.
- *Stenting*: Patients with gastric outlet obstruction who have persistent vomiting may benefit from the endoscopic placement of a self-expanding metallic stent although the results are unpredictable.
- *Palliative surgery*: Options include a gastric bypass (often done laparoscopically) for distal tumours, or a palliative resection. The latter is a big undertaking for patients with incurable disease and should only be considered in those with distal tumours who have not benefitted from lesser interventions and who are fit (Fig. 13.27).

Prognosis

When the tumour is confined to the mucosa or submucosa without lymph node or distant metastases, a 5-year survival of the order of 95–100% can be achieved. With increasing penetration of the tumour through the stomach wall and increasing numbers of nodes involved, the 5-year survival

Table 13.4 Examples of stages of gastric cancer and their prognosis.

Stage	5-year survival (%)
$T_1N_0M_0$	95+
$T_1N_1M_0$	70–80
$T_2N_1M_0$	45–50
$T_3N_2M_0$	15–25
M_1	0–10

decreases. A further deterioration occurs when distant metastases are present, in which case 5-year survival is unusual (Table 13.4).

Other gastric tumours

Lymphomas

The stomach represents the most common site for gastrointestinal lymphomas, which are malignant aggregations of lymphatic tissue. Many lymphomas are thought to arise from mucosa-associated lymphoid tissue and are therefore frequently referred to as MALT lymphomas. In such cases, there is a frequent association with the presence of *H. pylori* infection, which, it is thought, may bring about a lymphomatous change. Such lymphomas are usually low-grade and may respond to eradication of the *H. pylori* infection. Occasionally, lymphomas may transform to a high-grade type of tumour that carries a poorer prognosis. Such tumours are more likely to require more aggressive treatment with chemotherapy. Surgery is reserved for specific indications such as perforation or bleeding.

Carcinoid tumours

These are tumours of neuroendocrine origin that vary enormously in their malignant potential. The majority encountered are benign, but occasionally malignant carcinoids can behave aggressively. When associated with liver metastases, they can result in the carcinoid syndrome, which is related to the over-production of 5-hydroxytryptamine.

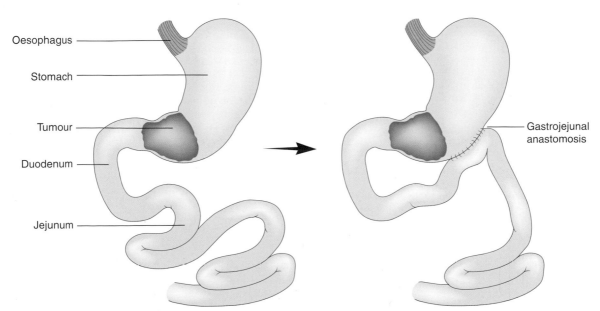

Fig. 13.27 Palliative bypass procedure (gastrojejunostomy) for obstructing distal gastric cancer.

13

Gastric cancer

- Curable if detected early
- Early symptoms similar to peptic ulcer
- Don't wait for 'alarm symptoms' to investigate – it's usually too late
- Multi-modal therapy for advanced disease
- Good palliation for incurable disease can be challenging
- Rare inherited cases prevented by prophylactic gastrectomy.

MISCELLANEOUS DISORDERS OF THE STOMACH

Ménétrier's disease

This is a condition of gastric mucosal hypertrophy, in which the mucosal rugal folds are grossly enlarged in the fundus and body of the stomach; the antrum is usually spared. Mucosal hypertrophy may lead to abnormally large secretions of mucus or acid. Over-secretion of acid and protein-rich mucus may contribute to symptoms of epigastric pain and hypoproteinaemia.

Ménétrier's disease is associated with an increased incidence of malignancy in the stomach and once it has been diagnosed total gastrectomy should be considered in an otherwise fit patient.

Gastritis

This common condition is due to inflammation of the gastric mucosal lining. It may be caused by a variety of injurious agents, both chemical and bacteriological. It is frequently associated with over-indulgence in alcohol. Biliary gastritis is seen in the presence of bile in the stomach (frequently seen after Polya-type partial gastrectomy).

Gastritis may arise as a consequence of extreme stress resulting from shock, and this form is therefore more frequently encountered in the intensive care situation. Such gastritis is thought to be a consequence of mucosal hypoperfusion and acidosis secondary to a shock-like state. This combination leads to mucosal ischaemia and resulting stress gastritis, which can cause loss of mucosa resulting in erosions that may on occasion bleed profusely. Gastritis may be lessened or prevented by resuscitation, administering mucosal protective agents, and neutralizing or minimizing gastric acid secretion. Surgery is undertaken rarely to control massive haemorrhage resulting from gastritis.

Dieulafoy's lesion

A condition of profuse bleeding from an abnormal vessel situated in the gastric mucosa and not associated with ulceration, Dieulafoy's lesion is usually found in the upper stomach. Such bleeding is treated initially by injection sclerotherapy, but may require open gastrotomy and over-sewing of the bleeding point.

Bezoars

Accumulations of hair (trichobezoars) or vegetable matter (phytobezoars) or combinations of the two (trichophytobezoars), these may on occasion form a complete cast of the stomach, and the ensuing reduced nutritional intake contributes to malnourishment. The diagnosis is made by barium examination and surgical removal is advisable.

MISCELLANEOUS CONDITIONS OF THE DUODENUM

Duodenal obstruction

Common causes of duodenal obstruction are pyloric stenosis and carcinoma of the pancreas. Rarer causes include blockage by mesenteric lymph nodes, duodenal diverticulum, duodenal atresia, annular pancreas and chronic duodenal ileus. If surgical treatment is required, bypass by duodenojejunal or gastrojejunal anastomosis is often appropriate. Symptomatic diverticula may have to be excised. Chronic duodenal ileus is an ill-defined entity that may affect visceroptotic females and rapidly growing, thin children. It has been suggested that the duodenum is obstructed by the superior mesenteric vessels as they cross its third part, but most surgeons are sceptical about this explanation. The condition is usually self-limiting in children, but in adults surgical bypass may have to be considered.

Duodenal diverticula

The duodenum is the second most common site for diverticulum formation in the gastrointestinal tract. The diverticula rarely develop before the age of 40 years, and are often found at the point of entry of the common bile duct. They are frequently discovered incidentally at endoscopy or on barium meal examination, but can cause obstruction, bleeding and inflammation (diverticulitis). Symptomatic diverticula should be excised if it is certain that they are the cause of problems.

Duodenal trauma

Duodenal damage may follow severe crush injury of the upper abdomen. Retroperitoneal air may be seen on abdominal X-ray.

Surgery for obesity

Obesity is an increasing problem world-wide. It is defined as a body mass index (BMI) greater than 32; morbid obesity represents a BMI greater than 38. (Until recently, the cut-offs were 30 and 35 respectively.) The effect of obesity on the respiratory, cardiovascular, locomotor and metabolic systems, as well as on mental health, can be severe. Patients with morbid obesity have a significantly reduced life expectancy; for example, a person with a BMI of 45 at the age of 25 will have a reduction in life expectancy of 11 years.

Prevention is better than cure and indeed there is no current 'cure' for obesity. Weight reduction programmes combining reduced calorie intake with increased exercise have variable results. Weight loss is slow and the programme often requires to be followed for many, many months. Furthermore, a change in eating and exercising behaviour is necessary if the weight loss is to be maintained long-term.

Patients who are morbidly obese can benefit from obesity or bariatric surgery. Such patients need to be assessed very carefully, taking account of their mental state, physical fitness, and the presence of medical conditions that lead to obesity but can be corrected by treatment (e.g. hypothyroidism). The careful selection of patients involves a multidisciplinary team approach.

A number of operations have been performed for obesity in the past. Many of the intestinal bypass operations and jaw wiring procedures are relegated to history. Current obesity surgery is designed to be restrictive or malabsorptive:

- *Restrictive*: decreases food intake, as the patient suffers early satiety even after small meals. Overeating causes upper abdominal pain, and vomiting may be required to relieve it
- *Malabsorptive*: alters digestion, leading to food intake being poorly absorbed and eliminated in the stool. Overeating typically leads to excessive diarrhoea and flatulence.

Operations for obesity

Current options include gastric banding, vertical banded gastroplasty, gastric bypass and duodenal switch. All these operations can be performed laparoscopically. However, the technical difficulty of such surgery increases in the order that these operations are listed above. The more complex operations are more likely to lead to better excess weight loss in the short term. However, there is increasing evidence to show that the percentage of excess weight loss at 3 years is similar for gastric banding and gastric bypass. The procedures can be combined; for example, gastric banding is technically easier to perform in the very obese patient who has a BMI greater than 55. Once excess weight loss has plateaued, removing the band and performing a gastric bypass may allow further excess weight loss.

The gastric band is a ring with an inflatable inner cuff, which is placed laparoscopically a short distance below the oesophagogastric junction, creating a small (approximately 50 ml) gastric pouch (Fig. 13.28A). The cuff can be inflated or deflated via injections into a port site located in the subcutaneous tissues, in order to tighten or relax the cuff around the stomach. The tighter the cuff, the longer foodstuffs entering the gastric pouch will take to exit through the ring into the remainder of the stomach and intestinal tract, prolonging the feeling of satiety.

Gastric bypass involves stapling the stomach closed a short distance below the oesophagogastric junction (Fig. 13.28B). A Roux limb is then brought up and anastomosed to the small proximal gastric remnant. Depending on the size of the pouch and calibre of the anastomosis, there will be a degree of restrictive activity, as well as a major malabsorptive element, as food will enter the distal jejunum and proximal ileum without exposure to bile or pancreatic and other digestive enzymes.

Vertical banded gastroplasty is now rarely performed. Duodenal switch is a complex operation reserved for a minority of obese patients.

Most patients with restrictive-type surgery find that they can eat more with time as the gastric remnant dilates. Hopefully, however, the target weight loss will have been achieved and improved eating habits established to allow maintenance of a healthier weight.

Complications of obesity surgery

Obesity per se increases the risk of all types of surgery: in particular, chest infection, deep venous thrombosis and wound infection.

Careful follow-up of patients by the multidisciplinary team is necessary, not only to monitor weight loss, but also to ensure that malnutrition of vitamins, trace elements,

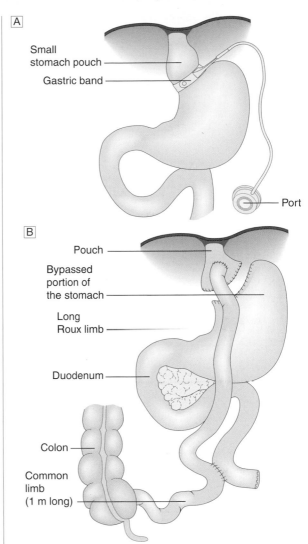

Fig. 13.28 **A** Gastric banding. **B** Gastric bypass.

Labels, panel A: Small stomach pouch; Gastric band; Port

Labels, panel B: Pouch; Bypassed portion of the stomach; Long Roux limb; Duodenum; Colon; Common limb (1 m long)

essential fatty acids and other important constituents of the diet does not occur. Patients who continue to eat chocolate and ice-cream to excess may not lose weight with the restrictive-type operations.

Most patients who lose significant weight will develop gallstones and, in some, cholecystectomy may be indicated at the same time as obesity surgery. Following significant weight loss, plastic surgery procedures may be necessary to remove excess skin, especially from the abdomen, thighs and arms.

SUMMARY BOX 13.5

Obesity surgery

- Different approaches (restrictive vs. malabsorptive)
- Mostly laparoscopic now
- Clinically effective and cost efficient
- Extends life expectancy and improves quality of life
- Can 'cure' diabetes.

13

14

O.J. Garden

The liver and biliary tract

CHAPTER CONTENTS

THE LIVER

Anatomy

The liver is the largest abdominal organ, weighing approximately 1500 g. It extends from the fifth intercostal space to the right costal margin. It is triangular in shape, its apex reaching the left midclavicular line in the fifth intercostal space. In the recumbent position, the liver is impalpable under cover of the ribs. The liver is attached to the undersurface of the diaphragm by suspensory ligaments that enclose a 'bare area', the only part of its surface without a peritoneal covering. Its inferior or visceral surface lies on the right kidney, duodenum, colon and stomach.

Topographically, the liver is divided by the attachment of the falciform ligament into right and left lobes; fissures on its visceral surface demarcate two further lobes, the quadrate and caudate (Fig. 14.1A). However, it is the liver segmental anatomy, as defined by the distribution of its blood supply, that is important to the surgeon.

Segmental anatomy

The portal vein and hepatic artery divide into right and left branches in the porta hepatis. Occluding either branch at surgery produces an easily visible line of demarcation that runs from the gallbladder bed behind and to the left of the inferior vena cava, thus separating the two hemilivers. Each hemiliver is further divided into four segments corresponding to the main branches of the hepatic artery and portal vein. In the left hemiliver, segment I corresponds to the caudate lobe, segments II and III to the left lobe (or left lateral section), and segment IV to the quadrate lobe. The remaining segments (V–VIII) comprise the right hemiliver (Fig. 14.1B).

Blood supply and function

The liver normally receives 1500 ml of blood per minute and has a dual blood supply, 75% coming from the portal vein and 25% from the hepatic artery, which supplies 50% of the oxygen requirements. The principal venous drainage of the liver is by the right, middle and left hepatic veins, which enter the vena cava (Fig. 14.1B). In 25% of individuals, there is an inferior right hepatic vein, and numerous small veins drain direct into the vena cava from the caudate lobe (segment I). The functional unit of the liver is the hepatic acinus. Sheets of liver cells (hepatocytes) one cell thick are separated by interlacing sinusoids through which blood flows from the peripheral portal tract into the hepatic acinus to the central branch of the hepatic venous system. Bile is secreted by the liver cells and passes in the opposite direction along the small canaliculi into interlobular bile ducts located in the portal tracts (Fig. 14.2).

The liver has an important role in nutrient metabolism and is responsible for storing glucose in the form of glycogen, or converting it to lactate for release into the systemic circulation. Amino acids are utilized for hepatic and plasma protein synthesis or catabolized to urea. The liver has a central role in the metabolism of lipids, bilirubin and bile salts, drugs and alcohol. It is the principal organ for storage of a number of minerals and vitamins, and is responsible for the production of the coagulation factors I, V, XI, the vitamin K-dependent factors II, VII, IX and X as well as proteins C and S and antithrombin. The liver is also the largest reticuloendothelial organ in the body and its Kupffer cells play a role in the removal of damaged red blood cells, bacteria, viruses and endotoxin, much of which enter the body from the gut.

 SUMMARY BOX 14.1

Surgical anatomy

- The liver is divisible into right and left hemilivers (each having four segments) using a line running from the gallbladder fossa to the inferior vena cava
- Each hemiliver receives a branch of the hepatic artery and portal vein; 75% of liver blood flow and 50% of its oxygen supply are provided by the portal vein
- The hepatocytes are arranged in lobules, each of which has a central branch of the hepatic vein and peripheral portal tracts (containing a branch of the hepatic artery, portal vein and bile duct)
- Liver anatomy allows the surgeon to perform right hepatectomy, left hepatectomy and extended right hepatectomy (i.e. resecting all of the liver to the right of the falciform ligament). Resection of individual segments is also possible.

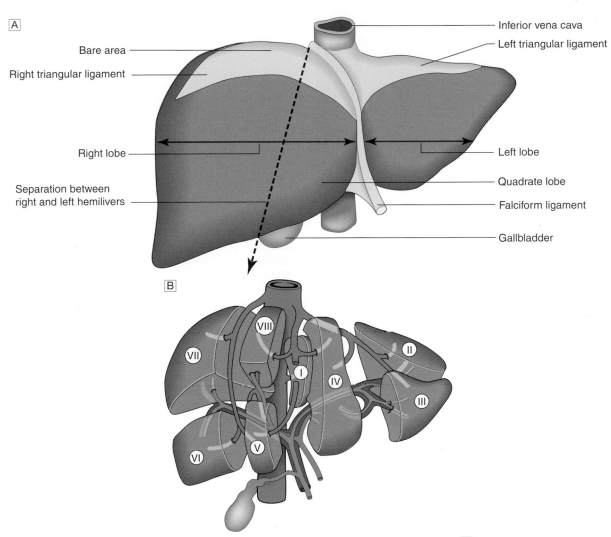

A

Inferior vena cava

Bare area

Left triangular ligament

Right triangular ligament

Right lobe

Left lobe

Separation between right and left hemilivers

Quadrate lobe

Falciform ligament

Gallbladder

B

14

VIII

VII

II

I

IV

III

V

VI

Fig. 14.1 Anatomy of the liver. A The broken line represents the separation between right and left hemilivers. B Segmental anatomy and venous drainage.

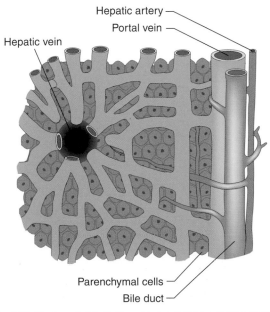

Hepatic artery

Portal vein

Hepatic vein

Parenchymal cells

Bile duct

Fig. 14.2 The hepatic lobule. Sinusoids drain into the central hepatic vein.

Jaundice

Jaundice is caused by an increase in the level of circulating bilirubin and becomes obvious in the skin and sclera when levels exceed 50 μmol/l (Fig. 14.3). It may result from excessive destruction of red cells (*haemolytic jaundice*), from failure to remove bilirubin from the blood stream (*hepatocellular jaundice*), or from obstruction to the flow of bile from the liver (*cholestatic jaundice*) (Fig. 14.4). Congenital non-haemolytic hyperbilirubinaemia (Gilbert's syndrome) is a relatively rare cause of jaundice due to defective bilirubin transport; the jaundice is usually mild and transient, and the prognosis is excellent.

To the surgeon, the most important type of *haemolytic jaundice* is that caused by hereditary spherocytosis, in which splenectomy may be necessary (Ch. 15). Haemolytic jaundice may also occur after blood transfusion and after operative or accidental trauma, when haematoma formation produces a pigment load that exceeds hepatic excretory capacity.

Hepatocellular jaundice is usually a medical rather than a surgical condition, although its recognition in patients presenting with abdominal pain is important, as surgical intervention may aggravate the hepatocellular injury.

Cholestatic jaundice due to intrahepatic obstruction of bile canaliculi may be a feature of acute and chronic liver disease

193

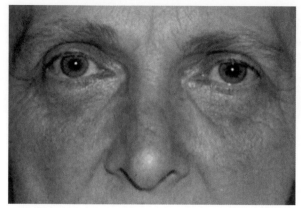

Fig. 14.3 Patient demonstrating the features of jaundiced skin and sclera.

and can be caused by drugs (e.g. chlorpromazine). This form of jaundice must be differentiated from that due to extrahepatic obstruction, the cause of which has most surgical relevance. Extrahepatic obstruction most commonly results from gallstones or cancer of the head of the pancreas. Other causes include cancer of the periampullary region or major bile ducts, extrinsic compression of the bile ducts by metastatic tumour, iatrogenic biliary stricture and choledochal cyst.

Diagnosis

History and clinical examination

An accurate, rapid diagnosis of the cause of jaundice allows prompt institution of appropriate treatment (Fig. 14.5). The age, sex, occupation, social habits, drug and alcohol intake, history of injections or infusions, and general demeanour of the patient must be considered.

A history of intermittent pain, fluctuant jaundice and dyspepsia suggests calculous obstruction of the common bile duct, whereas a history of weight loss and relentless progressive jaundice favours a diagnosis of neoplasia. Obstructive jaundice is likely if there is a history of passage of dark urine and pale stools, and if the patient complains of pruritus (owing to an inability to secrete bile salts into the obstructed biliary system). Hepatocellular jaundice is likely if there are stigmata of chronic liver disease, such as liver palms, spider naevi, testicular atrophy and gynaecomastia. The abdomen must be examined for evidence of hepatomegaly or gallbladder distension, and for signs of portal hypertension such as splenomegaly, ascites and large collateral veins (caput medusae) in the abdominal wall.

Biochemical and haematological investigations

Haemolytic jaundice is suggested if there are high circulating levels of unconjugated bilirubin but no bilirubin in the urine. Serum concentrations of liver enzymes are normal in these circumstances and the appropriate haematological investigations should be set in train.

In jaundice due to biliary obstruction, the circulating bilirubin is conjugated by the liver and rendered water-soluble; it can then be excreted in the urine and gives it a dark colour. As bile cannot pass into the gastrointestinal tract, the stool becomes pale and urobilinogen is absent from the urine. Obstruction increases the formation of alkaline phosphatase from the cells lining the biliary canaliculi, producing raised serum levels. This rise precedes that of bilirubin and its fall is more gradual once obstruction is relieved. Serum transaminase and lactic dehydrogenase levels may rise in obstruction. Conversely, swelling of the parenchyma in hepatocellular jaundice frequently produces an element of intrahepatic biliary obstruction and a modest rise in serum alkaline phosphatase concentration.

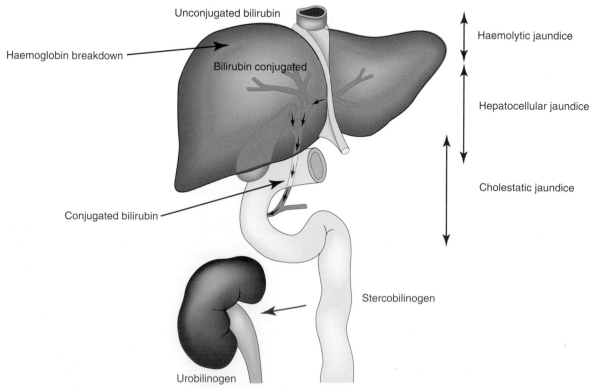

Fig. 14.4 Types of jaundice.

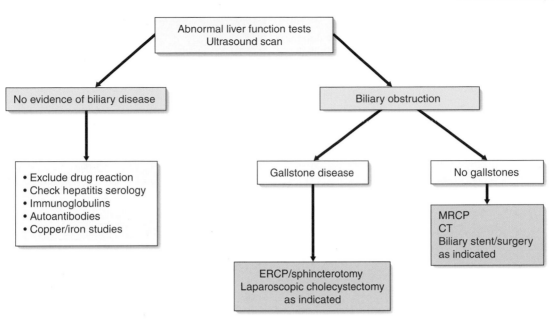

Fig. 14.5 Investigation of the jaundiced patient.

Full blood count and coagulation screen should be undertaken as a matter of routine and viral status should be determined. Anaemia may signify occult blood loss, and a low white cell or platelet count may indicate hypersplenism due to portal hypertension. Prolongation of the prothrombin time may be present in both hepatocellular and cholestatic jaundice, but should readily correct within 36 hours with the administration of parenteral vitamin K when jaundice is cholestatic.

Radiological investigations

If the clinical picture and biochemical investigations suggest that jaundice is obstructive, radiological techniques can be used to define the site and nature of the obstruction.

Ultrasonography

In skilled hands, this key investigation is safe, non-invasive and reliable. It is used to define whether the patient has bile duct dilatation or gallbladder distension due to obstruction, and to confirm the need for more invasive investigations. Ultrasonography will also detect gallstones and space-occupying lesions in the liver and pancreas, although overlying bowel gas may prevent a clear view of the pancreas.

Magnetic resonance imaging (MRI)

Magnetic resonance cholangiopancreatography (MRCP) has largely replaced other forms of invasive radiological imaging of the bile duct and pancreas. MRI has the advantage that it does not introduce infection into an obstructed biliary system or the pancreatic duct; it also enables assessment of the vascular anatomy and the parenchyma of the liver and pancreas. This is important in patients presenting with symptoms suggestive of malignant obstructive jaundice.

Endoscopic retrograde cholangiopancreatography (ERCP)

ERCP outlines the biliary and pancreatic systems by injecting contrast through a cannula inserted into the papilla of Vater by means of an endoscope passed into the duodenum. It gives more detailed information than ultrasonography and allows endoscopic treatment of gallstones, biopsy of periampullary tumours, and relief of obstructive jaundice by stent insertion. The investigation may be complicated by acute pancreatitis, and prophylactic antibiotics should be administered to reduce the risk of cholangitis for complex interventions. Haemorrhage and perforation are less frequent complications.

Percutaneous transhepatic cholangiography (PTC)

Used less often than formerly to assess obstruction of the upper biliary tree, PTC provides a clear outline of the biliary system by the injection of contrast through a slim flexible needle passed percutaneously into the liver. The technique may cause bleeding or bile leakage and can be complicated by bacteraemia and septicaemia; coagulation status must be checked and antibiotic cover should be given. It is almost exclusively undertaken before placement of a biliary drain or stent to relieve obstruction of the proximal biliary tree.

Computed tomography (CT)

Contrast enhanced CT can be used to identify hepatic, bile duct and pancreatic tumours in jaundiced patients. It often demonstrates the dilated biliary tree to the level of the obstruction, vascular abnormality or invasion and may show dissemination to adjacent lymph nodes. It is also used to assess viability of pancreatic tissue in severe pancreatitis.

Other radiological investigations

Positron emission tomography (PET-CT) has found an increasing role in staging hepatobiliary and pancreatic (HBP) malignancy. Isotopic liver scanning has been superseded by ultrasonography and CT. Selective angiography has been largely superseded by CT and MRI assessment of vascular anatomy but may be used for embolization of tumours or hemorrhagic complications of HBP disease.

Liver biopsy

Liver biopsy may be considered in patients with unexplained jaundice, in whom an obstructing lesion has been excluded radiologically. 'Targeted' liver biopsy can be conducted under ultrasound or CT guidance. Prothrombin time, platelet count and hepatitis B surface antigen (HBsAg) status must always be determined, and clotting abnormalities should be corrected before biopsy is undertaken.

Laparoscopy

Laparoscopy under general anaesthesia may be used in the evaluation of liver disease. In selected patients with malignancy of the liver, pancreas and biliary tree, it may have a role in the staging of the tumour to exclude peritoneal or hepatic dissemination.

Laparotomy

Laparotomy is no longer necessary to establish the cause of jaundice and is only undertaken to remove the causal lesion or relieve biliary obstruction. Intraoperative ultrasonography and operative cholangiography may give useful additional information in patients with neoplasia and biliary obstruction. Appropriate preoperative preparation is particularly important in jaundiced patients.

Congenital abnormalities

Up to 5% of the population has simple liver cysts. They are lined by biliary epithelium and contain serous fluid, but never communicate with the biliary tree. They rarely produce symptoms, are associated with normal liver function, and on ultrasound or CT have no discernible wall (Fig. 14.6). In the few patients who develop symptoms, cysts tend to recur following aspiration, and sclerosis by alcohol injection is of little value for large symptomatic cysts. Surgical management consists of deroofing and may be undertaken by laparoscopic means. Polycystic disease is a rare cause of liver enlargement and may be associated with polycystic kidneys as an autosomal dominant trait. In symptomatic patients, it may be necessary to combine a deroofing procedure with hepatic resection or to consider liver transplantation.

SUMMARY BOX 14.2

Jaundice

- Jaundice is a yellowish discoloration of the tissues that becomes clinically apparent when serum bilirubin levels exceed 50 μmol/l (normal < 20 μmol/l)
- It may be due to excessive haemolysis, hepatic insufficiency or cholestasis; cholestatic (obstructive) jaundice is the type encountered in surgical practice
- The two most common causes of surgical obstructive jaundice are cancer of the head of the pancreas and stones in the common bile duct (choledocholithiasis)
- In cholestatic jaundice, the bilirubin has been conjugated by the hepatocytes and is therefore soluble in water and can be excreted in the urine; patients with obstructive jaundice typically have dark urine and pale stools and may have pruritus (thought to be due to the accumulation of bile salts)
- Obstructive jaundice is characterized by elevated serum alkaline phosphatase levels in addition to hyperbilirubinaemia, and may be accompanied by modest elevations in transaminase (aminotransferase) levels, reflecting liver damage.

Cavernous haemangiomas are one of the most common benign tumours of the liver (up to 5% of population) and may be congenital. Women are affected six times more frequently than men. Most haemangiomas are small solitary subcapsular growths found incidentally at laparotomy or autopsy, but they are sometimes detected on ultrasound examination as densely hyperechoic lesions that mimic

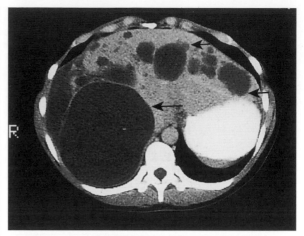

Fig. 14.6 CT demonstrating multiple biliary cysts appearing as hypodense areas within both lobes of the liver (arrowed).

hepatic tumours. These lesions rarely give rise to pain. Resection may be considered for symptomatic lesions exceeding 5 cm in diameter.

Liver trauma

After the spleen, the liver is the solid organ most commonly damaged in abdominal trauma, particularly following road traffic accidents. Stab injuries and gunshot wounds of the liver are also increasing in incidence. These are considered in Chapter 7.

Hepatic infections and infestations

Liver abscesses can be classified as bacterial, parasitic or fungal. Bacterial abscess is the most common type in Western medicine, but parasitic infestation is an important cause world-wide. Fungal abscesses are found in patients receiving long-term broad-spectrum antibiotic treatment or immunosuppressive therapy, and may complicate actinomycosis.

Pyogenic liver abscess

Infection from the biliary system is now more common due to the increasing use of radiological and endoscopic intervention. Infection may spread through the portal vein from abdominal sepsis (e.g. appendicitis, diverticulitis), via the hepatic artery from a septic focus anywhere in the body, or by direct spread from a contiguous organ (e.g. empyema of the gallbladder). Abscess formation may follow blunt or penetrating injury, and in one-third of patients the source of infection is indeterminate (cryptogenic). Common organisms are:

- *Streptococcus milleri*
- *Escherichia coli*
- *Streptococcus faecalis*
- *Staphylococcus aureus*
- anaerobes (*Bacteroides* spp).

Clinical features

The onset of symptoms is often insidious and the patient may present with pyrexia of unknown origin. There is sometimes a history of sepsis elsewhere, particularly within the abdomen, and pain in the right hypochondrium. Other patients present with swinging pyrexia, rigors, marked toxicity and jaundice. The liver is often enlarged and tender.

Investigations

Plain radiographs may show elevation of the diaphragm, pleural effusion and basal lobe collapse. Leucocytosis is usually present and liver function tests are deranged. Ultrasonography or CT is used to define the abscess (which is often irregular and thick-walled) and to facilitate percutaneous aspiration for culture. ERCP may be useful if biliary obstruction is thought to be responsible.

Management

Untreated abscesses often prove fatal because of spread within the liver to multiple sites, and because of septicaemia and debility. The principles of treatment are percutaneous drainage of accessible abscesses under ultrasound or CT guidance, and antibiotic therapy selected on the basis of culture of blood or pus. It is exceptional to resort to surgical drainage. Percutaneously or surgically placed drainage tubes are left in place and the size of the cavity is monitored by CT or serial X-rays following the injection of contrast material. Multiple small abscesses may require prolonged treatment with antibiotics for up to 8 weeks. Investigation is required to detect the source (e.g. colonoscopy, ERCP for stone removal).

Amoebic liver abscess

Entamoeba histolytica is a protozoal parasite that infests the large intestine and is endemic in many tropical regions. Trophozoites released by the cyst in the intestine may penetrate the mucosa to gain access to the portal venous system and so spread to the liver. The abscess is large and thin-walled, is usually solitary and in the right lobe, and contains brown sterile pus resembling anchovy sauce.

Clinical features

Right upper quadrant pain may be accompanied by anorexia, nausea, weight loss and night sweats. Tender enlargement of the liver is invariable, although jaundice is uncommon. Other signs include basal pulmonary collapse, pleural effusion and leucocytosis.

Investigations

Ultrasonography and CT are used to demonstrate the site and size of the abscess, which often has poorly defined margins. The stools should be examined for amoebae or cysts. Direct and indirect serological tests to detect amoebic protein are available.

Management

Early diagnosis is important, and treatment may be commenced empirically in areas where the problem is endemic. Treatment consists of the administration of metronidazole (800 mg 8-hourly for 5 days) and usually results in rapid resolution. The abscess should be aspirated by needle puncture, if there is no clinical response within 72 hours. If untreated, an amoebic abscess may rupture into the peritoneal cavity or into a bronchus.

Hydatid disease

This less common infestation is caused in humans by one of two forms of tapeworm, *Echinococcus granulosus* and *E. multilocularis*. The adult tapeworm lives in the intestine of the dog, from which ova are passed in the stool; sheep or goats serve as the intermediate host by ingesting the ova whereas humans are accidental hosts (Fig. 14.7). The condition is most common in sheep- and goat-rearing areas. Ingested ova hatch in the duodenum and the embryos pass to the liver through the portal venous system. The wall of the resulting hydatid cyst is surrounded by an adventitial layer of fibrous tissue and consists of a laminated membrane lined by germinal epithelium, on which brood capsules containing scolices develop.

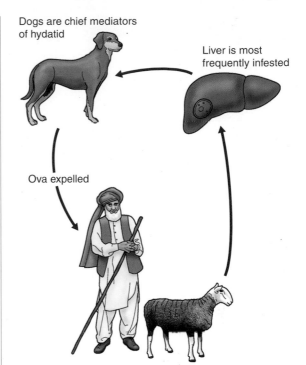

Dogs are chief mediators of hydatid

Liver is most frequently infested

Ova expelled

Fig. 14.7 Life cycle of *Echinococcus granulosus*.

Clinical features

The disease may be symptomless, but chronic right upper quadrant pain with enlargement of the liver is the common presentation. The cyst may rupture into the biliary tree or peritoneal cavity, the latter sometimes causing an acute anaphylactic reaction due to absorption of foreign hydatid protein. Other complications include secondary infection and biliary obstruction with jaundice.

Investigations

Eosinophilia is common and serological tests, such as complement fixation, are available to detect the foreign protein. Hydatid cysts commonly calcify and may be seen on a plain film of the abdomen. Alternatively, they can be detected by ultrasound or CT of the liver and are recognizable by their thick wall, which may contain multiple daughter cysts.

Management

In asymptomatic patients, small calcified cysts may require no treatment. Patients can be treated successfully with albendazole or mebendazole but this may be prolonged. Large symptomatic cysts are best managed by complete excision, together with the parasites contained within. A laparoscopic approach is possible for simple accessible cysts.

Portal hypertension

Portal hypertension is caused by increased resistance to portal venous blood flow, the obstruction being prehepatic, hepatic or posthepatic (Table 14.1). Rarely, it results primarily from an increase in portal blood flow. The normal pressure of 5–15 cmH_2O in the portal vein is consistently exceeded (above 25 cmH_2O). Portal vein thrombosis is a rare cause and is most commonly due to neonatal umbilical sepsis. The most common cause of portal hypertension is cirrhosis resulting from chronic liver disease and is characterized by liver cell damage, fibrosis and nodular regeneration.

Table 14.1 Causes of portal hypertension

Obstruction to portal flow:
Prehepatic
- Congenital atresia of the portal vein
- Portal vein thrombosis
  Neonatal sepsis
  Pyelophlebitis
  Trauma
  Tumour
- Extrinsic compression of the portal vein
  Pancreatic disease
  Lymphadenopathy
  Biliary tract tumours

Intrahepatic
- Cirrhosis
- Schistosomiasis

Posthepatic
- Budd–Chiari syndrome
- Constrictive pericarditis

Increased blood flow (rare)
- Arteriovenous fistula
- Increased splenic blood flow in hypersplenism

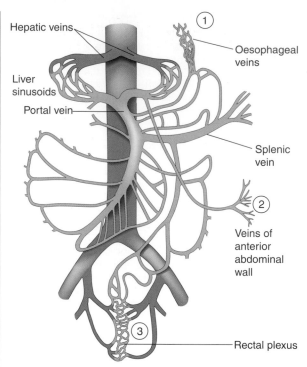

Fig. 14.8 The portal venous system. Sites of portosystemic shunting are marked 1–3. Retroperitoneal communications also exist.

The fibrosis obstructs portal venous return and portal hypertension develops. Arteriovenous shunts within the liver also contribute to the hypertension.

Alcohol is the most common aetiological factor in developed countries, whereas in North Africa, the Middle East and China, schistosomiasis due to *Schistosoma mansonii* is a common cause. Chronic active hepatitis and primary and secondary biliary cirrhosis may result in portal hypertension, but in a large number of patients the cause remains obscure (cryptogenic cirrhosis).

Post-hepatic portal hypertension is rare. It is most frequently due to spontaneous thrombosis of the hepatic veins and this has been associated with neoplasia, oral contraceptive agents, polycythaemia and the presence of abnormal coagulants in the blood. The resulting Budd-Chiari syndrome is characterized by portal hypertension, caudate hypertrophy, liver failure and gross ascites.

Effects of portal hypertension

As a result of gradual chronic occlusion of the portal venous system, collateral pathways develop between the portal and systemic venous circulations. Portosystemic shunting occurs at three principal sites (Fig. 14.8). The most important is the development of varices in the submucosal plexus of veins in the lower oesophagus and gastric fundus. Oesophageal varices may rupture, to cause acute massive gastrointestinal bleeding in about 40% of patients with cirrhosis. The initial episode of variceal haemorrhage is fatal in about one-third of patients, and recurrent haemorrhage is common. Bleeding from retroperitoneal and periumbilical collaterals ('caput medusae') is troublesome during abdominal surgery, and collaterals may develop and cause bleeding at the site of stomas. Anorectal varices are not uncommonly found at proctoscopy but rarely cause bleeding.

Progressive enlargement of the spleen occurs as a result of vascular engorgement and associated hypertrophy. Haematological consequences are anaemia, thrombocytopenia and leucopenia (with the resulting syndrome of hypersplenism). Ascites may develop and is due to increased formation of hepatic and splanchnic lymph, hypoalbuminaemia, and retention of salt and water. Increased aldosterone

and antidiuretic hormone levels may contribute. Portosystemic encephalopathy is due to an increased level of toxins such as ammonia in the systemic circulation. This is particularly likely to develop where there are large spontaneous or surgically created portosystemic shunts. Gastrointestinal haemorrhage increases the absorption of nitrogenous products and may precipitate encephalopathy.

Clinical features

Patients with cirrhosis frequently develop anorexia, generalized malaise and weight loss. Clinical manifestations include hepatosplenomegaly, ascites, jaundice and spider naevi. Slurring of speech, a flapping tremor or dysarthria may point to encephalopathy, and this may be precipitated or intensified by the accumulation of blood in the gastrointestinal tract. The serum bilirubin may be elevated and the serum albumin depressed. Anaemia may be present and the leucocyte count raised (or depressed if there is hypersplenism). The prothrombin time and other indices of clotting may be abnormal. Clinical and biochemical parameters are used as the basis of the modified Child's classification (Table 14.2). Patients allocated to grade A have a good prognosis, whereas those in grade C have the worst prognosis.

Patients with portal hypertension may be referred to a surgeon because of active uncontrolled bleeding from oesophageal varices, or for consideration of elective surgery for varices that have been resistant to non-surgical management.

Acute variceal bleeding

Patients presenting with acute upper gastrointestinal bleeding are examined for evidence of chronic liver disease (EBM 14.1). The key investigation during an episode of active bleeding is endoscopy. This allows the detection of varices and defines whether they are or have been the site of bleeding. It is important to remember that peptic ulcer and gastritis are common complaints that occur in 20% of patients with varices.

Table 14.2 Assessment of patients with portal hypertension using a modification of Child's grading system

Points scored

Criterion	1	2	3
Encephalopathy	None	Minimal	Marked
Ascites	None	Slight	Moderate
Bilirubin (μmol/l)	< 35	35–50	> 50
Albumin (g/l)	> 35	28–35	< 28
Prothrombin ratio	< 1.4	1.4–2.0	> 2.0

Grade A = 5–6 points; grade B = 7–8 points; grade C = 10–15 points.

EBM 14.1 Variceal bleeding in cirrhosis: assessment and prophylaxis

'Severity of cirrhosis is best described using the Child-Pugh score. If grade 3 varices are diagnosed, patients should have primary prophylaxis, irrespective of the severity of the liver disease. Pharmacological therapy with propranolol is the best available modality for primary prophylaxis, with variceal band ligation recommended in cases of intolerance or contraindication to propranolol.'

Jalan R, Hayes PC, British Society of Gastroenterology. Gut 2000; 46 suppl 3–4:III 1–III 15.

Management

The priorities in the management of bleeding oesophageal varices are summarized in Table 14.3.

Table 14.3 Priorities in the management of bleeding oesophageal varices

Active resuscitation
- Group and cross-match blood
- Establish i.v. infusion line(s)
- Monitor
  Pulse
  Blood pressure
  Hourly urine output
  Central venous pressure

Assessment of coagulation status
- Prothrombin time
- Platelet count

Urgent endoscopy
Control of bleeding
- Endoscopic banding or injection sclerotherapy
- Tamponade (Minnesota tube) if bleeding uncontrolled
- Pharmacological measures (e.g. vasopressin/octreotide)

Treatment of hepatocellular decompensation
Treatment/prevention of portosystemic encephalopathy
Prevention of further bleeding from varices
- Endoscopic banding or injection sclerotherapy
- Stapled oesophagogastric junction
- Portosystemic shunting/transjugular intrahepatic portosystemic stent shunting (TIPSS)
- Liver transplantation

Active resuscitation

The aim is to replace blood loss quickly with a view to urgent endoscopy. Many patients have coagulation defects from the outset, and thrombocytopenia is a common manifestation of hypersplenism. Fresh blood is preferred for transfusion purposes and the advice of the haematologist is sought regarding the use of fresh-frozen plasma (FFP) or platelet transfusion.

Endoscopy and control of bleeding

Endoscopy will reveal tortuous varices in three columns most prominent in the lower third of the oesophagus. Haemorrhage usually occurs from varices at the lowest few centimetres of the oesophagus. Rarely, bleeding occurs from varices in the gastric fundus. Although the synthetic form of somatostatin, octreotide, can be used to lower portal venous pressure and arrest bleeding, the injection of a sclerosant such as ethanolamine, or the application of bands is now used to arrest the bleeding at endoscopy (EBM 14.2). If haemorrhage is torrential and prevents direct injection, balloon tamponade may be used to stop the bleeding. The four-lumen Minnesota tube (Fig. 14.9) has largely replaced the three-lumen Sengstaken–Blakemore tube. The four lumina allow:

- aspiration of gastric contents
- compression of the oesophagogastric varices by the inflated gastric balloon
- compression of the oesophageal varices by the inflated oesophageal balloon

---

EBM 14.2 Control of variceal bleeding

'Variceal band ligation is the method of choice for control of variceal haemorrhage, with endoscopic variceal sclerotherapy as second choice. If endoscopy is unavailable, vasoconstrictors such as octreotide or glypressin, or a modified Sengstaken tube may be used while more definitive therapy is arranged. In case of bleeding that is difficult to control, a modified Sengstaken tube should be inserted until further endoscopic treatment, transjugular intrahepatic portosystemic stent shunting (TIPSS) or surgical treatment, with the mode of treatment (surgical intervention such as oesophageal transection or TIPSS) determined by the specialist centre.'

Jalan R, Hayes PC, British Society of Gastroenterology. Gut 2000; 46 suppl 3–4:III 1–III 15.

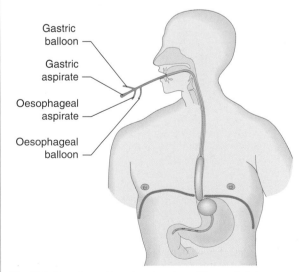

Gastric balloon
Gastric aspirate
Oesophageal aspirate
Oesophageal balloon

Fig. 14.9 Oesophageal tamponade using a Minnesota tube.

- aspiration of the oesophagus and pharynx to reduce pneumonic aspiration.

Balloon tamponade arrests bleeding from varices in over 90% of patients, but the tube is not left in place for more than 24–36 hours for fear of causing oesophageal necrosis. Tamponade should be regarded as a holding measure that allows further resuscitation and treatment of hepatic decompensation before more definitive measures are used.

Prevention of further bleeding

A number of methods are now available to reduce the risk of further variceal bleeding (EBM 14.3). Injection sclerotherapy is repeated at weekly or fortnightly intervals until the varices are completely sclerosed but excessive intervention may cause ulceration and necrosis.

EBM **14.3 Prevention of further variceal bleeding and infection**

'Following control of active variceal bleeding, the varices should be eradicated using variceal band ligation. TIPSS may be used in certain centres with particular expertise; it is more effective than endoscopic treatment in reducing variceal rebleeding but does not improve survival and is associated with more encephalopathy.'

'Infection is common after upper gastrointestinal bleeding in cirrhotic patients and is a major cause of morbidity and mortality All patients presenting with an episode of variceal bleed should have antibiotic prophylaxis with ciprofloxacin 1 g/day for 7 days.'

Jalan R, Hayes PC, British Society of Gastroenterology. Gut 2000; 46 suppl 3–4:III 1–III 15.

Endoscopic banding is favoured since there is a reduced risk of complication. Surgical disconnection (*stapled oesophageal transection*) is used rarely. The gastric vein and short gastric veins are ligated, and the distal oesophagus is transected and reanastomosed just above the cardia using a stapling gun (Fig. 14.10) to occlude flow into the varices. It carries considerable morbidity and mortality when employed as a last resort in the emergency situation.

Emergency portosystemic shunting

Shunt surgery carries a high mortality and has been abandoned in most centres. Elective portosystemic shunting is still used occasionally to decompress the portal system and reduce the risk of further variceal haemorrhage in patients with preserved liver function, but portosystemic encephalopathy can be troublesome. In severe liver disease, transplantation is more likely to be considered if there is no contraindication.

Types of shunt procedure

Most portosystemic shunts have been replaced by non-surgical approaches to treatment. In transjugular intrahepatic portosystemic stent shunting (TIPSS, Fig. 14.11), a metal stent is inserted via the transjugular route using a guidewire passed through the hepatic vein to the intrahepatic branches of the portal vein. The technique is a relatively safe means of decompressing the portal system as general anaesthesia and laparotomy are avoided. The risk of encephalopathy is similar to that of a surgical portosystemic shunt, but the procedure is now considered routinely before surgical intervention in both the acute and elective setting.

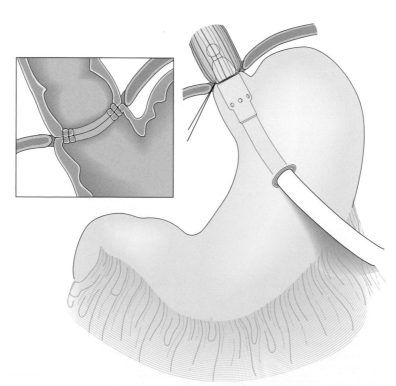

Fig. 14.10 Oesophageal stapling. The gun is inserted through an anterior gastrostomy. A ligature is tied just above the cardia, invaginating a flange of oesophageal wall between the two parts of the gun. Inset: the gun has been fired, simultaneously resecting a full-thickness ring of oesophageal wall and anastomosing the cut ends with staples.

SUMMARY BOX 14.3

Portal hypertension

- Portal hypertension is almost always due to obstruction to portal flow (rather than increased inflow), and may be prehepatic, hepatic or posthepatic
- Cirrhosis of the liver is the most common cause of portal hypertension in developed countries, and alcoholic cirrhosis is most often responsible
- Portosystemic shunts develop between gastric and oesophageal veins, in the retroperitoneum and periumbilical area, and occasionally in the anorectum. Varices in the submucosa of the lower oesophagus are a common source of major bleeding, but gastritis (portal gastropathy) can be responsible
- Child's grading (A, B or C) is based on encephalopathy, ascites, prothrombin time, bilirubin and albumin levels, and is a valuable prognostic index
- Variceal bleeding may be controlled by endoscopic banding or injection sclerotherapy, although balloon tamponade (four-lumen Minnesota tube) may sometimes be needed
- Surgical portosystemic shunts effectively decompress oesophageal varices and reduce rebleeding, but can cause encephalopathy and have been largely replaced by transjugular intrahepatic portosystemic stent shunting (TIPSS)
- Although banding (or injection sclerotherapy) reduces the risk of rebleeding and may improve survival rates, long-term outcome is determined by the nature and severity of the underlying liver disease.

Ascites

Ascites can be controlled by bed rest, salt and water restriction, and the aldosterone inhibitor spironolactone. If refractory, ascites can be treated by inserting a peritoneojugular (LeVeen) shunt, which allows one-way flow between the peritoneum and the jugular vein (Fig. 14.12). It is unusual for the shunt to remain patent for more than 12 months, but this may suffice for patients with refractory ascites and advanced liver disease who are not candidates for liver transplantation.

Tumours of the liver

Hepatic tumours can be benign or malignant, and primary or secondary. Primary tumours may arise from the parenchymal cells, the epithelium of the bile ducts, or the supporting tissues.

Benign hepatic tumours

Cavernous haemangioma

This is the most common benign liver tumour (see above). These lesions rarely reach a sufficient size to produce pain, abdominal swelling or haemorrhage. Heart failure rarely develops, if there is a large arteriovenous communication. Lesions discovered incidentally at laparotomy should be left alone; needle biopsy can be hazardous. Large symptomatic lesions should normally be resected only by an experienced surgeon.

Biliary hamartoma

These are small fibrous lesions that are often situated beneath the capsule of the liver. They can be mistaken for a small metastatic tumour unless a biopsy is obtained.

Focal nodular hyperplasia (FNH)

This is more common in females. The lesion is generally asymptomatic and may regress with time or on withdrawal of the contraceptive pill. Hyperplasia can be differentiated from adenoma by the central fibrous scar, which is often visible on ultrasound or CT (Fig. 14.13). Such lesions do not undergo malignant transformation and do not require excision unless symptomatic.

Liver cell adenoma

This is relatively uncommon and is found almost exclusively in women. The use of contraceptives containing high levels of oestrogen have been implicated causally. The majority present as solitary, well-encapsulated lesions, but

14

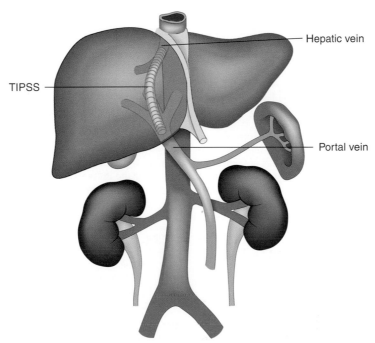

Fig. 14.11 Transjugular intrahepatic portosystemic stent shunting (TIPSS).

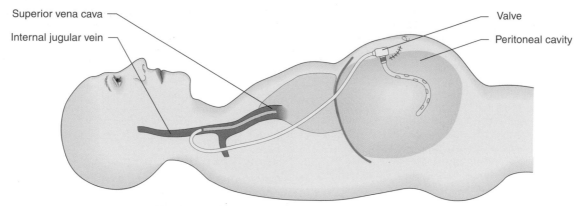

Fig. 14.12 Peritoneovenous (Le Veen) shunt to relieve ascites.

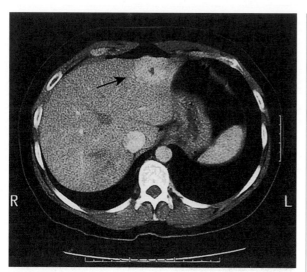

Fig. 14.13 Intravenous enhanced CT scan demonstrating a hypervascular lesion in the left lobe of the liver (arrowed).
This symptomatic focal nodular hyperplastic lesion was removed by left lobectomy.

malignant transformation has been reported. They may be asymptomatic but generally present with right hypochondrial pain as a result of haemorrhage within the tumour. Superficial tumours may bleed spontaneously and present with symptoms of haemoperitoneum. Adenomas may be detected by ultrasonography or CT. LFTs and serum α-fetoprotein levels are usually normal.

Treatment consists of formal hepatic resection because of the difficulties of distinguishing adenoma from a well-differentiated hepatoma, concerns that lesions may undergo malignant transformation, and the known risk of spontaneous haemorrhage. There is recent evidence to suggest that cytokeratin 7 and 19 immunostains along with neuronal adhesion molecule taken from liver biopsy can help in differentiating hepatic adenoma from FNH when radiological imaging is inconclusive.

Primary malignant tumours of the liver

Hepatocellular carcinoma (hepatoma)

Hepatocellular carcinoma (HCC) is relatively uncommon in the developed world but is common in Africa and the Far East. HCC is more common in males and it is thought to result in over 600,000 deaths worldwide each year. In the West, about two-thirds of patients have pre-existing cirrhosis and many others have evidence of hepatitis B or C

infection. In Africa and the East, 'aflatoxin' (derived from the fungus, *Aspergillus flavus*, which contaminates maize and nuts) is an important hepatocarcinogen.

Clinical features

The diagnosis is usually made late in the course of the disease. In non-cirrhotic patients, the tumour may have grown to a considerable size before giving rise to abdominal pain or swelling. In cirrhotic patients, hepatoma may become manifest as sudden deterioration in liver function, often associated with extension of the tumour into the portal venous system. Common presenting features would involve progression of existing liver disease symptoms, and may include abdominal pain, weight loss, abdominal distension, fever and spontaneous intraperitoneal haemorrhage. Jaundice is uncommon unless there is advanced cirrhosis. Examination may reveal features of established liver disease and hepatomegaly is invariable.

Investigations

LFTs are generally deranged. Although early detection of hepatocellular carcinoma in susceptible individuals can be pursued by a policy of serial measurement of α-fetoprotein (an oncofetal antigen) and ultrasound scanning, this tumour marker is present in only one-third of the white population with hepatocellular carcinoma, compared to 80% of African patients with this disease.

The lesion may be detected and characterized by abnormal ultrasound scanning. Percutaneous needle aspiration cytology and needle biopsy for histological confirmation should be reserved for patients who are not being considered for hepatic resection, as these investigations carry a small but significant risk of tumour dissemination and haemorrhage. There are accepted criteria based on radiology and tumor marker levels that accept a diagnosis of HCC without the need for biopsy (EBM 14.4).

Abdominal CT or MRI is valuable in planning resection and excluding the presence of nodal involvement. Hepatocellular carcinoma is seen as an extremely vascular lesion on

---

EBM 14.4 **Diagnosis of HCC established**

- *if two imaging modalities show a coincidental nodule with arterial hypervascularization regardless of AFP levels*
- *if a single modality shows a lesion when the AFP is > 400 ng/ml*
- *histological diagnosis is required if the nodule is less than 2 cm in diameter.*

Bruix J, Sherman M, Hepatology 2005; 42: 1208–1236.

arteriography, and propagation of tumour thrombus along the portal vein or its branches may be apparent. Pulmonary metastases may not be evident on chest X-ray and their presence should be excluded by a thoracic CT. Peritoneal dissemination may only be excluded by laparoscopy.

Management

In non-cirrhotic patients, large tumours (particularly those of the fibrolamellar type) are likely to be amenable to liver resection. Cirrhotic patients have less hepatic functional reserve, and even those with well-preserved liver function may only tolerate limited segmental resection if there is significant portal hypertension. In cirrhotic patients, multicentricity is common and satellite lesions often surround the primary tumour, so that cure is uncommon.

For advanced tumours, systemic chemotherapy with doxorubicin (adriamycin), methotrexate or 5-fluorouracil may have palliative value, although response rates of less than 20% are the norm. Sorafenib, a multitargeted oral kinase inhibitor, has recently been shown in a phase II trail to prolong survival in patients with HCC. Encouraging results have been reported following local embolization with chemotherapy by selective arteriography (transarterial chemo-embolization – TACE) and percutaneous ablation using radiofrequency and microwave energy have been used to useful effect for small lesions not amenable to surgery. Future efforts may involve a combination of these methods.

The disease is usually advanced at presentation and the 5-year survival rate is less than 10%. Liver transplantation has been used in the treatment of this tumour, but the best results have been reported in cirrhotic patients in whom an incidental hepatoma has been found on examination of the resected specimen following the transplant. If transplantation is not otherwise contraindicated, eligibility criteria have been extended for cirrhotic patients with a single tumour of 5 cm or less in diameter, or with no more than three tumour nodules each one 3cm or less in size (Milan criteria).

Cholangiocarcinoma

This adenocarcinoma may arise anywhere in the biliary tree, including its intrahepatic radicles. It accounts for less than 10% of malignant primary neoplasms of the liver in Western medicine, although its incidence is rising. Risk factors include chronic parasitic infestation of the biliary tree in the Far East, and choledochal cysts (see below).

Jaundice, pain and an enlarged liver are the common presenting features, although there may be co-existing biliary infection causing the tumour to masquerade as a hepatic abscess. Resection offers the only prospect of cure but is seldom feasible when cholangiocarcinoma arises in the liver substance. Cholangiocarcinoma arising from the extrahepatic bile ducts is considered below.

Other primary malignant tumours

- *Angiosarcoma* (Fig. 14.14). This rare tumour of the liver may arise after industrial exposure to vinyl chloride or exposure to the previously used radiological contrast medium, Thorotrast
- *Haemangioendothelioma*. This presents as a diffuse multifocal tumour and is rarely resectable at presentation
- *Biliary cystadenoma*. This rare condition of the liver, with a marked female predominance, has a 1:4 risk of malignant transformation and should be resected.

Metastatic tumours

The liver is a common site for metastatic disease; secondary liver tumours are 20 times more common than primary ones. In 50% of cases, the primary tumour is in the gastrointestinal tract; other common sites are the breast, ovaries, bronchus and kidney. Almost 90% of patients with hepatic metastases have tumour deposits in other sites.

Hepatomegaly and tenderness are distinctive features, and individual deposits may be palpable in advanced disease. The patient may be cachectic, and ascites or jaundice may be present. Pyrexia occurs in up to 10% of patients. The alkaline phosphatase and γ-glutamyl transpeptidase are often raised. Ultrasound and CT may demonstrate multiple filling defects. The diagnosis can be confirmed by aspiration cytology or needle biopsy undertaken under ultrasound control. Such invasive investigation may be unnecessary when resection is being considered.

There is no effective treatment for most patients with hepatic metastases due to the extent of liver involvement and the presence of extrahepatic disease. Nonetheless, for

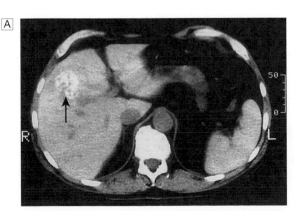
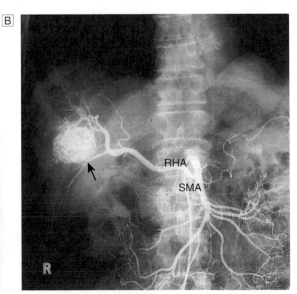

Fig. 14.14 Angiosarcoma. **A** CT demonstrating a lesion in segment V (arrowed). **B** Angiography shows an extremely vascular lesion (arrowed) taking its blood supply mainly from an aberrant right hepatic artery (RHA) arising from the superior mesenteric artery (SMA).

some tumours, notably those arising from the colon and rectum, disease may be confined to the liver and there is strong evidence of survival benefit if these are resected. Assessment of resectability will require a careful search to exclude or assess extrahepatic disease. This may necessitate colonoscopy and CT of chest, abdomen and pelvis. A more radical approach to resection of liver metastases has resulted from advances in chemotherapy and has been combined with staged resection of liver disease and preoperative portal embolization to induce hypertrophy of the intended residual liver. In well-selected patients, 5-year survival rates of 30–40% have been reported following resection. Non-curative resection may be considered exceptionally as a means of palliation in patients with symptomatic hepatic metastases such as a carcinoid or other neuroendocrine tumours.

Liver resection

Resection involves mobilization of the liver from its peritoneal attachments. Following isolation, ligature and division of the appropriate vessels, the devascularized lobe or segment is separated by careful dissection, which may be facilitated by the use of an ultrasonic dissector. Intervening biliary and vascular channels can be defined and divided between ligatures. The hepatic veins or tributaries are controlled by suture ligation following removal of the resected specimen.

Modern techniques of hepatic resection have greatly reduced operative blood loss, with a subsequent reduction in morbidity and mortality. Enhanced recovery programmes after liver surgery are associated with reduced use of abdominal drains, immediate restitution of oral intake and early mobilization in the postoperative period. Postoperative monitoring is undertaken in a high dependency environment and should include early blood gas, glucose and lactate measurement. Hepatic dysfunction may be evident from prolongation of the prothrombin time in major liver resectional surgery but complications such as postoperative haemorrhage and intra-abdominal/wound infection are less common.

Liver transplantation

This is considered in Chapter 25.

THE GALLBLADDER AND BILE DUCTS

Anatomy of the biliary system

The biliary tree consists of fine intrahepatic biliary radicles that drain individual liver segments before forming the right and left hepatic ducts. The left hepatic duct runs a mainly extrahepatic course and joins the right hepatic duct to form the common hepatic duct. This is joined at a variable position by the cystic duct to form the common bile duct, which ends at the ampulla of Vater, usually in the second part of the duodenum (Fig. 14.15). The common bile duct is approximately 8 cm long and up to 10 mm in diameter. It lies in the free edge of the lesser omentum before passing behind the first part of the duodenum and through the head of the pancreas. It is usually joined by the pancreatic duct just before entering the duodenum.

The gallbladder lies in a bed on the undersurface of the liver between its right and left halves. It is a muscular structure with a fundus, body and neck. Hartmann's pouch is a dilatation of the gallbladder outlet adjacent to the origin of the cystic duct, in which gallstones frequently become impacted. The gallbladder is supplied by the cystic artery, a branch of the right hepatic artery.

Physiology

Bile salts and the enterohepatic circulation

Bile acids are synthesized by the liver from cholesterol. The primary bile acids, chenodeoxycholic and cholic acid, are conjugated with glycine or taurine to increase their solubility in water, and the conjugates (e.g. glycocholic and

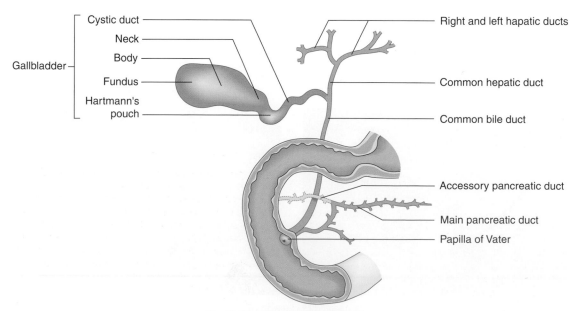

Fig. 14.15 Anatomy of the biliary tree.

taurocholic acid) form sodium and potassium bile salts. In the intestine, bacterial action produces the secondary bile salts, deoxycholic and lithocholic acid.

Bile salts can combine with lipids to form water-soluble complexes called micelles, within which lecithin and cholesterol can be transported from the liver. Bile salts are also detergents and a reduction in surface tension allows fat to be emulsified in the intestine, thus facilitating its digestion and absorption. On reaching the distal ileum, 95% of the bile salts are reabsorbed, transported back to the liver and passed once again into the biliary system. This enterohepatic circulation (Fig. 14.16) allows a relatively small bile salt pool (2–4 g) to circulate through the intestine some 6–12 times a day. The daily faecal loss equals that of hepatic synthesis (0.2–0.6 g/24 hrs). When bile is excluded from the intestine, 25% of ingested fat may appear in the faeces and there is marked malabsorption of fat-soluble vitamins, including vitamin K.

The gallbladder has a capacity of 50 ml and can concentrate bile by a factor of 10. It contracts in response to cholecystokinin (CCK), which is released from the duodenal mucosa by the presence of food, notably fatty acids. Gallbladder contraction is accompanied by reciprocal relaxation of the sphincter of Oddi. The secretion of bile is promoted by the hormone secretin. The vagus nerve also stimulates bile secretion and gallbladder contraction. Some 1–2 litres of bile are produced by the liver daily.

SUMMARY BOX 14.4

Bile salts

- The primary bile acids, chenodeoxycholic and cholic acid, are conjugated with glycine or taurine and form sodium or potassium bile salts (e.g. sodium taurocholate)
- Bile salts are vital for the excretion of cholesterol in bile; cholesterol is insoluble in water and must be transported in water-soluble complexes (micelles) with bile salts and lecithin
- Bile salts are detergents, and on reaching the intestine they emulsify fat and facilitate the digestion and absorption of fat and fat-soluble vitamins
- Bile salts must not be confused with bile pigments (e.g. bilirubin), which are waste products and excreted in bile. The small bile salt pool (2–4 g) is conserved by reabsorption of bile salts from the terminal ileum
- Disease or resection of the terminal ileum prevents the enterohepatic circulation of bile and is associated with a high incidence of cholesterol gallstones and diarrhoea (owing to the cathartic action of bile salts on the colon).

14

Congenital abnormalities

Congenital abnormalities of the gallbladder and bile ducts are common. The gallbladder may be absent (agenesis), double, intrahepatic, partitioned with a fold in the fundus (Phrygian cap), or multiseptate. The cystic duct may be absent or join the right hepatic duct rather than the common hepatic duct, and accessory ducts may be present. The cystic artery may be duplicated or may arise from the common hepatic or left hepatic artery. These anomalies are important in that great care must be taken to avoid the inappropriate division of major ducts and arteries in the course of cholecystectomy.

Biliary atresia

Failure of development of the duct system occurs once in every 20 000–30 000 births and is the most common cause of prolonged jaundice in infancy. Jaundice usually becomes apparent in the first 2–3 weeks of life and the liver and spleen usually enlarge. LFTs show an obstructive pattern. Liver biopsy reveals cholestatic jaundice, but differentiation from neonatal hepatitis is often surprisingly difficult.

In extrahepatic biliary atresia, a Roux loop of jejunum is anastomosed to the intrahepatic duct system in the hilum of the liver (Kasai operation). A delay in treatment will result in jaundice and cholangitis, allowing cirrhosis to develop, with portal hypertension and ascites.

Choledochal cysts

Cystic transformation of the biliary tree (choledochal cyst) is rare. The most common type results in a saccular dilatation of the common bile duct, which often has an abnormal termination that enters the pancreatic duct within the head of the pancreas. This may allow reflux into the biliary system, resulting in pain, inflammation, calculus formation and malignant transformation. The abnormalities are probably congenital, although diagnosis may be delayed until adult life.

In the neonate, the cyst may present with jaundice or spontaneous perforation. The adult patient usually presents with intermittent pain and jaundice, and may have attacks of pancreatitis. LFTs show a cholestatic pattern, and

Hepatic synthesis 0.2–0.6 g/24 h

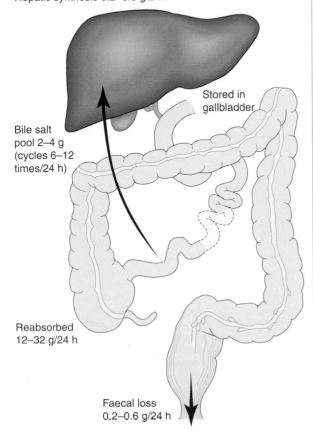

Stored in gallbladder

Bile salt pool 2–4 g (cycles 6–12 times/24 h)

Reabsorbed 12–32 g/24 h

Faecal loss 0.2–0.6 g/24 h

Fig. 14.16 The enterohepatic circulation.

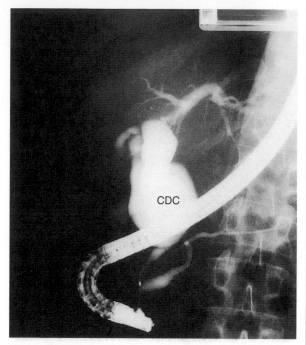

Fig. 14.17 ERCP demonstrating the common type of choledochal cyst (CDC) involving the common bile duct.

ultrasonography and cholangiography (MRCP or ERCP) establish the diagnosis (Fig. 14.17). In view of the significant risk of malignant transformation, excision of the cyst is indicated.

Caroli's disease consists of cystic biliary dilatation that is more marked in the peripheral intrahepatic ducts. Recurring infection may progress to cirrhosis and liver failure. When Caroli's disease is found in association with congenital hepatic fibrosis, portal hypertension is often present. Endoscopic, percutaneous and surgical manipulation of the biliary tree is best avoided, and liver transplantation may have a valuable role in management.

Gallstones

Pathogenesis

Gallstones are common in Europe and North America but less so in Asia and Africa. Their incidence increases with age. In developed countries, they occur in at least 20% of women over the age of 40; the incidence in males is about one-third of that in females. The disease has increased markedly in frequency and cholecystectomy is the most common elective abdominal operation in many Western countries.

Gallstone formation results from an imbalance of the constituents of bile. The majority of stones result from an inability to keep cholesterol in micellar form in the gallbladder; pigment stones are less common. Most cholesterol stones become mixed with bile pigments as they increase in size; such 'mixed' stones are much more common than pure cholesterol stones.

Cholesterol stones

Cholesterol stones are particularly common in middle-aged obese multiparous women. Stone formation is encouraged if bile becomes supersaturated with cholesterol (i.e. lithogenic), either by excessive cholesterol excretion or by a reduction in the amount of bile salt and lecithin available for micelle formation. Supersaturation is most likely to occur as the bile is concentrated in the gallbladder, and is favoured by stasis or decreased gallbladder contractility. The formation of cholesterol crystals is the key event, and this 'nucleation' may be due to coalescence of cholesterol molecules or their precipitation around particles of mucus, bacteria, calcium bilirubinate or mucosal cells. Pure cholesterol stones are yellowish-green with a regular shape but rough surface. They are usually solitary, whereas mixed stones are darker and are usually multiple.

Cholesterol stones are particularly common in some tribes of North American Indians, where more than 75% of women over 40 are affected. Such individuals have a small bile salt pool. Conversely, the high incidence of stones in Chilean women reflects high levels of cholesterol excretion. Obesity and high-calorie or high-cholesterol diets favour cholesterol stone formation by producing highly supersaturated gallbladder bile. Drastic weight reduction and diets designed to lower serum cholesterol levels may also promote stone formation by mobilizing cholesterol and increasing its excretion.

Disease or resection of the terminal ileum and drugs such as cholestyramine favour cholesterol nucleation by reducing the bile salt pool. Hormonal influences are reflected in an increased incidence of stone formation in women taking oral contraceptives or post-menopausal oestrogen replacement. Pregnancy may also have an effect by increasing stasis within the gallbladder.

Pigment stones

Pigment stones consist of calcium bilirubinate and are usually multiple and small. They are more prevalent in those areas of the world where haemolytic blood disorders are most common: for example, Mediterranean countries and malarial regions. Stones found in Western patients are usually composed of black pigment, whereas brown pigment stones are common in people from the Far East. Pigment stones account for 25% of all gallstones in Western patients, but for 60% of those in some Far Eastern countries such as Japan.

Chronic haemolysis favours pigment stone formation by increasing pigment excretion, and stone formation is common in congenital spherocytosis, haemoglobinopathy and malaria. Cirrhosis and biliary stasis are also important associations. Some patients with brown pigment stones have increased amounts of unconjugated bilirubin in the bile. In Far Eastern patients, this may be due to the action of β-glucuronidase produced by *E. coli,* an organism that invades duct systems infested with *Clonorchis sinensis* or *Ascaris lumbricoides.*

Pathological effects of gallstones
Acute cholecystitis and its complications

This is usually produced by obstruction of the neck of the gallbladder or cystic duct by a stone resulting in a chemical inflammatory reaction. Bacteria are cultured from the bile in approximately one-half of patients with gallstones, and unrelieved obstruction in the presence of this infected bile may produce an empyema. The thickened gallbladder becomes intensely inflamed, oedematous and occasionally gangrenous. The fundus of the distended, inflamed gallbladder may perforate, giving rise to localized abscess formation and occasionally to biliary peritonitis. The common organisms implicated in inflammation of the gallbladder are *E. coli, Klebsiella aerogenes* and *Strep. faecalis.* Staphylococci, clostridia and salmonella are occasionally present. These organisms may be cultured from the blood if there is bacteraemia.

Chronic cholecystitis

Repeated bouts of biliary colic or acute cholecystitis culminate in fibrosis, contraction of the gallbladder and chronic inflammatory change with marked thickening of the wall. The gallbladder ceases to function. Chronic inflammatory change may be present in the absence of gallstones, as is the case in the gallbladders of typhoid carriers. The incidence of carcinoma of the gallbladder is increased in patients with long-standing gallstones.

Mucocoele

A mucocoele develops when the outlet of the gallbladder becomes obstructed in the absence of infection. The imprisoned bile is absorbed, but clear mucus continues to be secreted into the distended gallbladder.

Choledocholithiasis

When gallstones enter the common bile duct, they may pass spontaneously or give rise to obstructive jaundice, cholangitis or acute pancreatitis. Gallstone pancreatitis most commonly occurs when a small stone becomes temporarily arrested at the ampulla of Vater.

Gallstone ileus

This uncommon form of intestinal obstruction occurs when a large gallstone becomes impacted in the intestine. Stones large enough to block the gut generally gain access by eroding through the wall of the gallbladder into the duodenum.

 SUMMARY BOX 14.5

Gallstones

- Most gallstones form because of failure to keep cholesterol in solution. This can result in pure cholesterol stones, but more commonly the stones also acquire a content of bile pigment as they enlarge, forming 'mixed' stones
- Pigment stones are the most common type of stone in some Far Eastern countries, but are less common in Western society, where they are associated with chronic haemolysis, biliary stasis and cirrhosis
- Only 15% of stones contain enough calcium to be seen on a plain film
- The majority of individuals with gallstones are asymptomatic and remain so; the presence of gallstones is not in itself an indication for cholecystectomy
- Gallbladder stones may cause flatulent dyspepsia, biliary colic, acute cholecystitis and gallbladder cancer (although the latter is so rare that this consideration does not affect the decision not to treat asymptomatic stones)
- Gallstones that migrate into the bile duct can cause obstructive jaundice, cholangitis and acute pancreatitis, although they often remain asymptomatic
- Gallstone ileus is a rare form of intestinal obstruction; stones large enough to obstruct the gut are usually too large to pass through the ampulla of Vater and have gained access to the gut by an internal fistula involving the gallbladder.

Common clinical syndromes associated with gallstones

The majority of individuals with gallstones are asymptomatic or have only vague symptoms of distension and flatulence. Less than a fifth of such patients develop symptoms or complications from their gallstones within 10 years.

Biliary colic

Biliary colic is due to transient obstruction of the gallbladder from an impacted stone. There is severe gripping pain, often developing after meals or in the evening, which is maximal in the epigastrium and right hypochondrium with radiation to the back. Despite being continuous, the pain may wax and wane in intensity over several hours, and vomiting and retching are common. Resolution occurs when the stone falls back into the gallbladder lumen or passes onwards into the common bile duct. The patient then recovers rapidly, but repeated bouts of colic are common. In some cases, the obstruction does not resolve and the patient develops acute cholecystitis.

Acute cholecystitis

Acute cholecystitis is a more prolonged and severe illness. It usually begins with an attack of biliary colic, although its onset may be more gradual. There is severe right hypochondrial pain radiating to the right subscapular region, and occasionally to the right shoulder, together with tachycardia, pyrexia, nausea, vomiting and leucocytosis. Abdominal tenderness and rigidity may be generalized but are most marked over the gallbladder. Murphy's sign (a catching of the breath at the height of inspiration while the gallbladder area is palpated) is usually present. A right hypochondrial mass may be felt. This is due to omentum 'wrapped' around the inflamed gallbladder.

In 85–90% of cases, the attack settles within 4–5 days. In the remainder, tenderness may spread and pyrexia and tachycardia persist or worsen. The development of a tender mass, associated with rigors and marked pyrexia, signals empyema formation. The gallbladder may become gangrenous and perforate, giving rise to biliary peritonitis. Jaundice can develop during the acute attack. Usually, this is associated with stones in the common bile duct, but compression of the bile ducts by the gallbladder may be responsible.

Acute cholecystitis must be differentiated from perforated peptic ulcer, high retrocaecal appendicitis, acute pancreatitis, myocardial infarction and basal pneumonia. Acute cholecystitis can develop in the absence of gallstones (acalculous cholecystitis), although this is rare.

 SUMMARY BOX 14.6

Acute cholecystitis

- In the great majority of cases acute cholecystitis is associated with gallstones and results from obstruction of gallbladder outflow
- In contrast to biliary colic, which results from obstruction alone, acute cholecystitis is associated with infection and is a systemic illness
- The patient appears unwell, has pyrexia and tachycardia, and is tender in the right hypochondrium; Murphy's sign is almost always positive
- In 90% of cases, acute cholecystitis will settle with conservative treatment (nil by mouth, intravenous fluids, antibiotics, nasogastric suction if appropriate)
- In 10% of cases, disease progression leads to life-threatening complications: notably, empyema, gangrene and perforation
- Given that the gallbladder is permanently diseased and that complications may supervene, most surgeons now advocate early cholecystectomy (i.e. within 5 days) for acute cholecystitis.

14

Chronic cholecystitis

Chronic cholecystitis is the most common cause of symptomatic gallbladder disease. The patient gives a history of recurrent flatulence, fatty food intolerance and right upper quadrant pain. The pain is worse after meals and is often associated with a feeling of distension and heartburn. The differential diagnosis includes duodenal ulcer, hiatus hernia, myocardial ischaemia, chronic pancreatitis and gastrointestinal neoplasia. Symptoms for mucocoele are the same as those for chronic cholecystitis but a non-tender piriform swelling may be palpable in the right hypochondrium. There is little systemic upset and no pyrexia.

Choledocholithiasis

Stones may be present in the common bile duct of some 5–10% of patients with gallstones. There is little muscle in the wall of the bile duct, and pain is not a symptom unless the stone impedes flow through the sphincter of Oddi. The vast majority of stones in the common bile duct originate in the gallbladder. 'Primary' duct stones are extremely rare.

Impaction of a stone at the sphincter obstructs the flow of bile, producing jaundice, pale stools and dark urine. Obstruction commonly persists for several days but may clear spontaneously, as a result either of passage of the stone or of its disimpaction. Small stones may pass through the common bile duct without causing symptoms. In longstanding obstruction the bile ducts become markedly dilated and the diameter of the common bile duct may exceed its upper limit of 10 mm. A totally obstructed duct system becomes filled with clear 'white bile', as back pressure on the hepatocytes prevents clearance of bilirubin and mucus secretion is increased.

Infection of an obstructed biliary tract causes cholangitis, which is characterized by attacks of pain, pyrexia and jaundice ('Charcot's triad'), frequently in association with rigors. Long-standing intermittent biliary obstruction may lead to secondary biliary cirrhosis. Obstructive jaundice due to stones in the common bile duct has to be distinguished from other causes of obstructive jaundice, notably malignant obstruction and cholestatic jaundice. Acute viral or alcoholic hepatitis may occasionally be confused with obstructive jaundice.

Acute pancreatitis may be associated with a stone in the common bile duct (Ch. 15).

Courvoisier's law

Fibrosed gallbladders that contain stones cannot distend when pressure increases in the obstructed biliary tree. Courvoisier's law states that if the gallbladder is palpable in the presence of jaundice, the jaundice is unlikely to be due to stone. This law is not inviolate. Distended gallbladders are not always easy to feel but can be detected readily by ultrasound.

Other benign conditions of the gallbladder

Cholesterosis

Cholesterosis or 'strawberry gallbladder' is a condition in which the mucous membrane of the gallbladder is infiltrated with lipid and cholesterol. It affects middle-aged and elderly patients of either sex. Cholesterol stones are found in the gallbladders of half of these patients. Macroscopically, the mucosa is brick-red and speckled with bright yellow nodules. Management is as for chronic cholecystitis.

Adenomyomatosis

This rare condition is characterized by mucosal diverticula (Rokitansky–Aschoff sinuses) that particularly affect the fundus and penetrate the muscular layers to the serosa.

Muscular hypertrophy and inflammatory cell infiltrates are present. The diagnosis may be made on careful imaging but is often only made following cholecystectomy, as the gallbladder normally contains stones.

Acute acalculous cholecystitis

Few patients with acute cholecystitis have acalculous inflammation. The condition may be precipitated by major surgery, bacteraemia, trauma, pancreatitis or other serious illness, and may complicate parenteral nutrition. The inflammatory reaction in the gallbladder wall may be intense and severe, leading to gangrene and perforation. In ill patients, percutaneous drainage (cholecystostomy) under ultrasound guidance may be considered, but urgent cholecystectomy is often advisable.

Investigation of patients with suspected gallstones

Blood tests

A full blood count may reveal a neutrophilia in acute cholecystitis or its complications. An elevated serum bilirubin or alkaline phosphatase may signify the presence of common duct stones. Prothrombin time should be measured if there has been a history of jaundice.

Plain abdominal X-ray

As only 15% of gallstones contain enough calcium to be seen on a plain radiograph, this investigation is not used in diagnosis. Gas is rarely seen outlining the biliary tree if there is a fistula between the biliary tract and the gut, as in gallstone ileus or following endoscopic sphincterotomy.

Ultrasonography

Ultrasonography permits inspection of the gallbladder, its wall and its contents, and demonstrates dilatation of the intrahepatic and extrahepatic biliary tree. Stones reflect the ultrasonic wave and are thrown into prominence by the acoustic shadow they produce (Fig. 14.18). The technique is extremely accurate in skilled hands. As it does not depend on hepatic excretion of contrast, it can be used in both jaundiced and non-jaundiced patients, and therefore has supplanted oral cholecystography.

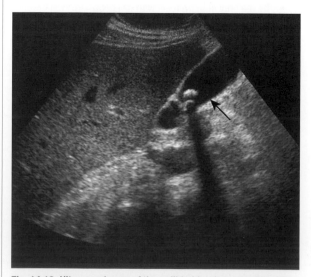

Fig. 14.18 Ultrasound scan of the gallbladder demonstrating the hyperechoic features of a solitary gallstone (arrowed) along with the typical acoustic shadow.

Cholangiography

Intravenous cholangiography has been replaced by MRCP which is used increasingly to assess the biliary tree non-invasively whereas ERCP is reserved for removing common bile duct stones by endoscopic sphincterotomy. Complications occur in up to 7% of patients and may include cholangitis and pancreatitis.

Surgical treatment of gallstones

Patients with symptomatic gallstones are usually advised to undergo cholecystectomy to relieve symptoms and avoid complications (EBM 14.5). Patients with asymptomatic gallstones are treated expectantly, particularly if they are elderly or suffering from medical conditions likely to increase the risk of surgery. In younger patients, there may be a stronger case for surgery despite the absence of symptoms, particularly if the stones are multiple and likely to cause complications, such as acute pancreatitis.

The principles of surgical treatment involve removal of the gallbladder and the stones it contains, while ensuring that no stones remain within the ductal system. 'Open' cholecystectomy has largely been replaced by laparoscopic cholecystectomy, but is still undertaken in up to 10% of patients with symptomatic gallstones and in patients in whom laparoscopic surgery cannot be completed safely. A laparoscopic procedure may not be possible in the patient who has previously undergone multiple abdominal operations but contraindications to laparoscopic surgery are few.

EBM 14.5 **Surgical treatment of gallstones**

'Asymptomatic gallstones do not require treatment by laparoscopic cholecystectomy unless there is a high risk of gallbladder cancer. Once a patient with gallstones becomes symptomatic, elective cholecystectomy is indicated. Laparoscopic cholecystectomy is associated with less pain, shorter hospital stay, faster return to normal activity and less abdominal scarring than open cholecystectomy. These advantages are also evident when the procedure is used in acute cholecystitis.'

NIH Consensus Statement 1992 Sep 14–16; 10(3):1–20. Kiviluoto T, et al. Lancet 1998; 351:321–325.

Conversion from a laparoscopic procedure to open cholecystectomy should be seen as a limitation of the minimally invasive technique and not as a failure of the surgeon. Laparotomy is mandatory when the anatomy in the area of the cystic duct and artery cannot be defined readily, if uncontrolled bleeding occurs, or if the bile duct is injured (EBM 14.6).

EBM 14.6 **Complications of cholecystectomy**

'Conversion to an open procedure from a laparoscopic procedure should be considered in the presence of adhesions, difficulty in delineating the anatomy or a suspected complication. Injury to the bile duct during cholecystectomy requires immediate referral to a surgeon or service specialised in the management of such a complication.'

Connor S, Garden OJ. Br J Surg 2006; 93(2):158–168.

Open cholecystectomy

The gallbladder is usually approached through a right subcostal incision. Following careful inspection and palpation of the abdominal contents to exclude other pathology, the cystic duct and artery are identified. Intraoperative cholangiography is performed under image intensification by cannulating the cystic duct and following the injection of contrast. The cholangiogram displays the anatomy of the duct system, identifies ductal stones, and confirms that dye passes freely into the duodenum (Fig. 14.19). The cystic duct and artery are ligated and divided and the gallbladder is removed. A retrograde approach, in which the gallbladder is mobilized 'fundus first', can be used when inflammation makes visualization of the biliary anatomy difficult, and in difficult cases a subtotal cholecystectomy may avoid damage of vital structures. Some surgeons pursue a policy of selective cholangiography, obtaining a cholangiogram only in patients at high risk of having ductal stones. The presence of such stones may be suspected if there is a history of jaundice or pancreatitis, if preoperative LFTs are abnormal, or if dilatation of the common bile duct or the presence of multiple gallbladder stones has been detected on ultrasound.

Following removal of the gallbladder, haemostasis is secured and the wound closed. The value of routinely placing an abdominal drain has been questioned although its use in difficult surgery may prevent the development of a collection and identify leakage of bile.

Laparoscopic cholecystectomy

Access to the peritoneal cavity is obtained through three or four cannulae inserted through the anterior abdominal wall and following insufflation of the peritoneal cavity with CO_2. The gallbladder is retracted by grasping forceps

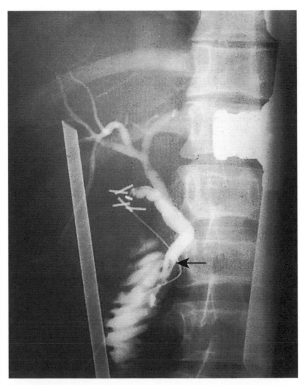

Fig. 14.19 Operative cholangiogram undertaken at laparoscopic cholecystectomy (note the radio-opaque ports). The extrahepatic ducts are seen and there is flow of contrast into the duodenum. A small radiolucent calculus is present at the lower end of the common bile duct (arrow).

14

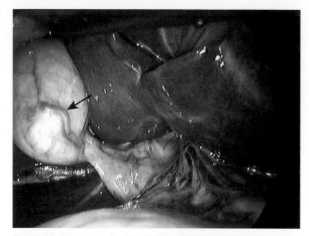

Fig. 14.20 Laparoscopic view of the gallbladder attached to the main bile duct beneath the liver and showing the branches of the cystic artery (arrow) on the gallbladder surface.

inserted to display the structures at the porta hepatis. An excellent view of the operating field is obtained with the laparoscope (Fig. 14.20), and the cystic duct and artery are isolated by dissection with instruments passed through the remaining cannulae. Some surgeons have found it difficult to undertake operative cholangiography routinely with this approach, and have either abandoned its use or relied upon MRCP or selective ERCP in the pre- or postoperative period to exclude the presence of common bile duct stones.

The cystic duct and artery are divided between metal clips and the gallbladder is dissected from the liver using diathermy. Extraction of the gallbladder through a cannula site may require extension of the incision or the tedious removal of individual stones from the gallbladder. Care must be taken to secure haemostasis and ensure the absence of bile leakage at the end of the procedure.

↻ SUMMARY BOX 14.7

Cholecystectomy

- Cholecystectomy is the standard treatment for symptomatic gallbladder stones; alternatives (stone dissolution, extracorporeal lithotripsy) are now seldom used
- Open cholecystectomy has been largely superseded by laparoscopic cholecystectomy, but conversion to open operation is still sometimes needed
- Cholecystectomy now has a low operative mortality (0.2%); inadvertent injury to the bile duct (0.2% incidence) remains the main source of major morbidity
- Some 5–10% of patients undergoing cholecystectomy have ductal stones, many of which are unsuspected. Opinions vary as to whether intraoperative cholangiography should be undertaken routinely to detect such stones
- In the era of laparoscopic cholecystectomy, there is a growing tendency not to perform routine operative cholangiography, and to extract symptomatic duct stones by non-operative means (i.e. at endoscopic papillotomy)
- If ductal stones cause symptoms, they frequently give rise to cholangitis and Charcot's triad of pain, jaundice and fever (often with rigors).

Exploration of the common bile duct

This is undertaken much less often with the free availability of ERCP and sphincterotomy (EBM 14.7). At open surgery, if stones are present in the duct system, the common bile duct is opened between stay sutures (*choledochotomy*) and the stones are extracted with forceps or a balloon catheter. Following exploration, further check cholangiogram films are obtained, or the interior of the duct can be inspected with a fibreoptic choledochoscope. The opening in the common bile duct is closed around a T-tube, the long limb of which is brought out through a stab incision in the abdominal wall (Fig. 14.21). This serves as a safety valve to allow the escape of bile if there is a temporary obstruction to flow into the duodenum following duct exploration. It also facilitates a T-tube cholangiogram some 7–10 days following surgery. If this shows free flow of dye into the duodenum and no residual duct stones, the T-tube can be clamped before removal.

EBM 14.7 **Exploration of the common bile duct**

'Patients undergoing cholecystectomy do not require ERCP preoperatively if there is a low probability of choledocholithiasis. Laparoscopic common bile duct exploration and postoperative ERCP are both safe and reliable in clearing common bile duct stones.'

Nathanson L, et al. Ann Surg 2005; 242:188–192.

If, at operation, a stone is firmly impacted at the lower end of the common bile duct, it may have to be removed through the duodenum. Transduodenal sphincterotomy and sphincteroplasty increase the risk of postoperative morbidity and mortality, and are undertaken rarely. With the reluctance of some surgeons to perform operative cholangiography during laparoscopic cholecystectomy, increasing reliance has been placed on removing common bile duct stones at ERCP. Other surgeons continue to adhere to the principles employed at open cholecystectomy and explore the common bile duct by means of a choledochotomy or through the dilated cystic duct.

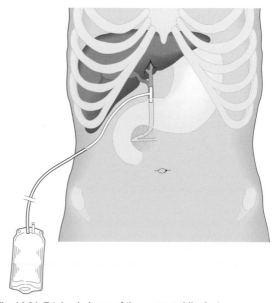

Fig. 14.21 T-tube drainage of the common bile duct.

Retained stones can be removed with the aid of a small-diameter fibreoptic choledochoscope under direct vision, or by means of a wire basket or an inflatable balloon catheter using the image intensifier. The surgeon can suture or leave a drain in the cystic duct, or can oversew the choledochotomy over a T-tube or stent.

Complications of cholecystectomy

The postoperative stay of patients undergoing open cholecystectomy may exceed 7 days. Respiratory complications are not uncommon and there is a significant risk of wound infection (see below). Operative mortality following elective open cholecystectomy is low (0.2%), but is increased tenfold if there is obstructive jaundice or if the common bile duct has to be explored.

Postoperative stay is reduced greatly with laparoscopic cholecystectomy, which in some centres is undertaken as a day-case procedure. Complications resulting from a major abdominal wound are undoubtedly avoided, but there is concern regarding the apparent increased incidence of injury to the bile duct. Failure of the patient to recover quickly following the procedure, the development of abdominal pain or the need for additional analgesia in the immediate postoperative period should cause the surgeon to consider the complications of haemorrhage or bile leakage, and mandates further assessment by LFTs, abdominal imaging or repeat laparoscopy. Mortality and morbidity related to the laparoscopic procedure have also been reported. Nevertheless, the advantages to the patient of this minimally invasive technique have led to its widespread adoption by surgeons.

Haemorrhage

This may originate from the cystic artery or the gallbladder bed. Significant intra-abdominal bleeding should be suspected from the development of pain or if the patient exhibits early features of hypovolaemic shock. Blood may issue from the drain, if one is present, and re-exploration is mandatory.

Infective complications

Wound infection from organisms present in the bile (notably *E. coli, Klebsiella aerogenes* and *Strep. faecalis)* can be reduced following cholecystectomy by the intravenous administration of a cephalosporin at the time of induction of anaesthesia, although the routine use of this group of drugs at laparoscopic cholecystectomy has recently been questioned (EBM 14.8). A longer course of antibiotics may be prescribed when significant bile contamination of the peritoneal cavity has occurred at surgery. Collections of bile and/or blood readily become infected after cholecystectomy. Formal drainage may be needed if this progresses to the formation of a subhepatic or subphrenic abscess.

EBM	14.8 Antibiotic prophylaxis in laparoscopic cholecystectomy
	'Routine prophylactic administration of antibiotics is unnecessary in patients at low risk of wound or postoperative infection.'
	Al-Ghnaniem R, et al. Br J Surg 2003; 90(3):365–366.

Bile leakage

This may be due to a ligature or clip slipping off the cystic duct, the accidental division of an unrecognized accessory duct, damage to the common bile duct, or retention of a duct stone after exploration. Bile leakage may be evidenced by the development of abnormal LFTs and localized or generalized abdominal pain. It may be contained if a drain is in place. In the absence of biliary peritonitis, a persistent leak requires investigation by means of endoscopic cholangiography. Surgery may be needed if biliary peritonitis develops.

Retained stones

Following bile duct exploration, any retained small stones evident on the postoperative T-tube cholangiogram (see above) may be flushed into the duodenum by irrigating the T-tube with saline. Their passage may be facilitated if glucagon is given to relax the sphincter of Oddi. If the duct cannot be cleared by irrigation, delayed extraction of the stones may be undertaken under radiological control. The patient is discharged with the T-tube in place. This is removed 4–6 weeks later and a steerable catheter passed along its track into the bile duct. A wire (*Dormia*) basket can be passed along the catheter to catch and withdraw the retained calculus (Fig. 14.22).

In some patients, unsuspected stones may be left in the bile duct at cholecystectomy. Such stones usually give rise to complications such as jaundice, cholangitis and pancreatitis in the months and years following cholecystectomy. Ultrasonography and MRCP can be used to confirm the presence of such retained stones (Fig. 14.23) and endoscopic retrograde cholangiography and sphincterotomy are performed to recover them (Fig. 14.24). In this technique, a diathermy wire attached to a cannula is passed through the duodenoscope and used to divide the sphincter of Oddi. The stones can then be extracted with a Dormia basket or balloon catheter. This same method can be used to extract stones detected in the immediate postoperative period. If the stones are too large to be withdrawn or the patient is unwell, a stent or a catheter can be left in the biliary

14

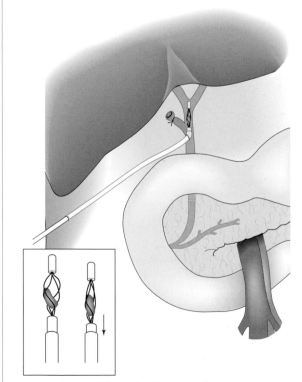

Fig. 14.22 Removal of a retained common bile duct stone.

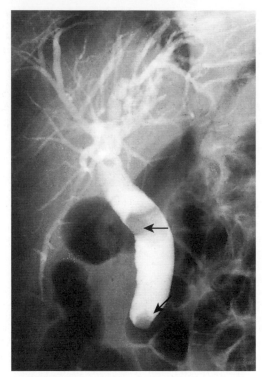

Fig. 14.23 Endoscopic retrograde cholangiography demonstrating multiple stones (arrows) within the biliary tree. These calculi were removed from the dilated bile duct by balloon extraction following sphincterotomy.

system (nasobiliary catheter). The stones can be crushed (lithotripsy) and removed at a later date by means of a repeat endoscopic examination. Surgery may be required to retrieve retained bile duct stones that cannot be dealt in this way.

Bile duct stricture

About 90% of benign duct strictures result from damage during cholecystectomy, in which the duct is divided, ligated or devascularized. This last mechanism appears to be a common cause of injury at laparoscopic cholecystectomy. Other causes of injury include division of a ligated common bile duct that has been mistaken for the cystic duct, division of the right hepatic duct below the point of anomalous insertion of the cystic duct, and encirclement of the common bile duct by the ligature or clip used to close off the cystic duct. Strictures only occasionally result from abdominal trauma or erosion of the bile duct by a gallstone impacted in the gallbladder (Mirizzi's syndrome).

If the common bile duct is completely occluded, progressive obstructive jaundice develops in the postoperative period. If there is a partial stricture, attacks of pain, fever and obstructive jaundice signal the development of cholangitis. The serum alkaline phosphatase and transaminase concentrations are usually elevated, and blood cultures may be positive during attacks of fever. If left untreated, persistent cholangitis and obstruction progress to hepatic abscess formation and rarely to secondary biliary cirrhosis.

The site and extent of the stricture must be defined radiologically. After ultrasonography has been performed, MRCP, ERCP and/or PTC are undertaken. Reconstructive surgery is carried out in a specialist centre and usually necessitates bringing up a Roux loop of jejunum and anastomosing this to the distended biliary system above the stricture (Fig. 14.25).

Post-cholecystectomy syndrome

This term is used to embrace a group of complaints such as post-prandial flatulence, fat intolerance, epigastric and right hypochondrial discomfort, and heartburn, which may follow cholecystectomy. The complaints tend to be more troublesome when cholecystectomy has been performed in the absence of gallstones. Investigations are usually negative, but some patients prove to have retained stones or other alimentary disorders such as peptic ulceration, gastritis and chronic pancreatitis. It is possible that some patients develop pain because of functional abnormalities of the sphincter of Oddi (see below).

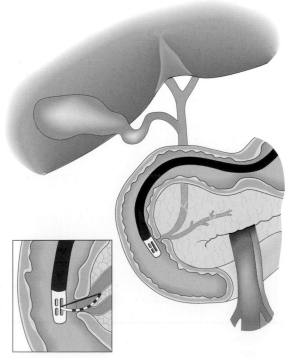

Fig. 14.24 Endoscopic papillotomy to remove retained stones.

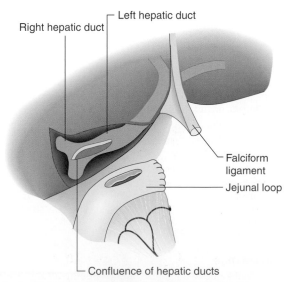

Left hepatic duct

Right hepatic duct

Falciform ligament

Jejunal loop

Confluence of hepatic ducts

Fig. 14.25 Relief of bile duct stricture by anastomosis of a limb of jejunum to the distended biliary tree above the stricture (hepaticojejunostomy Roux en Y).

Management of acute cholecystitis

Patients with acute cholecystitis are admitted to hospital, to be monitored, and analgesics, intravenous fluid and a broad-spectrum antibiotic such as a cephalosporin are prescribed. Patients are given nothing by mouth and a nasogastric tube is passed only if they are vomiting. The majority of patients settle within a few days on this regimen. Failure to settle suggests the presence of an empyema.

Some surgeons delay operation for 2–3 months after the attack in the expectation that the acute inflammatory reaction will have resolved by then, but most now prefer to perform cholecystectomy during the same admission and within 72 hours of the onset of the attack (EBM 14.9). Provided the operation is carried out by an experienced surgeon and under antibiotic cover, 'early' cholecystectomy is not associated with an increased incidence of complications. The duration of the illness and hospitalization is reduced, and further attacks of acute cholecystitis during the waiting period for elective surgery are averted. It should be noted that this is a planned procedure carried out after appropriate investigation (ultrasonography) and with all facilities, on a scheduled list. Laparoscopic cholecystectomy is more difficult to perform in the acute setting, but is the method preferred by most surgeons.

EBM 14.9 **Timing of cholecystectomy**

'Early cholecystectomy for acute cholecystitis is associated with a better outcome than delayed cholecystectomy.'

Papi C, et al. Am J Gastroenterol 2004; 99(1):147–155.
Shikata S, et al. Surgery 2005; 35:553–560.

If surrounding inflammation makes identification of the relevant anatomical structures difficult, drainage of the gallbladder with removal of stones (cholecystostomy) may be performed as an interim measure. Elective cholecystectomy is usually performed approximately 2 months later.

Atypical 'biliary' pain

More difficulty arises with patients who have attacks of pain consistent with biliary colic but in whom investigations such as ultrasonography, oral cholecystography and ERCP reveal no abnormality. Some of these patients with 'acalculous biliary pain' may eventually prove to have non-biliary disease, such as peptic ulceration, chronic pancreatitis or 'irritable' colon. In the majority, no explanation for the symptoms can be found, although recent evidence suggests that some may be suffering from a functional disorder of the sphincter of Oddi (Fig. 14.26). Endoscopic manometry may be useful in identifying patients who may benefit from endoscopic sphincterotomy.

Non-surgical treatment of gallstones

Dissolution therapy with bile salts is no longer popular in the management of gallstone disease. Percutaneous extraction or dissolution of gallstones is possible, but the efficacy of this approach has been questioned. Destruction of stones by extracorporeal shock-wave lithotripsy has been used in selected patients but, like the previous treatments, has largely been made redundant with the advent of laparoscopic cholecystectomy.

Management of acute cholangitis

This condition is caused by incomplete obstruction of the biliary tree and is more often due to common bile duct stones. It is not frequently observed as a presenting feature of malignancy, but may result from instrumentation of the

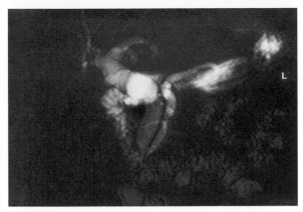

Fig. 14.26 MRCP in a patient who underwent laparoscopic cholecystectomy 5 years before the development of recurrent right upper quadrant pain. The bile and pancreatic ducts are dilated secondary to biliary dyskinesia.

biliary tree during the investigation or treatment of malignant obstructive jaundice.

The patient is often extremely unwell, with evidence of septic shock. Treatment involves resuscitation, the administration of appropriate antibiotics, and decompression of the biliary tree. Given the high associated morbidity and mortality of surgical intervention, decompression is normally achieved by endoscopic means. When common bile duct stones are responsible, it may be necessary to drain the biliary tree temporarily by means of a stent, even if sphincterotomy and stone extraction have apparently been successful.

Other benign biliary disorders

Asiatic cholangiohepatitis

There has been a decline in the incidence of this condition, which occurs in the Far East and is particularly common in coastal Chinese communities. Suppurative cholangitis develops and pigment stones form in the intrahepatic and extrahepatic biliary tree. Deconjugation of bilirubin glucuronide by bacteria may be implicated in stone formation, and *E. coli* and *Strep. faecalis* can often be isolated from the bile and portal blood.

The clinical features are those of obstructive jaundice, pain and fever, and liver abscesses may form. Cholangitis is treated with antibiotics, and stones in the duct can be removed by percutaneous, endoscopic and operative means. Ductal obstruction may be treated by choledochoduodenostomy or hepaticojejunostomy. A limb of the Roux loop of jejunum may be left in a subcutaneous position to facilitate subsequent percutaneous manoeuvres to treat residual or recurrent calculi. Hepatic resection may be indicated if suppuration and obstruction have led to regional destruction of liver tissue.

Primary sclerosing cholangitis

In this condition, both intrahepatic and extrahepatic bile ducts may become indurated and irregularly thickened. There is a marked chronic inflammatory cell infiltrate and fibrous narrowing of the biliary tree. Its aetiology is unknown, but it may have an immunological basis since most patients have evidence of autoantibodies. Over three-quarters of patients also suffer from ulcerative colitis; other associated conditions include retroperitoneal fibrosis, immunodeficiency syndromes and pancreatitis. Bile duct carcinoma can develop, and obstruction can give rise to bacterial cholangitis and secondary biliary cirrhosis.

The condition frequently affects young adults and gives rise to intermittent attacks of obstructive jaundice, pruritus and pain. ERCP and liver biopsy are the mainstays of diagnosis. Medical treatment is generally unsatisfactory, and the outlook is extremely variable. Duct strictures can sometimes by treated by surgical bypass or the insertion of stents, but such manoeuvres may compromise the ability to undertake successful liver transplantation, which offers the only prospect of cure.

Tumours of the biliary tract

Carcinoma of the gallbladder

Carcinoma of the gallbladder is rare and almost invariably associated with the presence of gallstones. The condition is four times as common in females as in males. About 90% of lesions are adenocarcinomas; the remainder are squamous carcinomas.

Direct invasion commonly obstructs the bile duct or porta hepatis, and early lymphatic and haematogenous dissemination is common. Initial symptoms are indistinguishable from those of gallstones but jaundice, if present, is unremitting. A mass may be palpable. Many tumours are detected incidentally at cholecystectomy for the treatment of gallstones. Some surgeons recommend an aggressive approach of resection of segments IV/V of the liver and dissection of the regional lymph nodes. Tumours presenting with jaundice cannot be cured by resection, and palliation by endoscopic or percutaneous insertion of a stent or surgical bypass is required. The 5-year survival rate is less than 5%.

Carcinoma of the bile ducts

Cholangiocarcinoma is a relatively uncommon cancer that affects the elderly and which is increasing in frequency. Such lesions may arise at any site within the biliary tree and can be multifocal. Tumours can be classified based on the level of involvement of the biliary tree (Fig. 14.27) and are most common at the hilus. Polypoidal tumours are uncommon but carry a more favourable outlook. Sclerotic lesions involving the confluence of the hepatic ducts (Klatskin tumour) pose considerable problems in management. The lesions are said to be slow-growing, but this has been over-emphasized. Cholangiocarcinoma may develop in patients with underlying primary sclerosing cholangitis or choledochal cyst.

Clinical features

Progressive obstructive jaundice, often preceded by vague dyspeptic pain, is the usual presenting feature. The gallbladder may become obstructed because of cystic duct involvement, and mucocoele or empyema can develop, but generally it is impalpable. Anorexia and weight loss are common. Pruritus is often particularly distressing.

Management

The diagnosis may be made on the history and clinical findings. The presence of intrahepatic duct dilatation and a collapsed gallbladder on ultrasound scan are highly suggestive of a tumour involving the common hepatic duct. Resectability is best assessed by CT or MRI to exclude the presence of hepatic metastases and nodal involvement and to determine vascular invasion.

Carcinoma of the lower common bile duct is treated by the Whipple operation (p. 227) if the tumour is localized and the patient is fit for radical resection. Long-term survival following this procedure is better in patients with cholangiocarcinoma than in those with carcinoma of the head of the pancreas.

Carcinoma of the upper biliary tract is resectable in only 10% of patients, some of whom may require hepatic resection to achieve satisfactory clearance of the tumour. Following resection, the divided intrahepatic ducts are anastomosed to a Roux limb of jejunum. Operative mortality is reported in as many as 10% of patients. In the majority of patients not submitted to resection, palliation can be achieved by insertion of a stent by endoscopic or percutaneous transhepatic techniques (Fig. 14.28). Most stents are liable to occlusion, exposing the patient to repeated attacks of cholangitis and/or jaundice. Quality of life is poor and few patients with cholangiocarcinoma survive for more than 18 months. The role of systemic chemotherapy and/or radiotherapy has yet to be established.

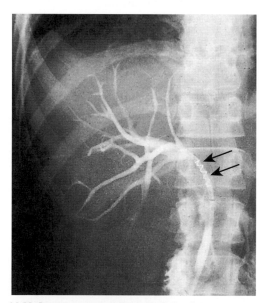

Fig. 14.28 Percutaneous transhepatic cholangiogram demonstrating a stricture at the confluence of the hepatic ducts. This lesion has the typical appearance of a cholangiocarcinoma and has been managed by percutaneous insertion of a stent (arrowed).

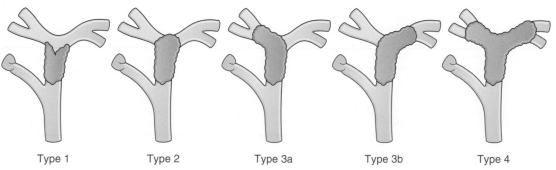

Type 1   Type 2   Type 3a   Type 3b   Type 4

Fig. 14.27 Classification of hilar cholangiocarcinoma.

C.J. McKay
C.R. Carter

15

The pancreas and spleen

THE PANCREAS

Surgical anatomy

The pancreas develops from separate ventral and dorsal buds of endoderm that appear during the fourth week of fetal life. The ventral pancreas develops in association with the biliary tree, and its duct joins the common bile duct before emptying into the duodenum through the papilla of Vater (Fig. 15.1). During gestation, the duodenum rotates clockwise on its long axis, and the bile duct and ventral pancreas pass round behind it to fuse with the dorsal pancreas. Most of the duct that drains the dorsal pancreas joins the duct draining the ventral pancreas to form the main pancreatic duct (of Wirsung); the rest of the dorsal duct becomes the accessory pancreatic duct (of Santorini) and enters the duodenum 2.5 cm proximal to the main duct. In fetal life, the common bile duct and main pancreatic duct are dilated at their junction to form the ampulla of Vater. In extra-uterine life, only 10% of individuals retain this ampulla, although most retain a short common channel between the two duct systems.

The pancreas lies retroperitoneally, behind the lesser sac and stomach. The head of the gland lies within the C-loop of the duodenum, with which it shares a blood supply from the coeliac and superior mesenteric arteries (Fig. 15.2). The superior mesenteric vein runs upwards to the left of the uncinate process, and joins the splenic vein behind the neck of the pancreas to form the portal vein. The body and tail of the pancreas lie in front of the splenic vein as far as the splenic hilum, and receive arterial blood from the splenic artery as it runs along the upper border of the gland. The intimate relationship of the friable pancreas to these major blood vessels is the reason that bleeding is problematic after pancreatic trauma. The close association between the common bile duct and the head of pancreas explains why obstructive jaundice is so common in cancer of the head of the pancreas, and why gallstones frequently give rise to acute pancreatitis.

Surgical physiology

Exocrine function

The exocrine pancreas is essential for the digestion of fat, protein and carbohydrate. The pancreas secretes 1–2 litres of alkaline (pH 7.5–8.8) enzyme-rich juice each day. The enzymes are synthesized by the acinar cells and stored there as zymogen granules. Trypsin is the key proteolytic enzyme; it is released in an inactive form (trypsinogen) and is normally only activated within the duodenum by the brush border enzyme, enterokinase. Once trypsin has been activated, a cascade is established whereby the other proteolytic enzymes become activated in turn. Lipase and amylase are secreted as active enzymes. The alkaline medium required for the activity of pancreatic enzymes is provided by the bicarbonate secreted by the ductal epithelium.

Pancreatic secretion is stimulated by eating. Hormonal and neural (vagal) mechanisms are involved. Food entering the duodenum (notably fat and protein digestion products) releases cholecystokinin (CCK), which stimulates pancreatic enzyme secretion, while at the same time causing the gallbladder to contract and increase bile flow into the intestine. Acid in the duodenum releases the hormone secretin, which stimulates the pancreas to secrete watery alkaline juice.

Endocrine function

The islets of Langerhans are distributed throughout the pancreas. Although they account for only 2% of the weight of the gland, they receive 10% of its blood supply. Interaction between the endocrine and the exocrine pancreas is facilitated by the close proximity of islets and acini, and by a local 'portal' system in which blood draining from the islets enters a capillary network around neighbouring acinar cells before entering the tributaries of the portal vein. Four types of islet cell are recognized: A cells produce glucagon; B cells, insulin; D cells, somatostatin; and PP cells, pancreatic polypeptide. Glucagon and insulin have well-established physiological roles; the function of the other islet products is uncertain, but somatostatin and pancreatic polypeptide

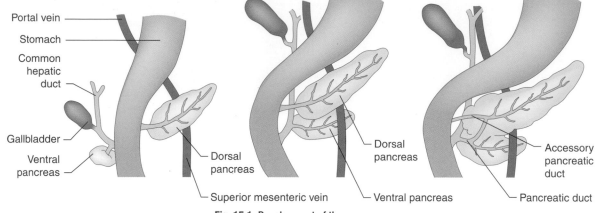

Fig. 15.1 Development of the pancreas.

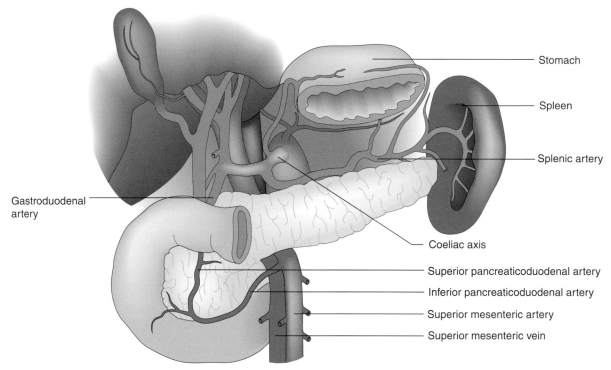

Fig. 15.2 Anatomical relationships of the pancreas.

may serve as local (paracrine) regulators, rather than as circulating (endocrine) messengers. Gastrin-producing (G) cells are not normally found in the pancreas, except in the rare Zollinger–Ellison syndrome.

Pancreatic pain

The parasympathetic nervous system has no role in the perception of pancreatic pain. Painful stimuli from the pancreas are transmitted by sympathetic fibres that travel along the arteries of supply to the coeliac ganglion, and from there to segments 5–10 of the thoracic spinal cord via the greater, lesser and least splanchnic nerves.

Congenital disorders of the pancreas

Annular pancreas is a rare cause of duodenal obstruction, resulting from failure of rotation of the ventral pancreas. In approximately 5% of individuals, the ducts draining

the dorsal and ventral pancreas fail to fuse, giving rise to pancreas divisum. This means that the secretions of the larger dorsal pancreas have to drain to the duodenum through the smaller accessory duct. There is no evidence to suggest a strong association between pancreas divisum and acute or chronic pancreatitis. Rests of pancreatic tissue may be found at a variety of sites within the gut wall, but are most common in the duodenum, stomach and proximal small bowel. Such heterotopic tissue is usually asymptomatic, but can become a focus of inflammation in the rare condition of cystic duodenal dystrophy ('groove' pancreatitis) causing pain and duodenal obstruction.

Pancreatitis

Pancreatitis may be acute or chronic. After an attack of acute pancreatitis, the gland usually returns to anatomical and functional normality, whereas chronic pancreatitis is associated with a permanent derangement of structure and function. Some patients suffer from recurrent acute pancreatitis but enjoy relatively normal health between attacks.

Acute pancreatitis

Acute pancreatitis is a common cause of emergency admission to hospital. There are 100–400 new cases per million of the population each year in the UK, and the incidence continues to rise, possibly because of an increase in gallstone disease, alcohol misuse and obesity in the population. The disease is relatively rare in children, but all adult age groups may be affected.

Aetiology

Conditions associated with the development of acute pancreatitis are listed in Table 15.1 – gallstones and alcohol are by far the most important.

Gallstone pancreatitis

Gallstones are present in some 40% of patients in the UK who develop acute pancreatitis, but tiny gallstones or even microscopic crystals (so called microlithiasis) are thought to account for the majority of 'idiopathic' cases. Transient impaction of a gallstone within the common channel between the common bile duct and pancreatic duct causes obstruction of the pancreatic duct (Fig. 15.3) and a sequence of events within the pancreatic acinar cells resulting in intracellular activation of pancreatic enzymes, acinar cell damage and pancreatic inflammation.

Alcohol-associated pancreatitis

The proportion of cases of acute pancreatitis linked to alcohol varies in different parts of the world. In Scotland the figure is around 30%, whereas in some parts of France and North America it may be as high as 50–90%. The mechanism responsible is uncertain. Although there is no direct relationship between the quantity of alcohol consumed and the risk of pancreatitis (in contrast with alcoholic liver disease) alcohol consumption normally exceeds 50 g day (or 5 standard drinks).

Other causes

Acute pancreatitis occurs in approximately 5% of patients undergoing ERCP. Such cases are usually mild but can be life threatening. Trauma, particularly blunt abdominal trauma,

Table 15.1 Causes of acute pancreatitis	
Class	**Specific causes**
Toxic	Alcohol
	Medication
	Tropical
Genetic	Cystic fibrosis
	Hereditary pancreatitis
	SPINK1 mutation
Metabolic	Hypercalcaemia
	Hyperlipidaemia
Obstructive	Stone disease
	Macrolithiasis (bile duct stone)
	Microlithiasis (sludge)
	Stricture (incl. Post AP, trauma)
	Neoplasm
	Infection
	Parasites
	Worms
	Anatomical
	Biliary cystic disease
	Choledochal cyst/(coele)
	Duplication cyst
	Duodenal obstruction
	Afferent limb obstructed
	Diverticulum
	Congenital anomaly
	Annular pancreas
	Anomalous pancreatobiliary junction
	Pancreas divisum
	Atresia
Inflammatory	Autoimmune disease
	Crohn's
	Polyarteritis nodosa
	SLE
	Vasculitis
	Autoimmune pancreatitis
	Infection
	Viral
Physiological	Sphincter of Oddi dysfunction

15

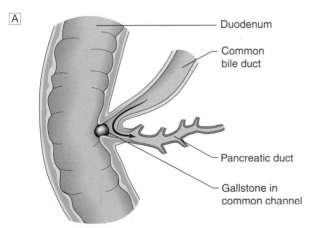

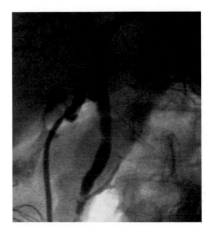

Fig. 15.3 **A** Common channel shared by the bile duct and the pancreatic duct may allow gallstone pancreatitis. **B** Operative cholangiogram showing a stone in the distal common bile duct and reflux of contrast into the pancreatic duct.

Labels in Figure A: Duodenum; Common bile duct; Pancreatic duct; Gallstone in common channel

may cause pancreatitis or pancreatic duct disruption. Hypercalcaemia is a rare cause of pancreatitis and is usually secondary to hyperparathyroidism. Hyperlipidaemia, due to familial hypertriglyceridaemia, is another rare cause of pancreatitis and in both of these metabolic conditions treatment is directed at the underlying cause. A small number of patients may have a family history of acute pancreatitis. Hereditary pancreatitis is a rare condition caused by mutations of the cationic trypsinogen gene and leads to the development of chronic pancreatitis at a young age.

Viral infections, including mumps, Coxsackie virus, rubella, measles and cytomegalovirus are the most common cause of pancreatitis in children. Bacterial infections are a very rare cause of pancreatitis. Ascaris worms are a relatively common cause of pancreatitis in areas of high prevalence, due to migration through the duodenal papilla from the common bile duct. Many drugs have been associated with acute pancreatitis although it is often difficult to prove a causal association and other causes always need to be considered. Azathioprine, mesalazine and simvastatin are responsible for the best documented cases.

Pancreatic neoplasms may cause obstruction of the pancreatic duct and lead to acute pancreatitis. Such neoplasms can be small and thus easily missed, even by CT. The presence of unexplained pancreatic duct dilatation or other suspicious clinical or radiological appearances should prompt further investigation, usually by endoscopic ultrasound.

Clinical features of acute pancreatitis

Constant, severe or agonizing pain in the epigastrium, with radiation through to the back, is usually prominent. Pain can also be experienced in either hypochondrium. Nausea, vomiting and retching are often marked. Clinical examination often reveals much less tenderness, guarding and rigidity than might have been expected from the patient's history and the presence of generalized peritonism may warrant further investigation by CT to exclude other intra-abdominal pathology. Signs of systemic disturbance include tachycardia, hypotension or tachypnoea and are indicative of severe pancreatitis. Obstructive jaundice may be apparent in patients with pancreatitis due to an impacted gallstone, and if present should raise awareness of the possibility of co-existent cholangitis.

Diagnosis

The key to the diagnosis of acute pancreatitis is a high index of suspicion and measurement of the serum amylase concentration. Serum lipase is an alternative and has some advantages but is rarely available in UK hospitals. The usual diagnostic cut-off for serum amylase is three times the upper reference limit but the diagnosis should be considered in any patient with a relevant history, even where there is a non-diagnostic rise in serum amylase. A high serum amylase can be seen in patients with abdominal pain due to other pathology. The most common of these is mesenteric ischaemia due either to mesenteric vascular occlusion or small bowel strangulation, and when there is diagnostic doubt, an urgent CT is indicated to clarify the diagnosis. High serum amylase levels are also seen in some patients with perforated ulcer or ruptured aneurysm but rarely above the diagnostic threshold for pancreatitis. In all cases, if the history or clinical examination is atypical for acute pancreatitis, CT should be carried out to clarify the diagnosis.

Serum amylase levels fall rapidly in acute pancreatitis and have no relationship to the severity of the attack or the resolution of the disease. Patients who present some days after the initial onset of abdominal pain may have normal or near-normal serum amylase levels and although urinary

amylase or serum lipase can be helpful in such cases, the diagnosis is again best clarified by CT.

Radiology

Initial diagnosis of acute pancreatitis is based on clinical features combined with serum amylase levels. The role of radiology in initial assessment is confined to cases where there remains diagnostic doubt, as when serum amylase is non-diagnostic or where the clinical history or examination findings are atypical (for example when there is evidence of generalized peritonitis). In these cases urgent contrast-enhanced CT is mandatory. In patients with acute pancreatitis, changes will be identified ranging from mild peripancreatic oedema through to extensive pancreatic necrosis (Fig. 15.4) but more importantly at this stage, other diagnoses which require urgent operative intervention, such as mesenteric ischaemia or perforated viscus, will be excluded.

Differentiation between gallstone- and alcohol-associated pancreatitis

It is important to clarify the aetiology of acute pancreatitis, primarily so that further attacks can be prevented where possible. In the UK, the majority of cases are due to gallstones and these may be present even where there is a clear history of alcohol excess. Therefore, all patients with acute pancreatitis should have an abdominal ultrasound carried out. Even when no stones are identified on ultrasound, other factors may suggest a gallstone diagnosis. In particular, elevated alanine transaminase (ALT) at admission of more than twice the upper reference limit is highly suggestive of a gallstone aetiology. In patients where no cause is found, further investigation by endoscopic ultrasound may detect microlithiasis or rare causes such as a small pancreatic neoplasm. This is best performed once the acute attack has resolved.

Assessment of severity

Approximately 80% of patients with acute pancreatitis will have a self-limiting illness which resolves within 48–72 hours. In such cases the main issue is identification and treatment of the underlying cause. The major challenge faced in the management of this condition is the 20% of patients who have a severe episode of pancreatitis in whom life-threatening complications can occur. Much effort has been directed at the early recognition of severe acute pancreatitis, the aim being to ensure these patients are adequately managed and placed in an appropriate high-dependency or intensive care environment. Many systems have been proposed of which the Glasgow Prognostic Score, APACHE II score

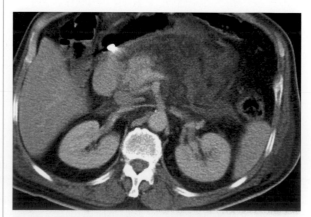

Fig. 15.4 Early CT with oedema and tail necrosis.

and C-reactive protein have been most widely studied. None of these however have proved sufficiently accurate to influence management decisions, particularly in the crucial first 24 hours after hospital admission. Other attempts with serum or urine markers of severity have either proved disappointing or have not yet been tested in prospective studies. When faced with a patient with acute pancreatitis, the challenge therefore is to *recognize* the development of a severe attack which necessitates a clear understanding of the natural history of the illness.

The most important feature of severe acute pancreatitis is the development of multiple organ dysfunction syndrome (MODS). In most patients who develop severe acute pancreatitis this is identified by the presence of hypoxia, shock or more rarely, renal dysfunction around the time of admission to hospital. A minority of patients will develop such complications over the course of the next 48 hours and in these cases the presence of SIRS (systemic inflammatory response syndrome) characterized by a tachycardia, raised white cell count and/or tachypnoea is almost always present. It is very rare for a patient without SIRS at admission to develop MODS. Where SIRS persists for more than 48 hours, the risk of further deterioration is very high and such patients need close monitoring for the development of respiratory and renal complications. It is the group of patients with early persistent SIRS or MODS who are also at greatest risk of developing septic and other local complications of acute pancreatitis.

Contrast enhanced CT is used in some institutions to identify severe acute pancreatitis, as the presence of pancreatic necrosis or extensive fluid collections identifies a group at high risk of further complications. However it is increasingly recognized that the main determinant of outcome is early systemic organ dysfunction and the role of early CT is now mainly confined to cases of diagnostic doubt.

Management

Most attacks of acute pancreatitis will settle with conservative management involving intravenous fluids, analgesia and gradual re-introduction of diet when nausea and vomiting have settled. All patients with SIRS or early systemic organ dysfunction should be managed in a high-dependency or intensive care environment where adequate monitoring and specialist care is available.

Conservative treatment

- *Pain relief.* Severe pain requires the administration of opiates; there is no evidence to support the use of pethidine rather than morphine.
- *Fluid resuscitation.* Patients with severe acute pancreatitis often require large volumes of fluid to maintain adequate urine output and blood pressure. Adequate early resuscitation in such cases is the most important consideration in early management and where systemic organ dysfunction is present will necessitate invasive monitoring of venous and arterial pressure. Patients with MODS or SIRS will need oxygen therapy and continuous monitoring of oxygen saturation as well as urine output.
- *Suppression of pancreatic function.* There is no evidence that suppression of pancreatic function improves the outcome in acute pancreatitis. Nasogastric tubes are not routinely used. Fluids and diet are withheld until nausea and vomiting settle and in cases where systemic complications or other factors prevent recommencement of normal diet, nasoenteric feeding is commenced at an early stage. Suppression of pancreatic secretion by drugs such as octreotide or somatostatin is of no benefit in acute pancreatitis.

- *Prevention of infection.* Antibiotic prophylaxis has been advocated by some as a means of reducing the risk of infected pancreatic necrosis. Others have been concerned that the more widespread use of antibiotics will result in an increased incidence of severe fungal infection. The most recent consensus is that there is no evidence that prophylactic antibiotics reduce the incidence of infected pancreatic necrosis or mortality (EBM 15.1). It is important to recognize that patients with severe acute pancreatitis often have evidence of SIRS and the presence of a fever and raised white cell count are to be expected, even in the absence of infection. The only definite indication for early antibiotic therapy is when patients are suspected of having cholangitis, which may co-exist with gallstone pancreatitis. Jaundiced patients with SIRS are therefore managed with appropriate broad spectrum antibiotics while arrangements are made for urgent ERCP as described below.

15

> **EBM** 15.1 **Prophylactic antibiotics in severe acute pancreatitis**
>
> 'There is no evidence that prophylactic antibiotics (in acute pancreatitis) reduce the incidence of infected pancreatic necrosis or mortality.'
>
> Bai Y, Gao J, Zou DW, Li ZS. Prophylactic antibiotics cannot reduce infected pancreatic necrosis and mortality in acute necrotizing pancreatitis: evidence from a meta-analysis of randomized controlled trials. Am J Gastroenterol 2008; 103(1):104–110.

- *Inhibition of inflammatory response.* Severe acute pancreatitis is one of many conditions where systemic organ dysfunction is driven by the systemic inflammatory response and there has been much experimental and clinical interest in the role of down-regulation of this response as a potential treatment for acute pancreatitis. The only agent that has been studied in large, prospective clinical trials was the platelet-activating factor (PAF) antagonist, lexipafant. Despite encouraging experimental data and promising results from initial clinical trials, a large international trial, recruiting 1500 patients, showed no difference in mortality.
- *Nutritional support.* Patients with severe acute pancreatitis who are unable to resume normal diet within 48–72 hours require nutritional support. This is best delivered by an enteral rather than parenteral route as meta-analyses of randomized trials (EBM 15.2) have demonstrated that TPN has a higher rate of complications and mortality. There are also sound experimental reasons to believe that enteral nutrition has additional benefits by potentially reducing the risk of bacterial translocation from the gut. There is no evidence that nasojejunal feeding is better or safer than nasogastric feeding but the nasojejunal route will be required where gastric stasis or outlet obstruction prevent effective nasogastric delivery.

> **EBM** 15.2 **Nutritional support in severe acute pancreatitis**
>
> 'In patients with severe acute pancreatitis who are unable to return to diet in 48-72 hours nutrition is best given by enteral rather than parenteral (TPN) route.'
>
> Petrov MS, Whelan K. Comparison of complications attributable to enteral and parenteral nutrition in predicted severe acute pancreatitis: a systematic review and meta-analysis. Br J Nutr 2010; 103(9):1287–1295.

- *Other measures.* A recent randomized trial assessed the role of probiotic therapy as an adjunct to early enteral feeding in the hope that this might reduce bacterial translocation from the gut more than enteral nutrition alone, thus potentially preventing later septic complications. Unfortunately, probiotic therapy actually increased mortality due to gut ischaemia and should no longer be used in these patients. Other proposed treatments which have been found to be of no benefit in prospective clinical trials include antiprotease therapy and peritoneal lavage.

Endoscopic treatment

Gallstone pancreatitis is due to the transient impaction of a stone at the papilla causing pancreatic duct obstruction. There is good experimental evidence that the duration of this obstruction is an important determinant of the severity of an attack and so early removal of an impacted gallstone by ERC and sphincterotomy has long been proposed as a potential treatment option for patients. Unfortunately the results from randomized trials have been conflicting, and differences in study design have made direct comparisons difficult. Patients with evidence of obstructive jaundice and SIRS within the first 24 hours are suffering from or are at least at risk of developing cholangitis and there is broad consensus that these patients should have urgent ERC with sphincterotomy. However the majority of patients will pass the gallstone spontaneously and in this situation ERC carries additional risk and no potential benefit (EBM 15.3). The most recent meta-analysis of randomized trials shows no benefit from early ERC in patients with severe acute pancreatitis where cholangitis is not present. Early ERC with stone removal can however be life-saving in the patient with cholangitis and it is important to be alert to this possibility in patients diagnosed as having severe acute pancreatitis. Our own practice is to perform urgent ERC and sphincterotomy only in patients with acute pancreatitis associated with obstructive jaundice and SIRS but there is considerable variation in practice across the UK.

EBM **15.3 ERCP and sphincterotomy in severe acute pancreatitis**

'There is no evidence that early ERC and sphincterotomy gives benefit to those patients with acute severe pancreatitis unless cholangitis is present (evidence of obstructed biliary system and SIRS).'

Ayub K, Imada R, Slavin J. Endoscopic retrograde cholangiopancreatography in gallstone-associated acute pancreatitis. Cochrane Database Syst Rev 2004;(4):CD003630.

Surgical treatment

There is no role for surgical intervention in the first 1–2 weeks of an attack of acute pancreatitis, even in the face of deteriorating multiple organ failure. Complications that were managed surgically in the past are now being managed by radiological or endoscopic treatments. Acute pancreatitis is managed conservatively whenever possible, but surgery is indicated under the following circumstances:

1. Where an alternative diagnosis is suggested by CT following initial assessment.
2. Where gallstones are considered the likely cause, cholecystectomy is carried out after recovery from the acute attack. In patients with mild acute pancreatitis this is best carried out during the index hospital admission but following a severe attack, cholecystectomy is delayed until resolution of the inflammatory process. Even after severe

acute pancreatitis it is usually possible to perform cholecystectomy by the laparoscopic route. In patients who have had no prior imaging of the common bile duct by MRCP or ERC, it is important to carry out operative cholangiography to exclude bile duct stones. In patients considered unfit for cholecystectomy, ERC with endoscopic sphincterotomy is carried out to protect against further attacks.

3. When certain complications develop (see below).

Complications

Infected pancreatic necrosis

Pancreatic necrosis itself is not an indication for surgical intervention, even when complicated by MODS. However, infected pancreatic necrosis is the most challenging complication of acute pancreatitis and management is complex, requiring the input of surgeons, interventional radiologists and endoscopists, as well as the critical care team. Infection occurs in up to 40% of patients with pancreatic necrosis and usually presents more than 2 weeks after symptom onset. The development of infection may be suspected where there is deterioration in systemic organ failure or where new organ failure develops in a patient more than 2 weeks after admission. However, infected pancreatic necrosis is not always complicated by organ failure and may present with worsening pain and fever associated with a rise in inflammatory parameters but with little evidence of systemic illness.

The development of infected pancreatic necrosis may be associated with evidence of gas within a pancreatic collection seen on CT, but this is not always the case and it can be difficult to make this diagnosis on radiological grounds alone. In some centres, if infected pancreatic necrosis is suspected, fine needle aspirates are taken from pancreatic collections under CT or ultrasound guidance to establish whether or not infection is present, with early surgical intervention where infection is proven. Others prefer to act on clinical grounds and where infection is suspected place a percutaneous drain under CT guidance prior to definitive surgical, endoscopic or radiological management.

There is much variation in practice in the management of this life-threatening complication of acute pancreatitis and the variety of approaches reflects variation in local expertise and experience and a lack of good evidence supporting any one approach over another. Where infected pancreatic necrosis is confirmed or strongly suspected, the common approaches to management are briefly described below.

Surgical debridement. Conventional management of infected pancreatic necrosis involves wide debridement of devitalized pancreatic and peripancreatic tissue and either placement of wide-bore drains for postoperative lavage or abdominal packing and planned re-exploration. This is clearly a major undertaking in the critically-ill patient and there has been an increasing trend towards measures to delay surgery until patients are stabilized and organ failure has resolved.

Percutaneous drainage/debridement. Following initial percutaneous drainage of infected pancreatic necrosis, patients will commonly show signs of initial improvement but subsequently deteriorate as drains block with necrotic debris. Rather than proceeding to conventional surgical debridement, several approaches have been described to facilitate removal of necrotic debris via the percutaneous drain track by radiological, laparoscopic or endoscopic means. A minimally-invasive surgical approach through a small flank incision has also been described. Retrospective studies tend to support the view that initial percutaneous drainage followed by conventional surgery or one of these minimally invasive techniques is associated with lower mortality and severe systemic complications than conventional surgery alone.

Endoscopic drainage. The retrogastric position of the pancreas allows endoscopic transgastric drainage of infected pancreatic necrosis, usually under control of endoscopic ultrasound. There is less experience with this approach than open surgery or percutaneous approaches but it is increasingly utilized in selected patients. More than one approach may be used at different times in an individual patient and the importance therefore of management within a specialist multidisciplinary environment cannot be over-emphasized.

Pancreatic pseudocyst

A pancreatic pseudocyst is a collection of pancreatic secretions and inflammatory exudate enclosed in a wall of fibrous or granulation tissue. It differs from a true cyst in that the collection has no epithelial lining and is surrounded by inflammatory tissue. Pseudocysts form most commonly in the lesser sac or in the adjacent retroperitoneum, and by consensus are differentiated from acute fluid collections in that they persist for 4 or more weeks from the onset of acute pancreatitis (Fig. 15.5). Small pseudocysts are usually asymptomatic and resolve spontaneously. In about 10% of patients, larger collections persist and can pose problems.

Pseudocysts typically do not declare themselves for some weeks after the episode of pancreatitis. Persistent or intermittent abdominal discomfort and mild to moderate hyperamylasaemia usually signal their presence, and larger collections may compress neighbouring structures to cause vomiting and obstructive jaundice. Some cysts become so large that they are palpable and, in some cases, visible.

The presence of a pseudocyst is not in itself an indication for surgical treatment. Approximately 50% of asymptomatic pseudocysts will resolve up to 12 weeks following the onset of acute pancreatitis. Treatment is indicated only if the pseudocyst is enlarging or symptomatic, and aims to prevent infection of the contents, haemorrhage or rupture. Simple percutaneous drainage carries a high risk of recurrence and

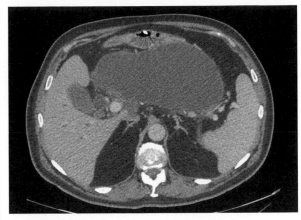

Fig. 15.5 Axial CT with a large retrogastric postacute inflammatory collection approximately 8 weeks after initial presentation.

some form of internal drainage is usually preferred. The conventional surgical approach consists of drainage of the pseudocyst into the stomach (pseudocyst-gastrostomy), a Roux loop of jejunum (pseudocyst-jejunostomy), or duodenum (pseudocyst-duodenostomy); whichever appears most appropriate (Fig. 15.6). As the tissues holding the sutures must be firm, it is desirable to avoid surgery until at least 6 weeks after the onset of the acute attack to allow the walls of the pseudocyst to 'mature'. Endoscopic cyst-gastrostomy or cyst-duodenostomy offers an alternative to surgery, and is now usually carried out under endoscopic ultrasound guidance. Laparoscopic cystgastrostomy or cyst-enterostomy is also described but the relative roles of conventional surgical, laparoscopic and endoscopic drainage have yet to

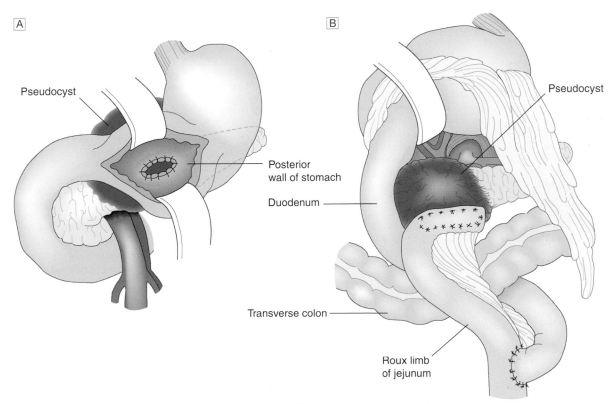

Pseudocyst

Posterior wall of stomach

Pseudocyst

Duodenum

Transverse colon

Roux limb of jejunum

Fig. 15.6 Treatment of pancreatic pseudocyst. A Transgastric cyst gastrostomy. B Roux cyst jejunostomy.

be determined. The selection of the appropriate procedure is often determined by the clinical presentation, anatomical features of the fluid collection, the extent of necrosis present and of course, local expertise. A multidisciplinary approach is mandatory.

Pancreatic abscess

A pancreatic abscess is a circumscribed intra-abdominal collection of pus, usually in proximity to the pancreas, containing little or no pancreatic necrosis. In effect, this is the result of infection of a pseudocyst and is an indication for drainage as described above. This is a later complication than infected pancreatic necrosis, usually many weeks after the initial attack and is rarely complicated by severe systemic illness. Where MODS is present or where the patient presents less than six weeks after onset of acute pancreatitis, there is some overlap with the treatment algorithm for infected pancreatic necrosis and initial percutaneous drainage may therefore be preferred.

Progressive jaundice

Jaundice at the time of presentation with acute pancreatitis suggests that a gallstone is impacted at the lower end of the biliary tree. Such patients may develop ascending cholangitis and early ERC with endoscopic sphincterotomy is therefore indicated as discussed above. Where jaundice develops later in the course of acute pancreatitis, this is usually a consequence of compression of the distal bile duct by an inflammatory pancreatic head mass. In such circumstances treatment is directed towards the underlying pathology, usually infected pancreatic necrosis or a large pseudocyst. In such patients ERCP is often impossible due to the degree of duodenal oedema and distortion.

Persistent duodenal ileus

Protracted ileus usually reflects continuing pancreatic inflammation. In the absence of an indication for operation (e.g. pancreatic necrosis, pseudocyst formation), conservative management is instituted and nutritional status maintained by nasoenteric feeding.

Gastrointestinal bleeding

Severe acute pancreatitis may be complicated by bleeding from gastritis, erosions or duodenal ulceration, and prophylactic PPI therapy is advisable. Bleeding which occurs following treatment of infected pancreatic necrosis is usually a consequence of erosion of a retroperitoneal vessel, often the splenic artery or a major branch of this vessel. Control is best achieved by mesenteric angiography with embolization where possible but surgical control may be necessary. Mortality from such bleeding remains high, particularly where surgical intervention is required. In patients with pseudocysts, bleeding may occur into the cyst causing sudden pain and often collapse. This is due to rupture of a false aneurysm within the wall of the pseudocyst and again is best managed by mesenteric embolization where possible. Overt evidence of gastrointestinal bleeding in a patient with infected pancreatic necrosis or pancreatic pseudocyst commonly indicates a communication between the retroperitoneal collections and the lumen of the GI tract (commonly stomach or colon) and urgent mesenteric angiography (or CT angiography if the patient is sufficiently stable) (Fig. 15.7) rather than endoscopy is the appropriate course of action.

Gastrointestinal ischaemia/fistulae

Acute mesenteric ischaemia can result in an acute abdomen with a raised amylase, and should be considered as part of the differential diagnosis at initial presentation. Segmental colonic ischaemia requiring resection may be encountered at open necrosectomy and exteriorization

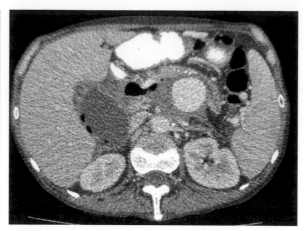

Fig. 15.7 Late CT with splenic artery pseudoaneurysm.

of the ends following resection recommended rather than an attempted anastomosis. Local areas of enteric ischaemia do occur, particularly around large necrosis-associated peripancreatic collections. Rupture of the collection into the intestine can either be associated with a clinical deterioration, where the collection remains inadequately drained and the fistulous connection results in secondary infection, or a clinical improvement when fistulation results in decompression of an infected collection. The presence of gas within a collection therefore does not necessitate intervention, which should be based on clinical parameters. Open surgical or percutaneous drainage of a collection prior to fistulation will result in an external enteric fistula. Colonic fistulation usually necessitates a defunctioning stoma, whereas gastric or duodenal fistulae may be managed by proximal gut rest, supplemented feeding, and adequate local drainage.

Prognosis

Most patients with acute pancreatitis suffer a self-limiting illness and can be expected to make a full recovery. Further treatment is directed at preventing further attacks by definitive management of gallstones or advising against further alcohol abuse. Unfortunately, many patients are unwilling or unable to abstain from drinking, and suffer further attacks of acute pancreatitis with progression to chronic pancreatitis.

Patients with severe acute pancreatitis may be expected to have a more protracted illness and may require many months of hospital care. Overall mortality for such patients is in the region of 10–20%, usually as a consequence of multiple organ failure. Death within the first two weeks of acute pancreatitis accounts for approximately 50% of all mortality in this condition and is more common in patients with extensive necrosis and in the elderly. Late deaths are usually due to complications arising from infected pancreatic necrosis, with mesenteric ischaemia or severe retroperitoneal bleeding being common terminal events. Following recovery from severe acute pancreatitis, return to normal activities can be expected but full recovery can take many months, requiring nutritional support, management of persistent or recurrent sepsis and definitive management of wound or gastrointestinal complications.

Chronic pancreatitis

Chronic pancreatitis is a chronic inflammatory condition characterized by fibrosis and the destruction of exocrine pancreatic tissue.

Aetiology

Chronic pancreatitis is a relatively rare disease but its incidence may be increasing with the growing problem of alcohol misuse. Although alcohol is by far the most common aetiological factor, being implicated in some 60–80% of cases, the factors that predispose some patients to develop chronic pancreatitis are poorly understood, however cigarette smoking appears to be an important co-factor. The risk of chronic pancreatitis appears to increase when alcohol consumption is greater than 50 g of alcohol (or 5 standard drinks) per day.

Hereditary pancreatitis is a rare form of chronic pancreatitis with onset in early adult life and is due to one of a variety of identified mutations of the trypsinogen gene. In addition, many cases of idiopathic chronic pancreatitis are now believed to be associated with other gene mutations, such as that of the cystic fibrosis gene, CFTR. In some cases however, the cause remains unknown. Even where there is evidence of alcohol aetiology, there may be complex genetic factors which predispose to the development of chronic pancreatitis.

Pathophysiology

The secretion of an unduly viscid pancreatic juice may allow protein plugs to form in the duct system, and these plugs subsequently calcify to form duct stones. Impaired flow of pancreatic juice then leads to inflammation, stricture formation in the duct system, and progressive replacement of the gland by fibrous tissue. Loss of acinar tissue is eventually reflected by steatorrhoea and, in time, loss of islet tissue may lead to diabetes mellitus.

Clinical features

Pain is the outstanding feature in most cases. It is characteristically epigastric with marked radiation through to the back, and is often eased by leaning forward or getting down on all fours. In some cases, the pain is precipitated by eating, or the patient learns to avoid certain foods, notably fatty ones. The application of heat sometimes brings relief, and permanent discoloration of the skin may reflect the continued use of heat pads or hot water bottles. The progressive use of powerful opioid analgesics can result in drug dependency.

Weight loss is usual and reflects a combination of inadequate intake, a poor diet and malabsorption. Steatorrhoea is common, the bowel motion being pale, bulky, offensive, floating on water, and difficult to flush. Diabetes mellitus develops in about one-third of patients, but islet function is often preserved for some years following the onset of exocrine insufficiency.

Other less common manifestations of chronic pancreatitis include transient or intermittent obstructive jaundice, duodenal obstruction and splenic vein thrombosis (leading to splenomegaly, hypersplenism and gastric and oesophageal varices). Many patients also have other comorbidity related to cigarette and alcohol consumption which, particularly when combined with nutritional failure, can make management challenging.

Investigations and diagnosis

The initial investigation for suspected chronic pancreatitis is CT. This may reveal the speckled calcification typical of chronic pancreatitis or may show evidence of inflammatory changes or pancreatic duct dilatation or pseudocyst formation (Fig. 15.8). MRCP is of value to reveal the architecture of the pancreatic duct, particularly if surgery or endoscopic therapy is contemplated. When investigating these patients, it must be borne in mind that cancer of the pancreas may block the duct system and cause pancreatitis, and that

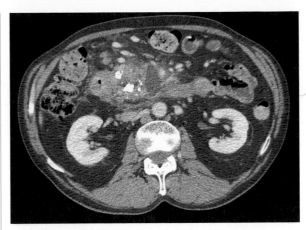

Fig. 15.8 Axial CT showing extensive calcification and cyst formation within the pancreatic head, duodenal wall thickening and narrowing of the superior mesenteric veins with extensive venous collaterals.

the two conditions can co-exist. Endoscopic ultrasound is increasingly utilized where diagnostic uncertainty exists, allowing pancreatic fine needle biopsy where appropriate.

Pancreatic endocrine function is assessed by measurement of random blood glucose levels, supplemented if necessary by a glucose tolerance test. Exocrine function can be measured in a multitude of ways, but insufficiency may not be detectable until 90% of the pancreatic parenchyma is destroyed. If necessary, faecal fat excretion can be measured over 3–5 days while the patient's fat intake is controlled at 100 g/day (normal individuals excrete less than 5 g/day). Faecal elastase is a more convenient method of assessment of exocrine pancreatic function but is less accurate. Where assays of exocrine function are not readily available, a trial of oral pancreatic supplements may be attempted.

Management

The diagnosis of chronic pancreatitis is not in itself an indication for treatment. Considerable clinical judgment is needed to determine the need for, and timing of, intervention. In most cases, pain is the most important indication for surgery but complications resulting from biliary obstruction or gastric outlet obstruction may also necessitate intervention. Many patients have complex problems and need a multidisciplinary approach to treatment.

Conservative management

This consists of encouraging abstinence from alcohol, relief of pain, treatment of exocrine and endocrine insufficiency, and attempts to improve nutritional status. Opiates are avoided, if possible, but their use may prove essential to relieve pain. Diabetes mellitus is treated by appropriate means (diet, oral hypoglycaemic agents or insulin). Nutritional failure is treated by pancreatic exocrine supplements, and modern position-release preparations (e.g. Creon) minimize the enzymic degradation of the supplements by acid and pepsin during their passage through the stomach. The involvement of an experienced dietician is important, particularly where, as is common, patients have a combination of diabetes mellitus, fat malabsorption and poor diet.

Endoscopic treatment

For many patients, endoscopic management is considered in the first instance. Pancreatic duct stents may be placed where there is evidence of a dominant pancreatic duct stricture or where there is a pancreatic duct disruption with pseudocyst formation or pancreatic ascites. Aggressive endoscopic treatment with stricture dilatation and stone removal has some advocates. Although endoscopic management can be successful in selected patients, results from randomized trials suggest where feasible, a surgical solution is preferable to repeated attempts at endotherapy.

Surgical treatment

This is indicated if pain is intractable; when neighbouring structures, such as the common bile duct, duodenum, portal or splenic vein, are sufficiently compressed to produce symptoms; when pseudocysts or abscesses develop; when endoscopic therapy has failed; or when cancer cannot be excluded.

In general, the objective is to relieve pain or compression, while at the same time conserving as much healthy pancreatic tissue and function as possible. Surgery involves drainage of the obstructed pancreatic duct into a Roux loop of jejunum, usually combined with some form of duodenum preserving pancreatic head resection. The two most commonly performed procedures are those described by Beger and Frey (Fig. 15.9), the difference between them being the greater extent of pancreatic parenchymal excision and need for formal division of the pancreatic neck in the Beger procedure. No one procedure has been proven to be superior. Approximately 70% of patients remain pain-free or substantially improved when assessed 5 years after surgery for chronic pancreatitis. As with all aspects of chronic pancreatitis treatment, the results of surgery are better in patients who manage to abstain from alcohol.

Neoplasms of the exocrine pancreas

Pancreatic tumours are epithelial in origin, and 80% of these are pancreatic ductal adenocarcinoma (PDAC). It is of importance that although the majority of tumours of the pancreas are PDAC, there are nearly 20 different histological types of pancreatic tumour (intraductal papillary mucinous neoplasm (IPMN), cystic mucinous or serous tumours, solid-pseudo papillary tumours, acinar cell carcinoma) or tumours with roughly similar clinical presentation (cholangiocarcinoma, ampullary, or duodenal carcinomas) with much better prognosis.

Careful assessment and staging of the individual patient is therefore required, to avoid inappropriate management pathways, based on the assumption that a pancreatic mass is a PDAC. Advances in cross sectional imaging (CT/MR) and the widespread availability of endoscopic ultrasound will allow accurate pre-treatment confirmation of the diagnosis in the majority of cases.

Adenocarcinoma of the pancreas

Aetiology

Ductal adenocarcinoma of the pancreas is the 10th (male)/11th (female) most common cancer in the UK, but the fifth commonest cause of cancer related death. There are about 7600 new cases in the UK per annum (or 20/day), and the incidence has been consistent over the last 40 years, with a lifetime risk of about 1 in 95. Male and females are equally affected. Only 15–20% are resectable, and in these there is only 20% 5-year survival. As with most tumours there is an increasing incidence with age but 20% of patients are less than 60 years of age. Whilst the aetiology is unknown, there is an association with tobacco smoking (20–30% thought to be smoking related), race (African–Americans > Hispanics or Caucasians), diabetes, chronic pancreatitis (particularly hereditary pancreatitis) and familial pancreatic cancer.

Pathology

Pancreatic ductal adenocarcinoma (PDAC)

The majority of adenocarcinomas arise from ductal rather than acinar tissue, 60% arising in the head of the gland. The histology (Fig. 15.10) is characterized by groups of infiltrating carcinoma cells often some (histological) distance apart, interspersed by a fibrous stroma, with involvement of nerves, vessels, lymphatics and lymph nodes, at a relatively early phase. Metastatic spread is most commonly to the liver and lung; 80% of patients present with either locoregional or metastatic dissemination.

Intraductal papillary mucinous neoplasm (IPMN)

This is a relatively recently recognized entity (1996) comprising a group of lesions characterized by a papillary growth of the ductal epithelium with rich mucin production and cystic expansion of the affected duct, and differ from cystic mucinous neoplasms because of a direct communication with the

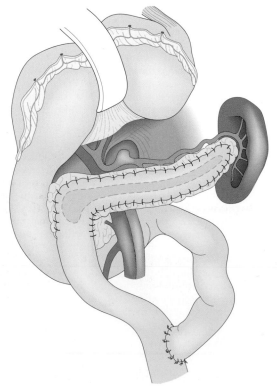

Fig. 15.9 Longitudinal pancreaticojejunostomy

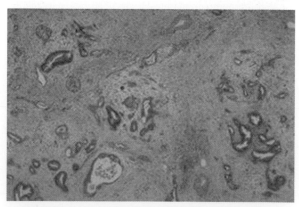

Fig. 15.10 Histology of pancreatic cancer with small groups of epithelial cells attempting to form glands, interspersed with fibrous stoma.

Wirsung duct and the absence of ovarian-type stroma. The recent widespread availability of cross-sectional imaging has resulted in many being picked up as incidental findings. There is a broad separation into two types, main duct and branch duct types. Main duct IPMN has a definite malignant potential whereas branch type IPMN commonly follows a more benign course. Resection is therefore recommended for main duct IPMN where clinically appropriate whereas many branch duct lesions may be observed (when small (< 3 cm), without septae or nodularity of the walls). Natural history of this tumour is different from PDAC in that the majority are resectable, with survival reaching 80–90% for in situ carcinoma, and 50–70% in the presence of invasive carcinoma.

Mucinous cystic neoplasm

Mucinous cystic tumours of the pancreas predominate in the body and tail of the pancreas and have a strong female predilection. They are multiloculated tumours with a characteristic smooth glistening surface, a dense fibrous wall and occasional calcification (Fig. 15.11). They arise from oversecretion of the mucus by the hyperplastic columnar lining of the ducts and therefore contain thickened viscous material, which can also be haemorrhagic. These tumours should be considered potentially malignant but are classified histologically as benign, borderline, or malignant based on degree of dysplastic changes.

Serous cystic neoplasm

Serous cystic neoplasms are most commonly microcystic, but can present in an 'oligocystic' or 'macrocystic' form when differentiation from other cystic neoplasms can be difficult. In the presence of multiple serous cysts Von Hippel–Lindau syndrome should be considered. They often present as incidental findings or with pressure symptoms or a palpable mass when large. The microcystic adenoma has a characteristic radiological appearance with a pancreatic mass characterized by a dense, internal, lacelike, honeycombed matrix composed of fibrous septae, and often a central scar. When the diagnosis can be confirmed preoperatively, resection is usually not required as serous cystic tumours have virtually no malignant potential.

Metastases

Isolated metastases in the pancreas are rare, the most common site of origin being renal cell carcinoma, followed by lung, lobular breast carcinoma, melanoma and gastric carcinoma. Localized SMA or celiac lymphadenopathy can often mimic a pancreatic primary radiologically. Some

may benefit from resection in certain circumstances and histological confirmation should be sought in all patients where possible.

Solid pseudopapillary tumour of the pancreas

Solid pseudopapillary tumour, otherwise known as solid-cystic tumour, or Frantz tumour of the pancreas, is an unusual form of pancreatic carcinoma (Fig. 15.12). Its natural history differs from the more common pancreatic adenocarcinoma in that it is almost always in female patients (10:1), often at a young age (20–30 years), is more indolent, and carries a better prognosis. Pathologically, the tumour is usually well circumscribed with regions of necrosis, haemorrhage, and cystic degeneration. Metastatic disease can occur, usually involving the liver, and resection is the preferred treatment.

Acinar cell carcinoma of the pancreas

Acinar cell carcinoma is a rare tumour accounting for 1% of pancreatic tumours, and arises from the acinar cells of the pancreas. Normal acinar cells are the primary cells of the exocrine pancreas and are responsible for secreting various enzymes; the tumour cells also may secrete pancreatic enzymes, most commonly lipase. Presentation may therefore be confused with acute pancreatitis

Ampullary tumours

Tumours may arise from the Ampulla of Vater, where the pancreatic duct (of Wirsung) and common bile duct merge and exit into the duodenum. They are relatively uncommon accounting for approximately 7% of all periampullary carcinomas, but because of their relationship to the common bile duct, obstruction and therefore jaundice can result relatively early. These tumours therefore account for a higher proportion of pancreatic resections, with a correspondingly better prognosis.

Cholangiocarcinoma

These tumours are adenocarcinomas that arise in the biliary duct system and may be intrahepatic, extrahepatic (i.e. perihilar), and distal extrahepatic. Those in the distal (intrapancreatic) portion of the biliary tree may be indistinguishable clinically and radiologically from pancreatic carcinomas, although a normal pancreatic duct on imaging is suggestive. These are relatively rare tumours with about 1000 cases in the UK per annum. Most are sporadic but inflammatory bowel disease, congenital abnormalities of the bile ducts (choledochal cysts), and chronic infection (parasitic liver fluke – *Clonorchis sinensis* – in Africa and Asia) are thought to increase the risk of developing bile duct cancer. Many proximal tumours are irresectable at presentation but early duct obstruction can again improve the prognosis for lesions situated in the distal bile duct.

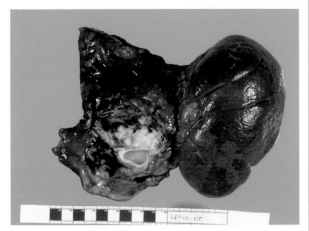

Fig. 15.11 Distal pancreatectomy / splenectomy specimen (transected) with mucinous cystic neoplasm (MCN showing cystic and solid components).

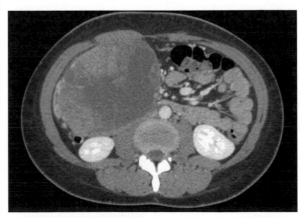

Fig. 15.12 Solid pseudopapillary tumour of the pancreatic head.

Clinical features of pancreatic neoplasms

Presenting symptoms are dependent on the site of the tumour within the pancreas. For *tumours in the head of the pancreas*, painless jaundice, associated with weight loss is the classical presentation. Involvement of the common bile duct as it runs through the head of the pancreas, results in a block to the flow of bile from the liver to the intestine, resulting in obstructive jaundice where the urine is dark and the interruption of the enterohepatic circulation results in pale stools due to the lack of bile pigments The gallbladder may become dilated and palpable (although non-tender) and this is a worrying sign in a jaundiced patient (Courvoisier's Law; Table 15.2). Intense itching may result in skin excoriation from scratching. Loss of taste, poor appetite and weight loss are common.

For *tumours of the body and tail*, biliary obstruction occurs late, and symptoms are often vague, with anorexia, weight loss and with subsequent involvement of the retroperitoneum, the development of back pain. New onset diabetes may predate the diagnosis. Delay in diagnosis is common, although increasing numbers are being diagnosed through cross sectional imaging studies. Steatorrhoea may result in initial investigations for an alteration in bowel habit. A late manifestation is a malignancy-associated hypercoagulable state, resulting in intravascular clots with vasculitis, named thrombophlebitis migrans (Trousseau's sign, Table 15.2).

Investigations and multidisciplinary management (MDM) planning

Patients should be managed by specialist multidisciplinary teams with an interest in pancreatic cancer. Transabdominal ultrasound, along with biochemical confirmation of cholestasis, is the initial investigation for the jaundiced patient, which will confirm intra- and extrahepatic biliary dilatation, exclude gallstones, and may show the mass lesion in the pancreas or liver metastases.

High quality multidetector CT scanning (Fig. 15.13), ± MR/MRCP can noninvasively define the site of the lesion and the extent of local or distant involvement. Diagnostic endoscopy may allow biopsy of an ampullary lesion. Endoscopic ultrasound can provide information on local staging, and also provide cytological confirmation of the diagnosis (EUS-FNA) without compromising resectability. Circulating tumour markers (e.g. CA 19–9) lack sufficient sensitivity and specificity for diagnosis but may be useful in the follow-up of treated patients.

Assessment of co-morbidity and fitness may be required prior to management planning at a Regional Pancreatic Multidisciplinary meeting. Early drainage of the biliary tree (ERCP/PTC), before MDM discussion is to be avoided where possible, as optimum treatment pathways may be compromised in some patients, through introduction of infection or procedure associated morbidity.

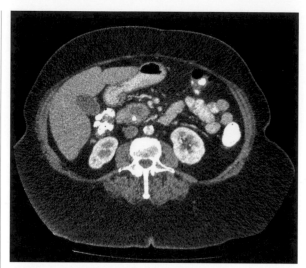

Fig. 15.13 Axial CT showing a 2 cm hypovascular lesion within the head of the pancreas, apparently clear of the mesenteric vessels. A biliary stent lies within the common bile duct.

Curative management

Surgical resection currently offers the only potential for cure in pancreatic tumours. Tumours localised to the pancreatic parenchyma, or with limited involvement of the peripancreatic fat or lymph nodes may be considered for resection. Many adenocarcinomas of the body and tail are unresectable at diagnosis, but when identified early may be removed by distal pancreatectomy and splenectomy.

For tumours sited in the head of the pancreas the standard operation is a pancreaticoduodenectomy (Whipple's procedure) (Fig. 15.14), which entails block resection of the head of the pancreas, the distal half of the stomach, the duodenum, gallbladder and common bile duct. Reconstruction is achieved by anastomoses of the pancreatic tail remnant to the jejunum (or stomach) and anastomosing the common hepatic duct and the stomach to the jejunum. The procedure used to carry a prohibitively high operative mortality, but in specialist hands this should now be less than 5%. Attempts to improve prognosis through escalating the radicality of resection by removing all of the pancreas or by extending the lymphadenectomy have proved disappointing. A standard pancreaticoduodenectomy combined with adjuvant chemotherapy, remains the standard of care, and is associated with a median survival of 24 months, although long-term cure remains a rarity. The prospects for patients with cancer of the periampullary region, distal common bile duct or duodenum are less gloomy, with 5-year survival rates ranging from 20% to 40%.

Palliative treatment

Only about 15–20% of patients are candidates for resection through a combination of advanced stage or co-morbidity. The objective is the optimization of quality of life through relief of obstructive symptoms (jaundice or duodenal obstruction), pruritus, and pain control. Effective preoperative staging has reduced the number of patients found to have inoperable disease at exploratory laparotomy, although when this occurs a double (biliary and gastric) bypass is appropriate.

Where inoperability is confirmed at the pretreatment planning meeting, surgical bypass can be avoided by achieving biliary drainage endoscopically at ERCP, or radiologically

Table 15.2 Named signs and laws in pancreatic malignancy	
Courvoisier's Law	**Trousseau's Sign**
In the presence of a non-tender palpable gallbladder, painless jaundice is unlikely to be caused by gallstones	Thrombophlebitis migrans in a patient with pancreatic carcinoma, a non-metastatic manifestation of malignancy

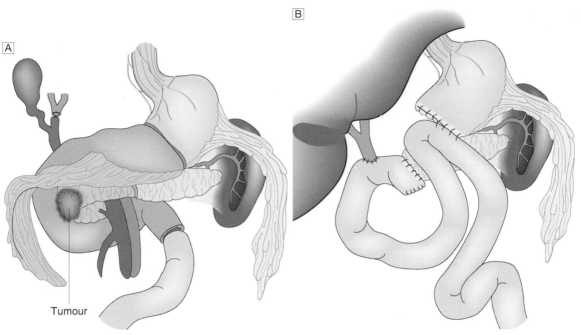

Tumour

Fig. 15.14 Classic pancreaticoduodenectomy (Kausch–Whipple).

by percutaneous transhepatic cholangiography (PTC), along with brush cytology for histological confirmation. This is particularly important if surgery is not contemplated, as a number of benign lesions (e.g. autoimmune pancreatitis, chronic pancreatitis) can masquerade as malignancy and, as discussed above, a number of pancreatic mass lesions may have a significantly better prognosis than pancreatic ductal adenocarcinoma. In those with negative brush cytology at the time of biliary drainage, cytology may be obtained by EUS-FNA. This is of importance in that quality of life can be improved through palliative chemotherapy and most oncologists will not proceed without histological evidence of malignancy.

Patients often benefit from proactive nutritional support with the addition of pancreatic exocrine supplements to alleviate steatorrhoea, dietary advice and antiemetics. Dexamethasone can be of benefit, but close glucose control is needed. Pain is often a late manifestation, but can often be effective controlled through an analgesic ladder or occasionally coeliac plexus block or thoracoscopic splanchnicectomy.

Pancreatic neuroendocrine tumours (PET)

Pancreatic neuroendocrine tumours are rare tumours (approximately 1/100 000 population/year) of which 60% are non-functioning or secrete peptides with low biological impact such as PP or neurotensin. In contrast to insulinoma, the majority of which are benign, approximately 50% of gastrinomas and the majority of non-functioning pancreatic neuroendocrine tumours are malignant (Table 15.3). They are usually sporadic but they may also appear among other features of genetic syndromes like multiple endocrine neoplasia type I or von Hippel–Lindau disease. In multiple endocrine neoplasia (MEN)1, pancreatic neuroendocrine tumours occur in 40–80% of patients and are mostly non-functioning tumours or gastrinomas. Pancreatic neuroendocrine tumours occur in 10–15% of patients with Von Hippel–Lindau (VHL) and are frequently multiple (> 30%).

Non-functioning PET

Many non-functional PETs are already metastatic by the time of diagnosis with the liver being the most common site of metastasis. Regional lymph node spread is also common, and PET may have a 5-year survival as low as 30%. Presentation is related to the mass effect of the tumour – symptoms are therefore often non-specific. Surgery with curative intent is the mainstay of treatment for localized or locoregional disease (Fig. 15.15). Non-functioning tumours should also be resected if sporadic and if > 2 cm in MEN1 or > 2–3 cm in VHL. Debulking surgery as well as other forms of local treatment like transarterial chemo-embolization or radiofrequency ablation can improve prognosis, even in patients with liver metastases. Systemic therapies have also been better defined and include radionuclide therapy against somatostatin receptors or MIBG and chemotherapy especially for poorly differentiated tumours. Cytotoxic therapy with compounds like streptozotocin, 5-fluorouracil or doxorubicin can achieve modest outcome.

Functioning PET

The functioning tumours and syndromes are named according to the hormones they produce: insulinoma, gastrinoma (most gastrinomas are found in the duodenum), VIPoma, glucagonoma, and somatostatinoma. The first two (insulinomas and gastrinomas) are the most frequent functioning pancreatic tumours. Unlike the non-functional tumours, presentation of functional PETs is more specific and related to the secretion of biologically active peptides like insulin, gastrin, glucagon, somatostatin, vasoactive intestinal polypeptide (VIP). The non-functional tumours also express and secrete peptides like neurotensin or chromogranin A, which are not active.

Insulinomas

Insulinomas arise from the beta cells within the pancreas and secrete excessive insulin. Insulinomas are benign in approximately 90% and solitary in 95% of sporadic cases. Beta cells should secrete insulin in response to an increase in blood sugar but the secretion of insulin by insulinomas is

Table 15.3 Clinical features of PETs

Tumour	Symptoms	Malignancy	Survival
Insulinoma	Confusion, sweating, dizziness, weakness, unconsciousness, relief with eating	10% of patients develop metastases	Complete resection cures most patients
Gastrinoma	Zollinger–Ellison syndrome or severe peptic ulceration and diarrhoea	Metastases develop in 60% of patients; likelihood correlated with size of primary	Complete resection results in 10-year survival of 90%; less likely if large primary
Glucagonoma	Necrolytic migratory erythema, weight loss, diabetes mellitus, stomatitis, diarrhoea	Metastases develop in 60% or more patients	More favourable with complete resection; prolonged even with liver metastases
VIPoma	Werner–Morrison syndrome of profuse watery diarrhoea with marked hypokalaemia	Metastases develop in up to 70% of patients; majority found at presentation	Complete resection with 5-year survival of 95%; with metastases, 60%
Somatostatinoma	Cholelithiasis; weight loss; diarrhoea and steatorrhoea. Diabetes mellitus	Metastases likely in about 50% of patients	Complete resection associated with 5-year survival of 95%; with metastases, 60%
Non-syndromic pancreatic neuroendocrine tumour	Symptoms from pancreatic mass and/or liver metastases	Metastases develop in up to 50% of patients	Complete resection associated with 5-year survival of at least 50%

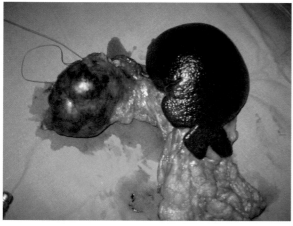

Fig. 15.15 Distal pancreatectomy / splenectomy specimen with non-functioning PET.

not properly regulated by glucose and the tumours continue to secrete insulin causing glucose levels to fall further than normal. As a result patients present with symptoms of low blood glucose (hypoglycaemia), which may be improved by eating. The diagnosis of an insulinoma is usually made biochemically: blood glucose $\leq 2.2\,\mathrm{mmol/L}$ ($40\,\mathrm{mg/dL}$), associated with an insulin level $\geq 6\,\mu U/mL$ ($36\,\mathrm{pmol/L}$), C-peptide levels $\geq 200\,\mathrm{pmol/L}$, proinsulin levels $\geq 5\,\mathrm{pmol/L}$. Further controlled testing includes the 72-hour fast, which is the criterion standard for establishing the diagnosis of insulinoma, as 98% of patients with insulinomas will develop symptomatic hypoglycaemia within 72 hours. Localization of the tumour is most commonly achieved with contrast enhanced CT and endoscopic ultrasound. The definitive treatment is surgery.

Gastrinomas

For gastrinomas (Zollinger–Ellison syndrome), two measurements are critical: fasting serum gastrin ($1000\,\mathrm{pg/ml}$) and basal gastric acid output. Fasting serum gastrin (FSG)

alone is not enough because of its lack of specificity, making it impossible to distinguish hypergastrinaemia caused by a gastrinoma from that caused by achlorhydric states (i.e. type 1 gastric NETs, use of PPIs, pernicious anaemia, atrophic gastritis). For these measures, a washout period from PPI treatment of 1–4 weeks is recommended. The 2006 European Neuroendocrine Tumour Society guidelines had cut-off values of greater than 10-fold elevation for FSG and gastric pH ≤ 2. Over 90% of gastrinomas are found in the 'gastrinoma triangle' bounded by the third part of the duodenum, the neck of the pancreas and the portahepatis. Gastrinomas are multiple in 20–40% of patients and often extra-pancreatic, with 20% found in the duodenum. Gastrinomas are frequently malignant with metastatic spread occurring to the liver and local lymph nodes. They tend to be small: 38% of pancreatic and all duodenal tumours are less than 1 cm in diameter at diagnosis. One-third of cases are associated with MEN type I in which multiplicity is the rule and there is a tendency to recurrence. Most gastrinomas are small lesions and therefore, localizing the tumour may be difficult. Investigations to localize the tumour include CT scan, octreotide scan, MRI and endoscopic ultrasonography.

Miscellaneous PETs

For VIPomas, glucagonomas, somatostatinomas, and PPomas, the biochemical markers are vasoactive intestinal peptide (VIP), glucagon, somatostatin, and PP, respectively, and the clinical features are detailed in Table 15.3. These tumours are malignant in the vast majority of patients and may present as large tumours at the time of diagnosis. Up to 70% of patients have evidence of spread of the tumour at the time of diagnosis. Aggressive surgical removal of as much tumour as possible is often indicated to relieve some of the severe symptoms that these tumours may cause because of secretion of hormones.

Multiple endocrine neoplasia type 1

Multiple endocrine neoplasia type 1 is characterized by hyperplasia and/or neoplasm of the parathyroid glands, enteropancreatic NETs, and pituitary adenomas. The gene for type 1 MEN has been localized to chromosome band 11q13. It is a tumour suppressor gene that encodes menin, a nuclear protein. Some patients do not present with all these tumours, so it has been agreed that diagnosis is made when a patient presents with two of these concomitantly. To diagnose familial MEN-1 syndrome, a first-degree relative has to manifest at least one of the tumours previously mentioned. Hyperparathyroidism occurs in about 90% of patients; endocrine pancreatic tumours in 60% of patients, usually they are small and non-functional, and the most common hormonally active ones are insulinomas or gastrinomas. In contrast to sporadic insulinoma these are multiple in 90% of MEN 1 patients. Pituitary adenomas are present in 40% of patients, and in 60% of the patients, skin manifestations can also be present. Biochemical screening for pancreatic NETs, in the presence of suspected MEN 1 syndrome, should include gastrin, insulin/pro-insulin, PP, glucagon, and CgA, which together have a sensitivity of approximately 70% that can be increased if α- and β-HCG subunits, VIP, postprandial gastrin, and PP measurements are added. It is recommended that carriers of MEN-1 mutation are screened biochemically every 1–3 years for hyperparathyroidism, prolactinoma, gastrinoma, insulinoma, and other enteropancreatic tumours. MEN 2 is not associated with pancreatic endocrine tumours.

THE SPLEEN

Surgical anatomy

The spleen is a vascular organ lying in the left upper quadrant of the abdomen alongside the 9th, 10th and 11th ribs, and is usually impalpable. It weighs 75–150 g in the adult, is between 8 cm and 13 cm in length, and is ellipsoid in shape. The convex outer surface and superior pole lies against the diaphragm, the concave inner surface is related to the fundus of the stomach, the tail of the pancreas and the upper pole of the right kidney, and its lower pole rests on the splenic flexure of the colon below. It has a fibrous capsule and, except at its hilum, is covered by peritoneum, which is reflected as supporting ligaments running to adjacent organs; the lienorenal, lienogastric and lienocolic ligaments. The phrenicocolic ligament, which runs between the splenic flexure of the colon and the under-surface of the diaphragm, provides additional support.

Arterial inflow is primarily through the tortuous splenic artery arising from the coeliac axis, which carries 40% of the splanchnic blood flow into the spleen. Venous blood drains into the portal venous system via the splenic vein. The splenic vessels are closely related to, and may run within the pancreas entering the spleen at the splenic hilum, the only part of the spleen without a peritoneal covering. The spleen has a secondary vascular inflow and outflow via the short gastric vessels that run within the lienogastric ligament to the upper part of the greater curvature of the stomach, which assume importance when the main splenic vessels are occluded through surgical division, radiological embolization or spontaneous thrombosis.

Normally, the spleen is impalpable and cannot be percussed. When enlarged, it extends downwards and medially below the costal margin. It is then best palpated bimanually, with the patient lying on the right side with the left side turned slightly forward. The distinctive notch on the antero-inferior border of the spleen may then be felt. On percussion, an enlarged spleen causes dullness over the ninth rib in the mid-axillary line. Splenomegaly is normally confirmed by abdominal ultrasound or CT scan.

Physiology

Circulatory filtration

The cut surface of the spleen reveals areas of red and white pulp surrounded by fibrous trabeculae. The red pulp is a loose honeycomb of reticular tissue that contains the splenic sinusoids, lined by macrophages, and blood vessels pass into the pulp along the trabeculae. As erythrocytes age, the normal lifespan being about 120 days, the cell membrane becomes less flexible and because erythrocytes are required to deform to pass through the sinusoids, senescent cells being trapped within the spleen and therefore removed from the circulating population of cells. Following phagocytosis iron is split from the haem portion, and stored as haemosiderin before being transported to the bone marrow bound to transferrin to be incorporated into a new population of erythrocytes.

Erythrocytes move in and out of the pulp tissue, so that 1% of the body's red cells and 20–30% of its platelets are sequestrated at any given moment. Unlike in some mammals (e.g. dogs), in humans the spleen is not a site of significant blood pooling except in pathological conditions with splenomegaly, where the spleen may contain more than a litre of blood. Following splenectomy, there is an increased number of mis-shapen red cells in the peripheral blood, some containing nuclear remnants (Howell-Jolly bodies) and others containing clumps of iron (siderocytes).

Immunological function

The spleen is an important site for promoting both cell-mediated and humoral immunity. The spleen represents the largest aggregation (~25%) of lymphoid tissue in the body forming the white pulp, which consists of lymphoid follicles (Malpighian bodies) and lymphatic tissue, containing lymphocytes, macrophages and plasma cells, these cells having migrated from the bone marrow and 30–50% of them are thymus-dependent. Antigens entering the spleen are engulfed by macrophages, promoting antigen presentation, with subsequent antibody production in the germinal centres. Following splenectomy, immunological responses are impaired.

Haemopoiesis

In utero in the second and third trimester the spleen is an important source of erythrocyte and granulocyte production for the fetus. Although at birth this function usually ceases, in some disease processes with a high turnover of erythrocytes the spleen may continue to contribute to this process (extramedullary haemopoiesis).

Technique of splenectomy

Preoperative preparation

As many of the indications (Table 15.4) are for haematological conditions, preparation requires multidisciplinary management to ensure preoperative optimization of full blood count and coagulation status, and usually involves a further course of steroids or administration of blood products. Vaccines are best administered two weeks before surgery.

Open technique

For an elective splenectomy, access is usually gained via a left subcostal incision. Rarely, a thoracoabdominal incision is necessary to remove a large spleen. A normal-sized

15

229

15

Table 15.4 **Indications for splenectomy.**

Traumatic	Blunt / penetrating trauma
	Iatrogenic intraoperative / endoscopic trauma
Haematological	The purpuras
	Haemolytic anaemia
	Hypersplenism
	Proliferative disease
Miscellaneous	Distal pancreatectomy (for benign or malignant disease)
	Proximal gastrectomy
	Splenorenal shunt

non-adherent spleen is approached by initial division of the diaphragmatic attachments and the lienorenal ligament allowing the spleen to be folded forward, improving access to the organ. Division of the short gastric vessels exposes the splenic hilum and the vessels divided either between ligatures or using a vascular stapling device, taking care to avoid injury to the tail of the pancreas. Division of the remaining peritoneal attachments allows removal of the organ.

When the spleen is enlarged or adherent to surrounding organs or the diaphragm, preliminary mobilization may not be possible and the vascular pedicle is dissected first. Alternatively, the splenic artery may first be ligated in continuity so that the spleen shrinks in size, allowing it to be mobilized and the vessels to be ligated close to the splenic hilum. Drains are not routinely used (as they may actually increase the incidence of subphrenic sepsis), unless there is a possibility that the tail of the pancreas has been injured or there is persistent oozing due to a coagulation defect.

Laparoscopic splenectomy

Laparoscopic splenectomy is now favoured by many surgeons, and a preoperative estimation of splenic size (15 cm longitudinal length) is helpful in ensuring a minimally invasive approach is appropriate. Mobilization is facilitated by a right decubitus position with a reverse Trendelenberg tilt. An epigastric midline cutdown with insertion of a blunt port, followed by left subcostal dissection ports triangulating on the splenic hilum. The splenic flexure is mobilized to expose the inferior pole of the spleen, access to the short gastric vessels can be facilitated by leaving the diaphragmatic attachments intact, the stomach falling away from the spleen on division of the short gastric. Having exposed the splenic hilum, the splenic vessels are divided using a vascular cartridge laparoscopic stapling device, taking care to avoid injury to the tail of the pancreas. The remaining peritoneal attachments can them be divided, freeing the organ. The spleen is then placed in an impervious bag specifically designed for the removal of tissue and the open ends of the bag brought out beyond the abdominal surface through a slightly extended port site. The spleen is then morcellated within the bag and removed piecemeal.

Postoperative course and complications

Left lower lobe collapse or atelectasis is the most frequent complication of splenectomy but usually responds to conservative measures. Any bleeding tendency increases the likelihood of postoperative haemorrhage, but meticulous haemostasis at the time of surgery and continued correction of coagulation defects are usually preventative. Serum amylase levels should be monitored in the immediate postoperative period, since pancreatitis may result from intraoperative manipulation of the pancreatic tail during mobilization of the spleen. Pancreatic or gastric fistula formation is fortunately uncommon, but can occur from inadvertent injury to either organ. Subphrenic abscess may arise from pancreatic or gastric injury, inadequate haemostasis or inappropriate use of drains.

Traumatic splenectomy

In the majority of situations which require an emergency splenectomy for trauma (Table 15.5), the potential for injury is relatively obvious through a history of blunt or penetrating trauma. Delayed presentation, an unusual mechanism (e.g. post-colonoscopy) or the absence of a history through intoxication make a high index of suspicion essential. In addition, in patients with splenic enlargement, the mechanism may be relatively trivial. The cardinal features are those of significant blood loss, and local signs of peritoneal irritation (peritonitis or left shoulder tip pain).

Patients that do not respond to initial resuscitation require an emergency laparotomy and usually a splenectomy along with a careful exploratory laparotomy to exclude injury to other structures. In the responding patient, cross-sectional imaging is advised.

Approximately 80% of splenic injuries may be managed conservatively, and of these the requirement for intervention is apparent within 72 hours in 95%. In the unstable patient, control of haemorrhage and restoration of circulating volume are paramount and consideration regarding organ preservation is of secondary importance. Unlike an elective splenectomy a midline laparotomy is usually performed with packing of the left upper quadrant which will normally control the splenic haemorrhage to allow the remainder of the abdomen to be examined. Having excluded other sources of haemorrhage, if examination of the spleen reveals bleeding from the splenic hilum, preservation is not appropriate and a splenectomy should be performed.

Splenic conservation

Because of the immunologic function of the spleen, interest over the last century has turned to salvage of the spleen rather than splenectomy. Minor lacerations may respond to topical haemostatic agents (Floseal, Baxter Healthcare, UK; or Surgicel, Johnson & Johnson, UK) coupled with enhanced haemostatic technology (argon diathermy, harmonic scalpel,

Table 15.5 **The American Association for the Surgery of Trauma classification of splenic trauma.**

Grade	Injury	Description
I	Haematoma	Subcapsular, < 10% of surface area
	Laceration	Capsular tear < 1 cm parenchymal depth
II	Haematoma	Subcapsular, 10–50% of surface area, Intraparenchymal, < 5 cm in diameter
	Laceration	1–3 cm parenchymal depth which does not involve a trabecular vessel
III	Haematoma	Subcapsular, > 50% of surface area, or expanding Ruptured subcapsular or parenchymal haematoma
	Laceration	Intraparenchymal haematoma > 5 cm or expanding
IV	Laceration	Laceration involving segmental or hilar vessels producing major devascularization (> 25% of spleen)
V	Laceration Vascular	Massive disruption of pancreatic head Hilar vascular injury which devascularizes spleen

Ethicon UK; or Ligasure, Covidien, UK) may allow haemorrhage to be controlled or a partial splenectomy to be performed. The role of interventional radiological embolization of the splenic artery has been reported, however it is dependent on the availability of appropriately skilled radiologists. As the majority of patients can be managed conservatively without embolization, care needs to be taken that in striving to avoid laparotomy inappropriate delay in haemostasis does not occur in those with ongoing bleeding. In those who are being managed conservatively, awareness and ongoing careful observation are critical, as 'delayed rupture' of a subcapsular haematoma can occur.

Indications for splenectomy (non-traumatic)

Although the recommendation to remove the spleen often comes from the haematologist, the surgeon must be aware of the indications for splenectomy and the criteria that should be fulfilled before accepting a patient for operation. The common indications are outlined below.

The purpuras

Idiopathic thrombocytopenic purpura (ITP)

There are two types of ITP. One type affects children, and the other type affects adults. In children, the usual age for getting ITP is 2–4 years, may be post-viral and most recover with no treatment. Most adults with ITP are young women, but it can occur in anyone. IgG antibody develops against platelet membrane antigen, resulting in the premature destruction of platelets. The low platelet count is associated with reactive megakaryocytosis within the bone marrow. Epistaxis, bleeding from the GI tract and other sites is associated with petechiae and ecchymoses. Platelet counts are below $50 \times 10^9/l$, and bleeding time is prolonged but clotting time is normal. The spleen is usually not overly enlarged, making it particularly suitable for laparoscopic removal.

Treatment is indicated in patients with platelet counts less than $20–30 \times 10^9/l$ and in patients who have counts less than $50 \times 10^9/l$ and have substantial mucous membrane bleeding (or risk factors for bleeding, such as hypertension, peptic ulcer disease, or the potential for substantial trauma to the body). Initial therapy with glucocorticoids, such as prednisone, is appropriate and may be augmented with intravenous immunoglobulin, and platelet transfusions. In patients with persistent thrombocytopenia (< $30 \times 10^9/l$ after 4–6 weeks of medical treatment) splenectomy is often appropriate.

Secondary thrombocytopenia

Secondary thrombocytopenia may occur secondary to a number of conditions and comprises about 40% of all cases of TTP. Predisposing factors include cancer, pregnancy, drugs (e.g. cyclosporine), HIV infection and bone marrow transplantation. Splenectomy is in general contraindicated in secondary purpuras, although it may be advised if hypersplenism is associated with symptomatic secondary thrombocytopenia.

Haemolytic anaemias

Hereditary spherocytosis

In this autosomal dominant disorder, the red blood cells are spherical rather than biconcave, are fragile, and are destroyed when trapped within the splenic sinusoids in the spleen. Excess haemolysis results in anaemia, jaundice and splenic enlargement. It is a disease of remissions and relapses, with 'haemolytic crises' requiring transfusion. Pigment gallstones occur in 30–60% of cases. Mild HS can be managed without folate supplements and does not require splenectomy. Moderately and severely affected individuals are likely to benefit from splenectomy which should be performed after the age of 6 years and with appropriate counselling about the infection risk. If gallstones are present, cholecystectomy is carried out simultaneously.

Acquired haemolytic anaemias

Excess haemolysis may occur following exposure to agents such as chemicals, drugs or infection, and with extensive burns, or it may be an immune phenomenon (e.g. *Mycoplasma pneumoniae* infection, SLE, chronic lymphatic leukaemia). In the latter, the red cells are coated with an autoantibody, which can be detected by agglutination when antihuman globulin is added to a suspension of the patient's erythrocytes (positive Coombs' test). Treatment consists of steroid therapy. Splenectomy is indicated if treatment fails from the outset or if there is a fall in the haemoglobin following the reduction or cessation of steroids.

Hypersplenism

This syndrome consists of splenomegaly and pancytopenia in the presence of an apparently normal bone marrow and the absence of an autoimmune disorder. There is sequestration and destruction of blood cells in the spleen, affecting predominantly white cells and platelets. Hypersplenism may complicate a number of inflammatory conditions (e.g. rheumatoid arthritis), infections (e.g. malaria), and myeloproliferative and lymphoproliferative disorders. In portal hypertension, splenic congestion frequently leads to splenomegaly and hypersplenism.

The enlarged spleen results in an expansion of the total blood volume to fill the increased vascular spaces of the enlarged spleen with pooling of cells and increased destruction within the sinusioids. This results in anaemia, leucopenia and thrombocytopenia, with reticulocytosis and leucoerythroblastosis in the marrow. Increased haemoglobin turnover results in increased amounts of urobilinogen in the urine. Splenectomy may be appropriate but the potential morbidity, the risks of late septic complications and the prognosis of the underlying cause of the hypersplenism require to be balanced with the potential alleviation of the pancytopenia.

Segmental portal hypertension

A localized form of portal hypertension associated with hypersplenism and oesophagogastric varices may follow occlusion of the splenic vein. Thrombosis may result from acute or chronic pancreatitis, or the vessel may become compromised by direct invasion from a carcinoma of the pancreas. Gastric varices are particularly prominent in this condition and often communicate directly with short gastric veins. Acute variceal haemorrhage in this situation is however relatively rare but may be best managed by splenectomy with ligation of the vessels on the greater curvature of the stomach, as endoscopic control can be difficult. Recurrent haemorrhage is unusual following surgery and the prognosis is favourable, given that there is often no associated liver disease.

Proliferative disorders

Myelofibrosis

It is recognized that this condition is due to an abnormal proliferation of mesenchymal elements in the bone marrow, spleen, liver and lymph nodes, and that extramedullary haemopoiesis occurs at many sites. Most patients present over the age of 50 years. The spleen may be grossly enlarged and splenic infarcts may occur. Splenectomy decreases transfusion requirements and, by relieving the discomfort of a grossly enlarged spleen, also improves symptoms.

15

Lymphomas

In non-Hodgkin's lymphoma, splenectomy is only indicated in the rare event that a primary neoplasm is confined to the spleen or, in both myelo- and lymphoproliferative conditions, to reduce transfusion requirements when hypersplenism is a problem.

Other tumours

Of the other rare tumours, haemangiomas (capillary or cavernous) may reach sufficient size to cause splenic enlargement, with a consumptive coagulopathy and haemorrhagic tendency.

Miscellaneous conditions

Cysts of the spleen

Cysts of the spleen are uncommon. They are usually single but occasionally multiple. *Congenital* cysts are due to an embryonic defect and result in a dermoid-like lesion. *Degenerative* cysts result from liquefaction of an infarct or haematoma. There may be a past history of minor trauma. The wall is fibrous and often calcified, and the cyst is filled with brownish fluid or paste-like material. Pancreatic pseudocysts may extend to involve the spleen and *parasitic* cysts may occur due to infection with *Echinococcus granulosus* (hydatid disease). Splenic cysts normally cause no symptoms and are often discovered fortuitously. Symptomatic cysts may present with left upper quadrant pain radiating to the back or left shoulder. The lesion may be recognized by CT or ultrasound scan, investigations that are usually sufficient to characterize the nature of the cyst. Intervention is not indicated for small congenital or degenerative cysts. Large symptomatic cysts are treated by partial or complete splenectomy.

Splenic infarct

Splenic infarct may present with acute onset of left upper quadrant pain in a patient with known hypersplenism. Asymptomatic infarcts may be observed in patients following a severe attack of pancreatitis or following a spleen-preserving distal pancreatectomy. These may resolve with the formation of a splenic cyst, but do not require surgical intervention.

Abscess of the spleen

A splenic abscess is rare. It should be suspected when progressive splenic enlargement is associated with bacteraemia and abscess formation at other sites. Splenectomy, although desirable, may not prove feasible and drainage may be preferable.

Splenic artery aneurysm

This may occur primarily as a complication of atherosclerosis in elderly patients where the calcified wall of the aneurysm may be visible on X-ray or secondary to acute or chronic pancreatitis. The presence of a small, uncomplicated primary aneurysm is not necessarily an indication for intervention, particularly as they often affect elderly, frail patients. Bleeding can occur, however, and angiography is the treatment of choice. Bleeding is more common in secondary aneurysms and again the treatment of choice is radiological if possible as surgery in an actively bleeding patient is associated with a high mortality rate.

Other indications for splenectomy

Removal of the spleen may be required as part of other surgical procedures, such as distal pancreatectomy and radical gastrectomy for carcinoma and, less frequently, for certain types of splenorenal shunt.

Post-splenectomy immunization

Loss of lymphoid tissue reduces immune activity and impairs the response to bacteraemia. The risk of overwhelming post-splenectomy sepsis is greatest when splenectomy is performed in childhood.

The British Committee for Standards in Haematology recommends that all splenectomized patients and those with functional hyposplenism should receive pneumococcal immunization and patients not previously immunized should receive haemophilus influenza type b vaccine. Patients not previously immunized should receive meningococcal group C conjugate vaccine. Influenza immunization should be given. Life long prophylactic antibiotics are still recommended (oral phenoxymethylpenicillin or erythromycin). Elective splenectomy should be preceded by the administration of vaccines 2–3weeks prior to surgery, but are still effective if given postoperatively.

M.G. Dunlop

16

The small and large intestine

CHAPTER CONTENTS

INTRODUCTION

Disorders of the intestine are common in the general population. Infective diarrhoea most commonly affects the young; inflammatory conditions those in early and middle adulthood; cancer, diverticular disease and ischaemia in middle and old age. Many intestinal disorders present with similar symptoms, meaning that it is not possible to differentiate diagnoses on clinical assessment alone. Thus, self-resolving disorders – in which watchful waiting is appropriate – may be difficult to distinguish from those that require rapid investigation and active management. Furthermore investigation frequently involves investigations such as colonoscopy and radiation exposure which can be potentially harmful. Careful history and examination, informed by knowledge of the hierarchy of likely age-related diagnoses is essential when assessing patients with intestinal problems.

SURGICAL ANATOMY AND PHYSIOLOGY

Anatomy and function of the small intestine

The small bowel extends from the pylorus to the ileocaecal valve and ranges in length from 3 to 9 metres. The jejunum, which comprises two-fifths of the small intestine, is of wider calibre than the ileum, and the diameter of the gut lumen narrows progressively from the duodenojejunal flexure to the ileocaecal valve. The small bowel mucosa is supported on a

 SUMMARY BOX 16.1

Clinical assessment of a patient with gastrointestinal symptoms

- Gastrointestinal symptoms are very common
- Most symptoms are due to self-resolving illness
- Patient age is an important factor when considering the differential diagnoses
- Duration of symptoms is an important arbiter of the need for investigation
- Careful assessment of the nature and severity of symptoms is important and may indicate peritonitis, obstruction or severe inflammation
- Symptoms of self-resolving intestinal disorders that are managed conservatively are often indistinguishable from major problems
- Investigation usually involves endoscopy and imaging, as well as stool culture.

strong submucosa and comprises a single layer of columnar cells in a villiform structure that dramatically increases the absorptive surface area. Columnar glandular epithelium is interspersed with mucus-secreting cells, Paneth cells and amine precursor uptake and decarboxylation (APUD) cells derived from the neural crest. Between the inner layer of circular muscle and the outer longitudinal layer runs Auerbach's myenteric plexus, which comprises vagal parasympathetic fibres and sympathetic fibres from the lesser and greater splanchnic nerves. This plexus controls orderly propulsive contractions of the muscular layers of the gut

233

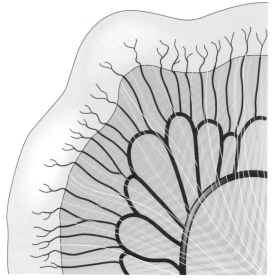

Fig. 16.1 Arterial arcades supplying the small intestine from the superior mesenteric artery.

wall. The sympathetic nervous system mediates the sensation of visceral pain, and a submucosal plexus (Meissner's plexus) of autonomic nerves innervates the glandular cells in the epithelium.

The small intestine is supplied by the superior mesenteric artery, which runs in the root of the small bowel mesentery, supplying the bowel by a series of arterial arcades (Fig. 16.1). These midgut vessels communicate with the coeliac axis through the pancreaticoduodenal arcade. The superior mesenteric supply also communicates with that of the inferior mesenteric artery by contributing to the colonic marginal artery through the left branch of the middle colic artery, which joins to the ascending branch of the left colic artery. Venous blood drains via the superior mesenteric vein to the portal vein. Lymphoid aggregates in the submucosa (Peyer's patches) are more numerous in the ileum, and lymph drains to regional nodes in the root of the mesentery before passing to the cisterna chyli.

The principal function of the small bowel is absorption of amino acids, short peptides, sugars and fats, as well as minerals, vitamins and other micronutrients. Its secretory and digestive functions supplement those of the upper gastrointestinal tract. The mucosa is thrown into circular folds (plicae semilunares) and is carpeted by finger-like villi, giving an absorptive area of 200–500 m². Some 5–8 litres of fluid enter the jejunum each day, of which only 1–2 litres normally pass to the colon.

Anatomy and function of the large intestine and appendix

The principle function of the large intestine is water absorption, particularly the proximal colon. The left colon and rectum act as a reservoir until defaecation is appropriate. Mucus is secreted as a lubricant. The large bowel mucosa consists of columnar epithelium interspersed with mucus-secreting goblet cells. The villi are shorter than those of the small intestine, and crypts pass down to the muscularis mucosa, which is supported by a strong submucosa. The large bowel extends from the ileocaecal valve to the upper anal canal (approximately 1.6 metres). The caecum is a blind pouch at the most proximal part of the large bowel.

The transverse and sigmoid colon are mobile because they have a mesentery, whereas ascending and descending colon are only partially peritonealized. The true rectum is demarcated by coalescence of the taeniae coli of the sigmoid colon to form a continuous outer muscular tube. The upper third of the rectum has peritoneal cover on its front and sides, the middle third is peritonealized only anteriorly and the lower third is wholly extraperitoneal.

The inferior and superior mesenteric arteries supply the colon and anastomose via a marginal artery (Fig. 16.2) that allows collateral supply in the event of arterial occlusion, but at the splenic flexure this arterial communication may be tenuous. The superior rectal artery is the continuation of the inferior mesenteric artery, supplying the rectum and anastomosing with the middle and inferior rectal arteries (branches of the internal iliac arteries). The inferior mesenteric vein drains into the splenic vein. Lymph channels run along the course of the arterial supply, draining to epicolic and paracolic nodes close to the bowel wall, and to regional nodes at the origin of the superior and inferior mesenteric vessels (Fig. 16.2). Lymph from the rectum drains upwards to superior rectal and inferior mesenteric nodes, whereas anal canal lymph drains to inguinal nodes. Knowledge of the lymphatic drainage has considerable relevance to surgical lymphadenectomy performed as part of radical cancer clearance, as well as to radiotherapy for rectal and anal cancers.

The appendix is lined by colonic epithelium but has no known function in humans. The submucosa contains prominent lymphoid follicles in childhood that regress in adolescence. In older patients, the lumen may be obliterated by fibrosis. The appendix projects from the medial wall of the caecum some 2 cm below the ileocaecal junction as the taeniae coli converge on the root of the appendix.

CLINICAL ASSESSMENT OF THE SMALL AND LARGE INTESTINE

History

Painful contraction of the midgut (supplied by the superior mesenteric artery: small bowel, right and part transverse colon) due to obstruction or inflammation results in periumbilical colic. Disorders affecting the large bowel, i.e. hindgut (supplied by the inferior mesenteric artery: from distal transverse colon to rectum), are frequently associated with ill-defined lower abdominal colicky pain. Nausea, vomiting and pain are early and predominant features of many small bowel disorders, particularly obstruction. In contrast, large bowel conditions may present with poorly defined features including abdominal distension and altered bowel habit; vomiting is a late feature. Normal bowel frequency ranges from one motion in 3 days, up to 3 motions/day. The passage of blood or mucus per rectum is a common feature of large bowel disease. It is important to differentiate 'outlet-type' bleeding from sinister blood loss, when the blood is mixed with the stool and there may be associated altered bowel habit or tenesmus. Outlet bleeding is typically bright red and may be present only on toilet paper or spattered in the pan, separate from the stool. There may be associated perianal pain, due to fissure or prolapsed piles. Blood originating from the distal bowel is usually bright red, whereas blood coming from the upper gastrointestinal tract is usually altered by gut bacteria and becomes black (melaena). Weight loss, malaise and anaemia are common non-specific features of intestinal disease.

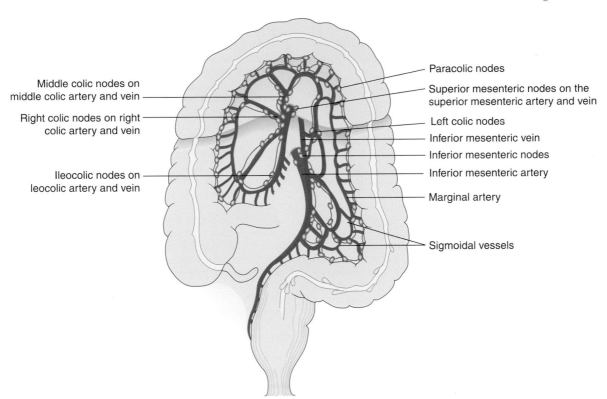

Middle colic nodes on middle colic artery and vein

Right colic nodes on right colic artery and vein

Ileocolic nodes on leocolic artery and vein

Paracolic nodes

Superior mesenteric nodes on the superior mesenteric artery and vein

Left colic nodes

Inferior mesenteric vein

Inferior mesenteric nodes

Inferior mesenteric artery

Marginal artery

Sigmoidal vessels

16

Fig. 16.2 Blood supply of the large intestine from the branches of the superior and inferior mesenteric arteries, with the lymphatic drainage of the colon and rectum.

Examination

The oral mucous membrane, hands, fingernails, eyes and conjunctiva should be inspected. Examination of the abdomen may reveal distension, a mass or visible peristalsis. In thin subjects, the caecum is often palpable, and the descending and sigmoid colon may be palpable when loaded with faeces. Hepatomegaly due to metastatic disease should be excluded. Abdominal auscultation determines the presence and pitch of bowel sounds and occasionally reveals an arterial bruit. Digital rectal examination is essential to detect a tumour and may also reveal blood or mucus. In patients with lower gastrointestinal symptoms, there is no rationale for checking the faeces for occult blood, as the sensitivity of the guaiac faecal occult blood (FOB) test is low. Investigation should not be influenced by FOB testing in the assessment of *symptomatic* patients.

Investigation of the luminal gastrointestinal tract

Investigation of diarrhoeal illnesses should include stool culture with sensitivities, tests for *Clostridium difficile* toxin as well as cysts, ova and parasites. Imaging modalities for small bowel investigation comprise plain radiography, magnetic resonance imaging (MRI) enteroclysis, barium follow-through, small bowel enema, computed tomography (CT), fibreoptic enteroscopy, capsule video-endoscopy, labelled white cell radionuclide scanning and labelled red cell radionuclide scanning. The terminal ileum can be inspected at colonoscopy, double-contrast barium enema frequently allows visualization of the terminal ileum, and a pneumocolon technique can also be used with barium follow-through to obtain double-contrast views of the terminal ileum. Duodenal biopsy undertaken at upper gastrointestinal video-endoscopy to identify the characteristic subtotal villous atrophy is the gold standard investigation of suspected coeliac disease. However, coeliac disease is frequently diagnosed by serum ELISA assays for auto-antibodies, including anti-endomysial, IgA anti-gliadin or tissue transglutaminase (tTG) antibodies. Tests of absorptive capacity are now rarely used. Bacterial overgrowth can be assessed using the glucose breath test, ^{14}C-xylose and ^{14}C-glycocholate breath tests. Small bowel aspiration can be carried out by nasojejunal tube or at enteroscopy for bacterial culture. Faecal calprotectin is a nonspecific test of intestinal inflammation that can be used to monitor inflammatory bowel disease activity.

Direct inspection of the large bowel includes proctoscopy, rigid sigmoidoscopy, flexible sigmoidoscopy and colonoscopy. These techniques allow biopsy and snare removal of colorectal polyps using cauterizing diathermy. Plain radiography is used extensively in the emergency situation but is seldom of value in elective investigation. CT double contrast radiography of the large bowel has largely superseded double contrast barium enema to allow inspection of the mucosa. CT also has considerable utility in the assessment of the acute abdomen. CT of chest, abdomen and pelvis is routinely used in staging of colon and rectal cancer, along with MRI for rectal cancer. Positron emission tomography (PET) after administering a fluoride[18] labelled tracer (fluorodeoxyglucose) that is metabolized by tumours (FDG-PET CT) has recently been introduced, although it is generally reserved for staging of complex colorectal cancer cases being considered for more major multiorgan resections. Colonic transit can be assessed in cases of suspected megacolon or slow-transit constipation by administering radio-opaque markers to estimate large bowel transit.

235

16

PRINCIPLES OF OPERATIVE INTESTINAL SURGERY

The crucial role of the small bowel in maintaining nutrition requires that resectional surgery should aim to retain the maximum possible length of bowel. Ileocaecal resection for Crohn's disease may result in gallstone formation and megaloblastic anaemia, owing to poor absorption of bile salts and vitamin B_{12}. Conversely, loss of the entire large bowel can be tolerated with little impact on nutritional status, but occasionally water and salt depletion can occur, especially in hot climates.

Small intestinal anastomoses heal well, owing to their excellent blood supply and rich submucosal arteriolar plexus. Small bowel content clears after 12 hours of fasting and so no specific bowel preparation, apart from fasting, is required for planned small bowel resection. The large intestine microcirculation consists of a series of small end-arteries, which, combined with the presence of faeces with a high density of bacterial colonization, results in poor anastomotic healing compared to those of the small intestine. This produces a higher anastomotic leak rate for colocolic or colorectal anastomoses.

In the emergency setting there is an increased risk of anastomotic leakage and so there is a lower threshold for the formation of a stoma. In specialist centres, every effort is made to reconstitute large bowel continuity in both elective and emergency resectional surgery. In emergency surgery for left-sided colonic obstruction or perforation, a total colectomy with anastomosis of the ileum to the rectum may be considered to avoid a colorectal anastomosis in the presence of faecal loading. Segmental left-sided resection and the formation of a colostomy (Hartmann's operation) avoids an anastomosis, but many specialist colorectal surgeons prefer left-sided resection with primary anastomosis.

There has been a move away from mechanical bowel preparation for elective large bowel resections because of lack of beneficial effect in research trials. Low-residue diet prior to surgery has an important place, while antibiotic prophylaxis is essential, comprising a single dose of a broad-spectrum antibiotic to cover coliform bacteria, in combination with metronidazole to cover anaerobic bacteria.

DISORDERS OF THE APPENDIX

Appendicitis

Acute appendicitis remains the most common acute abdominal emergency in childhood, adolescence and early adult life and is discussed in Chapter 12.

Appendiceal tumours

Benign tumours of the appendix

The appendix is the most common site for carcinoid tumours, which arise from argentaffin cells of the APUD system and are usually distinct yellow submucosal lesions located near the tip of the appendix. They account for 85% of all appendiceal tumours and are found in 0.5% of all appendices removed surgically. The vast majority are benign, but tumours larger than 2 cm can infiltrate the wall of the appendix and spread to the mesenteric and regional lymph glands. It is very rare for appendiceal carcinoid tumours to give rise to liver metastases and the carcinoid syndrome. Appendicectomy is sufficient treatment for most appendiceal carcinoid tumours, but right hemicolectomy is necessary if the tumour is larger than 2 cm, if it involves the caecum, or if the lymph nodes are affected

Benign tumours of the appendix include adenoma and cystadenoma. A mucocoele of the appendix may be confused with a tumour and arises due to chronic obstruction of the appendix base and accumulation of mucin in the lumen. Such simple mucocoeles are cured by appendicectomy.

Pseudomyxoma peritonei

This rare condition (~50 new cases per year in the UK) results from seeding of the peritoneal cavity with mucus-secreting cells from a mucin-secreting cystadenoma of the appendix. The resultant peritoneal tumour has a low mitotic rate but causes pressure symptoms owing to the amount of mucin produced. In a substantial proportion of cases, death results from the need for repeated excisions to palliate symptoms. Occasionally, the underlying basis of the condition is a true malignant mucus-secreting adenocarcinoma of the appendix. Median survival is 2.5 years and few patients are alive at 5 years. Surgical debulking is frequently necessary but rarely curative, and the lesions respond poorly to chemotherapy and radiotherapy. Surgical debaulking and peritoneal stripping along with intra-peritoneal instillation of hot chemotherapy has been used with some success.

Adenocarcinoma of appendix

This is an uncommon, but highly malignant, neoplasm that frequently presents with involved regional lymph nodes at diagnosis. The clinical presentation may mimic acute appendicitis or appendix mass. Right hemicolectomy is the treatment of choice, even in cases where the diagnosis is only apparent at histological assessment of an appendicectomy specimen. In cases with involved lymph nodes, adjuvant chemotherapy with standard large bowel regimens (see below) should be considered. Appendix adenocarcinoma often affects younger patients, and may arise in association with the autosomal dominant Lynch syndrome (see below).

 SUMMARY BOX 16.2

Tumours of the appendix

- Around 85% of all appendiceal tumours are carcinoids, the appendix being the most common site of carcinoid tumour in the gastrointestinal tract
- Carcinoid tumours are found in 0.5% of surgically removed appendices
- Size > 2 cm indicates increased risk of malignancy, but lymph node involvement is rare and metastases are extremely rare
- Appendix adenocarcinoma is rare and may be associated with hereditary non-polyposis colorectal cancer (HNPCC)
- Mucin-secreting cystadenoma, if ruptured, may lead to pseudomyxoma peritonei
- Pseudomyxoma peritonei is a rare, capricious condition that causes pressure symptoms on intestine and other intra-abdominal organs, and for which there is no curative therapy.

INFLAMMATORY BOWEL DISEASE

In view of the similarities in clinical presentation and in some aspects of management, it is useful to discuss Crohn's disease and ulcerative colitis together (Table 16.1). Ulcerative colitis affects the colon and rectum exclusively, whereas Crohn's disease may affect any part of the gastrointestinal tract. Inflammation is restricted to the mucosa in ulcerative

Table 16.1 Clinical features of Crohn's disease and ulcerative colitis.

	Crohn's disease	Ulcerative colitis
Incidence	5–7 per 100 000 and rising	10 per 100 000 and static
Extent	May involve entire gastrointestinal tract	Limited to large bowel
Rectal involvement	Variable	Almost invariable
Disease continuity	Discontinuous (skip lesions)	Continuous
Depth of inflammation	Transmural	Mucosal
Macroscopic appearance of mucosa	Cobblestone, discrete deep ulcers and fissures	Multiple small ulcers, pseudopolyps
Histological features	Transmural inflammation, granulomas (50%)	Crypt abscesses, submocosal chronic inflammatory cell infiltrate, crypt architectural distortion, goblet cell depletion, no granulomas
Presence of perianal disease	75% of cases with large bowel disease; 25% of cases with small bowel disease	25% of cases
Frequency of fistula	10–20% of cases	Uncommon
Colorectal cancer risk	Elevated risk (relative risk = 2.5) in colonic disease	25% risk over 30 years for pancolitis
Relationship with smoking	Increased risk, greater disease severity, increased risk of relapse and need for surgery	Protective, first attack may be preceded by smoking cessation within 6 months

16

colitis but transmural inflammation is a hallmark of Crohn's disease. There are also important implications for prognosis, as surgery for ulcerative colitis is curative, whereas Crohn's disease frequently follows a relapsing course, despite medical or surgical intervention.

Crohn's disease

Although originally described as a disease affecting the terminal ileum, any part of the gastrointestinal tract can be involved, from mouth to anus. In 50% of cases both small and large bowel are involved, whereas in 25% of cases large bowel alone is affected. The incidence is increasing in developed countries and the annual incidence rate is currently 5–7 cases per 100 000 in the UK population. At the time of initial clinical presentation, the features of Crohn's disease may be indistinguishable from those of ulcerative colitis. Indeed, in cases of colonic Crohn's disease, it may be difficult to differentiate the two conditions, even after resection and histological assessment.

Cigarette smoking is the single most important risk factor for developing the disease, and is associated with increased disease severity and frequency of relapse, as well as the need for surgical intervention. However there is a substantial heritable component to the disease. There is also evidence for the involvement of immunological factors and the gut bacterial flora in the pathogenesis of Crohn's disease. Recently, over 30 genetic loci have been identified that each contribute a small effect in host–bacteria interaction. These include CARD15 (NOD2), dysregulation of adaptive immunity (*IL23R*), and deficient autophagy (*ATG16L1*, *IRGM*).

Pathology

Macroscopically, Crohn's disease produces a cobblestone appearance, in which oedematous islands of mucosa are separated by crevices or fissures; these can extend through all coats of the bowel wall. Serpiginous ulceration is common so that fibrosis may result in multiple strictures of varying length. Multiple areas of inflammation are common with intervening normal bowel (skip lesions, Fig. 16.3). Full-thickness involvement of the bowel wall leads to serosal inflammation, adhesion to neighbouring structures, and

sinus or fistula formation. Microscopically, there are deep fissuring ulcers, oedema and inflammatory cell infiltrates with foci of lymphocytes and non-caseating granulomas in 50% of cases.

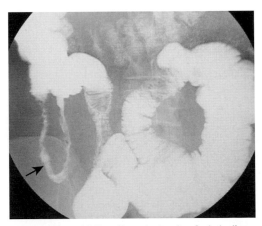

Fig. 16.3 Small bowel follow-through showing Crohn's disease strictures (arrow indicates long stricture).

Clinical features

Crohn's disease is a chronic disorder with exacerbations, remissions and a varied clinical presentation. Continuous or episodic diarrhoea is associated with recurring abdominal pain and tenderness, lassitude and fever. Declining general health, malabsorption and weight loss, with failure to thrive and to reach developmental milestones, are common in affected children.

Examination may reveal malnutrition and there may be a palpable abdominal mass. There may be features of subacute intestinal obstruction, and this may be due to active disease, stricturing of 'burnt-out' disease, or adhesions from previous surgical intervention. Fistula formation occurs in 20% of patients with small *and* large bowel disease, but less in those with disease restricted to the large bowel. Fistulae may communicate with adjacent loops of bowel, other viscera (e.g. bladder, vagina) or the skin. External fistulae may result

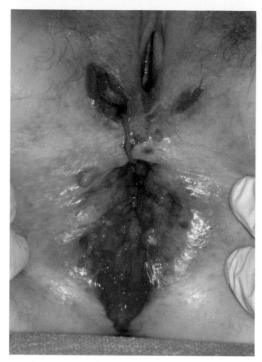

Fig. 16.4 Severe perianal Crohn's disease with fistulation.

from surgical intervention and commonly involve the anterior abdominal wall or perineum (Fig. 16.4). Abscesses can result from chronic bowel perforation, but free perforation is relatively uncommon because the inflamed segment usually adheres to surrounding structures. Although less common than in ulcerative colitis, toxic dilatation can complicate colonic disease. Fulminant Crohn's colitis is shown in

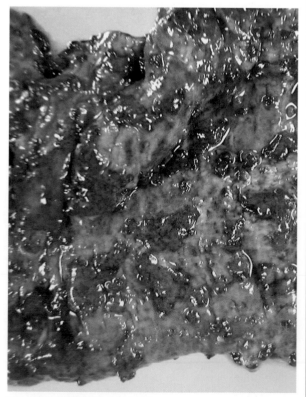

Fig. 16.5 Fulminant Crohn's colitis.

Figure 16.5; deep ulcers and fibrosis with mucosal oedema and inflammation can be seen.

It is essential to consider malignancy in patients with long-standing Crohn's disease, with or without symptoms. There is an elevated risk of colorectal adenocarcinoma: 2.5-fold overall and 4.5-fold for colonic disease, with a 10-year cumulative risk following diagnosis of 2.9%. Evidence is limited that surveillance provides protection and many patients with longstanding colonic Crohn's eventually come to colectomy. Crohn's disease is also associated with ~30-fold excess risk of small bowel adenocarcinoma, but because that cancer is rare, the absolute risk only amounts to 0.2% at 10 years and 2.2% at 25 years after diagnosis.

25% of patients with small bowel Crohn's disease and 75% with large bowel disease have troublesome anal lesions, including abscess, fistula, fissures, ulceration, oedematous skin tags, anorectal stricturing. Anal fissures are often multiple and indolent, and extend to involve any part of the perineum, including the vagina or scrotum. Systemic manifestations of Crohn's disease include anterior uveitis, iritis, polyarthropathy, ankylosing spondylitis, liver disease (e.g. sclerosing cholangitis) and erythema nodosum. Terminal ileal involvement may result in gallstones, with increased incidence following ileocaecal resection.

Investigations

Assessment of nutritional status, including serial weight measurement, is essential. Anaemia may be due to: iron deficiency from chronic blood loss and rarely due to malabsorption; a normocytic anaemia of chronic disease; macrocytic anaemia from vitamin B_{12} or folate malabsorption. Elevated acute-phase proteins such as C-reactive protein are useful in monitoring disease, though not specific for diagnostic purposes. Until recently, the diagnosis was most frequently made on barium follow-through: typical features are shown in Figure 16.6 – rose-thorn ulcers, long irregular terminal ileal stricture at the site of previous ileocaecal resection. Active disease produces radiological evidence of thickening, luminal narrowing and separation of loops, and is often associated with mucosal ulceration, deep fissuring ulcers and cobblestone appearance. Skip lesions and fistula formation may be apparent. However, MRI enteroclysis (image enhanced by administering oral osmotically active agent – e.g. PEG) has progressively become the investigation of choice (Fig. 16.7), which also has the advantage of limiting radiation exposure. Rectal examination, proctoscopy, sigmoidoscopy and colonoscopy determine disease extent and biopsy of inflamed bowel is mandatory. Newer investigative techniques include video-capsule endoscopy (Fig. 16.8), enteroscopy, and CT colonography. Double-contrast barium enema still has a place for assessing disease extent and delineation of fistulae.

Management

Medical management

Attention to general nutritional state is crucial. Anaemia should be corrected by transfusion, iron and/or vitamin supplements, as appropriate. Oral protein and calorie supplements may be required and patients with short bowel syndrome may require parenteral nutrition. Bile salt diarrhoea secondary to ileal disease or previous resection may benefit from cholestyramine.

Corticosteroids may be used to induce remission (prednisolone 30–60 mg daily by mouth), but long-term therapy should be avoided to reduce unwanted steroid side effects. Some patients with colonic disease may be maintained on 5-aminosalicylic acid agents (e.g. mesalazine, olsalazine) and some with relapsing terminal ileal disease, but there

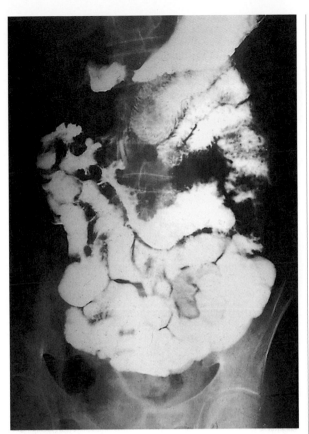

Fig. 16.6 Small bowel contrast enema in Crohn's disease, showing a long irregular stricture and typical rose-thorn ulceration.

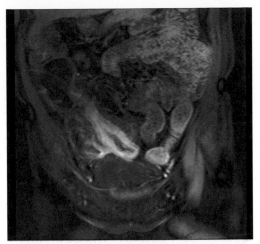

Fig. 16.7 Small bowel MRI showing thickened strictured small bowel in Crohn's disease.

16

used frequently in specialist centres and have a place in patients with resistant, relapsing or fistulating Crohn's disease. Newer agents such as anti-integrins have also been introduced.

Surgical management

Many patients with Crohn's disease undergo surgery at some stage of their disease course and multiple operations are common. There are four main categories of indications for surgical management of Crohn's disease:

1. Onset of complications of luminal disease: fulminant colitis, life-threatening haemorrhage, obstruction, abscess/sepsis, perforation, fistulation.
2. Acute or chronic failure of medical management to control symptoms/disease activity, failure to thrive, complications of medical therapy.
3. Treatment or prophylaxis of malignancy.
4. Perianal disease: abscess, fistula, anorectal stricture (EBM 16.1).

Modern surgical principles are to preserve bowel length whenever possible, by employing a conservative approach to bowel resection and liberal use of stricturoplasty (longitudinal enterotomy with transverse anastomosis of

is limited evidence that maintenance therapy reduces the risk of relapse. Immunosuppression using azathioprine or 6-mercaptopurine can be used in resistant cases to induce remission and for maintenance. There are concerns about complications of long-term immunosuppression – the agents are not generally continued beyond 2 years without review and are seldom used beyond 4 years. Monoclonal antibodies to tumour necrosis factor-α (TNF-α) are now

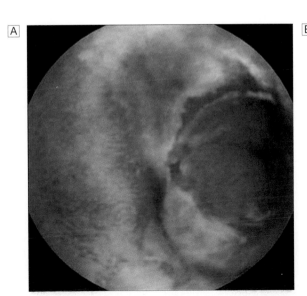

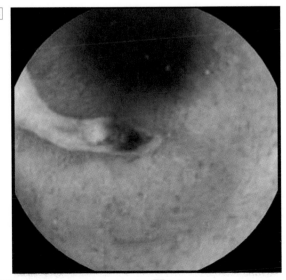

Fig. 16.8 Video-capsule enteroscopy of Crohn's disease. **A** Extensive ulceration and structuring. **B** A single deep ulcer.

EBM 16.1 Crohn's disease and ulcerative colitis

'Colonoscopic surveillance may reduce colorectal cancer risk in longstanding inflammatory bowel disease.

Surgical resection is required in patients resistant to medical management, those with complications of medical therapy and those developing complications.'

Guidelines for the management of inflammatory bowel disease in adults. Carter MJ, Lobo AJ, Travis SP; IBD Section, British Society of Gastroenterology. Gut. 2004 Sep;53 Suppl 5:V1-16. http://www.ncbi.nlm.nih. gov/pmc/articles/PMC1867788.

Guidelines for colorectal cancer screening and surveillance in moderate and high risk groups. Cairns SR, Scholefield JH, Steele RJ, Dunlop MG, Thomas HJ, Evans GD, Eaden JA, Rutter MD, Atkin WP, Saunders BP, Lucassen A, Jenkins P, Fairclough PD, Woodhouse CR; British Society of Gastroenterology; Association of Coloproctology for Great Britain and Ireland. Gut. 2010 May;59(5):666-89. http://gut.bmj.com/content/59/5/666.long

Colonoscopic surveillance for prevention of colorectal cancer in people with ulcerative colitis, Crohn's disease or adenomas. NICE Guideline. http://www. nice.org.uk/nicemedia/live/13415/53641/53641.pdf

strictured bowel) to enlarge the gut lumen. In all cases, length of small bowel remaining should be measured and documented. Radical surgery is not appropriate because the risk of recurrence is determined by the disease natural history rather than wide surgical clearance. Disease resurgence is common following small bowel resection but is less than 20% in colonic disease. In the initial phases of colonic Crohn's disease, segmental resection is preferred to bypass of affected segments. However, many such patients eventually undergo proctocolectomy and permanent ileostomy. In perianal Crohn's disease, loculated pus must be drained and radical surgery should be avoided, as the disease tends to recur. Simple fistulae may be laid open, but long-term drainage Setons are widely used for complex fistulae involving sphincter muscle. Complex reconstructions such as rectal advancement flaps tend to be avoided.

 SUMMARY BOX 16.3

Indications for surgery in Crohn's disease

Elective

- Chronic subacute obstruction due to fibrotic strictures, adhesions or refractory disease
- Symptomatic disease unresponsive to, or poorly controlled by medical management
- Chronic relapsing disease on discontinuation of medical management and steroid dependency
- Complications of medical management (e.g. osteoporosis)
- Concerns about long-term immunosuppression, risk of malignancy and viral/atypical infections
- Perianal sepsis and fistula
- Enterocutaneous fistula
- Onset of malignancy, including colorectal adenocarcinoma and small bowel lymphoma
- Rarely, control of debilitating extra-colonic manifestations such as iritis and sacroiliitis.

Emergency

- Fulminant colitis or acute small bowel relapse unresponsive to medical management
- Acute bowel obstruction
- Life-threatening haemorrhage
- Abscess or free perforation
- Perianal abscess.

Ulcerative colitis

The annual incidence of ulcerative colitis is ~10/100 000 population in Westernized countries but rare in developing countries. The aetiology is incompletely understood, but genetic, immunological and dietary factors all play a part. The disorder may affect any age group but peak incidence is in early adulthood. In the majority of cases, the disease is contiguous, affecting the rectum and extending proximally (see Table 16.1). In 5% of cases, it is segmental and the rectum is occasionally spared. There is substantial risk of colorectal adenocarcinoma in cases with pancolitis. Although ulcerative colitis is primarily a disease of the large bowel, systemic manifestations (iritis, polyarthritis, sacroiliitis, hepatitis, erythema nodosum, pyoderma gangrenosum) can occur. Primary sclerosing cholangitis (PSC) affects 2–5% of cases of ulcerative colitis; it tends to indicate severe disease and predicts complications. Patients with PSC may develop liver failure and require liver transplantation.

Pathology

The characteristic feature of ulcerative colitis is inflammation restricted to the mucosa and submucosa of the large bowel. In severe episodes, there may be full-thickness involvement with inflammatory infiltrate. Abscesses develop at the base of the colonic crypts, which burst and coalesce to form crypt abscesses. These undermine the mucosa, resulting in ulceration (Fig. 16.9) and oedema of the intervening mucosa, which may form inflammatory pseudopolyps. Histologically, as well as ulceration and crypt abscesses, there is chronic inflammatory cell infiltrate, crypt architectural distortion and goblet cell depletion, but granulomas are absent. The colon loses its haustrations and becomes thick and rigid. Stricturing is uncommon and its presence should raise the possibility of Crohn's disease. There can be difficulty in distinguishing ulcerative colitis from Crohn's colitis both pathologically and clinically, when the term 'indeterminate colitis' is used to denote uncertainty. There may even be migration from one disease entity to the other. There are important implications for surgical treatment, since ileo-anal pouch should be avoided in cases of Crohn's colitis.

Clinical features

Ulcerative colitis characteristically runs a relapsing/remitting course, although some patients may have a chronic continuous variant. In some cases, the initial attack is fulminant, and toxic dilatation with exacerbation of abdominal and systemic

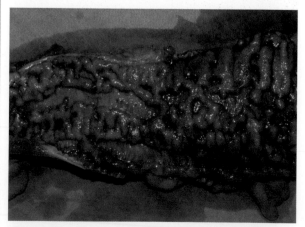

Fig. 16.9 Resected colonic specimen of fulminant ulcerative colitis showing denuded colonic epithelium.

symptoms may occur at any time. Diarrhoea with the passage of mucus and blood is typical of relapse. Abdominal pain and tenderness may be present and intermittent pyrexia is common. Passage of 10–15 or more stools each day is not unusual in acute severe exacerbations. As well as increased faecal frequency, incapacitating faecal urgency is a distressing problem degrading quality of life for many patients.

Careful rectal examination should detect anal complications such as fissure, fistula and haemorrhoids, which are present in 25% of cases. The rectal mucosa often feels thick and boggy. Sigmoidoscopy and biopsy is the key investigation and reveals a red, granular mucosa with contact bleeding. In the early stages of disease, the only sign on sigmoidoscopy may be loss of the rectal mucosal vessels. As the disease progresses, severe ulceration leads to fulminant colitis, the complications of which include dramatic nutritional depletion, toxic dilatation, perforation and severe bleeding. During an exacerbation, the dilated colon may become paper-thin. Recent population-based studies have revealed that the mortality for all inpatient admissions for ulcerative colitis is ~15% at 3 years, and this emphasizes the potential severity of the disorder.

Investigations

Expert colonoscopy is the mainstay of diagnosis and assessment of disease extent/severity. Endoscopic features of severe acute colitis are shown in Figure 16.10. Barium enema is infrequently used in modern inflammatory bowel disease practice and may risk perforation. Typical changes include loss of haustrations, fluffy granularity of the mucosa, and pseudopolyps. Undermining ulcers may create a double contour to the edge of the colon. Widening of the retrorectal space, due to perirectal inflammation and reduced distensibility of the rectum, is common. In longstanding colitis, the bowel may become short and featureless, resembling a smooth tube (lead-pipe colon). In an acute attack, plain films of the abdomen may reveal a dilated gas-filled colon in which pseudopolyps are evident. When toxic dilatation is suspected, daily plain X-rays are essential to monitor progress (Fig. 16.11). 'Backwash ileitis' may produce a dilated and featureless terminal ileum in which the mucosa appears granular. In the acute phase, it is essential to collect stool cultures to exclude supervening bacterial infection and especially *C. difficile*.

Surveillance colonoscopy has an important place in the management of long-standing colitis to detect dysplasia or supervening cancer.

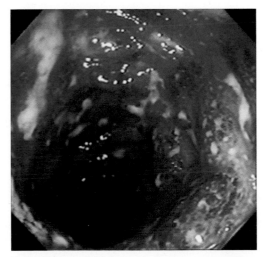

Fig. 16.10 Colonoscopic appearance of severe acute colitis.

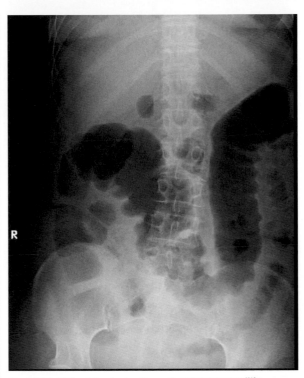

Fig. 16.11 Plain abdominal radiograph of fulminant colitis showing distension and mucosal oedema and thumbprinting.

Management

Medical management

Repeated clinical and laboratory assessment is key during an acute exacerbation to identify those with a severe episode that requires escalation of therapy and/or surgical resection. Daily stool charting, temperature and pulse, along with assays of C reactive protein and albumin are essential. Various criteria are used to identify those with a severe episode and these include Truelove and Witt's score: stool frequency > 6 × /24h *AND* any of Hb < 105 g/l, ESR > 30 mm/h, pulse > 90 bpm, T > 37.5°C

Fluid and electrolyte replacement, correction of anaemia, nutritional support, intravenous corticosteroid therapy, and timely surgical intervention are the mainstay of treatment of an exacerbation. High-dose systemic steroids (oral prednisolone, intravenous methylprednisolone or hydrocortisone) are needed during an acute relapse. In fulminant colitis, immunosuppression with ciclosporin A or anti-TNF therapy (e.g. infliximab) may be helpful. Topical steroids delivered by enema or suppository usually control mild attacks of proctocolitis. Long-term aminosalicylates, such as mesalazine or olsalazine, have been shown to reduce the risk of relapse when a patient is in remission. Azathioprine is used for maintenance therapy and may induce remission, though it is not used with such intent. Around 15% of all patients diagnosed with ulcerative colitis will eventually require surgery. The risk varies from 1 in 50 for those with mild proctitis, to 1 in 20 for moderately severe colitis, and 1 in 2 for those with extensive disease.

Surgical management

Indications for surgery in the emergency and elective setting include fulminant colitis that fails to respond to aggressive medical therapy, perforation and toxic dilatation. Patients presenting as an emergency are catabolic, malnourished, immunosuppressed, bacteraemic and septic. Hence,

16

surgical reconstruction in the acute phase is inadvisable and management comprises colectomy and ileostomy as a 'first-aid' operation. The rectum is closed over as a stump in the pelvis, or by bringing out the distal end as a mucous fistula. Completion proctectomy and the formation of an ileo-anal pouch are undertaken ~6 months following the emergency operation to allow general health improvements. It is important that patients understand that it is essential to remove the residual rectum because of the elevated risk of rectal cancer over the remaining lifetime.

Indications for surgery in the elective setting include failure of medical management or repeated relapses on medical treatment. Failure to thrive, as reflected in retardation of growth and sexual development in children, or malnourishment and anaemia in adults, is a common indication for operation. The onset of biopsy-proven dysplasia or carcinoma in chronic disease necessitates surgical intervention.

Modern surgical practice comprises restorative proctocolectomy with retention of the anal sphincters and reconstruction by formation of an ileal pouch anastomosed to the upper anal canal. This approach has the benefits of removing all but a tiny cuff of rectal mucosa in the upper anal canal, and also maintaining the ability to defaecate normally. A temporary ileostomy may be required. Median stool frequency is 4–6 liquid/soft motions/day, but the debilitating faecal urgency associated with colitis is eliminated and the overall quality of life is excellent. Where pouch anal anastomosis is not possible, a Koch's continent ileostomy may be considered. Proctocolectomy and permanent end ileostomy still has an important place in management.

 SUMMARY BOX 16.4

Indications for surgery in ulcerative colitis

Elective
- Symptomatic disease unresponsive to, or poorly controlled by, medical management
- Chronic relapsing disease on discontinuation of medical management and steroid dependency
- Complications of medical management
- Concerns about long-term immunosuppression, risk of malignancy and viral/atypical infections
- Severe dysplasia on surveillance biopsies of colorectal epithelium
- Onset of colorectal adenocarcinoma
- Rarely, control of debilitating extra-colonic manifestations such as iritis and sacroiliitis.

Emergency
- Fulminant colitis unresponsive to maximal medical management
- Toxic megacolon
- Free perforation
- Life-threatening haemorrhage
- Acute complications of medical management.

Cancer surveillance in ulcerative colitis

Colorectal cancer risk in long-standing ulcerative colitis is a major factor contributing to surgical decision-making. Carcinoma is typically difficult to detect in colitis, is usually poorly differentiated and has a poor prognosis. Around 2% of all patients will develop cancer at 10 years, 8% at 20 years and 18% at 30 years. In pancolitis, the overall risk is around 25% after 30 years. Early age at first onset (< 15 years), pancolitis, a family history of colorectal cancer and associated PSC are strong cancer risk factors. Cancer surveillance is recommended in the long-term management of patients with chronic ulcerative colitis, and colonoscopy should be performed at 2-yearly intervals (see EBM 16.1). Random biopsies are taken at surveillance colonoscopy, since dysplasia indicates a high risk of cancer. Dysplasia-associated lesion or mass (DALM) is a high-risk indicator of impending, or concurrent, cancer development. Cancer risk for patients with high-grade dysplasia or DALM is > 60% in the next 2 years and so restorative proctocolectomy is recommended. Patients with pancolitis may opt for prophylactic restorative proctocolectomy, especially when ulcerative colitis was diagnosed before the age of 15 years, rather than the uncertainty associated with life-long surveillance.

DISORDERS OF THE SMALL INTESTINE

Small bowel neoplasms

Small bowel tumours account for less than 5% of all gastrointestinal neoplasms.

Benign tumours

Solitary tumours include adenomatous polyps, hamartomas, lipomas and haemangiomas. Multiple hamartomas are found in the Peutz–Jeghers syndrome (see below). Benign tumours are rarely symptomatic and so the true incidence is unknown. Symptoms may arise as a result of intussusception or bleeding.

Malignant tumours

Malignant small intestinal tumours are rare and frequently diagnosed late because symptoms are non-specific and so initial presentation may be at laparotomy for small bowel obstruction. In symptomatic cases, imaging modalities include MRI enteroclysis, barium follow-through, CT scan, flexible enteroscopy and video-capsule endoscopy.

Gastrointestinal stromal tumours (GIST)

GISTs are the most common form of mesenchymal tumour of the intestinal tract. The lesions are derived from smooth muscle of the gut tube; 50–60% arise in stomach, 20–30% in small bowel, 10% in rectum and 5% in oesophagus. There is a spectrum from benign to malignant. Malignant lesions have a poor prognosis, tending to recur locally and to metastasize. Expression of the oncogene *c-Kit* differentiates malignant from benign characteristics. The Kit protein is a transmembrane tyrosine kinase receptor and malignant GISTs have a mutation in the *c-Kit* gene or the platelet-derived growth factor receptor alpha gene (PDGFRA) which causes up-regulation of tyrosine kinase activity and promotes tumour cell growth. Understanding the involvement of *c-Kit* in GIST development and progression has allowed the development of new effective tyrosine kinase inhibitor anticancer agents specifically designed to inhibit Kit or PDGFRA, such as imatinib mesylate.

Small bowel adenocarcinoma

The duodenum and upper jejunum are the most common sites of this rare tumour. Adenocarcinomas, which are usually poorly differentiated and are mucin-secreting, may be associated with FAP (familial adenomatous polyposis) or HNPCC (Lynch syndrome). Resection of the affected segment is carried out, but palliative bypass may be all that is possible, as the disease often presents late.

Lymphoma

Small bowel is the most common site for lymphoma to arise in the intestine and may present as intermittent obstruction, bleeding or perforation. Coeliac disease is associated with an increased risk of various types of non-Hodgkin's lymphomas but particularly enteropathy-type T-cell lymphoma (ETTL). Antigliadin, anti-TTG and anti-endomysial antibodies should be determined and a biopsy of adjacent normal small intestine or duodenum should always be assessed for villous atrophy in cases of lymphoma. Treatment is frequently surgical in the first instance because the diagnosis is made histologically after small bowel resection, but chemotherapy is required in most cases.

Carcinoid tumour

The small bowel is the second most common site for carcinoid tumour (after appendix). Metastasis to lymph nodes is common at presentation, and obstruction and bleeding are the usual modes of presentation. Abdominal CT typically reveals a small bowel mass lesion with prominent calcification (Fig. 16.12). There may be features of the carcinoid syndrome in the presence of liver metastasis. Tests for urinary 5-HIAA (hydroxy-indole-acetic acid) and blood levels of chromogranin A should be undertaken. The primary tumour should be resected where possible. Lesions are frequently multifocal and may require multiple resections.

Peutz–Jeghers syndrome

Peutz–Jeghers syndrome is an autosomal dominant inherited disorder with high penetrance. The disease is caused by mutations in the *LKB1* gene, located on the short arm of chromosome 19. Some cases are due to as yet unmapped genes. The clinical manifestations include gastrointestinal polyps and melanin pigmentation at mucocutaneous junctions, characteristically around the mouth and eyes. Occasionally there is pigmentation on the dorsum of the hands and feet. Affected individuals are at risk of colorectal, gastric, pancreatic, breast, and ovarian cancers. Small intestinal and gastric cancers occur in around 7% of patients and colorectal cancer in 10–20%.

Pathology

Polyps occur most commonly in the jejunum; they have a short pedicle with a lobulated surface resembling that of an adenomatous polyp or sometimes a villous tumour. On microscopy, the hamartomas consist of branches of muscularis mucosae covered by epithelium and lamina propria. There is a greatly increased risk of adenocarcinoma, but it is not clear whether this arises in a hamartoma or an adjacent area of normal epithelium.

Clinical features

Most cases present in childhood or adolescence. There are usually dark brown or bluish spots on the lips and inside the mouth. The face, palms, soles, arms and perianal region can also be affected, but patients without pigmentation have been described. The usual presentation is with abdominal pain or obstruction due to intussusception of a polyp, but rectal bleeding and iron deficiency anaemia are also common. The diagnosis may be made in childhood or early adulthood on clinical grounds due to the association of abdominal colic and typical pigmentation. The small bowel investigation of choice in suspected Peutz–Jeghers Syndrome is MRI enteroclysis (Fig. 16.13). This avoids the radiation dose associated with repeated barium small bowel follow-through or CT examinations.

16

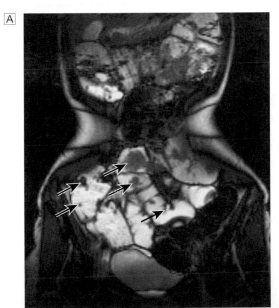

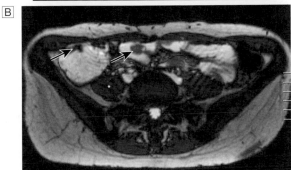

Fig. 16.13 Peutz–Jeghers syndrome. **A** Abdominal MRI (coronal view) showing multiple polypoid filling defects due to hamartomatous polyps. **B** Cross-sectional MRI of a large jejunal polyp.

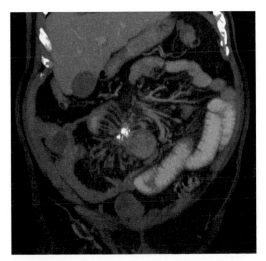

Fig. 16.12 CT showing small bowel carcinoid tumour with characteristic calcification and desmoplastic reaction. There is small bowel obstruction proximal to the lesion.

Management

Laparotomy, enterotomy and polypectomy are often required because an emergency admission with obstruction is the frequent mode of presentation. On-table enteroscopy can reduce the numbers of enterotomies and allows inspection of the whole length of the gastrointestinal tract from oesophagus to anus, with removal of all polyps. Upper and lower gastrointestinal surveillance endoscopy is recommended, as well as breast cancer screening, because the risk of cancer at these sites is high.

Meckel's diverticulum

This remnant of the vitello-intestinal duct is present in 2% of people and is the most common congenital abnormality of the gastrointestinal tract. The diverticulum may be ~5 cm long and arises from the antimesenteric border of the ileum some 50 cm from the ileocaecal valve. It is a true diverticulum and in 10% of cases its tip is connected to the umbilicus by a fibrous cord. Heterotopic mucosa is found in 50% of symptomatic diverticula; this is most often acid-secreting gastric mucosa although pancreatic tissue may be present. Only 5% of Meckel's diverticula cause symptoms, most frequently in childhood or early adult life. Peptic ulceration distal to a Meckel's diverticula is the most common cause of severe gastrointestinal bleeding in childhood. Intestinal obstruction may occur due to intussusception, or to a loop of bowel twisted around the band to the umbilicus (volvulus). Abdominal pain and tenderness, pyrexia and leucocytosis, due to peptic inflammation may mimic acute appendicitis.

Symptomatic Meckel's diverticula should be excised. Asymptomatic diverticula found incidentally at laparotomy should be left alone, unless the neck is narrow or nodularity suggests that the diverticulum contains abnormal mucosa. In patients with unexplained gastrointestinal bleeding, heterotopic mucosa within a Meckel's diverticulum can be detected by scintiscanning after injection of ^{99m}Tc-labelled sodium pertechnetate.

Jejunal diverticulosis

Jejunal diverticulae are acquired during adult life. Occasionally, only one or two diverticula are present but often diverticulosis is very extensive, with multiple wide-mouthed sacs caused by herniation of mucosa into the mesentery at the site of vessel penetration of the gut wall. Jejunal diverticulosis may be first diagnosed at laparotomy for complicated disease, or incidentally on imaging studies (Fig. 16.14). Diverticulae may cause

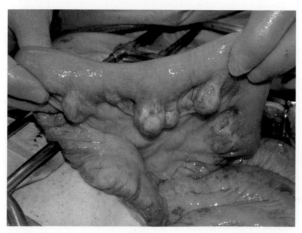

Fig. 16.14 Jejunal diverticulosis.

bleeding, inflammation, malabsorption (due to bacterial over-colonization) and perforation. Occasionally, fish bones or NSAID tablets can become trapped in a diverticulum and cause local perforation. In symptomatic disease the extensive nature of the disorder often necessitates a conservative approach with antibiotics and intravenous fluids. However, a bowel segment with complicated diverticulosis may require limited resection, leaving other affected areas in situ.

Radiation enteritis

External beam irradiation or radioactive implants can cause enteritis. The terminal ileum is the most commonly affected site within the small bowel. In the acute phase, oedema, inflammation and ulceration may produce watery diarrhoea, lower abdominal pain, tenesmus, mucous discharge and rectal bleeding. Subsequently, the bowel may thicken, with fibrosis and stricture which may require resection. The small bowel may fistulate to other loops, to large bowel or to the vagina. The involved segments require resection but anastomotic healing is frequently compromised because of the radiation damage.

Small bowel ischaemia

Small intestinal ischaemia is usually due to atheromatous occlusion with superadded thrombosis of the superior mesenteric artery. Factors predisposing to mesenteric thrombosis include thrombophilia, hyperviscosity syndromes, dehydration, hypovolaemia or hypoperfusion of the gut resulting from trauma, cardiogenic shock, cardiac arrhythmia and septic shock. Arterial embolism can result from atrial fibrillation or recent myocardial infarction. In a third of patients dying from acute ischaemic necrosis of the midgut, there is no demonstrable occlusion of a major vessel, and in these cases low perfusion is responsible. Other causes include polycythaemia, sickle cell disease and disseminated intravascular coagulation. Arteritis should be suspected where there are other stigmata or a history of disseminated arteritis, such as pre-existing renal failure. Impaired venous return from the gut can be due to hyperviscosity syndromes and prothrombotic tendency, but are also seen in the presence of malignancy and portal hypertension.

Ischaemic necrosis may progress to necrosis of all bowel layers with gangrene and perforation. Acute occlusion of the superior mesenteric artery (SMA) is predominantly a disease of the elderly and leads to complete midgut necrosis.

Clinical features

Early diagnosis is often difficult as the symptoms and signs are non-specific. There may be a preceding history of chronic or episodic abdominal pain associated with meals ('mesenteric angina'), diarrhoea and weight loss. Cardiac arrhythmias, notably atrial fibrillation, are often present on initial presentation. Abdominal pain is a predominant symptom and may be associated with vomiting. In a third of cases, there is watery or bloody diarrhoea. The pain varies in its location but is generally central, severe and constant in nature. Abdominal tenderness, guarding and rigidity are late signs denoting gangrene and perforation, and cardiovascular collapse signifies hypovolaemia and sepsis.

Investigations and diagnosis

Clinical suspicion is essential if the diagnosis is to be made before the situation is unsalvageable. Plain abdominal films may reveal calcified atheroma in the mesenteric arteries and aorta, and there may be dilated thickened gas-filled small bowel loops. Gas in the bowel wall or in the peritoneal cavity is a grave sign. Marked leucocytosis and hyperamylasaemia are common, but the finding of metabolic acidosis on blood gas analysis should raise strong suspicion of bowel ischaemia. Contrast enhanced CT is usually diagnostic and will show lack of gut enhancement. Formal arteriography is only occasionally helpful in practice because of the late presentation of most cases.

Management

Following vigorous resuscitation, gangrenous bowel requires resection, but this may be futile in elderly patients with extensive midgut involvement and a decision may be taken to limit intervention and keep the patient comfortable with palliative care. In some instances of acute occlusion, arterial flow can be restored by embolectomy or thrombectomy. A 'second-look' laparotomy 24 hours later may be useful. Massive resection is inevitable unless flow can be restored within 6 hours. Even if the patient survives, there may be substantial nutritional problems. The prognosis is poor, with an overall mortality of 70–90%. Survival is restricted almost exclusively to patients in whom a defined vascular occlusion is treated early. Mesenteric venous occlusion has an equally bleak prognosis, and treatment is usually confined to resection of the gangrenous bowel and anticoagulation.

Chronic mesenteric ischaemia

Chronic mesenteric ischaemia results in repeated bouts of ill-defined colicky central abdominal pain, typically commencing 20–30 minutes after eating, leading to 'fear of food' and almost universally resulting in weight loss. Diagnosis is often elusive and is usually preceded by extensive investigation to exclude other conditions of the small or large bowel, such as Crohn's disease and malignancy. Mesenteric arteriography may be diagnostic but must be taken in the context of symptoms because atheromatous change in mesenteric vessels is common. Mesenteric revascularization may be feasible in a minority of cases.

SMALL AND LARGE BOWEL OBSTRUCTION

Obstruction refers to a mechanical impedance to the normal propulsive action through the intestine. While the underlying mode of clinical presentation and underlying aetiology may differ between small and large intestine, a number of underlying principles can be considered together. The most common causes of small intestinal obstruction are adhesions (60%), obstructed hernia (20%) and malignancy (primary and secondary – 5–8%). In the large bowel, colorectal adenocarcinoma predominates (> 70%), followed by stricturing diverticular disease (10%) and sigmoid volvulus (5%). The aetiology of large and small bowel obstruction can be systematically classified as intraluminal, intramural and extramural (Table 16.2). Treatment should be focused on the underlying cause of obstruction and operation is frequently required.

The clinical presentation of bowel obstruction reflects the anatomical location of the lesion. The predominating features from proximal to distal are as follows.

Proximal jejunal obstruction – very short history of anorexia, vomiting, relatively severe upper abdominal pain and absent/minimal abdominal distension with limited, if any, change in bowel habit.

Table 16.2 Causes of small and large bowel obstruction

	Small intestine	Large intestine
Intramural (intrinsic)	Crohn's disease Radiation stricture Tuberculosis Ischaemic stricture (caecal carcinoma) Primary tumour – lymphoma, adenocarcinoma, carcinoid tumour Intussusception secondary to: hypertrophy of Peyer's patches, Peutz–Jeghers polyp	Colorectal adenocarcinoma Diverticular stricture Sigmoid volvulus Radiation stricture (rectum/sigmoid) Ischaemic stricture Caecal volvulus Crohn's disease
Extrinsic	Postoperative adhesions Adhesions from previous inflammatory condition Congenital band Hernia Compression by tumour mass Volvulus	Rare due to lumen diameter and retroperitoneal location Compression by tumour mass Massive inguinal hernia Incisional hernia
Intra-luminal	Foreign body Gallstone ileus Worm infestation Bezoar	Faecal concretion (very rare)

Distal small bowel obstruction – short history of colicky midgut (peri-umbilical pain, distension, vomiting and recent absolute constipation).

Colonic obstruction presents more insidiously with poorly defined hindgut abdominal pain/discomfort, weight loss, pronounced abdominal distension, history of altered bowel habit tending to constipation with little or no vomiting.

Initially the bowel proximal to obstruction contracts vigorously in an attempt to overcome the mechanical impedance. However, eventually peristalsis subsides and paralytic ileus ensues due to electrolyte imbalance and gross distension proximal to the obstruction. Patients with obstruction frequently present with profound dehydration due to a combination of vomiting, enforced fasting and 'third space' losses into the wall of the thickened intestine and peritoneal transudate. If the situation continues without decompression and resolution, there is progressive bacterial translocation into the portal circulation and the patient becomes increasingly toxic. Eventually bowel viability becomes compromised and may perforate. Features that indicate imminent perforation, strangulation or established peritonitis from perforation are: pyrexia, tachycardia, dehydration, hypotension, leucocytosis, peritonism on abdominal palpation and completely absent bowel sounds.

Full clinical history and examination is essential, along with immediate instigation of intravenous fluid and electrolyte therapy. Digital rectal examination may reveal rectal or extrinsic malignancy, empty rectum or constipation. Hernial orifices must be carefully inspected and any previous surgical abdominal scars noted. Abdominal X-ray will reveal distended small bowel or large bowel loops (Fig. 16.15) and may give an indication of the level of obstruction. Free gas under the diaphragm indicates perforation and mandates laparotomy and grossly distended bowel loops or evidence of a closed loop obstruction also merit early surgical intervention. Increasingly CT scan is used to assess bowel obstruction, because it allows interpretation of the

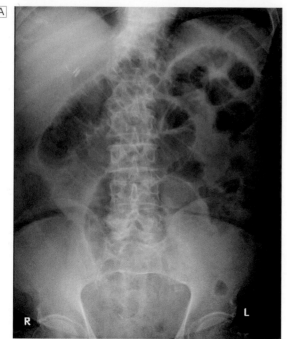

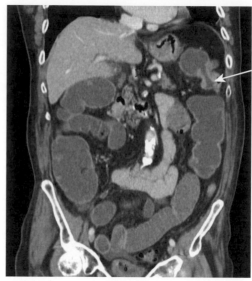

Fig. 16.16 CT of a large and small bowel obstruction proximal to a splenic flexure carcinoma (arrowed).

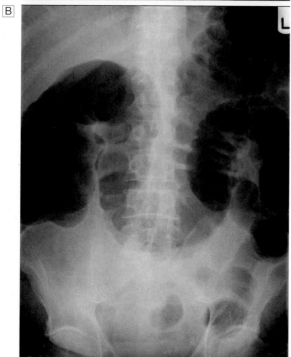

Fig. 16.15 Plain abdominal X-rays showing obstruction. **A** Small bowel obstruction. **B** Large bowel obstruction.

likely need for surgery, as well as identifying the underlying aetiology (Fig. 16.16). Right iliac fossa tenderness along with radiological evidence of gross caecal distension in the presence of distal colonic obstruction is a critical sign as it indicates imminent caecal perforation, which is a frequent complication of distal colonic obstruction. The reason that the caecum perforates even with obstruction due to sigmoid cancer is because the caecum is anatomically the largest diameter segment in the gut. Thus tension is greatest in the caecal wall, despite equalized intra-luminal pressure along the colon (practical relevance of the Law of Laplace).

Closed loop obstruction in either small or large bowel is more likely to strangulate and perforate. Closed loop obstruction can occur in small bowel due to adhesions or malignant involvement of two parts of the small bowel. If the ileocaecal valve remains competent in colonic obstruction, this acts as one end of a closed loop and the risk of perforation is high, typically at the caecum as described above.

Pseudo-obstruction and nonmechanical gut functional disorder

Paralytic ileus

Paralytic ileus should not be confused with mechanical obstruction, although it is a sequela of the end-stages of mechanical obstruction. The term refers to lack of propulsive contractions of both jejunum and ileum, although the ileus can be localized in some instances. It is common as a secondary feature of peritonitis due to any cause. It also may occur (1) after any surgical procedure due to handling of the bowel; (2) due to electrolyte abnormalities such as hypokalaemia, hyponatraemia, uraemia, diabetic ketoacidosis or; (3) secondary to drugs such as tricyclic antidepressant; lithium therapy, excessive opiate use. Management is conservative with bowel rest, nasogastric aspiration and fluid and electrolyte support. Treatment is otherwise focused on the underlying cause.

Pseudo-obstruction

The causes of pseudo-obstruction are shown in Table 16.3. The underlying mechanism is not fully understood but the pathogenesis involves autonomic imbalance resulting from decreased parasympathetic tone or excessive sympathetic output. It is essential to consider pseudo-obstruction in patients who present with signs and symptoms of bowel obstruction.

The majority of cases of pseudo-obstruction are due to large bowel dysfunction, although small bowel may be affected. It usually arises in the elderly and frail. Around 15% of all patients who present with signs and symptoms of large bowel obstruction in fact have pseudo-obstruction.

Table 16.3 Causes of non-mechanical bowel dysfunction/pseudo-obstruction

Systemic/metabolic
- Hypokalaemia
- Hyponatraemia
- Hypocalcaemia
- Hypoxia
- Diabetic ketoacidosis
- Uraemia
- Dehydration

Drugs
- Tricyclic antidepressants
- Lithium therapy
- General anaesthesia

Miscellaneous
- Idiopathic
- Retroperitoneal malignancy (Ogilvie's Syndrome)
- Spinal trauma
- Retroperitoneal haematoma
- Brain injury
- Pelvic surgery
- Postoperative ileus
- General debility from any wasting illness
- Extra-abdominal sepsis
- Peritonitis

Operative mortality in patients with pseudo-obstruction is > 15% and so surgery should be avoided wherever possible. Blood electrolyte estimation is essential, along with further imaging to ensure that mechanical obstruction is not present. For cases with large bowel distension, contrast radiography is essential using rectal contrast with fluoroscopy or in combination with computed tomography scanning to avoid unnecessary operation.

Management is conservative and involves stimulant enemas. Colonoscopic deflation may be required in cases where caecal distension causes concern about impending caecal perforation. Intravenous erythromycin can be effective in non-resolving cases and has been shown to stimulate motility by binding to colonic motilin receptors. Intravenous neostigmine has been shown to be effective when other measures fail to resolve the pseudo-obstruction. Progression of disease can lead to colonic perforation and so, in a small minority of cases, colectomy with ileorectal anastomosis, or with ileostomy, may be required.

NON-NEOPLASTIC DISORDERS OF THE LARGE INTESTINE

Colonic diverticular disease

Colonic diverticulosis is extremely common in developed countries, being apparent to some extent in more than 60% of people over the age of 70 years. The true population prevalence is unknown because estimates are based on indirect information from people who have undergone GI investigation for some reason. In most cases it is asymptomatic, often being noted incidentally on investigation for symptoms that are not due to the disease itself. Diverticulosis is the preferred term for such cases. Symptomatic diverticular disease can be classified as uncomplicated or complicated as discussed below. Diverticulosis is an acquired condition linked with a low-fibre diet, being rare in populations whose staple diet is high in fibre.

Although the whole colon can be affected, the sigmoid colon is most commonly involved, related to the high intraluminal pressure at this site caused by a low-residue diet. Muscular hypertrophy can be detected radiologically before diverticulae develop. Pulsion diverticulae emerge between the mesenteric and antimesenteric taeniae and result from herniation of mucosa through the circular muscle at the sites of penetration of feeding arteries. The true rectum is not affected because of differences in the arrangement of the blood supply and also because the outer longitudinal smooth muscle tube encompasses the full circumference of the rectum, contrasting with the colonic taeniae.

In addition to the common acquired diverticular change that may affect the caecum, there is a rare congenital solitary diverticulum of the caecum that can arise from the medial wall close to the ileocaecal valve and can extend upwards retroperitoneally. This may become obstructed by a faecolith and inflamed, producing a clinical picture indistinguishable from appendicitis.

Colonic diverticulae may give rise to intermittent lower abdominal/left iliac fossa pain, altered bowel habit, urgency of defaecation and episodic rectal bleeding. The sigmoid colon may be tender on examination. Barium enema reveals muscle thickening and multiple diverticula (Fig. 16.17). Abdominal CT, either as CT colonography or plain abdominal CT, is used increasingly and provides an assessment of the degree of surrounding inflammation and/or abscess formation, in addition to extent of the diverticular changes (Fig. 16.18). Colonoscopy reveals the ostia of diverticulae and may show surrounding inflammation.

In the management of uncomplicated diverticular change, patients should be advised to take a high-fibre diet, supplemented by bran or a bulk laxative such as methylcellulose. Stimulant laxatives and purgatives are to be avoided. Antispasmodics, such as propantheline or mebeverine, may be useful if there is smooth muscle spasm and colicky pain. There is evidence that NSAIDs increase

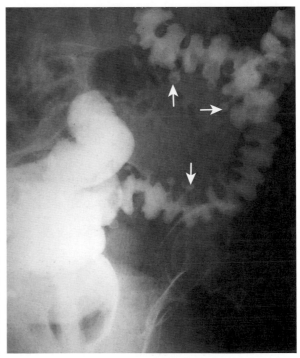

Fig. 16.17 Diverticular disease, barium contrast radiography.

16

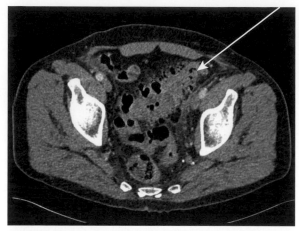

Fig. 16.18 Diverticular disease, CT showing local perforation and collection (arrowed).

Table 16.5 Hinchey classification of septic complications of diverticular disease	
Hinchey grade I	Localised para-colonic abscess
Hinchey grade II	Distant abscess (e.g. pelvic, sub-phrenic)
Hinchey grade III	Purulent peritonitis
Hinchey grade IV	Faecal peritonitis

the risk of complications and advice should be given to avoid these agents wherever possible. Surgical resection of the affected segment may be indicated if there are persistent symptoms, or when carcinoma cannot be excluded by radiology or colonoscopy (EBM 16.2).

EBM 16.2 Diverticular disease

'Surgery is required for complicated diverticular disease and acute cases failing to respond to antibiotics.'

Fozard JBJ, Armitage NC, Schofield JB, Jones OM. Association of Coloproctology of Great Britain & Ireland Position Statement on Elective Resection for Diverticulitis. http://www.acpgbi.org.uk/assets/documents/Position_Statemen___Elective_Resection_for_Diverticulis.pdf
Jacobs DO. Clinical practice. Diverticulitis. N Engl J Med. 2007 Nov 15;357(20):2057-66. http://www.nejm.org/doi/full/10.1056/NEJMcp073228
Shaikh S, Krukowski ZH. Outcome of a conservative policy for managing acute sigmoid diverticulitis. Br J Surg. 2007 Jul;94(7):876-9.

Complicated diverticular disease

Although most diverticular disease is asymptomatic, serious complications are a frequent cause for emergency admission to surgical wards and are life-threatening and debilitating. Complications of diverticular disease are causally linked to inflammation (Table 16.4). Faeces inspissated in a diverticulum produce stasis and a local inflammatory response. Infection spreads locally and results in peridiverticulitis, producing a low-grade pyrexia and left iliac fossa pain. Persistent infection may cause necrosis and the formation of a peridiverticular abscess. Septic complications are classified by Hinchey grade (Table 16.5). Patients presenting with established diverticular abscess are toxic. Free perforation of the peridiverticular abscess may result. Diverticulitis is also the underlying cause of diverticular bleeding as the feeding arteries are at the apex of each appendix.

Diverticulitis

Peridiverticulitis presents with pyrexia, leucocytosis, nausea and vomiting, and there is often a history of altered bowel habit. Pain and tenderness in the left iliac fossa are almost universal and a mass may be palpable. The initial diagnosis is primarily a clinical one, with the typical presentation being sufficient to treat the patient expectantly. In current practice the diagnosis is usually secured by CT scanning with or without gentle rectal contrast. Colonoscopy or flexible sigmoidoscopy and biopsy of inflamed segments are not usually necessary in the acute phase of illness and best left until the acute inflammation settles. Barium enema may reveal diverticular disease, but is best avoided for 4–6 weeks, to allow the inflammatory response to settle.

Treatment comprises fasting or clear fluids by mouth, bed rest, intravenous fluids and broad-spectrum antibiotics, such as a cephalosporin or gentamicin, along with metronidazole. Failure to settle suggests the development of pericolic abscess, and surgical resection and peritoneal toilet combined with abscess drainage may be required. In the absence of rapid improvement within 36–48 hours, intravenous and oral contrast-enhanced CT should be undertaken. CT scan with rectal contrast will reveal communication with the abscess cavity or free perforation. The presence of an abscess indicates the need for surgical resection. Such patients have a very high chance of ongoing sepsis and future surgery is almost certain due to chronic symptoms, even if the acute bout settles with antibiotics. Approximately one-third of all patients admitted with complicated acute diverticular disease require surgery during the index admission, while the remainder settle. Around 10% of these patients will eventually require surgical resection, preferably with primary colocolic anastomosis.

Perforation

Rupture of a pericolic abscess gives rise to purulent peritonitis, whereas free perforation of the bowel produces faecal peritonitis. The patient is usually profoundly ill, with septic shock, dehydration, marked abdominal pain, tenderness and distension. Intravenous broad-spectrum antibiotics and vigorous preoperative resuscitation are essential, followed by resection of the affected bowel and peritoneal lavage. Specialist colorectal surgeons may elect to perform an anastomosis in view of the fact that only 30% of colostomies are ever closed, and so the risk of a second laparotomy may be avoided. If peritoneal contamination is severe and there is poor bowel perfusion of the gut, a colostomy may be preferable. The most common approach is to bring the end of the proximal colon through the abdominal wall and close the rectal stump (Hartmann's procedure). The distal end may be exteriorized as a mucous fistula. Continuity can be restored once the patient has recovered, but this should not be for at least 3 months. Laproscopic peritoneal washout and drain replacement has gained much recent favour but is of unproven benefit. The mortality of perforated diverticular disease is 10–20% but may be as high as 50% in the elderly with faecal peritonitis.

Stricture formation and obstruction

Long-standing diverticular disease may cause stricture formation and intestinal obstruction. Such strictures are often very difficult to distinguish from malignancy, particularly as diverticular disease co-existing with a cancer is common. A resection may be undertaken to rule out a diagnosis of cancer.

Fistula

Diverticular disease can give rise to fistulae to other viscera, in particular the bladder. Colovesical fistula is more common in men because in women the uterus is interposed between bladder and sigmoid colon and prevents direct contact to some degree. The patient with a colovesical fistula usually complains of dysuria and the passage of cloudy urine, with bubbling on micturition (pneumaturia). The diagnosis may be confirmed by barium enema but may not reveal the fistula in every case, because it is often intermittent. Cystoscopy is frequently performed. Many patients present to the urology service with chronic bladder instability and infections. CT may reveal air in the bladder and show the fistulous tract itself. Treatment consists of resection of the affected segment, usually a sigmoid colectomy, with synchronous repair of the bladder.

Bleeding

Diverticular disease is the most common pathology responsible for lower GI haemorrhage. It may present with persistent fresh rectal bleeding or massive haemorrhage. Differential diagnosis includes angiodysplasia (which frequently co-exists with diverticular disease), haemorrhoids, polypoid colorectal tumours and, very occasionally, fulminant inflammatory bowel disease. Colonoscopy seldom allows the bleeding site to be identified. CT angiography is widely used. Angiography may be helpful but the bleeding must be at the rate of 1 ml/min to be visible. It may be possible to embolize the bleeding vessel using gel foam. In some cases of unremitting torrential haemorrhage, operation has to be undertaken when a source of bleeding has not been localized. On-table lavage and colonoscopy may be helpful in allowing a segmental resection of the affected bowel. However, in some cases, a blind total colectomy and ileorectal anastomosis may be required.

Large intestinal ischaemia

The aetiology of ischaemia of the large bowel is similar to that of the small intestine. Atheroma at the origin of the inferior mesenteric artery results in relative insufficiency of the arterial supply from the marginal artery (see Fig. 16.2). In rare cases where the inferior mesenteric artery is patent and an abdominal aortic aneurysm is present, colonic infarction may complicate aortic surgery if the inferior mesenteric artery is ligated. Untreated colonic ischaemia often progresses to gangrene and perforation. Some cases present with an acute bloody diarrhoeal illness known as ischaemic colitis, but others may declare symptoms from a chronic stricture.

Ischaemic colitis

In almost 50% of cases, ischaemia of the large intestine is transient and necrosis is confined to the mucosa and submucosa. The patient presents with lower abdominal pain, nausea, vomiting and bloody diarrhoea. Cardiovascular comorbidity should raise suspicion of the diagnosis. Examination reveals tenderness and guarding, often maximal in the lower left abdomen. There is usually a leucocytosis and pyrexia. Plain abdominal radiography may reveal a thickened segment of colon and thumb printing due to submucosal oedema, which may be evident on barium enema or CT (Fig. 16.19). Contrast studies should be carried out with water-soluble contrast such as gastrografin, because of the risk of perforation. The splenic flexure and sigmoid colon are most often affected (Fig. 16.20). Ischaemic colitis is treated conservatively in the first instance unless abdominal signs reveal peritonitis, but symptoms should resolve after a few days of

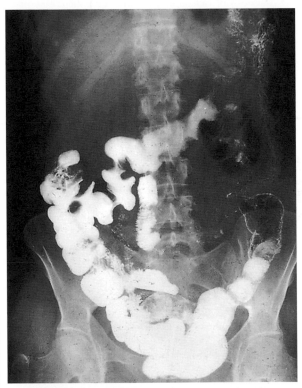

Fig. 16.19 Typical features of ischaemic colitis. Barium enema showing mucosal oedema and 'thumb printing'.

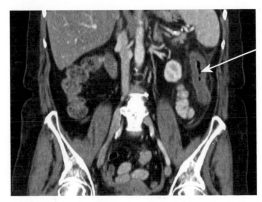

Fig. 16.20 CT scan showing gross mucosal thickening typically affecting the left side of the colon and sigmoid colon (arrowed).

supportive therapy. Further assessment by colonoscopy is indicated once the acute episode has settled, to exclude diverticular disease and colorectal cancer.

Gangrenous ischaemic colitis

The clinical presentation is localized or generalized peritonitis. Surgery is required for patients deemed sufficiently fit following consultation with the patient wherever possible, or with the family. Without surgery, death is virtually certain. However, surgical mortality is around 50%. Resection of the infarcted segment with colostomy formation is the rule, as poor blood supply usually militates against a primary anastomosis.

Ischaemic stricture of the colon

Colicky abdominal pain, constipation and abdominal distension, following a history of an attack of bloody diarrhoea or a documented episode of ischaemic colitis, may suggest the diagnosis of ischaemic stricture. The patient may present with frank large bowel obstruction. Contrast CT or enema reveals a smooth narrowing of a segment of bowel, with a funnelled appearance at either end but lacking the shouldered appearance of a malignant stricture (Fig. 16.21). Colonoscopy reveals a smooth, narrowed stricture with unremarkable biopsies, or occasionally histology may reveal evidence of chronic fibrosis. Resection is usually required, but some cases never come to medical attention.

Irritable bowel syndrome

Although not discussed here, irritable bowel syndrome is a common functional bowel disease that is highly relevant to surgical practice because it presents with symptoms that are indistinguishable from structural bowel disease, such as inflammatory bowel disease and cancer. Because of the lack of discriminatory clinical features, the diagnosis is largely one of exclusion, once appropriate investigation has ruled out other disorders.

Volvulus

Volvulus of the colon most commonly affects the sigmoid colon, and rarely the caecum, and is an important differential diagnosis of any cause of large bowel obstruction, such as

cancer and diverticular disease. Sigmoid volvulus is due to a twist around a narrow origin in the sigmoid mesentery. It is an acquired condition and is the most common cause of large bowel obstruction in countries with a high level of dietary fibre and those affected are frequently young adults. By contrast in the UK, patients are usually elderly and chronic constipation is associated. The clinical presentation is of a bowel obstruction with lower abdominal pain, abdominal distension, nausea, vomiting and absolute constipation. Occasionally, the patient may present with sepsis owing to an established visceral perforation. Plain radiography reveals a characteristic Y-shaped shadow surrounded by a grossly distended colon arising out of the pelvis on a plain radiograph ('coffee bean' sign) (Fig. 16.22). Water-soluble contrast radiography or CT may show the characteristic 'beaking' at the site of the twist.

Sigmoid volvulus can be treated conservatively in the emergency situation by reduction and deflation, using rigid or flexible sigmoidoscopy and the placement of a large-bore tube into the sigmoid. Elective sigmoid colectomy following full bowel preparation is curative in the fit patient. In frail and demented patients or those with significant cardiac or other comorbidity, a conservative approach may be taken, but a relapse of the twist is very likely and frequent readmission is the rule. Hence, surgery is the preferred option wherever possible (Fig. 16.23).

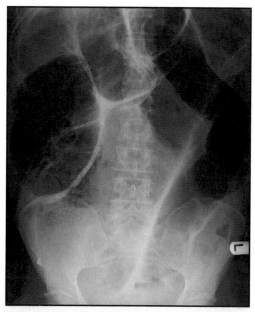

Fig. 16.22 Sigmoid volvulus. Plain abdominal radiograph showing characteristic 'coffee bean' sign.

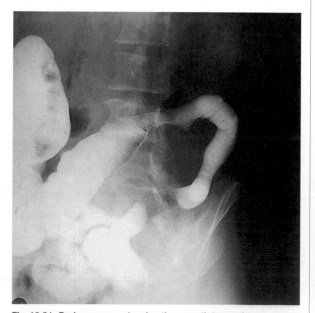

Fig. 16.21 Barium enema showing the smooth tapered appearance of a chronic benign stricture.

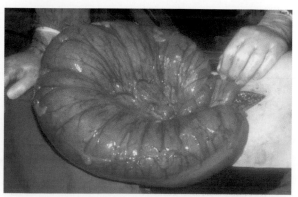

Fig. 16.23 Operative view of gross distension in sigmoid volvulus.

Caecal volvulus is a misnomer because it involves both the caecum and the small intestine, with the twist occurring around the superior mesenteric artery. The presence of a congenital intraperitoneal caecum predisposes to volvulus. It is usually suggested by plain radiography showing anticlockwise rotation of dilated small bowel loops around a grossly distended caecum. Caecal volvulus usually requires emergency laparotomy because of the danger of compromise to the arterial supply of substantial lengths of the small bowel.

Angiodysplasia

Angiodysplasia is an important cause of massive lower gastrointestinal haemorrhage, and may co-exist with diverticular disease. The acquired submucosal arteriovenous malformations commonly affect the caecum and sigmoid colon, but any part of the large bowel can be involved. The diagnosis may be secured by visualization of a bleeding point at colonoscopy. Bleeding angiodysplastic lesions can be treated by angiographic embolization, by laser treatment or injection sclerotherapy at colonoscopy, or by resection at emergency laparotomy.

Pseudomembranous colitis

Pseudomembranous colitis is almost always a healthcare associated infection (HAI) associated with the use of oral broad-spectrum antibiotics. C. difficile is the organism responsible in the vast majority of cases, and can be diagnosed by stool culture or by assays for the presence of C. difficile toxin in stool or blood. Necrosis of the colorectal mucosa causes watery diarrhoea, toxaemia, shock and collapse. The stools are watery, green, foul-smelling and blood-stained, and often contain fragments of mucosal slough. A typical pseudomembrane may be visible on sigmoidoscopy but is not a prerequisite. Biopsy confirms the diagnosis. The patient may be profoundly unwell, with dehydration and sepsis, and may require intensive resuscitation with intravenous fluid replacement. Treatment consists of oral metronidazole or vancomycin for 10 days. Severe cases may develop a toxic megacolon indistinguishable from that associated with inflammatory bowel disease. This surgical emergency requires colectomy and ileostomy. An ileorectal anastomosis can be performed at a later date when the patient is fully recovered.

Microscopic colitis

Other rare subtypes of colitis are collagenous and lymphocytic colitis (collectively known as microscopic colitis), characterized by chronic diarrhoea, normal endoscopic and radiological findings, and typical findings on histological examination of colonic tissue. Microscopic colitis occurs more commonly in females; it can affect people of all ages but mean age is in the seventh decade. Collagenous colitis is characterized by macroscopically normal colonic mucosa overlying a typically thickened subepithelial collagen band on histological examination. Lymphocytic colitis is characterized by an increased number of lymphocytes in the submucosa but lacks the features of either ulcerative or Crohn's colitis. It can have a segmental distribution and so differentiation from Crohn's colitis is important. There is a loose association with coeliac disease and measures should be taken to exclude this condition. There may be an association with a coexistent autoimmune disorder or the use of drugs such as non-steroidal anti-inflammatory drugs (NSAIDs). Treatment comprises avoidance of caffeine and other aggravating factors known to the patient. 5-ASA agents may have a place in those not responding. Anti-diarrhoeal agents may be helpful. The disorder tends to resolve with such measures, but some resistant cases may benefit from topical steroid.

Hirschsprung's disease

Hirschsprung's disease affects 1 in 5000 live births and is due to the absence of ganglion cells in Auerbach's and Meissner's plexuses. It is an inherited disorder showing incomplete penetrance and variable expressivity. In some cases, there is a strong familial component, and mutations of the RET oncogene on chromosome 10 are responsible for most of these. RET gene mutations are also associated with multiple endocrine neoplasia (MEN) type II. In most cases, 5–20 cm of the distal large bowel is affected. The disease usually presents in childhood, but late presentation in adult life is not unknown. Loss of peristalsis in the affected segment leads to large bowel obstruction with gross distension of the colon proximal to the aganglionic segment. The differential diagnosis in the neonate includes imperforate anus and meconium ileus, and in older children, megacolon acquired as a result of chronic constipation. Ischaemic colitis and, in children, necrotizing enterocolitis have been reported due to superinfection with Staphylococcus aureus.

MRI is replacing barium enema, but either will reveal dilated bowel above the narrowed aganglionic segment. Lack of ganglia is confirmed by full-thickness biopsy of the abnormal area. In neonates, treatment consists of irrigation of the bowel with saline, followed by operation at about 6 weeks to bring ganglionated bowel down to the anal verge. In older children, a preliminary colostomy may be needed to allow bowel decompression. In the rare instance where the disease is not diagnosed until adulthood, the proximal colon is usually dysfunctional due to chronic megacolon and proctocolectomy, and ileo-anal pouch reconstruction may be preferable to anterior resection.

Acquired megacolon and idiopathic slow-transit constipation

In some children, chronic constipation may result in megacolon and is associated with behavioural problems and difficulty with toilet training. The initial complaint is often faecal soiling, but a vicious cycle of constipation and anal fissure may ensue. In adults, defaecatory problems ranging from idiopathic slow-transit constipation to adult megacolon and megarectum may arise. Electrophysiological studies have shown changes reminiscent of Hirschsprung's disease affecting the whole of the large bowel, and there may be associated gastric motility dysfunction. Examination reveals gross faecal loading of the colon and rectum. Barium studies reveal a capacious and poorly contracting bowel with huge redundant loops. Transit studies with radio-opaque markers or a radiolabelled enema typically show delayed transit.

Initial conservative management with aperients, bulk laxatives and regular enemas is successful in many cases, but faecal disimpaction under general anaesthesia may be required. Colectomy may be indicated in resistant cases but specialist advice should be sought, as severe cases are often due to neuropathy of the whole gut and surgery may not be curative.

INTESTINAL STOMA AND FISTULA

Stoma

Intestinal stomas have an important place in the management of small and large intestinal disease. An ileostomy is formed by bringing out the ileum through the abdominal wall, usually through the rectus muscle in the right iliac fossa. Ileal bowel content is irritant to skin and a spout is fashioned to allow appliances to be fitted and so prevent

16

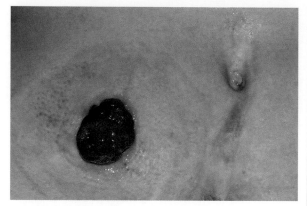

Fig. 16.24 Ileostomy sited in the right iliac fossa and demonstrating a spout.

skin contact with bowel content (Fig. 16.24). Ileostomy comprises either an 'end' stoma, or a 'loop' or 'defunctioning' stoma. It may be employed as an adjunct to resectional surgery when the disease process prevents re-anastomosis, or as a temporary stoma to allow a distal anastomosis to heal, such as for a low colorectal or ileoanal anastomosis. End-ileostomy is used when the colon has been removed, and occasionally when small intestine distal to the stoma has been removed, as in extensive Crohn's disease.

The colon can be brought out as an end or a loop colostomy, usually through the rectus muscle in the left iliac fossa. Transverse colostomy is seldom used in modern surgical practice but is brought out onto the right upper quadrant. A colostomy does not require a spout, as faeces are not usually irritant to the skin. End-colostomy is used as part of a Hartmann's procedure and is an integral part of an abdominoperineal resection for rectal cancer (see below). A loop colostomy of the sigmoid colon is used to divert faeces from a diseased anorectum, such as during the management of complex perianal fistula or faecal incontinence surgery. It may also be used as palliation for pelvic cancer or during radical radiotherapy for rectal cancer.

Intestinal fistula

A fistula is an abnormal communication between two epithelialized surfaces, and can manifest as a communication between intestine and other parts of the gastrointestinal tract, skin, urinary tract or vagina. Intestinal fistulae may arise as part of a disease process (Crohn's, complicated diverticular disease or radiation enteritis) or as an iatrogenic complication, such as leak from a surgical anastomosis. Anastomotic leak may result in a cutaneous fistula, with bowel content appearing through the wound several days after intestinal surgery. The overall leak rate from colorectal surgery is around 5%, but around 10% for colorectal anastomoses. Anastomotic leak may present as a rectovaginal fistula, when defunctioning stoma with conservative management may be the best option but laparotomy and drainage of pus combined with taking down of the anastomosis with the formation of a stoma may be required. Radiation fistula typically presents several months or years after the primary treatment, owing to the late development of endarteritis obliterans and chronic microvascular ischaemia. Malignant tumours of the upper and lower intestine can result in any combination of fistulation. Actinomycosis and tuberculosis are rare causes of cutaneous fistula. Treatment of disease-related fistula usually requires management of the primary problem.

POLYPS AND POLYPOSIS SYNDROMES OF THE LARGE INTESTINE

The terms 'polyp' and 'tumour' are not synonymous. A polyp is a descriptive term referring to an excrescence of the mucosa and is not a pathological definition. The histological classification of colorectal polyps into four groups is shown in Table 16.6. Polyps may be identified by rigid sigmoidoscopy, flexible sigmoidoscopy, colonoscopy, CT colonography (increasingly) or barium enema (now used increasingly less). Colonoscopy affords the opportunity for polypectomy and so enables histological assessment.

Colorectal adenoma

Neoplastic epithelial polyps are classified as tubular, tubulovillous or villous adenomas, depending on their histological architecture, and such classification has clinical relevance with respect to cancer risk. Adenomas affect 40% of people over 50 years of age and 70% of those aged 65–69 years. Tubular adenomas account for 75% of all adenomas and are frequently pedunculated but may be sessile. Villous adenomas account for 10% and tubulovillous types for 15% of all adenomas. However, villous adenomas account for 60% of lesions larger than 2 cm. Villous tumours are most commonly located in the rectum and may be very large, carpeting the rectum. Around 50% of such tumours have a focus of carcinoma at presentation. Villous adenomas greater than 1 cm in diameter have an approximately 30% chance of malignancy, whereas the risk in a similar-sized tubular adenoma is around 10%. Multiple adenomas are common, with 24% of patients having at least two tumours.

Clinical features

The vast majority of polyps are asymptomatic, but symptoms include rectal bleeding or large bowel colic (especially when a large polyp intussuscepts). Occasionally, a rectal

Table 16.6 **Classification of benign intestinal polyps**		
Type	**Solitary**	**Multiple**
Neoplastic	Adenoma (tubular, tubulovillous, villous)	Familial adenomatous polyposis (FAP)
Hamartomatous	Juvenile polyp	Juvenile polyposis syndrome (JPS)
	Peutz–Jeghers polyp	Peutz–Jeghers syndrome (PJS)
		Cronkhite–Canada syndrome
		Cowden's disease
Inflammatory	Benign lymphoid polyp	Benign lymphoid polyposis
		Pseudopolyposis in ulcerative colitis
Metaplastic	Metaplastic (hyperplastic)	*MYH*-associated polyposis (MAP)
	Serrated adenoma	Multiple metaplastic polyps

polyp may prolapse through the anus. Patients with giant villous adenoma of the rectum may present with severe watery diarrhea due to excessive mucus loss. This may result in dehydration and electrolyte depletion (profound hyokalaemia is typical). Rectal adenomas may be palpable, but villous tumors are soft and may be missed by the inexperienced finger. Distal polyps are detected readily by sigmoidoscopy, but there is a need for full colonoscopy in view of the risk of synchronous lesions (Fig. 16.25).

Management

Colonoscopic polypectomy using an electrocautery snare prevents future risk of malignant conversion as well as enabling histological assessment. Small adenomas can be biopsied and a current applied to destroy the entire polyp ('hot' biopsy). In many cases, polypectomy is the only treatment required, even when there is a malignant focus, so long as there are none of the following features: poor differentiation, stalk invasion at the resection margin or invasion of submucosal lymphatics or microvasculature (Fig. 16.26). Surgical resection (Fig. 16.27) is indicated following polypectomy if these histological features are noted, since there is a greatly increased risk of bowel wall invasion or lymphatic spread. Polypectomy may be technically impossible or the

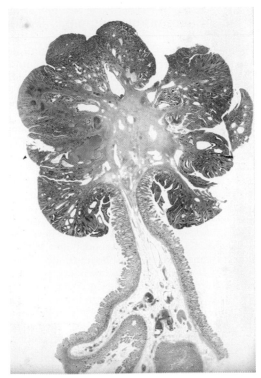

Fig. 16.26 Histological appearance of an adenomatous polyp, with malignant degeneration and early stalk invasion.

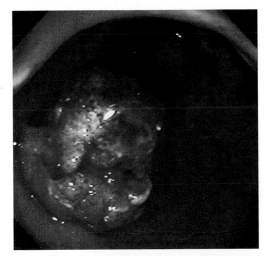

Fig. 16.25 Endoscopic appearance of a rectal adenomatous polyp.

risk of perforation too high (caecal lesions) and so bowel resection may be indicated for larger polyps. Transanal endoscopic microsurgery (TEM) allows resection of large rectal villous adenomas and repair of the rectal defect using an operating microscope. Advanced colonoscopic techniques such as lasering or submucosal resection are now well established for larger lesions when surgery is to be avoided.

Follow-up colonoscopy is recommended after 6–12 months and 2–3 years. The current view is not in favour of long-term follow-up once the colon has been shown to be clear of any further polyps, unless the polyps fulfilled high-risk criteria or there were recurrent lesions at the 3-year screen.

16

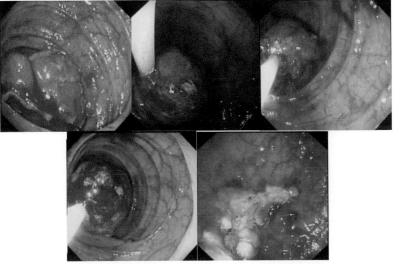

Fig. 16.27 Large adenoma of sigmoid colon resected endoscopically.

Familial adenomatous polyposis (FAP)

FAP is one of the most common single-gene disorders predisposing to cancer and is inherited as an autosomal dominant trait. The gene responsible is *APC*, which is located on the long arm of chromosome 5. In addition to germline changes resulting in FAP, almost every sporadic colorectal cancer has a somatic defect in the *APC* gene or in other components of the W nt signalling pathway. The annual incidence of FAP is 1 in 6670 live births and the population prevalence is 1 in 13 528. Around 25% of affected individuals have no family history of FAP, the disease arising in these sporadic cases as the result of a new germline mutation. Direct testing for the *APC* gene is now routine. Clinicopathological diagnosis requires the presence of > 100 adenomatous polyps of the large bowel (Fig. 16.28). Adenomatous polyps usually develop during teenage years and early adulthood, with > 90% chance of colorectal cancer by the third or fourth decade if prophylactic colectomy is not undertaken. Because of effective surgical prophylaxis, FAP now accounts for less than 0.2% of all cases of colorectal cancer in the UK. The prevalence of colorectal cancer at diagnosis is 65% for symptomatic 'sporadic' cases and < 5% for screened family members, emphasizing the effectiveness of prophylaxis and surveillance.

Extra-colonic features

Polyps are detected in 70% of FAP patients in the gastric fundus, but these are cystic gland polyps rather than adenomas. Gastric antral and duodenal adenomas are apparent in over 90% of cases and malignant degeneration of peri-ampullary adenoma is now the major cause of death – 7% of patients eventually develop peri-ampullary cancer. Ileal adenomas also occur in FAP, but the risk of progression to malignancy appears to be very low. Craniofacial and long bone osteomas occur in the majority of FAP patients, and when these are a predominant feature, especially when associated with epidermoid cysts, the term Gardner's syndrome is widely used. However, Gardner's syndrome is simply a subgroup of FAP.

Intra-abdominal desmoid tumours arise in around 10% of FAP cases. Although benign, these lesions expand and compress adjacent structures. Treatment with toremifene, tamoxifen, sulindac, indomethacin, chemotherapy and radiotherapy may provide benefit in non-resectable cases with problematical symptoms or complications.

An epidermoid cyst arising in a prepubescent child should raise suspicion of FAP. Bilateral asymptomatic pigmented retinal lesions, known as congenital hypertrophy of the retinal pigment epithelium (CHRPE) are a feature of FAP. There is an increased risk of papillary thyroid

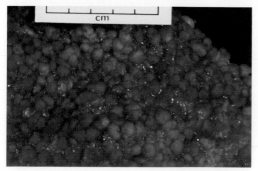

Fig. 16.28 Macroscopic features of dense polyposis due to familial adenomatous polyposis.

carcinoma in women (160-fold excess risk < 35 years), but no increased risk in men. Other rare associations with FAP include hepatoblastoma, carcinoma of the gallbladder, bile duct and pancreas, and an increased risk of brain tumours.

Diagnosis and management

The diagnosis can be established by sigmoidoscopy and biopsy. Screening of affected individuals by direct *APC* gene mutation analysis is used to define the optimal timing of prophylactic surgery. All FAP patients should be referred to a regional genetics service for registration and gene analysis. Pre-symptomatic detection of FAP allows prophylactic colectomy before malignancy supervenes (EBM 16.3). There is no general consensus on the preferred surgical strategy, as both restorative proctocolectomy with ileo-anal pouch formation and total colectomy with ileo-rectal anastomosis have particular advantages. The upper gastrointestinal tract should be screened for duodenal adenoma or carcinoma.

> **EBM** 16.3 **Colorectal adenomas**
>
> *'Prophylactic surgical resection of the large bowel is indicated for familial adenomatous polyposis and MUTYH associated polyposis.'*
>
> Guidelines for colorectal cancer screening and surveillance in moderate and high risk groups. Cairns SR, Scholefield JH, Steele RJ, Dunlop MG, Thomas HJ, Evans GD, Eaden JA, Rutter MD, Atkin WP, Saunders BP, Lucassen A, Jenkins P, Fairclough PD, Woodhouse CR; British Society of Gastroenterology; Association of Coloproctology for Great Britain and Ireland. Gut. 2010 May;59(5):666-89. http://gut.bmj.com/content/59/5/666.long

Peutz–Jeghers syndrome (PJS)

PJS is a colorectal polyposis syndrome associated with a greatly increased risk of colorectal cancer and is discussed in the section on small intestinal disorders.

Juvenile polyposis syndrome (JPS)

Juvenile polyps are usually classified as hamartomas, although some regard them as inflammatory, with blockage of crypts resulting in retention cysts. Single juvenile polyps occur in around 1% of populations in developed countries, but juvenile polyposis is rare (estimated population frequency ~1:50 000). JPS is an autosomal dominant genetic disorder characterized by the development of multiple hamartomatous polyps throughout the gastrointestinal tract, usually around age 10 years. Causal mutations of the SMAD4 or BMPR1A/ALK3 genes are responsible, indicating genetic heterogeneity. Penetrance is incomplete for polyposis and colorectal cancer. Estimates for gastrointestinal cancer risk range from 9% to 68%, but is probably ~50% lifetime risk of colorectal cancer. In JPS families, or individuals with a documented SMAD4 or BMPR1A mutation, colonoscopic surveillance is recommended 1–2-yearly from the age of 15–18 years. Surveillance intervals can be extended after the age of 35 years. Documented gene carriers or affected cases should, however, be kept under surveillance until the age of 70 years. Consideration should be given to prophylactic colectomy, much in the same way as in FAP. While it is essential that cases are recognized and managed appropriately, because of its rarity < 0.1% of all cases of colorectal cancer are attributable to JPS.

Metaplastic (hyperplastic) polyposis and MUTYH-associated polyposis (MAP)

Metaplastic (now more properly termed as hyperplastic) polyps are usually less than 5 mm in diameter and occur in increasing numbers with age, being present in some 75% of the population over the age of 40 years. Polyps tend to be pale, flat-topped, sessile plaques, found mainly in the rectum and often on the crest of mucosal folds. Histologically, the crypts are elongated, dilated and lined by columnar epithelium that has a sawtooth pattern. These polyps are often indistinguishable from adenomatous polyps, and are frequently removed because of the difficulties in differentiating them from adenomas. Some of the larger metaplastic polyps take on the features of a serrated adenoma and principally affect the caecum, where they are highly likely to progress to cancer.

A subset of individuals with multiple hyperplastic polyps early in life has a substantially elevated cancer. A gene involved in DNA base excision repair (MUTYH) has been shown to be responsible for colorectal hyperplastic polyposis in association with adenomatous polyps. The syndrome should be considered as a differential diagnosis of FAP, but with smaller numbers of adenomas. Mode of inheritance is autosomal recessive (cf. FAP which is autosomal dominant) and colorectal cancer risk is very high. The management of documented homozygous MUTYH mutation carriers is controversial. Some advocate colonoscopic surveillance in the same manner as FAP and JPS but others cite the penetrance for colorectal cancer > 90% and recommend prophylactic colectomy and ileorectal anastomosis.

Other rare polyposis syndromes

Turcot's syndrome

Turcot's is an adenomatous colorectal polyposis syndrome associated with astrocytoma (also medulloblastoma or glioblastoma) of brain or spinal cord.

Cowden's disease

This is a rare gastrointestinal hamartomatous polyposis with an autosomal dominant pattern of inheritance, due to inactivating mutations of the PTEN gene. There is an increased risk of colorectal cancer but benign and malignant disease of the breast and thyroid are the main risks. Peri-orbital warty tricholemmomas are pathognomonic in association with oral fibromas and keratoses of the hands and feet.

Cronkhite–Canada syndrome

A rare, non-heritable, syndrome comprising intestinal polyposis with alopecia, nail atrophy and brown macular hyperpigmentation. Histological examination shows cystic crypt dilatation similar to juvenile polyposis.

Miscellaneous colorectal polyps

Benign lymphoid polyps are round, smooth and sessile tumours comprising aggregates of lymphoid tissue lined by attenuated epithelium varying in diameter from a few millimetres to 3 cm. Other differential diagnoses of colorectal polyps include pseudopolyps in chronic ulcerative colitis; submucosal lipoma; lymphosarcoma; carcinoid tumour; leiomyoma. Neurofibromatosis rarely results in colonic polyps. Mucosal ganglioneuromatosis has been described in association with multiple adenomatous or juvenile polyps and in MEN type IIb.

MALIGNANT TUMOURS OF THE LARGE INTESTINE

Colorectal adenocarcinoma

Adenocarcinoma of the large bowel is the most common gastrointestinal malignancy. It is second only to lung cancer as a cause of cancer death in developed countries. There are ~36 000 new cases in the UK annually, accounting for around 15% and 12% of all cancer registration in males and females respectively. Lifetime risk is ~5%. It is third-ranked cancer overall after lung and prostate in males, and breast and lung in females. The male:female ratio for colon cancer is close to unity, whereas that for rectal cancer is 1.7:1. Incidence rates increase substantially with age. The rectum and sigmoid are particularly common sites for tumours (Fig. 16.29). However, in low-incidence countries, tumours are more evenly distributed. Around 3% of patients present with synchronous tumours, and another 3% develop a metachronous tumour.

Aetiology

The aetiology is multifactorial, but there is a substantial environmental aetiological contribution, as evidenced by comparison of incidence between populations and by migration studies that demonstrate how a migrant population takes on the risk of the host population within a generation. These include male gender (males' lifetime risk 1.5 times that of females), increasing age, a strong family history of the disease and consuming a 'Westernized' diet.

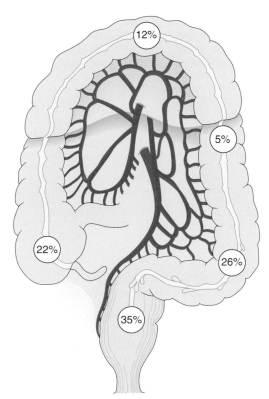

Fig. 16.29 Distribution of colorectal cancer in the large bowel in the UK.

16

Diet

Diet is a major environmental risk factor but no single dietary factor is solely responsible. Recently, dietary fibre has again gained favour as a protective factor. A diet high in fibre is associated with lower cancer rates in certain populations and within the UK population, whereas the consumption of a diet high in fat and red meat is associated with higher cancer rates. A high-energy diet is an associated risk factor. A low-fibre, high-fat diet appears to increase faecal pH, and this may enhance bile acid toxicity. Brassica vegetables, such as broccoli, contain antioxidants and other potential antineoplastic compounds. A deficiency of dietary calcium and vitamin D is associated with increased colorectal cancer risk. Despite strong supporting epidemiological evidence, intervention studies have not so far definitively shown that any dietary intervention reduces risk of colorectal adenoma or cancer. This suggests that a combination of various elements that make up a 'Western' diet is responsible.

Protective agents

Aspirin has been shown conclusively in case-control and cohort epidemiological studies and also recently in randomized trials to substantially reduce colorectal adenoma and cancer risk (variously 30–50% risk reduction). Other NSAIDs also appear to be protective. Dietary calcium supplements and vitamin D also are associated with a reduced risk. Hormone replacement therapy also seems to be protective (EBM 16.4).

EBM 16.4 **Prevention and detection of colorectal adenocarcinoma**

'Aspirin and non-steroidal anti-inflammatory drugs protect from colorectal neoplasia and are associated with reduced cancer mortality.

Population screening by faecal occult blood test reduces mortality by 18% in those accepting screening.

Population screening by 'once-only' flexible sigmoidoscopy may have a place in reducing colorectal cancer mortality.'

Rothwell PM, Fowkes FG, Belch JF, Ogawa H, Warlow CP, Meade TW. Effect of daily aspirin on long-term risk of death due to cancer: analysis of individual patient data from randomised trials. Lancet. 2011 Jan 1;377(9759):31-41. Epub 2010 Dec 6. PubMed PMID: 21144578.

Hewitson P, Glasziou P, Watson E, Towler B, Irwig L.Am J Gastroenterol. Cochrane systematic review of colorectal cancer screening using the fecal occult blood test (hemoccult): an update. 2008 Jun;103(6):1541-9. Epub 2008 May 13.

Atkin WS, Edwards R, Kralj-Hans I, Wooldrage K, Hart AR, Northover JM, Parkin DM, Wardle J, Duffy SW, Cuzick J; UK Flexible Sigmoidoscopy Trial Investigators. Once-only flexible sigmoidoscopy screening in prevention of colorectal cancer: a multicentre randomised controlled trial. Lancet. 2010 May 8;375(9726):1624-33. Epub 2010 Apr 27. PubMed PMID: 20430429.

Smoking, alcohol and exercise

Smoking and alcohol excess are risk factors for men but women appear not to be subject to the excess risk. An association between lack of physical exercise and colorectal cancer has been observed. Colonic transit time may be reduced by exercise, but alterations in the levels of prostaglandins and antioxidant enzymes may also occur.

Inflammatory bowel disease

The risk of colorectal cancer in ulcerative colitis and Crohn's disease is discussed above.

Genetic susceptibility

Genetic susceptibility contributes 35% to the overall incidence of colorectal cancer. This genetic component ranges from an ill-defined increased risk in individuals with a positive family history, to well-defined autosomal dominant genetic traits in which the responsible genes have been identified and mutations characterized. Three broad categories of genetic susceptibility trait have been defined at the clinical and/or molecular level: autosomal dominant heritable colorectal cancer susceptibility syndromes (HNPCC, FAP, PJS, JPS); recessive inheritance (MUTYH associated polyposis); common genetic inheritance.

Autosomal polyposis syndromes and MAP are described above. HNPCC (also known as Lynch syndrome) is the most common autosomal dominant cancer syndrome, accounting for 3–5% of all colorectal cancer cases. It is associated with only small numbers of adenomas, but the risk of colorectal cancer is very high, with 70% of males and 35% of females developing the disease over a lifetime. There is also an elevated risk of other malignancies, including endometrial, gastric ovarian, upper urinary tract and small intestinal.

HNPCC is of major interest because it is a relatively common definable genetic cause of colorectal cancer and thus lends itself to identification of gene carriers by DNA analysis of blood samples. Mutation analysis allows targeting of those at risk for colonoscopic screening and adenoma removal, and this has been shown to be an effective cancer control measure in HNPCC.

HNPCC is due to mutation of one of the genes that participate in DNA mismatch repair. Mutations are most common in *MSH2* on chromosome 2p, *MLH1* on chromosome 2q and *MSH6* on chromosome 2p. Around 90% of large dominant HNPCC families from research studies have identifiable mutations. In clinical genetics practice, however, only 30% of selected families have mutations in one of the genes responsible. Overall, causative mutations have been identified in ~3% of all colorectal cancer cases, but patients who develop colorectal cancer at an early age are more likely to have developed the disease because of an underlying DNA mismatch repair gene defect; 1 in 4 of patients aged < 40 years and 1 in 20 aged < 55 years at diagnosis of colorectal cancer carry a mutation, irrespective of family history.

Common genetic variance has been shown to contribute to colorectal cancer through genome-wide analysis. So far 14 common variants have been identified with allele frequencies in the general population in the range 10–50%. Many of the variants are in genes encoding proteins participating in cellular growth signaling pathways such as SMAD and TGF signaling pathways. However, the colorectal cancer risk associated with these variants is low (typically RR 1.05–1.2) and so they currently cannot be used for individual risk prediction.

Clinical features of established colorectal cancer

Intestinal symptoms are extremely common in the general population but there are no specific symptoms that discriminate cancer from benign intestinal diseases or from symptoms common in healthy individuals. Presentation may include intermittent rectal bleeding, blood mixed with mucus, altered bowel habit, iron deficiency anaemia and colicky lower abdominal pain. Tenesmus occurs in over 50% of patients with low rectal cancers. Massive lower gastrointestinal haemorrhage is rare and so is more likely to represent underlying benign disorders rather than colorectal cancer. Abdominal wall invasion may manifest as parietal pain and occasionally leads to abscess formation. Perianal or sciatic-type pain is an ominous sign suggesting locally advanced rectal cancer. Around 3% of presenting patients are under the age of 35, but sinister symptoms are often ignored by young patients. Around 15% of all patients present with obstruction and 3% have a perforation at presentation, complications which are associated with poorer stage-specific prognosis.

A full history is essential, as clinical examination is often negative. There may be signs of anaemia, and abdominal examination may reveal hepatomegaly or an abdominal mass, especially in right-sided colon cancer. There may be signs of bowel obstruction. Digital rectal examination is mandatory to detect low cancers and to assess fixity and sphincter involvement. Faecal occult blood (FOB) testing will not alter the decision to investigate the symptomatic patient and so is a superfluous investigation.

Population screening for colorectal cancer

Early detection of colorectal cancer by population screening in asymptomatic individuals aged 50–75 years has been shown to result in ~20% improvement in survival. The most extensively studied screening test is the faecal occult blood test (FOBT) using guaiac-impregnated paper – Haemoccult – but sensitivity is only 50–60%. The predictive value is around 10% for cancer and 50% for adenomas > 1 cm. Specificity is the main problem with the test, as it generates large numbers of people with positive slides but no cancer. Population screening using colonoscopy is widespread for those that can afford it in the USA, but it seems unlikely to be implemented in other countries in view of the massive cost implications. However, once-only flexible sigmoidoscopy at age 50–55 years has recently been shown to reduce colorectal cancer mortality by detecting early rectosigmoid cancers and identifying individuals prone to develop adenomas. Other screening modalities are also under assessment, including cancer-specific stool DNA testing, but these approaches are many years away from formal clinical evaluation.

Investigations

Colonoscopy is the investigation of choice (Fig. 16.30). However, increasingly CT colonography (Fig. 16.31) is employed in the investigation of altered bowel habit. It has similar diagnostic accuracy to colonoscopy, although clearly lacks the advantage of enabling diagnostic biopsy or snaring of adenomas. Barium enema (Fig. 16.32) still has a place but is becoming a somewhat obsolete test. Typical features of

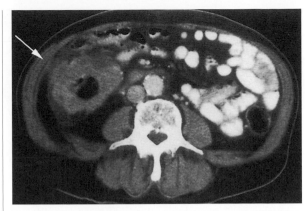

Fig. 16.31 CT showing a typical colorectal cancer with thickening, shouldering and mucosal ulceration.

colorectal cancer are shouldering and mucosal destruction, but biopsy is essential wherever possible. In some instances the diagnosis is only made at laparotomy for a perforated or obstructed viscus.

Preoperative staging

Staging is a central component of preoperative work-up, as it provides important information on prognosis, helps inform surgical strategy and indicates the need or otherwise for adjuvant radiotherapy for rectal cancer and adjuvant postoperative chemotherapy for colorectal cancer. All patients with colon or rectal cancer should undergo CT of the chest, abdomen and pelvis (Fig. 16.33). Liver ultrasound and chest X-ray have now been almost totally superseded by CT. For rectal cancer, digital examination and rigid sigmoidoscopy should be undertaken in every case (examination under anaesthetic – EUA – may be required) to assess the degree of tumour fixity. Pelvic MRI is essential to assess the degree of local invasion of rectal cancer. Endoanal ultrasound may also be useful for local staging of rectal cancer, but is somewhat operator-dependent and requires considerable

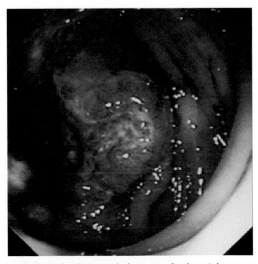

Fig. 16.30 Typical colonoscopic features of colorectal cancer.

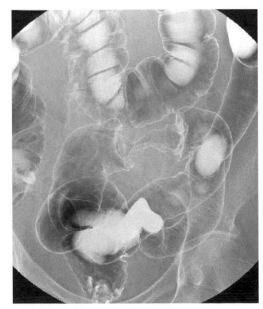

Fig. 16.32 Barium enema showing a malignant 'applecore' appearance in the sigmoid colon, due to stenosing colorectal cancer.

16

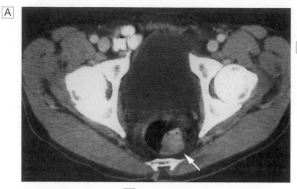
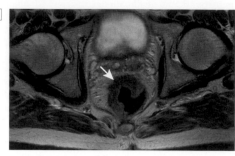

Fig. 16.33 Rectal cancer imaging. **A** CT features of early T_1 cancer (arrowed), restricted to the bowel wall. **B** Pelvic MRI showing T_3 cancer (arrowed), invading through the bowel wall and into the mesorectum.

experience and interpretational skill. In some cases being considered for major debilitating surgery with a view to cure, FDG positron emission tomography in combination with CT scanning (FDG-PET-CT) is indicated. PET-CT has the potential to detect unsuspected distant metastatic disease that can influence the decision to undertake major resectional surgery, rather than more limited procedures.

Management of colorectal adenocarcinoma

Surgery

Elective colorectal resection with curative intent

The mainstay of treatment comprises *en bloc* resection of the primary tumour and loco-regional nodes. This achieves cure in 75% of cases undergoing intended 'curative' resections. Excision of the colonic mesentery, ligation of the arterial supply at its origin, and excision of all accompanying lymph nodes achieve locoregional lymphadenectomy for the respective segment of bowel (Fig. 16.34). Resection offers cure for patients with localized disease; even for patients with lymph node metastases but no distant metastases, cure can be expected in 50% of cases with surgery alone. For rectal cancer, excision of the entire mesorectum can reduce local recurrence rates to < 5%. Wherever possible, bowel continuity should be restored. In specialist hands, low rectal cancer should be treated by low anterior resection and colo-anal anastomosis. A colonic J-pouch may be formed in an attempt to improve defaecatory function. However, for low rectal cancer involving the sphincter muscle, it may be necessary to remove the anal sphincter as part of an abdominoperineal resection and fashion a permanent end-colostomy. Laparoscopic colorectal resection is increasingly used and has been shown to provide short-term benefits, with less pain and shorter hospital stay. However, there is no definitive evidence of improved long-term outcomes over open surgery.

Rectal cancer can be excised per-anally under direct vision or using trans-anal endoscopic microsurgery (TEM). TEM is particularly applicable to small low-lying cancers (< 3 cm). Per-anal excision has a place for T_1 or T_2 tumours and may allow avoidance of major abdominal surgery. However, careful staging is essential because the recurrence rate is 25–30% if there are incomplete excision margins or if the lesion was staged inaccurately. Pathology assessment may indicate the need to proceed to formal resection and mesorectal excision.

Early polyp cancers removed at colonoscopic snare polypectomy may be treated without the need for formal trans-abdominal resection. However, where the pathology specimen of the snared polyp cancer shows poor differentiation or submucosal lymphatic or vascular invasion, or where the diathermized margin is involved, formal resection and regional lymphadenectomy are indicated. With the introduction of population colorectal cancer screening by FOBT, this is becoming a more common scenario.

In the elective setting, the patient should be fasted and have undergone full preoperative work-up to assess cardiac, respiratory and any other co-morbidity; reversible risk factors for major surgery should have been addressed. Bowel preparation has been radically reshaped in recent years. Fluid diet is instigated for 48 hours prior to surgery but mechanical bowel preparation is now avoided for the majority of resections and only a phosphate enema 2 hours prior to surgery is required for left sided resections. Recent meta-analyses indicate that there is no benefit for mechanical bowel preparation (comprising polyethylene glycol, sodium picosulfate or phospho-soda), and it may even be harmful. However bowel preparation does have a place for low rectal anastomoses, especially if a defunctioning ileostomy is planned. Antibiotic

---

EBM **16.5 Preparation for surgery in patients with colorectal adenocarcinoma**

'Preoperative staging is required to guide surgery and pre-operative adjuvant radiotherapy.

Bowel preparation is not required for colorectal resection.

Compression stockings and heparin are required thromboprophylaxis for patients undergoing colorectal surgery.

Patient should be fasted prior to surgery.

Co-morbidity should be addressed wherever possible to limit perioperative mortality risk.

Perioperative antibiotic prophylaxis is essential and should cover coliform and anaerobic organisms.'

The Association of Coloproctology of Great Britain and Ireland. Guidelines for the Management of Colorectal Cancer 3rd edition (2007). http://www.acpgbi.org.uk/assets/documents/COLO_guides.pdf
Güenaga KF, Matos D, Wille-Jørgensen P. Mechanical bowel preparation for elective colorectal surgery. Cochrane Database of Systematic Reviews 2011, Issue 9. Art. No.: CD001544. DOI: 10.1002/14651858.CD001544.pub4.
Prevention and management of venous thromboembolism. Scottish Intercollegiate Guideline Network. http://www.sign.ac.uk/pdf/sign122.pdf
Wille-Jørgensen P, Rasmussen MS, Andersen BR, Borly L. Heparins and mechanical methods for thromboprophylaxis in colorectal surgery. Cochrane Database of Systematic Reviews 2004, Issue 1. Art. No.: CD001217. DOI: 10.1002/14651858.CD001217.
Antibiotic prophylaxis in surgery. Scottish Intercollegiate Guideline Network. http://www.sign.ac.uk/pdf/sign104.pdf
Nelson RL, Glenny AM, Song F. Antimicrobial prophylaxis for colorectal surgery. Cochrane Database of Systematic Reviews 2009, Issue 1. Art. No.: CD001181. DOI: 10.1002/14651858.CD001181.pub3.

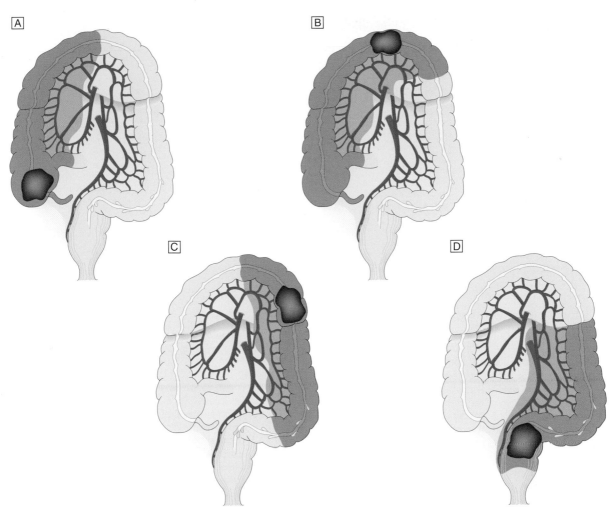

Fig. 16.34 Surgical resection for colorectal cancer arising at various locations within the large bowel. Radical tumour resection requires clearance of the primary tumour and also the arteries supplying that part of the colon. Lymphatic drainage follows the path of arterial supply, allowing a regional lymphadenectomy. **A** Excision of a right-sided tumour and the ileocaecal, right colic and right branch of middle colic arteries. **B** Tumours of transverse colon are usually treated by extended right hemicolectomy, again taking the feeding vessels at their origin from the superior mesenteric artery. **C** For left colonic lesions, the feeding vessels are taken. **D** Anterior resection is treated by high ligation of the inferior mesenteric artery.

prophylaxis comprises perioperative broad-spectrum anti-biotics (e.g. a third-generation cephalosporin, or gentamicin and ampicillin, and metronidazole). Chemical thrombo-prophylaxis (low molecular weight fractionated heparin or calcium heparin), along with compression stockings and intraoperative intermittent pneumatic calf compression (EBM 16.5) is indicated as the risk of deep venous thrombosis and pulmonary embolism is high in such cases.

Emergency colorectal resection

In cases of perforation or obstruction of colorectal cancer, there is a substantially increased risk of perioperative mortality. The patient should be resuscitated before laparotomy is undertaken. For obstructed right-sided colon cancer, right hemicolectomy is the operation of choice. An ileo-transverse anastomosis can be safely performed, as the ileum has an excellent blood supply and the distal colon is not obstructed. Treatment of obstructed left colon cancer is best achieved by a one-stage resection with anastomosis whenever possible. Measures that may be employed to reduce the risk of anastomotic leakage in such cases include on-table colonic lavage to remove faecal residue. Resection of the entire colon and ileorectal anastomosis avoid a colocolic anastomosis and also remove any synchronous tumour (3% of cases). Patients with gross faecal

peritonitis secondary to perforation of left colon cancer usually require resection with the creation of an end-colostomy (Hartmann's procedure). If contamination is minimal, a specialist surgeon may elect to carry out primary resection and anastomosis. As in the elective setting, surgery should be covered with perioperative antibiotics and DVT prophylaxis.

Pathology and staging

Macroscopically, colorectal cancer may be polypoidal, ulcerating or stenosing (Fig. 16.35). Two-thirds are ulcerating and a typical lesion has raised everted edges, a slough-covered floor and indurated base. Tumours of the caecum tend to be large exophytic growths. Tumour differentiation may be classified as good, moderate or poor. Around 10–20% of tumours have mucinous histology and this tumour type has a poor prognosis. There is an increasing proportion of proximal tumours in the UK, as right colonic cancer is more common in the elderly and the UK population is ageing.

Colorectal cancer may spread by lymphatic invasion, via the portal blood to the liver and/or by trans-peritoneal seeding. Once the peritoneum is breached, dissemination throughout the abdominal cavity is likely. Invasion of lymphatics results in regional lymph node involvement. Very low rectal tumours may also involve the inguinal nodes.

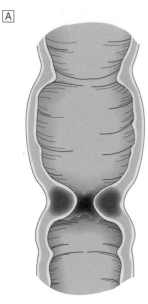 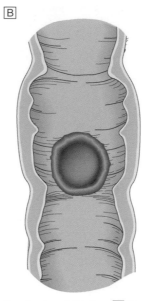 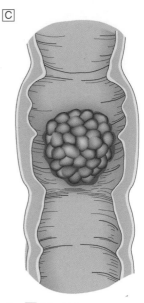

Fig. 16.35 Macroscopic characteristics of colorectal cancer. [A] Stenosing. [B] Ulcerating. [C] Polypoidal.

EBM 16.6 **Improving postoperative survival rates in colorectal adenocarcinoma**

'Improved surgical and anaesthetic management has had a major impact on overall survival. Preoperative adjuvant radiotherapy reduces local recurrence rates, but not overall survival. Postoperative adjuvant chemotherapy improves survival by 30% for stage III tumours and 2% for stage II tumours. Postoperative intensive follow-up is associated with a 9% survival improvement by identifying those with surgically salvageable relapse.'

The Association of Coloproctology of Great Britain and Ireland. Guidelines for the Management of Colorectal Cancer 3rd edition (2007). http://www.acpgbi.org.uk/assets/documents/COLO_guides.pdf
Management of colorectal cancer. Scottish Intercollegiate Guideline Network (and update). Management of colorectal cancer. Guideline No 67. http://www.sign.ac.uk/guidelines/fulltext/67/index.html
Wong RKS, Tandan V, De Silva S, Figueredo A. Pre-operative radiotherapy and curative surgery for the management of localized rectal carcinoma. Cochrane Database of Systematic Reviews 2007, Issue 2. Art. No.: CD002102. DOI: 10.1002/14651858.CD002102.pub2.
Midgley R, Kerr DJ. Adjuvant chemotherapy for stage II colorectal cancer: the time is right! Nat Clin Pract Oncol. 2005 Jul;2(7):364-9. Review. PubMed PMID: 16075796.
Gill S, Loprinzi CL, Sargent DJ, Thomé SD, Alberts SR, Haller DG, Benedetti J, Francini G, Shepherd LE, Francois Seitz J, Labianca R, Chen W, Cha SS, Heldebrant MP, Goldberg RM. Pooled analysis of fluorouracil-based adjuvant therapy for stage II and III colon cancer: who benefits and by how much? J Clin Oncol. 2004 May 15;22(10):1797-806. Epub 2004 Apr 5. PubMed PMID: 15067028.

Table 16.7 **Dukes' staging for colorectal cancer**

Dukes' stage	Description	Proportion of colorectal cancers (%)
A	Spread into, but not beyond, muscularis propria	10
B	Spread through full thickness of bowel wall	30
C	Spread to involve lymph nodes	30
D*	Distant metastases	20

*There is formally no D stage in Dukes' staging; this is a misnomer, as Dukes' staging refers only to degree of local invasion and to lymphatic spread. However, the term is widely used in clinical practice.

Table 16.8 **TNM staging of colorectal cancer**

T (Tumour)
- T_x — Primary tumour cannot be assessed
- Tis — Carcinoma in situ
- T_1 — Cancer invades submucosa
- T_2 — Cancer invades into muscularis propria
- T_3 — Cancer invades through muscularis propria and into subserosa or adjacent non-peritonealized tissues
- T_4 — Cancer perforates the visceral peritoneum or directly invades adjacent organs

N (Node)
- N_x — The regional lymph nodes cannot be assessed
- N_0 — No regional lymph nodes involved
- N_1 — Metastases in 1–3 pericolic or perirectal lymph nodes
- N_2 — Metastases in 4 or more pericolic or perirectal lymph nodes
- N_3 — Metastases in lymph node along the course of a major named blood vessel

M (Metastases)
- M_x — The presence of distant metastases cannot be assessed
- M_0 — No distant metastases
- M_1 — Distant metastases

Systemic metastases may occur in the later stages of the disease. Tumour staging systems include Dukes' and TNM staging (Tables 16.7 and 16.8). TNM stages can be grouped using the American Joint Committee on Cancer (AJCC) system (Table 16.9). Pathological staging has important implications for prognosis and also for directing clinical management (EBM 16.6). Staging information informs both predicted survival outcome and also decision-making on whether adjuvant chemotherapy is indicated.

Adjuvant therapy

Radiotherapy

Adjuvant preoperative radiotherapy has an important place in the management of rectal cancer, and so preoperative staging of rectal cancer is essential in order to plan optimal management. Radiotherapy has been shown to reduce local

Table 16.9 American joint committee on cancer (AJCC) stage groupings and equivalence with Dukes' staging

AJCC	TNM		Dukes
I	$T_1N_0M_0$ or $T_2N_0M_0$	Spread into submucosa or just into muscularis propria No lymph node or distant spread	A
IIA	$T_3N_0M_0$	Spread through bowel wall into outermost layers No lymph node or distant spread	B
IIB	$T_4N_0M_0$	Spread through bowel wall into other tissues or organs No lymph node or distant spread	B
IIIA	$T_{1-2}N_1M_0$	Spread into submucosa or just into muscularis propria Spread to ≤ 3 nearby lymph nodes but no distant spread	C
IIIB	$T_{3-4}N_1M_0$	Spread through bowel wall into other tissues or organs Spread to ≤ 3 nearby lymph nodes but no distant spread	C
IIIC	Any T N_2M_0	Any T stage and spread ≥ 4 lymph nodes but no distant spread	C
IV	Any T Any N M1	Any T and N stage but distant spread (e.g. liver, lung, peritoneum)	D*

*There is formally no D stage in Dukes' staging; this is a misnomer, as Dukes' staging refers only to degree of local invasion and to lymphatic spread. However, the term is widely used in clinical practice.

16

recurrence rates but there is no effect on overall survival (EBM 16.6). Most specialist centres in the UK offer selective preoperative radiotherapy for those at increased risk of local recurrence, because there is significant morbidity associated with pelvic irradiation and many patients will be cured by surgery alone. Risk factors include a low tumour, bulky fixed lesion, anterior lesion, evidence of T_3 or T_4 stage and/or involved lymph nodes on imaging. Either a 5-day short-course regimen of 45 Gy daily or a long-course regimen of 52 Gy given weekly over 3 months is administered. The former is reserved for patients with operable but tethered tumours or very low or anterior tumours, or if extra-rectal spread is evident. Fixed, inoperable tumours are best dealt with by radical radiotherapy over 3 months, and this may be combined with chemotherapy (capecitabine or 5-fluorouracil (5-FU)). Postoperative radiotherapy results in poor bowel function and may damage the small intestine, and hence the importance of preoperative staging to guide administration of radiotherapy before surgery whenever possible.

Adjuvant chemotherapy

Systemic adjuvant chemotherapy using 5-FU alone or in combination with other agents has been shown to improve survival for Dukes' C colorectal cancer after surgical resection (EBM 16.6). Intravenous regimens employing intravenous 5-FU has largely been replaced in current practice by targeting the same pathway through inhibition of thymidylate synthase using chemical inhibitors such as capecitabine. Capecitabine is less toxic than 5-FU and can be administered orally. There is an overall 30% improvement in survival for patients with Dukes' C tumours who receive chemotherapy, equating with an 11% absolute improvement in survival for that group and a 6% overall improvement in survival for patients with colorectal cancer of all stages. In the UK, it is now routine practice to offer chemotherapy based on 5-FU to all patients with stage C cancers who do not have significant comorbidity, particularly cardiovascular disease. Regimens now routinely combine capecitabine with oxaliplatin as first line therapy. Recently, it has also been shown that Dukes' B tumours gain modest survival benefit (~2%). However, adjuvant chemotherapy for Dukes' B tumours is restricted to poor-prognosis lesions (poor differentiation, venous or lymphatic invasion). Capecitabine (or 5-FU) chemotherapy is considered a conventional 'first-line' chemotherapeutic

regimen for colorectal cancer. Other newer agents, such as cetuximab (monoclonal antibody to epidermal growth factor receptor) and bevacizumab (antibody to vascular endothelial growth factor), have shown promise in patients with relapsed disease after first-line chemotherapy. Other agents such as temozolomide, used either alone or in combination with other standard agents are also used in relapsed disease and in trials. Although irinotecan (CPT-11) showed initial promise, a number of negative trials indicate it may only have a place in the management of a small selected subset of patients.

Palliative therapy

In addition to resection with curative intent, surgery can provide valuable palliation for patients with local disease relapse, hepatic or other distant metastases. This is achieved through ameliorating symptoms or by averting distressing features of advanced local disease. In some instances, diversion of the faecal stream through a defunctioning colostomy or ileostomy may be all that is feasible, but wherever possible it is preferable to resect the tumour and involved bowel in a formal way. Hence, the vast majority of patients undergo surgical resection, whether curative or palliative. In a small number of cases with poor functional status and/or extensive metastatic load and in whom surgical resection is relatively contraindicated, combined radiological and colonoscopic placement of an *intraluminal expanding stent* will palliate an obstructing colonic cancer.

Radiotherapy has an important role in palliation of locally advanced irresectable rectal cancer and can control pain, mucus discharge, disordered bowel habit, bleeding and faecal incontinence. It also has a value in palliation of rectal cancer recurrence and in alleviating bone pain from metastases. It may rarely be used to palliate locally invasive colonic cancer invading the abdominal wall, but this approach is restricted because the fields are difficult to define and damage to adjacent bowel is likely.

Palliative chemotherapy is now used extensively both to treat symptoms of disseminated disease, and to control disease progression and extend survival. This is especially the case with the introduction of oral capecitabine. Median life expectancy from diagnosis of hepatic metastases is now around 12–14 months.

Colorectal cancer

- Colorectal adenocarcinoma is the most common gastrointestinal malignancy, with 36 000 cases per annum in the UK
- It is second only to lung cancer as a cause of cancer death in developed countries, accounting for 15% of all cancers in males and 12% in females, with a 5% lifetime risk
- 2–3% of patients present with synchronous tumours, and a further ~3% develop metachronous tumours
- Risk factors include male gender, increasing age, family history of an affected relative, 'westernized' diet, inflammatory bowel disease and pre-existing adenomatous polyps
- Genes have been identified for a number of autosomal dominant colorectal cancer predisposition syndromes, accounting for ~3% of all cases.
- Around 35% of the aetiology of colorectal cancer is attributable to genetic factors and a number of common genetic variants have recently been identified, offering future potential for genetic profiling

- Two-thirds of all large bowel cancers occur in the rectum and sigmoid colon, and the most common clinical features are alteration in bowel habit and the passage of blood per rectum
- Diagnosis involves colonoscopy and biopsy, CT colonography, or barium enema (used less). Preoperative staging involves CT, MRI and PET-CT scanning
- Surgery is the mainstay of treatment, involving radical local clearance combined with regional lymphadenectomy
- Adjuvant therapy options include preoperative radiotherapy for rectal cancer and postoperative chemotherapy
- Pre-symptomatic diagnosis may be achieved by population screening using faecal occult blood testing or by surveillance colonoscopy in high-risk groups
- Overall 5-year survival is 55%. Staging systems provide useful prognosis to guide therapy and inform patients of expected outcome.

Prognosis

Systematic population data from cancer registry show that overall 1-year and 5-survival is 75% and 55% respectively, having improved by over 20% in both males and females in the last 10 years. The marked improvement in survival from colorectal cancer is due to a combination of earlier diagnosis across all stages, improved perioperative anaesthetic and surgical management, and improved adjuvant therapies, especially chemotherapy. However, overall prognosis is even better for patients who have no evidence of metastases on preoperative staging tests and who have undergone a resection with curative intent, with 5-year survival of 75% being achievable. This underscores the importance of preoperative staging in informing radical surgery. The 5-year survival by Dukes' stage is 90–95% for Dukes' stage A, 65–75% for Dukes' stage B and 40–50% for Dukes' stage C. Only a minority of patients with liver or lung metastases will survive to 5 years and most die within 2 years of diagnosis. Operative mortality is low (~4%) for elective resections but rises to 25% in patients with complications such as obstruction and perforation who require emergency surgery, emphasizing the importance of early detection and surgery prior to the development of complications. Patients with isolated hepatic metastases may be candidates for hepatic resection with a view to cure, and there is some evidence for long-term survival benefit in selected series.

Other malignant tumours of the large intestine

Colorectal adenocarcinoma dominates the incidence of large bowel cancer and all other malignant tumours are very rare in comparison.

Squamous cancer of the large bowel

Such tumours are not simply metastatic anal carcinomas, but may arise in the caecum and proximal colon from an area of squamous metaplasia in long-standing ulcerative colitis. In the absence of chronic inflammation, an adenosquamous pattern may be seen and the prognosis is poor.

Carcinoid tumour of the large bowel

Large bowel carcinoid tumours are very rare, but benign lesions may be found incidentally during rectal examination as solitary, spherical, hard, sessile, yellowish submucosal nodules. Malignant carcinoid tumors of the colon are frequently highly malignant and may give rise to the carcinoid syndrome. Around 60% have metastasized by the time of diagnosis.

Lymphoma of the large intestine

Primary lymphomas usually arise in the rectum or caecum but are occasionally multicentric. Secondary involvement of the large bowel in generalized disease is more common. Barium enema shows a long rigid segment with intramural thickening. The diagnosis is established by endoscopic or operative biopsy. Primary lymphomas are treated by resection, followed by chemotherapy and radiotherapy. Secondary malignant lymphoma and malignant lymphomatous polyposis are treated by systemic chemotherapy and targeted radiotherapy.

Gastrointestinal stromal tumours (including leiomyosarcoma)

These tumours are rare in the large bowel and are discussed above with respect to the small bowel. They arise from the muscle of the bowel wall, most usually the rectum, and are usually diagnosed by digital examination or by sigmoidoscopy. As discussed, there is a spectrum from benign to malignant and the tumours are often impossible to distinguish clinically; resection is therefore advisable. Metastases occur via the bloodstream to the liver and lungs.

M.G. Dunlop

17

The anorectum

CHAPTER CONTENTS

INTRODUCTION

Anorectal complaints are extremely common; approximately 2–3% of the population have anorectal symptoms at any given time. An understanding of the principles of applied anatomy and pathophysiology helps to differentiate patients who merit specialist assessment from those who can be treated symptomatically in the first instance. There remains a great deal of social taboo associated with anorectal disorders and so the symptoms are often ignored or hidden from relatives and doctors. It is important that the perianal symptoms are elicited without embarrassment to patient or clinician. The more common disorders of the anus and rectum that are encountered in clinical practice in the UK are described in this chapter. Symptoms due to anorectal conditions overlap with those due to conditions affecting the large bowel, and so documentation of a full gastrointestinal history is essential.

APPLIED SURGICAL ANATOMY

The anus enables the passage of stool or flatus (when socially convenient) but is also capable of maintaining continence to gas, fluid and solid at almost all other times in healthy individuals.

Anal musculature and innervation

The anal canal is 3–4 cm long in males and slightly shorter in females. It consists of two concentric muscle layers known as the internal and external sphincters (Fig. 17.1). The internal sphincter is a condensation of the circular smooth muscle of the rectum and is a continuation of the circular muscle of the gastrointestinal tract. It is controlled by the autonomic nervous system with fibres from the pelvic sympathetic nerves, the lower lumbar ganglia and the pre-aortic/inferior mesenteric plexus. Parasympathetic fibres arise from the sacral plexus. The smooth muscle of the internal sphincter maintains tone and contributes to resting pressure within the anal canal, so playing an important role in maintaining continence. The longitudinal muscle of the gut ends at the anus as a series of fibrous bands that radiate to the perianal skin, and is of little consequence to perianal disease. The striated muscle of the external sphincter is under voluntary control, being innervated bilaterally by the internal pudendal nerves and the fourth branch of the sacral plexus. The circular muscle tube of the external sphincter blends with the lower part of the levator ani, known as the puborectalis sling (Fig. 17.2). The puborectalis fibres of the levator ani originate from the posterior aspect of the pubic symphysis and pass posteriorly to join the external sphincter. The levator ani muscles themselves are also important in maintaining the relationship of the anus and rectum during defaecation.

Anal canal epithelium

The cell type of the anal canal epithelium determines why certain diseases, such as tumours and viral infections, affect only particular levels of the canal. The epithelium of the anal canal is specialized and contains three distinct zones. The external zone (from dentate line to anal verge) is keratinized, stratified squamous epithelium. There is a short, modified, anal transitional zone of non-keratinized squamous epithelium, which lies immediately proximal to the dentate line, separated from the columnar epithelial of the anal canal but continuous with the rectal epithelium. The anal valves are crescentic mucosal folds that form a serrated or dentate line on the luminal aspect of the mid-anal canal (Fig. 17.3). The dentate line represents the line of fusion between the endoderm of the embryonic hindgut and the ectoderm of the anal pit. Thus, the epithelium is innervated by the autonomic

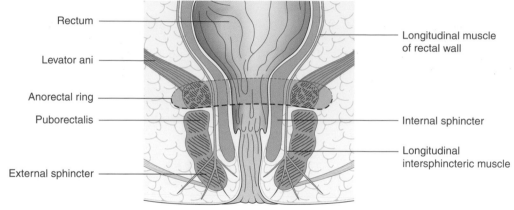

Rectum

Levator ani

Anorectal ring

Puborectalis

External sphincter

Longitudinal muscle of rectal wall

Internal sphincter

Longitudinal intersphincteric muscle

Fig. 17.1 Musculature of the anorectum.

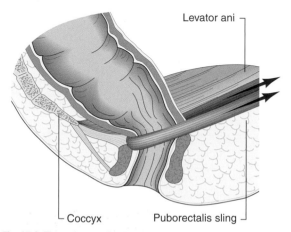

Levator ani

Coccyx

Puborectalis sling

Fig. 17.2 The puborectalis sling establishing the anorectal angle.

nervous system and is insensate with respect to somatic sensation. The canal lining below the dentate line is innervated by the peripheral nervous system and so conditions affecting this region, such as abscess, anal fissure or tumour, result in anal pain.

The composition of the epithelium of the anorectum determines the type of tumour that affects the region. Thus, squamous cell carcinoma of the anal canal arises from the epithelium *below* the dentate line or in the transitional zone of non-keratinized squamous epithelium. Because the canal above the anal transition zone contains columnar glandular epithelium, tumours of the upper anal canal are adenocarcinoma; they are best considered as a low rectal cancer and treated accordingly.

There are 4–8 specialized anal glands located within the substance of the internal sphincter or in the space between the internal and external sphincters at the level of the mid-anal canal; these glands have ducts that open directly on to the dentate line (Fig. 17.4). They are involved in the aetiology of perianal abscess and fistula-in-ano. The function of the anal glands is to secrete mucus, lubricating and protecting the delicate epithelium of the anal transition zone. The ducts from these glands open into the folds of mucosa at the dentate line. The relevance of these glands lies in the fact that they are the source of most perianal abscesses. When an anal gland duct becomes occluded, the obstructed gland may become infected with gut organisms such as coliforms, and anaerobic bacteria such as *Bacteroides*.

The anal (haemorrhoidal) cushions

Although the internal and external sphincters, the puborectalis sling and the anorectal angle play important roles in maintaining anal continence, fine control is aided by the anal 'cushions' that lie in the submucosa within the anal canal, above the dentate line. The anal cushions are specialized

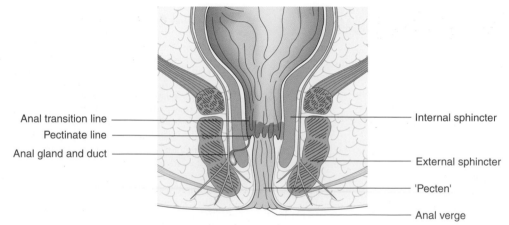

Anal transition line

Pectinate line

Anal gland and duct

Internal sphincter

External sphincter

'Pecten'

Anal verge

Fig. 17.3 The lining of the anorectal canal.

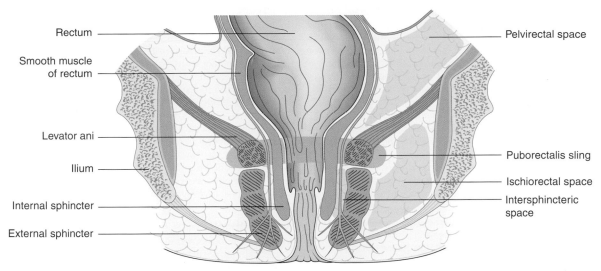

Fig. 17.4 Principal anorectal spaces in relation to the anal sphincters and rectum.

vascular structures comprised of fibroconnective tissue containing arteriovenous communications, fed by the terminal branches of the superior rectal artery with inconstant anastomoses to the middle and inferior rectal arteries. There are usually three anal cushions because there are three terminal branches of the artery (left, right posterior and right anterior, corresponding with the 3, 7 and 11 o'clock positions when the patient is in the lithotomy position). These positions determine the position of haemorrhoids, which are caused by distension and prolapse of the anal cushions. Haemorrhoids are not 'varicose veins' of the anal canal, but prolapse of the specialized anal cushions; indeed, haemorrhoids are uncommon in patients with portal hypertension, despite the fact that the anal canal represents a potential portosystemic anastomosis.

 SUMMARY BOX 17.1

Factors maintaining anal continence

- Intact anorectal and pelvic floor sensation
- Intact anal sphincters and levator ani
- Preservation of the anorectal angle
- The bulk provided by the anal haemorrhoidal 'cushions'.

Lymphatic drainage of the anal canal

Lymphatic drainage of the anus below the dentate line is to the inguinal lymph nodes. This contrasts with the lower rectum where lymphatic drainage passes superiorly through the mesorectum to follow the superior rectal artery and on to the inferior mesenteric and aortic chains. There are also some lymphatic channels that follow the course of the middle rectal arteries to drain to the nodes around the internal iliac arteries. This anatomical distinction between the lymphatic drainage of the anus and the rectum has important implications for the management of tumours of the rectum and anus. Anal cancer frequently metastasizes to inguinal lymph nodes, whereas rectal cancer metastasizes upwards to the mesorectum and onwards to the para-aortic chain. Thus, radiotherapy fields for anal squamous cancer normally incorporate the inguinal nodes.

SUMMARY BOX 17.2

Causes of severe acute anal pain

- Perianal abscess
- Anal fissure
- Thrombosed haemorrhoids
- Perianal haematoma
- Anorectal cancer.

ANORECTAL DISORDERS

Haemorrhoids

Despite haemorrhoids (colloquially known as piles) being very common, the aetiology remains obscure. Almost all haemorrhoids are primary, with only a tiny proportion due to other factors, such as a cancer in the distal rectum. Haemorrhoids are enlarged, prolapsed anal cushions and the pathophysiology involves degeneration of the supporting fibroelastic tissue and smooth muscle, with enlargement and protrusion of the cushions at the 3, 7 and 11 o'clock position. As the cushions prolapse, there is keratinization and hypertrophy of the overlying anal transitional zone and eventually prolapse of the columnar epithelial component in advanced stages. However, the underlying cause of the stretching of the fibroelastic support is unknown. Constipation and straining at stool are common features. These may be aggravated by a high anal sphincter pressure, with further entrapment of prolapsed piles. Haemorrhoids during pregnancy are very common and are probably due to hormonal effects inducing connective tissue laxity, combined with constipation and pressure from the baby's head. Sitting on the toilet for long periods, such as when reading, is also held to be an associated aetiological factor. However, as with other putative aetiological factors, there is no real evidence for cause and effect.

Clinical features

Bleeding and prolapse are the cardinal features and may occur in isolation or together. The bleeding is typically intermittent 'outlet-type' bleeding, separate from the stool and evident in the pan or only on wiping. There may also be aching or dragging discomfort on defaecation, and patients may self-reduce their piles to obtain relief after each bowel motion. Severe constant pain is unusual and in such cases other pathology should be suspected. In the later stages, haemorrhoids remain prolapsed at all times and there is staining of the underwear with mucus and faecal fluid. However, it is very unusual for patients to present with incontinence of solid faeces and a sphincter defect should be suspected in such cases. In cases of constant prolapse, there is often pruritus due to the discharge, with irritation of the perianal skin.

Haemorrhoids can be staged according to the degree of prolapse, but it is important to note that this classification does not necessarily relate to the amount of trouble that symptoms cause the patient:

- *First-degree* piles are those that bleed, are visible on proctoscopy but do not prolapse
- *Second-degree* piles are those that prolapse during defaecation but reduce spontaneously
- *Third-degree* piles are prolapsed constantly but can be reduced manually (Fig. 17.5)
- *Fourth-degree* piles are irreducibly prolapsed.

Patients may present as an emergency with a complication of haemorrhoids, such as thrombosed prolapsed piles or torrential haemorrhage. Prolapsing haemorrhoids may acutely thrombose and there is associated marked sphincter spasm. The thrombosed piles are large, swollen, irreducible haemorrhoids, which are dark blue or even black owing to necrosis and submucosal haemorrhage. They are acutely painful and tender and the diagnosis is easily made on inspection, but a rectal examination will be impossible because of pain. Major haemorrhage, resulting in significant hypovolaemia and anaemia, is unusual but should be excluded in any patient presenting with a major fresh rectal bleed.

History

Assessment of suspected piles must always include consideration of other potential differential diagnoses, as the symptoms of piles and colorectal cancer can be very similar. However, piles are very common and so it is important to

avoid indiscriminate large bowel investigation for such a common complaint as rectal bleeding. Careful history is essential to guide further clinical assessment and investigation. Outlet type bleeding comprises fresh red blood, dripping in the pan, on wiping and separate from the bowel motion in the toilet pan. If the bleeding is outlet type, there is no alteration in bowel habit and the patient is under 50 years of age, then the chance of rectal cancer is remote. In such cases, digital rectal examination, combined with proctoscopy and rigid sigmoidoscopy, should secure the diagnosis. If piles are confirmed, then treatment can be instigated without recourse to imaging the rest of the colon by colonoscopy. If no demonstrable cause is identified then further colonic investigation is essential. In older patients, if there is a change of bowel habit, then further colonic investigation is also indicated.

Examination

Examination of the perianal region should be carried out in the left lateral position. Prolapsed piles will be apparent at this stage and evidence of associated anal skin tags should be noted. Digital rectal examination is essential to assess sphincter tone and to exclude other anal conditions. First- or second-degree piles are rarely palpable, as they compress on pressure, and diagnosis is made by proctoscopy. The proctoscope should be gently inserted to the hilt and withdrawn, when bulging haemorrhoids will be visible at right anterior, right posterior and left lateral positions. Rigid sigmoidoscopy should be performed to exclude other rectal pathology.

Management

In many cases, reassurance after appropriate evaluation is all that many patients require. Specific treatment is not required for most cases, as symptoms are minor and intermittent. A high-fibre diet with plenty of vegetables is commonly recommended, although there is no good evidence that this actually provides any benefit at all. However, if constipation is a feature, it does seem reasonable advice; in some cases, bulk laxatives or stool softeners may be indicated. Patients often self-medicate with proprietary ointments and creams. There is no good evidence from controlled trials that these are effective, but if patients find that they help, then it seems reasonable to advise their intermittent use.

Non-operative approaches

There are many non-operative approaches to the treatment of haemorrhoids, the aim of which is to cause fibrosis and shrinkage of the protruding haemorrhoidal cushion in order to prevent bleeding and prolapse. Current outpatient clinic treatment approaches include application of small rubber bands to strangulate the pile (using a special Barron's bander); submucosal injection of sclerosant; and the application of heat by infrared photocoagulation. There is no strong evidence that any of these approaches is much better than doing nothing at all. In the long term, the symptoms of *untreated* piles tend to wax and wane, and the recurrence of symptoms after any of these procedures is much the same as without any treatment. However, of all the non-operative treatments, rubber band ligation (Fig. 17.6) may be the most effective in the short term. Where there is a significant cutaneous component to the piles, any of the outpatient treatments is likely to be painful because of the cutaneous nerve supply, and is also unlikely to succeed. In these circumstances, the decision should be to do nothing but reassure the patient, or to offer an operation.

Operative approaches

The principle of haemorrhoidectomy involves total removal of the haemorrhoidal mass and securing of haemostasis of the feeding vessel. The wound can be left open or can be closed,

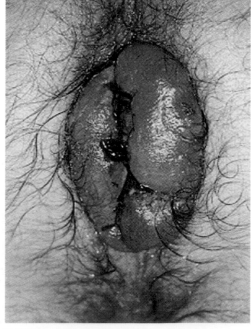

Fig. 17.5 Third-degree haemorrhoids.

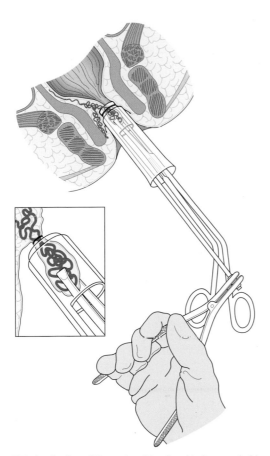

Fig. 17.6 Application of Barron's rubber band to haemorrhoids.

but there are rarely problems with healing or infection. In some cases, there are secondary haemorrhoids between the main right anterior, right posterior and left lateral positions, and these are also removed as part of the operation. Recently, a different surgical approach using a circular stapler has been developed, the stapled anopexy. This technique aims to divide the mucosa and haemorrhoidal cushions above the dentate line in order to transect the feeding vessels and hitch up the stretched supporting fibroelastic tissue, rather than removing the whole haemorrhoidal mass as in the standard haemorrhoidectomy. Stapled haemorrhoidectomy may have a place for the treatment of symptomatic first- and second-degree piles (EBM 17.1). With all surgical approaches to treating

---

EBM 17.1 **Haemorrhoids**

'Non-operative treatment is preferable wherever possible but surgery may be required for a small proportion of cases. Open haemorrhoidectomy is superior to stapled haemorrhoidectomy both in terms of symptom control and recurrence; rubber band ligation has similar efficacy to haemorrhoidectomy.'

Acheson AG, Scholefield JH. Management of haemorrhoids. BMJ. 2008 Feb 16;336(7640):380-3. http://www.ncbi.nlm.nih.gov/pmc/articles/PMC2244760
Lumb KJ, Colquhoun PH.D., Malthaner R, Jayaraman S. Stapled versus conventional surgery for hemorrhoids. Cochrane Database of Systematic Reviews 2006, Issue 4. Art. No.: CD005393. DOI: 10.1002/14651858. CD005393.pub2.
Shanmugam V, Hakeem A, Campbell KL, Rabindranath KS, Steele RJC, Thaha MA, Loudon MA.Rubber band ligation versus excisional haemorrhoidectomy for haemorrhoids. Cochrane Database of Systematic Reviews 2005, Issue 3. Art. No.: CD005034. DOI: 10.1002/14651858. CD005034.pub2.

Haemorrhoids

Haemorrhoids are common and best treated conservatively.
Classification:
- First-degree: visible in the lumen on proctoscopy but do not prolapse
- Second-degree: prolapse on defaecation but return spontaneously
- Third-degree: remain prolapsed but can be replaced digitally
- Fourth-degree: long-standing prolapse and cannot be replaced in the anal canal.

Symptoms:
- Outlet-type bleeding, prolapse, mucus discharge, discomfort and thrombosis.

Treatment:
- First-degree: advice on avoiding constipation and straining
- Second-degree: conservative management, banding, injection sclerotherapy, haemorrhoidectomy
- Third-degree: if symptomatic, haemorrhoidectomy
- Fourth-degree: thrombosed piles are usually treated conservatively in the first instance; interval haemorrhoidectomy may not be required.

17

piles, it is important to consider that the haemorrhoidal cushions contribute to fine control of continence. Hence, an element of anal incontinence can be one of the long-term sequelae of any haemorrhoidectomy. Surgery should not be considered lightly.

Fissure-in-ano

Fissure-in-ano is a common condition characterized by a linear anal ulcer, often with the internal sphincter visible in the base, affecting the anal canal below the dentate line from the anal transition zone to the anal verge (Fig. 17.7). There is often little in the way of granulation tissue in the ulcer base. Owing to failed attempts at healing, there may be a tag of skin at the lowermost extent of the fissure, known as a 'sentinel pile'. At the proximal extent of the fissure there may be a hypertrophied anal papilla. Sometimes fissures will heal incompletely and mucosa will bridge the edges of the fissure. This results in a low perianal fistula and may present years later. Fissures are most frequently observed in the posterior midline of the anal canal, although anterior fissures may occur in women following childbirth; they are rarely seen in males.

The condition most commonly affects people in their twenties and thirties, with a slight male preponderance. Most fissures are idiopathic, but it is clear that the pathophysiology involves ischaemia in the base of the ulcer, associated with marked anal spasm and a significantly raised resting anal pressure. Successive bowel motions provoke further trauma, pain and anal spasm, resulting in a vicious circle of anal pain and sphincter spasm that causes further trauma to the anal mucosa during defaecation. Fissures may be acute and settle spontaneously, but chronic anal fissure is defined as an ulcer that has been present for at least 6 weeks. Recurrent multiple or unusually extensive fissures affecting areas other than the midline should raise the suspicion of Crohn's disease, which can occasionally present with anal fissure as the sole initial complaint. Occasionally, anal fissure may be associated with ulcerative colitis. Fissure is an uncommon complication of haemorrhoidectomy and results from a non-healing wound combined with anal spasm.

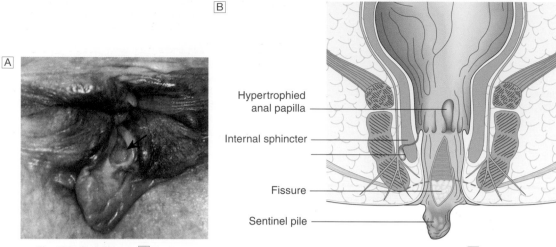

Fig. 17.7 Anal fissure. [A] The fissure (arrow) comprises a linear ulcer at the typical 6 o'clock position (arrow). [B] Explanatory diagram.

Fissure-in-ano is one of the most common causes of constipation in infants and children. The pain associated with the fissure leads to a pattern of behaviour in which the child tries to avoid defaecation. This results in stool retention and rectal stool bolus formation. The rectum becomes overdistended and the child becomes unaware of the need to pass stool. Overflow incontinence and soiling result.

Clinical features and diagnosis

The most common symptoms are pain on defaecation in a young patient. There is often associated rectal bleeding of the outlet type, with blood on the paper or dripping into the pan after passing the motion. The amount of bleeding is usually minor and there may be some staining or mucous discharge in the underwear. Patients often report that it is painful to wipe the anus after moving the bowels. Pain is the predominant symptom and may be burning, tearing or sharp in nature. It may last a few hours after defaecation. There may be a history of constipation, which could be aetiologically responsible for the tear, but is more likely a response to the pain.

The diagnosis should be suspected from the history alone and is confirmed by gently parting the superficial part of the anal sphincter with the gloved fingers to reveal the characteristic linear ulcer. There may be an associated 'sentinel pile', which consists of heaped-up skin at the lowermost extent of the linear ulcer (Fig. 17.7). It is often too painful to perform a digital rectal examination or a proctoscopy, and so this is best left until after treatment is instigated. However, it is important to complete clinical assessment with rigid sigmoidoscopy at a later date. A full history is important to exclude previous perianal surgery, perianal abscess, trauma during childbirth or symptoms consistent with Crohn's disease.

Management

Many acute fissures resolve spontaneously and so treatment should be reserved for chronic symptoms of 6 weeks' or more duration. Having established that the fissure is primary, treatment is aimed at alleviating pain and anal spasm in order to break out of the vicious circle. It is important to document reproductive history for females, as surgery may have implications for future anal continence.

The optimal approach is conservative in the first instance. Stool softeners may help, but rarely effect a cure as the sole treatment. Chemical sphincter relaxation is first-line treatment of choice using topical 0.5% diltiazem or nitrates (glyceryl trinitrate 0.2–0.5%) as a cream applied 12-hourly to the anal canal. Headaches can be a dose-limiting side effect

especially with topical nitrates, but healing can be achieved in 50–70% of chronic fissures. Other means of reduction in sphincter tone include direct injection of the sphincter with botulinum toxin, which temporarily paralyses the sphincter.

Until the relatively recent advent of chemical sphincterotomy as first-line treatment, surgery was the only option. Surgery still has a major role in the management of patients who have fissures resistant to medical treatment, or who have recurrence. Anal stretching has been abandoned, as it is associated with significant sphincter damage and the risk of incontinence (EBM 17.2). Lateral sphincterotomy is the most common operation for anal fissure and involves controlled division of the lower half of the internal sphincter at the lateral position (3 o'clock or 9 o'clock with the patient in the lithotomy position). There is a small but appreciable risk of late anal incontinence following lateral sphincterotomy. This is usually only to gas, but occasionally faecal incontinence to liquid or solid can occur, particularly in women who have had birth-related anal sphincter damage. In women, it may therefore be more appropriate to avoid further division of any sphincter muscle, and this can be achieved using an anal advancement flap or a rotation flap to cover the ulcerated base of the fissure and allow new, well-vascularized skin to heal the ulcer and reduce the associated anal spasm.

EBM 17.2 **Anal fissure**

'A step-wise hierarchical approach to treatment is optimal comprising medical therapy (diltiazem cream then botulinum toxin), internal sphincterotomy or anal advancement flap. Anal stretch is an outdated surgical treatment and is associated with a significant excess risk of faecal incontinence.'

Nelson RL. Non surgical therapy for anal fissure. Cochrane Database of Systematic Reviews 2006, Issue 4. Art. No.: CD003431. DOI: 10.1002/14651858.CD003431.pub2.
Nelson RL, Chattopadhyay A, Brooks W, Platt I, Paavana T, Earl S. Operative procedures for fissure in ano. Cochrane Database of Systematic Reviews 2011, Issue 11. Art. No.: CD002199. DOI: 10.1002/14651858.CD002199.pub4.

Perianal abscess

Perianal abscess is a nonspecific term encompassing abscesses in the perianal, intersphincteric, ischiorectal or pelvirectal spaces (Fig. 17.8). Perianal suppuration is common, affecting men three times more frequently than women.

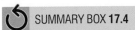

SUMMARY BOX 17.4

Anal fissure

Pain on defaecation and outlet type bleeding are the cardinal symptoms

Typically affects younger age groups (18–30 years)

In older age groups, Crohn's disease or cancer should be suspected.

Treatment:

- Medical treatment is preferred in the first instance
- Stool softeners
- Chemical sphincterotomy (0.5% diltiazem or 0.4% glycerol trinitrate cream)
- Botulinus toxin paralysis of anal sphincter
- Anal skin advancement flap (mainly reserved for females)
- Lateral internal anal sphincterotomy.

Conditions that predispose to perianal abscess include Crohn's disease and ulcerative colitis, as well as any cause of immunosuppression such as haematological disease, diabetes mellitus, chemotherapy and human immunodeficiency virus (HIV) infection. Most patients who present with perianal abscess have no predisposing factors and most abscesses are cryptoglandular, initiated by blockage of the anal gland ducts (see Fig. 17.3). The obstructed anal gland becomes secondarily infected with large bowel organisms such as *Bacteroides*, *Streptococcus faecalis* and coliforms. The fact that the anal glands are situated in the intersphincteric space (see Fig. 17.4) explains the routes that the infection may take as pus tracks along the line of least resistance through the tissue spaces. Rarely, patients with established sepsis elsewhere may develop metastatic suppuration in the perianal region.

Clinical features

In cases where the abscess remains localized within the intersphincteric space, the patient presents with acute anal pain and tenderness. There is usually no evidence of suppuration on inspection of the perianal region. Pain often prevents digital examination, and so general anaesthetic is required. The main differential diagnosis is acute anal fissure. The diagnosis is confirmed by demonstration of a localized pea-sized lump in the intersphincteric space. True perianal abscess is the most common type, in which pus tracks inferiorly to appear at the perianal margin between the internal and external sphincters (Fig. 17.8).

Symptoms are usually of 2–3 days' duration and the abscess may have discharged spontaneously. Systemic upset is minimal and anal pain is the predominant presenting complaint.

Infection may extend into the ischiorectal space resulting in ischiorectal abscess, which is a relatively uncommon but serious problem. Poorly controlled diabetes is a common underlying correlate and should be excluded in all cases. As the ischiorectal space is horseshoe-shaped and there are no fascial barriers within it, infection can track extensively, including posteriorly around the anus to affect the contralateral space. In such cases, the patient is toxic and pyrexial with a large, painful, fluctuant, brawny swelling affecting both buttocks, due to large volumes of pus. There is a history of perianal pain for several days, associated with difficulty in sitting.

Infection tracking upwards from the infected anal gland through the upper part of the intersphincteric space may result in a high intersphincteric (high intermuscular) abscess or a pelvirectal abscess. As these spaces encircle the anorectum above the levator muscles, abscesses can be bilateral and often present with a major systemic upset. These are complex problems meriting specialist management. With high abscesses, it is also important to consider intra-abdominal sepsis from Crohn's or diverticular abscess.

Management

An established abscess will not respond to antibiotics alone and requires surgical drainage. Treatment of perianal abscess is usually straightforward and involves drainage of the pus under general anaesthetic. Most cases are adequately dealt with by incising and deroofing the abscess at the point of maximal fluctuance. However, anatomical considerations are important, as inappropriate incision of sphincter muscle can result in incontinence in the long term. Furthermore, drainage of pus through the wrong space will create a perianal fistula (see below). At operation, pus should be sent for bacteriological assessment to determine the causative organism(s). In uncomplicated cases, antibiotics have no place after incision and drainage. Where there is extensive cellulitis, as is often the case with ischiorectal abscess, parenteral antibiotics, such as broad-spectrum cephalosporins and metronidazole, should be administered. Parenteral antibiotics are mandatory for diabetic patients with perianal sepsis. Unusually complex perianal sepsis or recurrent abscess should raise suspicion of underlying Crohn's disease. Sigmoidoscopy and rectal biopsy should be performed and the roof of the abscess sent for histology.

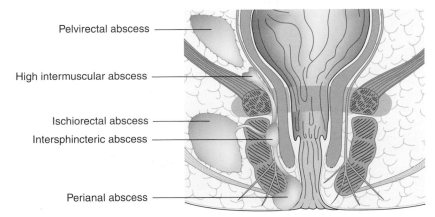

Pelvirectal abscess

High intermuscular abscess

Ischiorectal abscess

Intersphincteric abscess

Perianal abscess

Fig. 17.8 Spread of infection from the anal gland to the anorectal spaces and resultant abscess formation.

SUMMARY BOX 17.5

Anorectal sepsis

- Most anorectal sepsis is cryptoglandular
- Perianal and ischiorectal abscesses most common anorectal abscesses
- Recurrent abscess should raise suspicion of fistula and Crohn's disease
- Abscess requires incision and drainage.

Fistula-in-ano

The underlying pathogenesis of the vast majority of cases of perianal abscess or anal fistula is obstruction of the anal gland duct. This results in stasis and infection of the anal gland (cryptoglandular infection). Abscess precedes all such cases of fistula, although the sepsis is often subclinical. Inappropriate surgical drainage of perianal abscess is responsible for a small but significant proportion of fistulae. Figure 17.9 is a simplified diagram showing the classification of fistula-in-ano. A fistulous tract should be suspected

in all patients with recurrent perianal abscess. Typically the patient presents repeatedly with an abscess that intermittently points and discharges pus on to the perianal skin. However, there is no need to search routinely for a fistula when draining straightforward perianal abscesses. Inexpert probing may inadvertently induce a fistula.

In addition to cryptoglandular aetiology, perianal fistula may be due to Crohn's disease, anal trauma, inexpert surgical drainage and anorectal carcinoma. Other rare causes include ulcerative colitis, tuberculosis and actinomycosis. Around 10% of patients with small intestinal Crohn's disease without colorectal involvement, have perianal disease. Hence, it is important to exclude Crohn's disease in patients with recurrent perianal fistula or sepsis resistant to treatment.

Clinical features and assessment

In most cases, the patient presents with a chronically discharging opening in the perianal skin, associated with pruritus and perianal discomfort. A detailed clinical history is essential to determine any predisposing medical conditions or previous surgery. Investigation requires examination under anaesthetic (EUA) by a colorectal specialist when the fistula should be probed to trace the tract from external to the internal openings. Goodsall's Law is a rough rule of thumb as to the likely course of fistulous tracts. Thus, when the fistula opens on the perianal skin of the anterior anus, the tract usually passes radially directly to the anal canal. However, when the opening is posterior to a line drawn between the 3 o'clock and 9 o'clock positions (Fig. 17.10), then the tract usually passes circumferentially backwards and enters the anal canal in the midline (6 o'clock position). It is essential to avoid inducing further fistulae by ill-advised probing of the region. It is important to determine whether the fistula is low or high (Fig. 17.9), as the prognosis and treatment are different for each. Most fistulae can be delineated and treated at EUA, but complex cases may merit magnetic resonance imaging (MRI). MRI of a complex high fistula involving the pelvirectal space is shown in Figure 17.11. Endoanal ultrasound may be useful. Further investigation to exclude Crohn's disease may be appropriate, involving colonoscopy, small bowel MRI or small bowel follow-through.

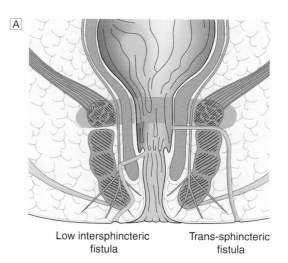

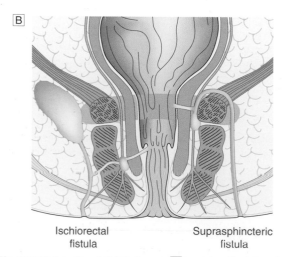

Low intersphincteric fistula   Trans-sphincteric fistula

Ischiorectal fistula   Suprasphincteric fistula

Fig. 17.9 Categories of fistula-in-ano. **A** Low intersphincteric and trans-sphinteric. **B** Ischiorectal and suprasphincteric.

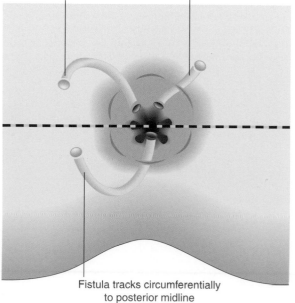

Anterior fistula tracks radially to dentate line

Fistula tracks circumferentially to posterior midline

Fig. 17.10 Goodsall's rule.

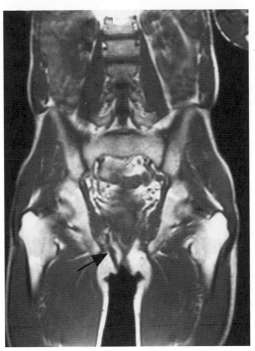

Fig. 17.11 Coronal MRI scan of complex pelvirectal fistula (arrow).

Management

Treatment is determined by the course of the fistula tract. Usually, low fistulae can simply be laid open and allowed to heal. However, where a significant proportion of the internal and/or external sphincter is involved, then laying open the tract will result in faecal incontinence. In such complex cases, the fistula tract can be probed and a seton passed along its length (Fig. 17.12) to allow the fistula to drain. Once it is drained, a tighter seton can be applied that will gradually cut out through the sphincters, allowing them to heal behind the seton. Applying such a cutting seton maintains the ends of the sphincters together and minimizes the risk of incontinence. High fistulae may be treated by an anorectal advancement flap. This involves raising a flap of rectal wall and upper internal sphincter. The flap is advanced distally to close the internal opening. The external opening and superficial part of the tract heals as there is no faecal stream to maintain the sepsis. In some complex cases, a defunctioning colostomy may be necessary.

 SUMMARY BOX **17.6**

Fistula-in-ano

Aetiology
- Idiopathic (cryptoglandular) due to blockage of anal gland duct
- Crohn's disease
- Anorectal trauma
- Iatrogenic (surgical)
- Anorectal carcinoma.

Rare causes
- Ulcerative colitis
- Tuberculosis
- Actinomycosis.

Treatment
- Low fistulae should be laid open
- Complex high fistulae require repair and/or seton insertion.

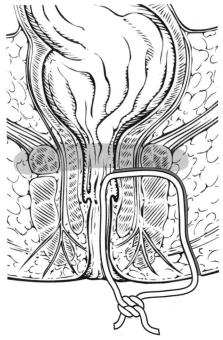

Fig. 17.12 **A seton encircling a trans-sphincteric fistula.** A seton is a piece of surgical thread, suture material or specialized tie that is passed through the fistula. It is tied in a loop to allow the fistula to drain (loose seton) and/or to cut slowly through the sphincter muscle, with the muscle healing behind the advancing seton (tight seton).

MISCELLANEOUS BENIGN PERIANAL LUMPS

Perianal haematoma

Perianal haematoma is a painful condition caused by subcutaneous haemorrhage and formation of thrombus in the superficial space between the anoderm and the anal sphincter. A localized lump forms at the anal verge, due to blood tracking subcutaneously from haemorrhoids after the passage of a hard bowel motion. It can also arise in patients with a bleeding diathesis or those on anticoagulants. It is important to recognize the condition because it is readily treated by surgical drainage under local anaesthetic, with almost instantaneous relief. The condition will settle eventually without surgical intervention, but recognizing the haematoma will spare the patient many days of an exquisitely tender anus.

Perianal haematoma is easily recognized by the presence of a well-circumscribed, bluish dome-shaped lump under the perianal skin. The main differential diagnosis is prolapsed, thrombosed haemorrhoids, and so it is essential to make an accurate diagnosis. Inappropriate incision of haemorrhoids will result in considerable bleeding. Perianal haematoma should be readily differentiated from perianal abscess by nature of the colour and by the surrounding erythema and induration.

Anal warts

Anal warts cause discomfort, pain, pruritus ani and difficulty with perianal hygiene. Warts are also associated with an increased risk of squamous carcinoma because they are usually associated with human papillomavirus (HPV). The lesions may be very extensive or relatively sparse.

After viral infection and the development of an initial crop of warts, they may be spread extensively by scratching, which is provoked by the associated pruritus ani. Many cases resolve spontaneously, but those requiring treatment can usually be managed effectively by the application of podophyllin. More extensive cases may require surgical excision, and very extensive cases associated with dysplasia may require excision and skin grafting, combined with a temporary colostomy.

Fibroepithelial anal polyp

Fibroepithelial anal polyp it is not a neoplasm, but hypertrophic epithelium arising on a stalk from the anal canal itself. Histologically, it comprises of keratinized squamous epithelium supported by scarred, fibrotic subcutaneous tissue. The clinical history may suggest haemorrhoids as the main differential diagnosis, but this is easily discounted by digital examination and proctoscopy, which reveals the polyp on a stalk. The main differential diagnosis is of a prolapsing rectal adenomatous polyp on a long stalk. However, rectal polyps arise above the dentate line. Excision biopsy confirms the nature of the polyp.

Patients with a fibroepithelial polyp may present with a prolapsing anal lesion, discomfort on defaecation, or pruritus ani associated with faecal-stained mucus causing irritation to the delicate perianal skin. Anal polyps are usually associated with a current or previous history of perianal disease, including haemorrhoids or fissure-in-ano. Treatment of symptomatic polyps is by simple excision under general anaesthetic.

Anal skin tags

Prolapse of haemorrhoids is usually followed by a degree of regression, and may leave irregular skin at the anal verge, known as anal skin tags. Haemorrhoids often present with minor anal skin tags, but it is important to stress that the tags themselves are not haemorrhoids. Although the anus may not look particularly tidy, there is no indication to operate unless the patient is having significant problems with perianal hygiene or the lesions are causing pruritus. Anal tags associated with haemorrhoids that merit surgery can be removed at the same time as haemorrhoidectomy.

ANAL CANCER

Anal cancer is rare in comparison with colorectal cancer. There are around 600 new cases annually in the UK. Over 85% of anal cancers are squamous in origin and arise from the keratinized squamous epithelium of the anal margin or from the non-keratinized squamous epithelium of the anal transitional zone immediately above the dentate line. Anal verge tumours often present earlier than canal tumours because the patient becomes aware of a mass or irregular area at the anal margin. Around 5% of tumours are adenocarcinomas and these arise from the glandular epithelium of the upper anal canal or rarely from the anal glands located in the intersphincteric space. These are distinct from low anorectal adenocarcinoma. Most patients with anal cancer present in the sixth or seventh decade, but younger cases are well recognized, particularly in those with HIV and high risk activities. Other rarer tumours include melanoma, lymphoma and sarcoma.

There is a strong association between anal cancer and infection with HPV types 16 and 18. HPV infection is responsible for the majority of anal carcinomas. Smoking is a risk factor and likely interacts with viral infection. Anogenital warts are also a risk factor, as is anoreceptive intercourse. HIV infection is also a predisposing factor, owing to immunosuppression and susceptibility to viral infection. The premalignant lesion, anal intraepithelial neoplasia (AIN), is probably the precursor of most anal carcinomas and is analogous to cervical intraepithelial neoplasia (CIN), the precursor lesion of cervical cancer. The level of AIN (1–3) is dependent on the degree of cytological atypia and the depth of that atypia in the epidermis. A high proportion of AIN 3 progresses to carcinoma and is shown in Figure 17.13. It is important to perform a cervical smear in patients with proven anal cancer. There is also an association with vulval intraepithelial neoplasia (VIN), which also has a common HPV aetiology.

Clinical features and assessment

Anal cancer is frequently misdiagnosed in the early stages because of its rarity and because symptoms of benign anal conditions are highly prevalent. Early cancer may be confused with fissures, piles and warts. Nevertheless, because of accessibility, anal tumours are readily detectable by careful clinical examination; anal pain/discomfort, bleeding or discharge into the underwear, and pruritus ani should be sought. Advanced tumours that have spread to the anal sphincters may present with incontinence. Clinical examination of anal cancer at the margin reveals an ulcerated discoid lesion at the anal verge (Fig. 17.14). Cancer of the anal canal may not be visible, although extensive lesions may protrude to the anal verge by direct spread. Careful examination under anaesthetic is required to allow tumour biopsy and sigmoidoscopy. Biopsy is essential to confirm the diagnosis, but also to determine the tissue of origin, as the treatment for squamous carcinoma varies from that for adenocarcinoma.

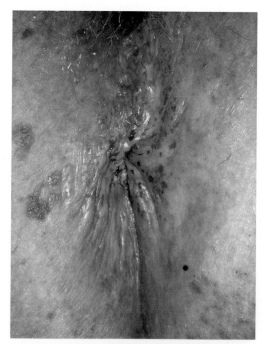

Fig. 17.13 The most severe degree of anal intraepithelial neoplasia (AIN 3), the precursor of most anal squamous cancer.

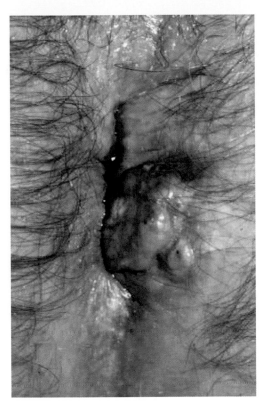

Fig. 17.14 Squamous carcinoma of the anal verge.

Staging

Staging is important for prognosis and also guides treatment approaches. The TNM staging system for anal cancer is shown in Table 17.1. The lymph nodes most commonly involved are the inguinal groups, particularly for anal verge cancers. Canal tumours may spread proximally to the mesorectal nodes or to the internal iliac nodes via the middle rectal lymph nodes. Lymphadenopathy alone is not sufficient to confirm lymph node spread, and accessible nodes should be biopsied because reactive changes due to infection are common. Examination under anaesthetic is an important part of clinical staging, as the tumour is often painful and the anus tender to digital examination. CT and MRI are essential; endoanal ultrasound may be helpful but usually needs to be performed under anaesthetic.

Management

It is important to detect anal cancer at an early stage, as extensive local invasion and metastatic disease are associated with a poor outcome. Multidisciplinary treatment of anal cancer is essential with surgeon and radiotherapist involved in assessment and treatment.

For early, well-circumscribed superficial (T_1N_0) carcinomas, wide surgical excision is the optimal treatment, as it avoids the morbidity of chemoradiotherapy. However, for T_2, T_3 and T_4 tumours, treatment comprises radiotherapy to the anal canal and inguinal lymph nodes, combined with 5-fluorouracil (5-FU) (recently capecitabine is preferred) and mitomycin C (EBM 17.3). Newer regimens of radiotherapy, combined with capecitabine and cisplatinum, are also being introduced. The usual approach is external beam radiotherapy, but radioactive implants such as selectron wires are also used in selected cases. Surgery has a limited role in the primary treatment of these lesions but does play an important part in the management of advanced disease. Surgery is reserved for radiotherapy treatment failures, when 'salvage' abdominoperineal excision of the anus and rectum may afford a cure in some cases and alleviate symptoms in others.

Modern multimodality approaches involving tailored surgery and chemoradiation have radically improved the morbidity of treatment by avoiding abdominoperineal resection and permanent colostomy for many patients; the 5-year survival rate is now around 65%.

Table 17.1 TNM staging of anal cancer

T (Tumour)
- TX — Primary tumour cannot be assessed
- T0 — No evidence of primary tumour
- T1 — < 2 cm
- T2 — 2–5 cm
- T3 — > 5 cm
- T4a — Invading vaginal mucosa
- T4b — Invading structures other than skin, or rectal or vaginal mucosa (i.e. local spread to muscle or bone)

N (node)
- NX — Regional lymph nodes cannot be assessed
- N0 — No regional lymph node metastasis
- N1 — Metastasis in perirectal lymph node(s)
- N2 — Metastasis in unilateral internal iliac and/or inguinal lymph node(s)
- N3 — Metastasis in perirectal and inguinal lymph nodes and/or bilateral internal iliac and/or inguinal lymph nodes

M (Metastases)
- MX — Distant metastasis cannot be assessed
- M0 — No distant metastasis
- M1 — Distant metastasis

EBM 17.3 Anal cancer

'*Combination chemoradiation is the primary treatment modality for anal canal and T2, T3 and T4 tumours. Abdominoperineal resection is reserved for salvage procedures in cases of relapse after chemoradiation.*'

Anal Cancer. Position Statement of the Association of Coloproctology of Great Britain and Ireland. http://www.acpgbi.org.uk/assets/documents/Anal_Cancer_Position_Statement.pdf
Glynne-Jones R, Northover JM, Cervantes A; ESMO Guidelines Working Group. Anal cancer: ESMO Clinical Practice Guidelines for diagnosis, treatment and follow-up. Ann Oncol. 2010 May;21 Suppl 5:v87-92. PubMed PMID: 20555110. *http://annonc.oxfordjournals.org/content/20/suppl_4/iv57.full*

SUMMARY BOX 17.7

Anal carcinoma

- Anal carcinoma is associated with human papillomavirus types 16 and 18
- Anal intraepithelial neoplasia (AIN) is a malignant precursor
- Local surgical excision is the treatment of choice for T1N0 lesions
- Chemoradiotherapy is treatment of choice for T2, T3, or T4 lesions
- Chemoradiotherapy is mandatory for those with involved lymph nodes
- Abdominoperineal resection is reserved for failures of chemoradiation.

RECTAL PROLAPSE

Rectal prolapse is a distressing condition that can affect young and older adults, as well as children. The term rectal prolapse encompasses three types of abnormal protrusion of all, or part of, the rectal wall:

- A *full-thickness* rectal prolapse (procidentia) includes the mucosa and the muscular layers.
- *Mucosal* prolapse, as the name suggests, involves only the mucosal lining of the rectum.
- *Occult* rectal prolapse refers to intussusception of the rectal wall but without the prolapse protruding through the anal canal. This term also refers to the much rarer condition of *solitary rectal ulcer syndrome.* This consists of a prolapse of the full thickness of the anterior rectal wall only, although the terms occult rectal prolapse and solitary rectal ulcer syndrome are not synonymous.

The pathological process that results in rectal prolapse is incompletely understood. However, certain factors are clearly implicated in predisposing to the condition. Mucosal prolapse should not be confused with full-thickness prolapse. It is often associated with a degree of haemorrhoids, but whether these are causal or simply the result of a common aetiology is not understood. The majority of cases of full-thickness rectal prolapse occur in elderly women, with no obvious aetiological basis. Weight loss in the elderly with loss of fat supporting the rectum, combined with degeneration of collagen fibres and weakness of the musculature of the pelvic floor, results in loss of the anorectal angle and laxity of the rectal wall (see Fig. 17.2). In many cases, there is a deep rectovaginal pouch with a long loop of sigmoid colon that pushes down into the rectovaginal pouch and contributes to the prolapse. Occasionally, there is a clear history of obstetric injury but most patients are nulliparous.

Chronic constipation and straining at stool are the most common aetiological factors in young adults, although spinal injury, psychiatric illness, multiple sclerosis, spinal injuries and spinal tumour are predisposing factors. In children, the lack of a sacral hollow, combined with constipation and excessive straining at stool, is responsible for evagination of the rectum and protrusion of the prolapse through the anus. In children with cystic fibrosis, excessive coughing contributes to elevated intra-abdominal pressure.

Clinical features and assessment

Patients present with an uncomfortable sensation of 'something coming down' the back passage. Initially, this is only on defaecation, but eventually the rectum remains constantly prolapsed and will not reduce spontaneously. The patient may be able to reduce the prolapse digitally. Constipation is usually an accompanying feature. There is often a degree of faecal incontinence and there may be mucous discharge into the underwear. Blood-stained mucus is also common when the rectum remains prolapsed. The prolapse may become ulcerated and may become strangulated. In extreme cases, there may be associated uterine prolapse, alluding to the fact that the underlying aetiology relates to weakness of the entire pelvic floor.

Examination confirms the diagnosis in most cases. If the prolapse is not apparent, it will usually appear when the patient strains on a commode. A typical example of a full-thickness rectal prolapse is shown in Figure 17.15. Digital examination reveals a patulous anus, poor sphincter tone and evidence of a weak pelvic floor on straining. Rigid sigmoidoscopy will reveal cases of occult prolapse. If the history is of short duration, consideration should be

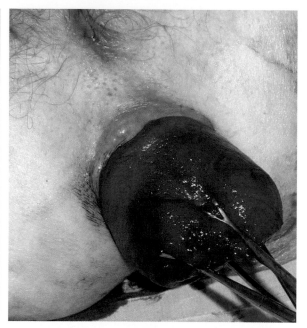

Fig. 17.15 Full-thickness rectal prolapse at operation prior to repair.

given to the presence of a spinal tumour, a spinal stenosis or a prolapsed intervertebral disc. In occult rectal prolapse, radiological assessment using a defaecating proctogram or dynamic MRI may help secure the diagnosis. Conditions that might be mistaken for a rectal prolapse include large fourth-degree haemorrhoids, prolapsing rectal neoplasia, anal warts, anal skin tags and fibroepithelial anal polyp. On the basis of symptoms alone, the differential diagnosis of rectal prolapse includes rectal cancer and inflammatory bowel disease, and these should be excluded by appropriate investigations.

Management

Childhood rectal prolapse

Rectal prolapse in children is usually treated effectively by attention to maintaining a regular bowel habit with stool softeners, combined with digital reduction of the prolapse by the parents. The condition is self-limiting and surgery is rarely indicated.

Mucosal rectal prolapse

In adults, mucosal rectal prolapse can be treated by submucosal injection of sclerosant, by photocoagulation or by applying Barron's bands to the prolapsed area. In resistant cases, a limited excision of the area, similar to a haemorrhoidectomy, is effective. Stapled anorectal rectopexy has gained favour in some centres.

Full-thickness rectal prolapse

Surgery is the only effective treatment for established full-thickness rectal prolapse. However, none of the available surgical options is wholly satisfactory. The aim of surgery is to treat the prolapse and improve any associated incontinence. Operations for rectal prolapse can be undertaken employing perineal or abdominal approaches:

- *Perineal approaches* aim to fixate or excise the prolapse surgically from below. 'Delorme's procedure' involves the excision of the mucosa lining the prolapse, with plication of the muscle tube, and 'perineal rectosigmoidectomy' entails excision through the anus of the prolapsed rectum and lower part of the sigmoid. The latter may be combined with a repair of the pelvic floor (Altmeier procedure)

- *Abdominal approaches* aim to fix the rectum to the bony pelvis using sutures or foreign material. Increasingly these procedures are performed laparoscopically. The abdominal approach may also include resection of the redundant sigmoid colon, particularly when constipation is a predominant feature, because rectal fixation usually aggravates the constipation.

Solitary rectal ulcer syndrome

This rare condition is difficult to treat effectively because the main aetiology is behavioural and there may be a psychological overlay. The peak age-group affected is 20–40 years. The condition is associated with an introspective and anxious personality. Patients with this condition spend an inordinate amount of time in the toilet attempting to defaecate. The diagnosis is confirmed by visualizing the anterior ulcer in the low rectum, and biopsy shows the typical features of submucosal fibrosis, hypertrophy of the muscularis mucosae and overlying ulceration. Management involves the use of stool softeners and other conservative measures, along with input from a psychologist. Biofeedback may have a place in suitable patients who are compliant. Various surgical procedures have been attempted including anterior or posterior rectopexy, and even low anterior resection. However, the results are usually poor and surgery should be avoided if at all possible.

SUMMARY BOX 17.8

Rectal prolapse

- Rectal prolapse may occur at any age but most common in the elderly
- Diagnosis is clinical
- Defaecating proctogram may be required to confirm the diagnosis in a minority
- Dynamic MRI delineates the extent of the entire pelvic floor problem.
- Treatment is usually surgical: either perineal or transabdominal.

ANAL INCONTINENCE

Several factors are involved in maintaining anal continence (see Box 17.1) and these may be adversely affected by any combination of structural damage to the musculature, disruption of the nerve supply, and marked intestinal hurry with defaecatory urgency (such as in ulcerative colitis). Damage to the internal or external sphincters may occur during childbirth. Peripartum nerve injury due to a prolonged 2nd stage of delivery due to pressure effects from the baby's head or due to forceps can affect the pudendal nerves, eventually leading to denervation and atrophy of the striated muscle of the external sphincter, the puborectalis sling and the levator ani. Neurodegenerative disease is also a recognized aetiological factor. Perianal sepsis or the surgery required to treat it, may result in structural damage to the sphincter complex.

Faecal incontinence is both distressing and socially disabling, but patients are often reluctant to discuss the issue with relatives or with medical professionals due to social stigma and embarrassment. Hence, the population prevalence of incontinence is probably underestimated. Nevertheless, it has been variously estimated at 2–5% in the general population and 10% of adult females. There are a variety of specific aetiological factors but the majority of cases are 'idiopathic', most commonly affecting older parous women. Aetiological factors associated with anal incontinence are listed in Table 17.2.

The majority of patients are women with a past history of obstetric problems and difficult deliveries. The underlying mechanism of subsequent incontinence in such cases is complex. Although full-thickness obstetric tears are rare, significant sphincter defects have been observed to occur in 10–30% of women after vaginal delivery. As well as structural sphincter defects, prolonged labour may lead to internal pudendal nerve damage. Denervation of the pelvic floor results in atrophy of the sphincter complex and the levator ani in later life. Most cases of incontinence involve a combination of sphincter muscle damage and the secondary effects of denervation.

Clinical features and assessment

A full history is essential, with particular reference to obstetric history and any past perianal operations. Incontinence should be graded using established scoring systems, such as the Cleveland Clinic Incontinence Score, which incorporate frequency and severity of episodes of incontinence to gas, liquid or solid stool. Such scores enable more objective assessment of any improvement or deterioration in incontinence. Coexisting disease should be documented and neurological symptoms sought. A defaecation history should be sought, including the degree of defaecatory urgency. It is important to enquire about co-existing urinary incontinence. Examination to determine sphincter tone, the presence of previous scars and the state of the rectovaginal septum should be undertaken. Poor anal sensation suggests

Table 17.2 **Aetiology of anal incontinence**
Trauma
• Obstetric sphincter injury (including episiotomy)
• Accidental trauma (e.g. road traffic accident, bicycle injury)
• Surgical trauma (injudicious fistula surgery, drainage of perianal abscess or haemorrhoidectomy)
• Perianal sepsis
Congenital
• Anorectal atresia (usually treated surgically in childhood)
• Spinal dysraphism (spina bifida)
Neurological
• Denervation of pelvic floor following childbirth
• Multiple sclerosis
• Low spinal or sacral tumour
• Spinal trauma
• Dementia
Miscellaneous
• Rectal prolapse
• Haemorrhoids
• Rectal cancer invading sphincter
• Perianal Crohn's disease
• Faecal impaction
• Relative incontinence due to intestinal hurry (e.g. inflammatory bowel disease)
• Psychiatric or behavioural disorders (including encopresis)

a neurogenic basis for the incontinence. Other anorectal causes of incontinence, as listed in Table 17.2, should be excluded where possible, and by rigid sigmoidoscopy in all cases. It is important to remember that any cause of intestinal hurry (such as colonic cancer, inflammatory bowel disease or even infective diarrhoea) can render incontinent a patient who had previously been coping with a more formed stool. Hence, colonoscopy is an important part of assessment. Endoanal ultrasound scanning of the sphincters delineates the presence and extent of any sphincter defect. Anorectal physiology studies document resting and squeeze anal sphincter pressures, and also define whether there is a predominant neurogenic element. Where there is any concern from the history or clinical examination regarding a spinal lesion, MRI should be performed.

Conservative management

Any remedial causes of incontinence (Table 17.2) should be addressed appropriately. However, women with 'idiopathic' faecal incontinence constitute the majority of cases. In older women, who almost universally have a combination of sphincter and nerve damage, conservative measures should be instigated in the first instance. Dietary advice is important to avoid exacerbating factors in the diet, such as caffeine, spicy foods and excessive alcohol. Stool-bulking agents such as Fybogel should be combined with loperamide to reduce the propulsive activity of the GI tract and induce a degree of constipation. In cases with a predominant neurogenic basis, rectal irritability resulting in faecal urgency may respond to therapy with amitriptyline (25–50 mg at night). Conservative measures should be combined with regular emptying of the rectum using stimulant suppositories or enemas. In many cases, these measures have a dramatic beneficial effect on quality of life even when minor degrees of incontinence persist.

Surgical management

Surgery is indicated only in a small minority of patients with idiopathic faecal incontinence. In a small subset of patients with a clear history of sphincter injury due to trauma or to surgical injury, overlapping sphincter repair is frequently highly successful. However, it is important to underline that overall the results of anterior sphincter repair are poor in the long term. Patients with evidence of denervation tend to have poor results. Complex total floor repairs have been performed with some success in a limited proportion of patients. Other surgical approaches include stimulated gracioplasty – transferring the gracilis muscle on a proximal pedicle to wrap it subcutaneously around the anal canal. An electrical stimulator is implanted, which delivers an electrical signal to maintain the muscle in a tonic state by conversion of muscle fibres to slow-twitch type. This allows long-term tonic contraction of the gracilis muscle to maintain continence. The procedure has an acceptable level of success in around 50% of patients, but at a cost of major surgery and potentially major complications.

Implantable artificial anal sphincters have also been developed and these are placed to encircle the anorectum. Results from the use of the available devices are encouraging but, as with any foreign material, there is a propensity for infection and many have to be removed. Nevertheless, prosthetic devices have a place in the management of a small subset of patients with anal incontinence. Sacral nerve stimulation has been introduced with good effect. This involves insertion of an electrode through the S3 sacral foramina and inducing a low-voltage electrical stimulus. The underlying mechanism is poorly understood but in substantial proportion of selected patients the effects are dramatic. Another surgical option for the patient with anal incontinence is the creation of a permanent colostomy. Although this might be seen as an admission of failure, a well-sited stoma and professional input from a stoma care specialist can transform a patient's life, from being afraid to leave the house to leading a virtually normal existence.

The management of anal incontinence remains imperfect, but it is clear that patients should be managed by specialist surgeons. This allows a full investigative work-up and tailoring of management for individual patients. In such a setting, the management of anal incontinence can be highly successful. Improvements in obstetric practice are reducing the incidence in sphincter and nerve damage during childbirth. Unfortunately, progress in this area is hampered by the fact that it is many decades after the initial insult before patients present with anal incontinence.

SUMMARY BOX 17.9

Faecal incontinence

- Faecal incontinence is most common in females
- Childbirth injury is a common aetiological factor
- Associated with neurological disorders, trauma and perianal sepsis or surgery.

Treatment:
- Most respond well to conservative management
- Stool bulking, antidiarrhoeal agents such as loperamide
- Enemas may be required to maintain the rectum free of faeces
- Surgery reserved for debilitating incontinence after failed conservative management:

  sphincter repair – excellent results for (rare) discrete
  sphincter injury, poor for majority
  artificial sphincter implant
  stimulated gracioplasty
  sacral nerve stimulation
  colostomy may be only option in debilitating cases.

PRURITUS ANI

The condition can be a minor, short-lived episode but may be an all-consuming obsession for some patients. It is a particular problem at night and some patients may unconsciously scratch the perianal region during sleep, resulting in further trauma and irritation. Pruritus ani is a common complaint and may be a symptom of many anorectal disorders, including haemorrhoids, fistulae, fissures, faecal incontinence, anal carcinoma and rectal prolapse. Dermatological conditions can also be associated with pruritus ani, and these include psoriasis, dermatitis, lichen planus and anal warts; skin infections can also be responsible. Fungal infections should be considered, including candida and tinea, especially in the diabetic patient.

Management

Underlying conditions, such as anal cancer, perianal fistula and haemorrhoids, should be treated and diabetes mellitus excluded. If there is evidence of fungal infection, this should be treated with antifungal creams. In cases where all other contributing disorders have been excluded and the condition is idiopathic, full explanation and support for the patient are essential. The cycle of trauma to the delicate perianal skin, followed by irritation and subsequent scratching, should be explained in detail. Advice on avoidance of scratching and a requirement for willpower is essential. In some cases, it may be necessary for the patient to wear cotton gloves in bed, to avoid nocturnal scratching. The use of perfumed soap and strong antiseptics or lotions should be discouraged. The avoidance of nylon undergarments is important to minimize sweating. Particular attention should be paid to the diet, as certain foods (e.g. spicy foods or alcohol) may be responsible. Explanation should be given of the need to avoid over-zealous cleansing of the perianal region after defaecation. Gentle cleaning with toilet paper, followed by washing with mild soap, may be necessary, but it is important to take care to avoid trauma during drying. A simple barrier cream such as is used for nappy rash may be appropriate in some patients, but generally it is best to avoid relying on creams. Although it may take several months to control, it is possible to improve the symptoms of idiopathic pruritus ani in almost all cases, providing there is the necessary commitment from the patient.

PILONIDAL DISEASE

Pilonidal disease is a common perianal disorder with a population incidence of 20–30 per 100 000. It is characterized by chronic inflammation in one or more sinuses in the midline of the natal cleft that contain hair and debris (Fig. 17.16). The superficial part of the midline sinus is lined with squamous epithelium, but the tracts themselves are lined with granulation tissue resulting from chronic infection. Pilonidal disease can also affect the digital clefts in hairdressers but this is not discussed here.

Perianal pilonidal disease is more common in males than females, and affects around 2% of the population between the ages of 15 and 35. However, it is very rare after the age of 40, suggesting that there is an aetiological relationship with age and skin character. The disease is vanishingly rare before puberty, when sex hormones act on hair follicles and sebaceous glands. There is enlargement of a hair follicle, which allows the accumulation of extraneous hairs that are caught in the natal cleft itself. A foreign-body reaction is set up, with the result that there is a chronic discharging sinus that attracts other debris and hairs. A sedentary occupation, particularly where sweating is common, is a predisposing factor. The condition was described in large numbers of American troops in the Vietnam war, owing to the use of Jeeps in the warm climate.

Clinical features

Many people have asymptomatic pilonidal sinuses and so it is important to treat the condition only if it is causing problems, in view of the high prevalence and the fact that it seldom presents after the fourth decade. Typical presentation comprises midline natal cleft pits discharging mucopurulent material which may smell mildly offensive and may be blood-stained. There is often tenderness on pressure and the patient may avoid long periods of sitting. When a sinus becomes infected and the pus is loculated, the disease presents as pilonidal abscess, with the abscess typically pointing just off the midline. However, there is invariably a communication with a midline sinus containing hair and granulation tissue. Occasionally, pilonidal sinus may present with extensive and complex branching sinus tracts. In these cases, it is important to consider perianal Crohn's disease, and careful examination of the anal canal is essential.

Management

The treatment of pilonidal disease may be conservative or surgical. Conservative management comprises attention to natal cleft hygiene and hair removal by depilatory creams or by careful shaving. Antibiotics have a place in the early stages of abscess formation and may avert the need for incision and drainage of an established abscess. Hair removal from the sinus tract itself on a regular basis allows the sinus to drain and avoids the collection of hair and debris.

Surgical drainage is indicated for established abscess and the incision should avoid the midline to minimize the likelihood of recurrence. Debilitating, chronically discharging sinus tracts also merit surgery and there are a number of surgical options. The tracts can be laid open, the granulations removed with a curette and the resultant defects dressed until they heal from the base. Tracts can also be excised and closed primarily with sutures, although the wound is prone to break down and heal by second intention. Unfortunately, the treatment of pilonidal disease is characterized by frequent recurrence, due partly to inadequate or inappropriate surgery in some cases, but mostly to the fact that the underlying aetiology is still present: namely, the natal cleft and a predisposed skin type. Recurrent disease can be treated using rotation flaps to replace the pitted skin with fresh skin from the buttock. For complex recurrent disease, ablation of the natal cleft using a flap procedure (cleft closure) is highly effective but leaves a fairly large unsightly scar. It is important to advise the patient to keep the natal cleft free of hair by depilation after any successful surgical treatment.

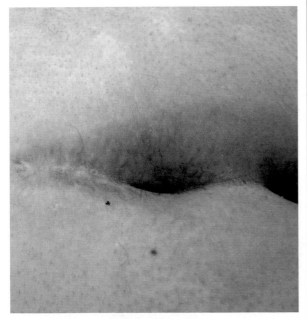

Fig. 17.16 Pilonidal sinus in the natal cleft.

SUMMARY BOX 17.10

Pilonidal disease

- Pilonidal disease is due to hair creating chronic inflammatory sinuses in the natal cleft
- Abscess should be drained
- Symptomatic tracts should be excised
- Recurrence is common and can be dealt with by closure of the natal cleft or other plastic surgical technique.

SECTION 3

Surgical specialties

18

Plastic and reconstructive surgery

INTRODUCTION

Plastic and reconstructive surgery is concerned with the restitution of form and function after trauma and ablative surgery. The techniques by which this is achieved are applicable to virtually every surgical subspecialty and are not limited to any single anatomical region or system. The 'reconstructive ladder' is broad, simple and widely applicable at its base, but narrow, technically demanding and complex at its top (Fig. 18.1). It is important to distinguish plastic and reconstructive surgery from cosmetic, or aesthetic, surgery. In the latter, the techniques of the former are applied to improve appearance but not physical function, although there may be considerable psychological benefit.

STRUCTURE AND FUNCTIONS OF SKIN

Skin consists of epidermis and dermis. The epidermis is a layer of keratinized, stratified squamous epithelium (Fig. 18.2) that sends three appendages (hair follicles, sweat glands and sebaceous glands) into the underlying dermis. Because of their deep location, the appendages escape destruction in partial-thickness burns and are a source of new cells for reconstitution of the epidermis. The basal germinal layer of the epidermis generates keratin-producing cells (keratinocytes), which become increasingly keratinized and flattened as they migrate to the surface, where they are shed. The basal layer also contains pigment cells (melanocytes) that produce melanin, which is passed to the keratinocytes and protects the basal layer from ultraviolet light.

The dermis is composed of collagen, elastic fibres and fat. It supports blood vessels, lymphatics, nerves and the epidermal appendages. The junction between the epidermis and the dermis is undulating where dermal papillae push up towards the epidermis.

The three types of epidermal appendage extend into the dermis and, in some places, into the subcutaneous tissues. Hair follicles produce hair, the colour of which is determined by melanocytes within the follicle. The sebaceous glands secrete sebum into the hair follicles, which lubricates the skin and hair. The sweat glands are coiled tubular glands lying within the dermis and are of two types; eccrine sweat glands secrete salt and water on to the entire skin surface, while apocrine glands secrete a musty-smelling fluid in the axilla, eyelids, ears, nipple and areola, genital areas and the perianal region. Hidradenitis suppurativa affects the latter.

The nails are flat, horny structures composed of keratin. They arise from a matrix of germinal cells, which can be seen as a white crescent (lunula) at the nail base. If a nail is avulsed, a new nail grows from this matrix. If the matrix is destroyed, nail regeneration is impossible, and the layer of epidermal cells covering the nailbed thickens to form a keratinized protective layer.

WOUNDS

A wound may be defined as disruption of the normal continuity of bodily structures due to trauma, which may be penetrating or non-penetrating. In both cases, inspection of the body surface may give little indication of the extent of underlying damage.

Types of wound

Wounds can be classified according to the mechanism of injury:

- *Incised wounds.* A sharp instrument causes these; if there is associated tearing of tissues, the wound is said to be lacerated
- *Abrasions.* These result from friction damage and are characterized by superficial bruising and loss of a varying thickness of skin and underlying tissue. Dirt and foreign bodies are frequently embedded in the tissues and can give rise to traumatic tattooing
- *Crush injuries.* These are due to severe pressure. Even though the skin may not be breached, there can be massive tissue destruction. Oedema can make wound closure impossible. Increasing pressure within fascial compartments can cause ischaemic necrosis of muscle and other structures (compartment syndrome)

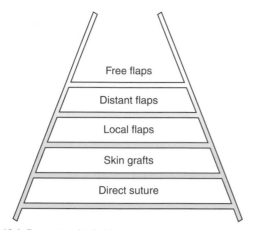

Fig. 18.1 Reconstructive ladder.

- *Degloving injuries.* These result from shearing forces that cause parallel tissue planes to move against each other: for example, when a hand is caught between rollers or in moving machinery. Large areas of apparently intact skin may be deprived of their blood supply by rupture of feeding vessels
- *Gunshot wounds.* These may be low-velocity (e.g. shotguns) or high-velocity (e.g. military rifles). Bullets fired from high-velocity rifles cause massive tissue destruction after skin penetration
- *Burns.* These are caused not only by heat but also by electricity, irradiation and chemicals.

Principles of wound healing

The essential features of healing are common to wounds of almost all soft tissues, and result in the formation of a scar. Soft tissue healing can be subdivided into three phases (Table 18.1) according to the development of tensile strength (Fig. 18.3).

Lag phase

The lag phase is the delay of 2–3 days that elapses before fibroblasts begin to manufacture collagen to support the wound. It is characterized by an inflammatory response to

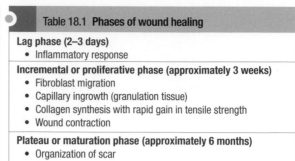

Table 18.1 Phases of wound healing
Lag phase (2–3 days)
• Inflammatory response
Incremental or proliferative phase (approximately 3 weeks)
• Fibroblast migration
• Capillary ingrowth (granulation tissue)
• Collagen synthesis with rapid gain in tensile strength
• Wound contraction
Plateau or maturation phase (approximately 6 months)
• Organization of scar
• Slow final gain in tensile strength (80% of original strength)

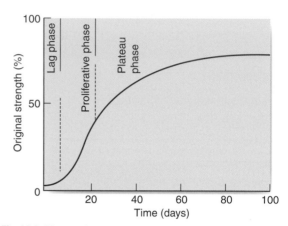

Fig. 18.3 Phases of wound healing.

injury, during which capillary permeability increases and a protein-rich exudate accumulates. It is from this exudate that collagen is later synthesized. Inflammatory cells migrate into the area, dead tissue is removed by macrophages, and capillaries at the wound edges begin to proliferate.

Incremental phase

During the incremental or proliferative phase, there is progressive collagen synthesis by fibroblasts and a corresponding increase in tensile strength. Increased collagen turnover

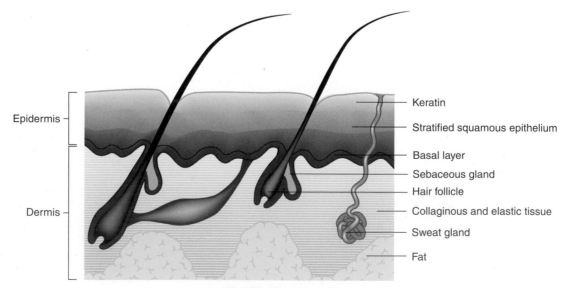

Fig. 18.2 Structure of skin.

in areas remote from the wound suggests that there may also be a systemic stimulus for fibroblast activity. Collagen synthesis increases over a period of about 3 weeks, during which the gain in tensile strength accelerates. Old collagen undergoes lysis and new collagen is laid down.

Plateau or maturation phase

After 3 weeks, the gain in tensile strength levels off as the rate of collagen breakdown first approaches and then temporarily surpasses its synthesis. Excess collagen is removed during this final clearing-up process and the number of fibroblasts and inflammatory cells declines. Orientation of collagen fibres in the direction of local mechanical forces increases tensile strength for some 6 months. However, skin and fascia usually recover only 80% of their original tensile strength.

At the time of suture removal, the edges of the newly healed wound should be directly apposed and flat. Thereafter, for up to 3 months, the scar may become progressively raised, red and thickened. It can then remain static for a further 3 months, before slowly improving to become narrow, flat and pale. These changes vary with age, race, the direction of scar and the degree of dermal damage.

In children, scars take longer to resolve, whereas in the elderly they tend to mature and fade very quickly.

Hypertrophic scars

This is an exaggeration of the normal maturation process. Such wounds are very raised, red and firm, but never continue to worsen after 6 months. They are particularly common in children and after deep dermal burns. Unless under tension, they eventually resolve, often after several years. Resolution can be hastened by elastic pressure garments, steroid injections or the application of silicone gel. These scars should not be excised.

Keloids

These are similar to hypertrophic scars, except that they continue to enlarge after 6 months and invade neighbouring uninvolved skin. They are most likely to occur across the upper chest, shoulders and earlobes, and are common in black patients. They are difficult to treat successfully. If the measures described above fail, intralesional excision followed immediately by low-dose radiotherapy is sometimes considered.

Epidermis

Epithelium heals by regeneration and not by scar formation. Epithelial cells at the edge of the wound lose their adhesion to each other and migrate across the wound until they meet cells from the other side. As they migrate, they are replaced by new cells formed by the division of basal cells near the wound edge. The cells that have migrated undergo mitosis and the new epithelium thickens, eventually forming normal epithelial cover for the scar produced by the dermis.

Primary and secondary intention

Wounds may heal by primary intention if the edges are closely approximated: for example, by accurate suturing. Epithelial cover is quickly achieved and healing produces a fine scar (Fig. 18.4). If the wound edges are not apposed, the defect fills with granulation tissue and the restoration of epidermal continuity takes much longer. The advance of epithelial cells across the denuded area may be hindered by infection. This is known as healing by secondary intention and usually results in delayed healing, excessive fibrosis and an ugly scar (Fig. 18.5). If a wound has begun to heal by

secondary intention, it may still be possible to speed healing by excising the wound edges and bringing them into apposition, or by covering the defect with a skin graft.

SUMMARY BOX 18.1

Classification of wound healing

- Healing by first intention is the most efficient method and results when a clean incised surgical wound is meticulously apposed and heals with minimal scarring
- Healing by second intention occurs when wound edges are not apposed and the defect fills with granulation tissue. In the time taken to restore epithelial cover, infection supervenes, fibrosis is excessive and the resulting scar is unsightly
- The term 'healing by third intention' describes the situation where a wound healing by second intention (e.g. a neglected traumatic wound or a burn) is treated by excising its margins and then apposing them or covering the area with a skin graft. The final cosmetic result may be better than if the wound had been left to heal by second intention.

Factors influencing wound healing

Many of the factors influencing healing are interrelated: for example, the site of the wound, its blood supply, and the level of tissue oxygenation. Although some adverse factors, such as advanced age, cannot be influenced, others, such as surgical technique, nutritional status and the presence of intercurrent disease, can be modified or eliminated.

Blood supply

Wounds in ischaemic tissue heal slowly or not at all. They are prone to infection and frequently break down. When this occurs, the wound may not be able to sustain the metabolic demands of healing by second intention. Arterial oxygen tension (P_aO_2) is a key determinant of the rate of collagen synthesis. Anaemia may not affect healing if the patient has a normal blood volume and arterial oxygen tension. Poor surgical technique, such as crushing tissue with forceps, approximating wound edges under tension and tying sutures too tightly, can make well vascularized tissue ischaemic and lead to wound breakdown.

Infection

The general risks of wound infection depend upon age, the presence of intercurrent infection, steroid administration, diabetes mellitus, disordered nutrition, and cardiovascular and respiratory disease. Local factors are also important. Bacterial contamination can be minimized by careful skin preparation and aseptic technique, but some wounds are more likely to be contaminated than others. Bacteria may enter wounds from the atmosphere, from internal foci of sepsis or from the lumen of transected organs. In some cases, contamination occurs in the postoperative period. Provided contamination is not gross and local blood supply is good, natural defences are usually able to prevent and contain overt infection. Devitalized tissues, haematomas and the presence of foreign material such as sutures and prostheses favour bacterial survival and growth. Common infecting organisms are staphylococci, streptococci, coliforms and anaerobes. Overcrowding of wards and excessive

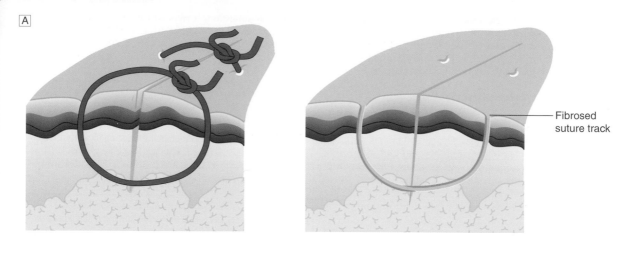

A

Fibrosed
suture track

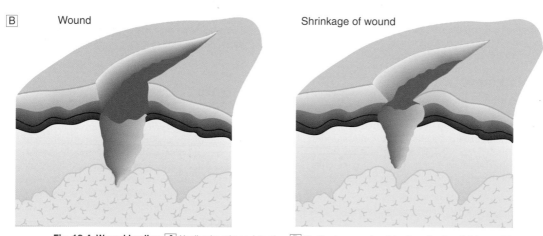

B   Wound   Shrinkage of wound

Fig. 18.4 Wound healing. A Healing by primary intention. B Healing by secondary intention, showing shrinkage of the wound.

use of operating theatres increase the bacterial population of the atmosphere and hence the risk of wound infection. The failure of medical and nursing staff to wash their hands before and after touching and examining each patient is perhaps the greatest source of cross-contamination.

When wound contamination is anticipated, topical antibacterial chemicals or topical and systemic antibiotics can be used prophylactically. For example, a single dose of systemic antibiotic is normally used to reduce the risk of infection during gastrointestinal surgery and when prosthetic material (hip joint, cardiac valves, arterial bypass) is being inserted. In acute traumatic wounds, tetanus prophylaxis is routine, but antibiotics are not normally necessary provided prompt and thorough surgical treatment is undertaken. However, if there has been a delay in the treatment of such a wound, antibiotic prophylaxis may be necessary.

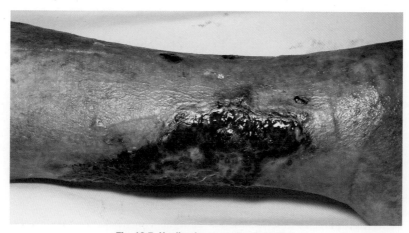

Fig. 18.5 Healing by secondary intention.

Age

Wounds in the elderly may heal poorly because of impaired blood supply, poor nutritional status or intercurrent disease. However, as mentioned above, they tend to form 'good' scars.

Site of wound

Surgical incisions placed in the lines of least tissue tension are subject to minimal distraction and should heal promptly, leaving a fine scar. On the face, these lines run at right angles to the direction of underlying muscles and form the lines of facial expression.

Nutritional status

Malnutrition has to be severe before healing is affected. Protein availability is most important, and wound dehiscence and infection are common when the serum albumin is low. Healing problems should be anticipated if recent weight loss exceeds 20%. Vitamin C is essential for proline hydroxylation and collagen synthesis. The number of fibroblasts is not reduced in scorbutic states. Zinc is a co-factor for important enzymes involved in healing, and its deficiency retards healing. Supplements of ascorbic acid and zinc are effective in patients with known deficiencies, but do not improve healing in normal subjects.

Intercurrent disease

Healing may be affected by the disease itself or by its treatment. Cachectic patients with severe malnutrition (as seen in advanced cancer) have marked impairment of healing. Diabetes mellitus impairs healing by reducing tissue resistance to infection and by causing peripheral vascular insufficiency and neuropathy. Haemorrhagic diatheses increase the risk of haematoma formation and wound infection. Obstructive airway disease lowers arterial PO_2 and so affects healing. Abdominal wound dehiscence is more common in patients with respiratory disease because of the strain put on the wound during coughing. Corticosteroid therapy reduces the inflammatory response, impairs collagen synthesis and decreases resistance to infection. The effect of steroids on wound healing is most marked if they are given within 3 days of injury. Immunosuppressive therapy and chemotherapy impair healing by reducing resistance to infection. As radiotherapy greatly reduces the vascularity of the tissues, the healing of wounds in irradiated areas is often impaired.

Surgical technique

Where possible, skin incisions are placed in the line of least tissue tension. Aseptic technique, gentle handling and accurate apposition of wound edges favour healing by first intention. Dead spaces must be avoided, as the accumulation of blood and exudate encourage infection. Correct suturing of the deeper layers avoids dead space and often allows the skin edges to fall together without tension, so that superficial sutures or adhesive tape can achieve skin apposition. Drains should be used in contaminated wounds and those where exudate is expected. Drains may be connected to a suction apparatus or allowed to empty by gravity. The drain site is a potential portal of entry for infection and drains should be removed as soon as possible, especially when prosthetic material has been implanted.

Choice of suture and suture materials

Foreign material in the tissues predisposes to infection. The finest sutures that will hold the wound edges together should be used. Whereas 5/0 or 6/0 sutures are appropriate for the face, stronger ones (3/0 or 4/0) are needed for incisions near joints and still stronger ones for the abdominal wall. The suture should be strong enough to support the wound until tensile strength has recovered sufficiently to prevent breakdown. Absorbable materials are preferred for buried layers.

Wound infection

Classification

Surgical procedures can be classified according to the likelihood of contamination and wound infection as 'clean', 'clean-contaminated' and 'contaminated':

- *Clean procedures* are those in which wound contamination is not expected and should not occur. An incision for a clean elective procedure should not become infected. In clean operations, the wound infection rate should be less than 1%.

 SUMMARY BOX 18.2

Factors affecting wound healing

The site of the wound and its orientation relative to tissue tension lines are major determinants of healing
Wounds with a good blood supply (e.g. head and neck wounds) heal well
Infection is a major adverse factor and the risk of infection is influenced by:
- general factors such as the patient's age, presence of intercurrent infection, nutritional status and cardiorespiratory disease
- local factors including bacterial contamination, antibacterial prophylaxis, aseptic technique, degree of trauma, presence of devitalized tissue, haematoma and foreign bodies.

Intercurrent disease may impair healing. Important factors include:
- malnutrition
- diabetes mellitus
- haemorrhagic diatheses
- hypoxia (e.g. obstructive airways disease)
- corticosteroid therapy
- immunosuppression
- radiotherapy.

Surgical technical factors that have a major influence on wound healing include:
- gentle tissue handling
- avoidance of undue trauma
- accurate tissue apposition
- meticulous haemostasis
- appropriate choice of suture material.

- *Clean-contaminated procedures* are those in which no frank focus of infection is encountered but where a significant risk of infection is nevertheless present, perhaps because of the opening of a viscus, such as the colon. Infection rates in excess of 5% may suggest a breakdown in ward and operating theatre routine.
- *Contaminated or 'dirty' wounds* are those in which gross contamination is inevitable and the risk of wound infection is high; an example is emergency surgery for perforated diverticular disease, or drainage of a subphrenic abscess.

Antibiotic prophylaxis is appropriate for the latter two types of operation.

18

18

Clinical features

Wound infection usually becomes evident 3–4 days after surgery. The first signs are usually superficial cellulitis around the margins of the wound, or swelling of the wound with some serous discharge from between the sutures. Fluctuation is occasionally elicited when there is an abscess or liquefying haematoma. Crepitus may be present if gas-forming organisms are involved. In some cases of deep infection, there are no local signs, although the patient may have pyrexia and increased wound tenderness. Systemic upset is variable, usually amounting to only moderate pyrexia and leucocytosis. Toxaemia, bacteraemia and septicaemia can complicate serious wound infection, especially where there is an accumulation of pus. The differential diagnosis includes other causes of postoperative pyrexia, wound haematoma and wound dehiscence. Wound haematoma may result from reactive bleeding during the first 24–48 hours after an operation. It causes swelling and discomfort, but only minimal pyrexia and few systemic signs.

Prevention

The risk of wound infection is reduced by careful patient preparation, the prophylactic use of antibiotics in high-risk patients, and meticulous attention to good operating theatre techniques. Severely contaminated wounds are sometimes best closed by delayed primary suture; most gunshot wounds are treated in this way. Skin sutures may be inserted at this time but are not tied for several days, by which time it should be clear that infection has been avoided. Antibiotic therapy is essential for grossly contaminated wounds. The aim is to achieve high tissue concentrations as soon as possible. The choice of antibiotic is determined by the nature of the infection. Topical agents such as povidone-iodine may also be used to combat infection in contaminated wounds. Radical excision of the wound margins, thorough mechanical cleansing and delayed suture may also be required.

Management

A wound swab or specimen of pus is routinely sent for bacteriological culture and sensitivity determination. In urgent cases, a Gram stain may be useful. The state of immunity against tetanus is assessed and appropriate action taken. Trivial superficial cellulitis can be managed expectantly. The area of redness is 'mapped out' with an indelible pen so that its extent can be monitored. Spreading cellulitis is an indication for antibiotic therapy. Many infected wounds heal rapidly without further surgery, particularly if the original skin incision is placed in the line of least tissue tension. The problem is often to keep the wound open, rather than to achieve closure. If it appears that spontaneous wound closure will take a long time, secondary suture or skin grafting can be considered to speed healing, but only once it is clear that infection has been eradicated. The presence of clean healthy granulation tissue in the wound is usually a good indication that closure can be undertaken.

Involvement of other structures

All wounds must be inspected carefully in good light to assess the extent of devitalization and injury to other structures. However, it is important to appreciate that a small, apparently innocent wound may conceal extensive damage to deeper structures. Body cavities may have been penetrated, or tendons, nerves and blood vessels divided. Damage to muscles, tendons or nerves is assessed by checking relevant motor and sensory function. If the injury

SUMMARY BOX 18.3

Principles of management of contaminated traumatic wounds

- Contaminated wounds should be debrided under general anaesthesia
- The contaminated wound and its margins must be cleansed thoroughly, and grit, soil and foreign bodies/materials removed
- Devitalized tissue is formally excised until bleeding is encountered
- Primary closure is avoided if there has been gross contamination and when treatment has been delayed for more than 6 hours. Inappropriate attempts to achieve primary closure increase the risk of wound infection and expose the patient to the risks of anaerobic infection (tetanus and gas gangrene)
- Wounds left open may be suitable for delayed primary suture after 2–3 days, or for later excision and secondary suture (with or without skin grafting)
- Appropriate protection against tetanus must be afforded and the use of antibiotics should be considered.

involves a limb, the distal circulation must be checked. Where appropriate, X-rays will help to establish whether peritoneal, pericardial or pleural cavities have been entered, and whether there is underlying bony injury.

Provided there is no deep damage, small, relatively uncontaminated wounds can be treated under local anaesthesia in the A&E department. The wound margins are cleaned with a mild antiseptic such as cetrimide and the wound is irrigated with sterile saline. Any devitalized tissue is removed, deep tissues are sutured with absorbable material and the skin margins are closed.

More extensive or severely contaminated wounds usually require inpatient treatment, with exploration and debridement under general anaesthesia. The wound and its margins are cleansed and all obvious foreign material picked out. Devitalized tissue is trimmed back until bleeding occurs. In areas of poor vascularity such as the leg, or if there is severe contamination, crushing or a fracture, the wound margins are formally excised (Fig. 18.6). Bleeding from the wound margin is not a certain indication of its ultimate survival, as impaired venous drainage can lead to progressive necrosis, particularly after a crushing or degloving injury. If there is any doubt, the wound should not be sutured and a 'second-look' dressing change should be undertaken under anaesthesia after 48 hours.

Primary closure should be avoided if there is significant delay in treating a grossly contaminated wound: that is, more than 6 hours without antibiotic cover. If primary closure is attempted, wound infection and breakdown are likely and there is a risk of anaerobic infection. It is also too late for formal excision but foreign bodies and dead tissue should be removed in the usual way. The wound is dressed and antibiotics are started. The dressing is changed daily, and if the wound is clean, delayed primary suture may be carried out after 48 hours. If closure is delayed, any granulation tissue is usually excised and secondary suture performed. If this is not possible, split-skin grafts (see below) can be applied to the granulations.

Provided that surgical treatment is carried out early, prophylactic antibiotics are only required for deeply penetrating wounds, especially those from dog and human bites or those caused by nails, where adequate debridement

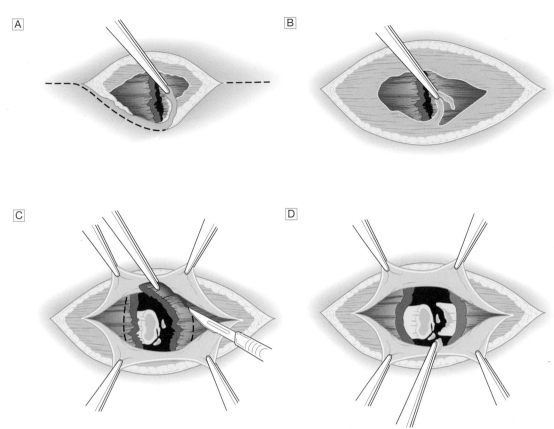

Fig. 18.6 Technique of wound debridement for a compound fracture. [A] Excision of skin edges. [B] Excision of fascial layer. [C] Excision of traumatized muscle. [D] Removal of small bone fragments.

may be impossible. However, the early use of antibiotics in situations where a delay in surgical treatment is anticipated may allow primary suture of wounds after 8–12 hours, an interval that is normally considered safe.

Devitalized skin flaps

A common emergency problem is posed by the patient, usually an elderly woman, who falls and raises a triangular flap over the surface of the tibia (pretibial laceration). In some cases, the flap is blue-black in colour and obviously non-viable, but in most cases viability is uncertain. Similar injuries can occur elsewhere in the body. The wound must be cleansed and non-viable tissue excised. No attempt should be made to suture the flap back into place; because of the post-traumatic oedema this would only be possible under tension, and would lead to death of the flap. A small defect can be treated conservatively on an outpatient basis by wound dressing and an elastic supporting bandage providing the arterial circulation is normal; Ch. 21) and the patient is kept ambulant. The wound will normally take several weeks to heal. A larger defect may require a split-skin graft, either immediately or as a delayed primary procedure.

Wounds with skin loss

If skin has been lost as a direct result of trauma, or following the excision of a tumour or necrotic tissue, direct suture may not be possible. A small skin defect at a functionally or aesthetically unimportant site may be allowed to heal by secondary intention. However, it is often better to speed healing by importing skin to close the wound by means of a skin graft, which requires a vascular bed as it has no blood supply of its own, or a flap.

Skin grafts

These may be split-skin or full-thickness. Split-skin grafts are cut with a special guarded freehand knife or an electric dermatome. The donor site heals by re-epithelialization from epithelial appendages in the dermis within 2–3 weeks, depending on the thickness of the graft. To cover very large areas, the graft can be expanded by 'meshing'. The thinner the graft, the more easily it will take on a bed of imperfect vascularity but the poorer the quality of skin will be and the more it will shrink. Split-skin grafts are used to cover wounds after acute trauma, granulating areas and burns, or when the defect is large. A full-thickness graft leaves a donor defect (which needs to be sutured or grafted) as large as the one to be filled and requires a well-vascularized bed to survive. However, such grafts are strong, do not shrink, and look better than a split-skin graft. They are rarely advisable after acute trauma but are commonly used in reconstructive surgery to close small defects where strength is needed (e.g. on the palm of the hand) or where a good functional and/or cosmetic result is important (e.g. on the lower eyelid). An area where there is skin to spare is chosen for the donor site (e.g. the groin for the former and the area behind the ear or upper eyelid for the latter).

18

Flaps

Whereas grafts require a vascular bed to survive, flaps bring their own blood supply to the new site. They can therefore be thicker and stronger than grafts and can be applied to avascular areas such as exposed bone, tendon or joints. They are used in acute trauma only if closure is not possible by direct suture or skin grafting, and are more usually reserved for the reconstruction of surgical defects and for secondary reconstruction after trauma. The simplest flaps use local skin and fat (local flaps), and are often a good alternative to grafting for small defects such as those left after the excision of facial tumours (Fig. 18.7). A flap may have to be brought from a distance (distant flap) and remain attached temporarily to its original blood supply until it has picked up a new one locally (Fig. 18.8). This usually takes 2–3 weeks, after which the pedicle can be divided. Advances in our knowledge of the blood supply to the skin and underlying muscles have led to the development of many large skin, muscle and composite flaps, which have revolutionized plastic and reconstructive surgery. One example is the use of the transverse rectus abdominis musculocutaneous (TRAM) flap for reconstruction of the breast. The ability to join small blood vessels under the operating microscope now allows the surgeon to close defects in a single stage, even when there is no local tissue available, by free tissue

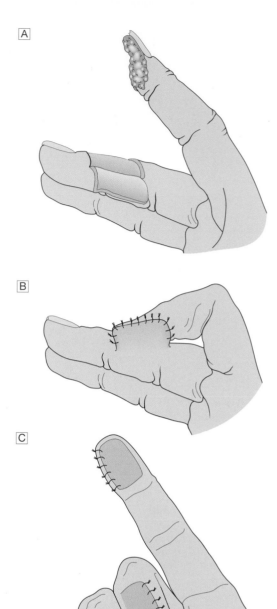

Fig. 18.8 Example of a pedicled (cross finger) skin flap used to cover a defect on the tip of the index finger. A Raised. B Inset. C Divided.

transfer (Fig. 18.9). Other tissues, such as bone, cartilage, nerve and tendon, can also be grafted to restore function and correct deformity after tissue damage or loss.

Crushing/degloving injuries and gunshot wounds

Wounds of this type should never be closed primarily due to the extensive tissue destruction. After thorough irrigation and the removal of any obviously dead tissue and

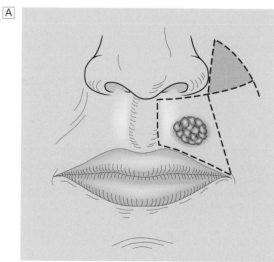

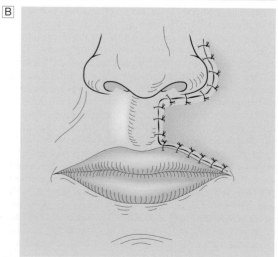

Fig. 18.7 Local skin flap used to repair a defect after the excision of a skin lesion. A Before surgery. B After surgery.

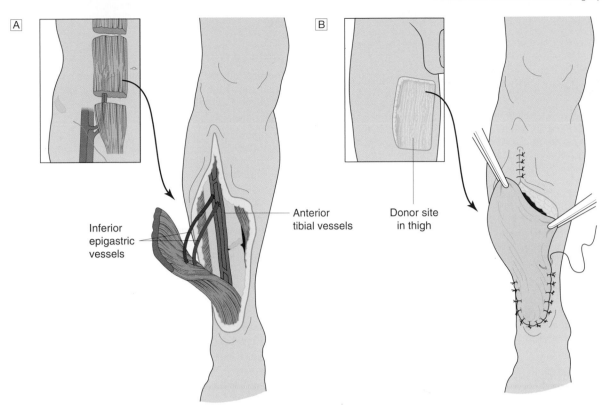

Inferior epigastric vessels

Anterior tibial vessels

Donor site in thigh

Fig. 18.9 Example of free tissue transfer based on inferior epigastric vessels. [A] Rectus abdominis muscle transferred to shin and its vessels (inferior epigastric vessels) anastomosed to anterior tibial vessels. [B] Muscle covered by split-skin graft.

foreign material, such wounds should be lightly packed and dressed. Dressings are removed 48 hours later under anaesthesia and further excision is carried out if necessary. The wound is closed by suture, skin grafting or flap cover, once it is clear that all dead tissue has been removed.

BURNS

Mechanisms

Burn injuries range from the trivial to severe burns that pose a threat to life, involve a long hospital stay, and carry the risk of permanent disfigurement or impaired function. They may be caused by flames, hot solids, hot liquids or steam, irradiation, electricity or chemicals. Toddlers are particularly liable to scalding by hot liquids in kitchen accidents, and unguarded fires are a threat to all children. Burns sustained in house fires are often accompanied by smoke inhalation, with injury to the lungs. Alcohol is a common contributing factor in burn injury. In the elderly and infirm, impaired mobility, poor coordination and diminished awareness of pain increase the incidence of burns. Industrial accidents account for most physiocochemical burns, although the accidental or deliberate ingestion of caustic or corrosive chemicals is still an occasional cause of domestic burns.

Local effects of burn injury

The local effects result from destruction of the more superficial tissues and the inflammatory response of the deeper tissues (Table 18.2). Fluid is lost from the surface or trapped in blisters, the magnitude of loss depending on the extent of injury. Loss is greatly increased by leakage of fluid from

Table 18.2 Effects of burn injury
Destruction of tissue
• (Depth depends on heat of causative agent and contact time)
• Loss of barrier to infection
• Fluid loss from surface
• Red cell destruction
Increased capillary permeability
• Oedema
• Loss of circulating fluid volume
• Hypovolaemic shock
Increased metabolic rate

the circulation (see below) where, instead of the normal insensible loss of $15\,\text{ml/m}^2$ body surface/hour, as much as $200\,\text{ml/m}^2$ may be lost during the first few hours. With deeper injuries, the epidermis and dermis are converted into a coagulum of dead tissue known as eschar. In its least severe form, the dermal inflammatory response consists of capillary dilatation, as in the erythema of sunburn. With deeper burns, the damaged capillaries become permeable to protein, and an exudate forms with an electrolytic and protein content only slightly less than that of plasma. Lymphatic drainage fails to keep pace with the rate of exudation and interstitial oedema leads to a reduction in circulating fluid volume. An increase of 2 cm in the diameter of the leg represents the accumulation of over 2 litres of excess interstitial fluid. Exudation is maximal in the first 12 hours, capillary permeability returning to normal within 48 hours.

Destruction of the epidermis removes the barrier to bacterial invasion and opens the door to infection. The burn surface may become contaminated at any time, and wound

18

care must commence when the patient is first seen. Sepsis delays healing, increases energy needs, and may pose a new threat to life, just when the early dangers of hypovolaemia have been overcome.

General effects of burn injury

The general effects of a burn depend upon its size. Large burns lead to water, salt and protein loss, hypovolaemia and increased catabolism. Circulating plasma volume falls as oedema accumulates, and fluid leaks from the burned surface. With large burns, the effect is compounded by a generalized increase in capillary permeability, with widespread oedema. Some red cells are destroyed immediately by a full-thickness burn, but many more are damaged and die later. However, red cell loss is small compared to plasma loss in the early period, and haemoconcentration, reflected by a rising haematocrit, is the norm. The shifts in water and electrolytes are ultimately shared by all body tissues, and if circulatory volume is not restored, hypovolaemic shock ensues. Large burns increase metabolic rate as water losses from the burned surface cause expenditure of calories to provide the heat of evaporation. In severe burns, some 7000 kcal may be expended daily, and a daily weight loss of 0.5 kg is not unusual unless steps are taken to prevent it.

Classification

Burns are classified according to depth as either partial- or full-thickness (Fig. 18.10).

Superficial partial-thickness burns

Superficial partial-thickness burns involve only the epidermis and the superficial dermis. Pain, swelling and fluid loss can be marked. New epidermal cover is provided by undamaged cells originating from the epidermal appendages. The burn will usually heal in less than 3 weeks, with a perfect final cosmetic result.

Deep partial-thickness burns

In deep partial-thickness (also known as deep-dermal) burns, the epidermis and much of the dermis are destroyed. Restoration of the epidermis then depends on there being

SUMMARY BOX 18.4

Consequences of burns

The morbidity and mortality of burns depend on the site, extent and depth of the burn and on the age and general condition of the patient

Early consequences
- hypovolaemia (loss of protein, fluid and electrolytes)
- metabolic derangements (hyponatraemia followed by risk of hypernatraemia, hyperkalaemia followed by hypokalaemia)
- sepsis, which may be both local and generalized
- haemolysis with anaemia and need for transfusion
- hypothermia.

Short-term consequences
- renal failure (acute tubular necrosis due to hypovolaemia, haemoglobinuria and myoglobinuria)
- respiratory failure (smoke inhalation, airway obstruction, acute respiratory distress syndrome)
- catabolism and nutritional depletion
- venous thrombosis
- Curling's ulcer and erosive gastritis.

Long-term consequences
- permanent disfigurement
- prolonged hospitalization
- psychological problems
- impaired function.

intact epithelial cells within the remaining appendages. Pain, swelling and fluid loss are again marked. The burn takes longer than 3 weeks to heal, as fewer epithelial elements survive, and often leaves an ugly hypertrophic scar. Infection often delays healing and can cause further tissue destruction, converting the injury to a full-thickness one.

Full-thickness burns

A full-thickness burn destroys the epidermis and underlying dermis, including the epidermal appendages. The destroyed tissues undergo coagulative necrosis and form an eschar that begins to lift after 2–3 weeks. Unless the raw area is grafted, epidermal cover can only occur through

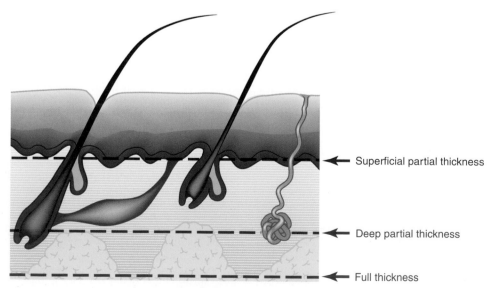

Superficial partial thickness

Deep partial thickness

Full thickness

Fig. 18.10 Depth of burn injury.

the inward movement and growth of cells from intact skin around the burn, and by contraction of its base. Fibrosis and ugly contracture are thus inevitable in all but small, ungrafted injuries.

Determination of burn depth

There is no infallible method for the early determination of burn depth; experienced plastic surgeons may not be able to make an accurate assessment for days or even weeks after injury.

Mechanisms

Burn depth is proportional to the temperature of the causal agent and to the length of contact time. Scalds from liquids below boiling point usually produce partial-thickness injury, whereas scalds from boiling water and burns due to prolonged contact with hot metal often produce full-thickness damage. Flame burns can be of mixed depth but nearly always include areas of full-thickness loss. Electrical burns are almost always full-thickness, and high-tension electricity can cause devastating necrosis of muscles and other deep tissues.

Appearance

Erythema means that epidermal damage is superficial, and blanching on pressure confirms that dermal capillaries are intact and that the injury is partial-thickness. Blisters are accumulations of fluid superficial to the basal layer of the epidermis and suggest partial-thickness injury. A dead-white appearance frequently indicates full-thickness injury, although at least some of these burns prove to be deep-dermal. A dry, leathery mahogany-coloured eschar with visible thrombosed veins denotes full-thickness destruction.

Sensation

Intact cutaneous sensation implies that the epidermal appendages have survived, as they lie at the same level as cutaneous nerve endings in the dermis. Superficial burns are thus very painful.

PROGNOSIS

Age and general condition

Infants, the elderly, alcoholics and those with other co-morbidity fare less well than healthy young adults (see EBM 18.1).

EBM 18.1 Burns

'Mortality is related to the size (% body surface area, BSA) and age of the patient.

$$\text{Mortality} = (\%BSA + age) / 100$$

Large burns > 15% in adults (> 10% in children) require intravenous resuscitation.'

This is a shorthand way of calculating actuarial survival based on Bull J P (1971) Revised analysis of mortality due to Burns. Lancet, 2, 1133-4.

Extent of the burn

The approximate extent of the burn can be quickly calculated in adults by using the 'rule of nines' (Fig. 18.11). Tables are available for more accurate estimations of burn area. The patient's hand and fingers together constitute about 1% of body surface area (BSA). Hypovolaemic shock is anticipated if more than 15% of the surface is burned in adults, or more than 10% in a child. The 'rule of nines' cannot be used in children because of the relatively large head size (about 20% of body surface at birth) and the relatively small limbs (legs are about 13%).

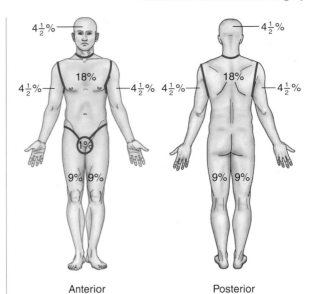

Fig. 18.11 Rule of nines for calculating surface areas of a burn.

18

Depth of the burn

Superficial burns of whatever size should heal without scarring within 3 weeks if properly managed. Deep-dermal burns take longer and produce hypertrophic scarring. Full-thickness burns inevitably become infected unless excised early, and in the case of large burns infection may prove life-threatening.

Site of the burn

Burns involving the face, neck, hands, feet or perineum are particularly liable to threaten appearance or function. They require inpatient management.

Associated respiratory injury

This is now extremely common in house fires and usually results from the inhalation of smoke from burning plastic foam upholstery. It is frequently fatal.

Management

First aid

Prompt effective action prevents further damage and may save life or prevent months of suffering. The key principles are to arrest the burning process, ensure an adequate airway and avoid wound contamination (Table 18.3).

Table 18.3 First aid for burns

- Arrest the burning process
  extinguish flames
  remove clothing
  cool with water
- Ensure adequacy of airway
- Avoid wound contamination
  Clingfilm
  Transfer for definitive treatment as soon as possible

18

Arrest the burning process

Burning clothing is extinguished by smothering the flames in a coat or carpet. The victim is laid flat to avoid flames rising to the head and neck, with inhalation of smoke and fumes. Heat within clothing can continue to cause damage for many seconds after flames have been extinguished or if soaked with scalding water; clothing must therefore be removed or doused with cold water. Cool water is an excellent analgesic and dissipates heat, but common sense must be applied; immersing a child in cold water or covering a patient with cold soaks can cause hypothermia. Cooling counteracts the heat of a burn only if applied immediately after injury. Chemical burns require copious irrigation particularly those involving the eyes. Electrical burning is arrested by switching off the current, not by pulling the patient free. If this is not feasible, the patient should be pushed free from the contact using a non-conductor such as a wooden chair.

Ensure an adequate airway

The patient must be moved as quickly as possible into a smoke-free atmosphere. Smoke and fumes can cause asphyxia, often contain poisons and can precipitate respiratory arrest. Mouth-to-mouth ventilation is commenced, if necessary. If cardiac arrest follows electrocution, resuscitation is instituted.

Avoid wound contamination

The burn should be covered with a clean sheet or clingfilm. Traditional household remedies must be avoided. At best they are messy and interfere with subsequent care; at worst they are destructive, converting a partial injury to a full-thickness one.

Transfer to hospital

The patient should be transferred to hospital as quickly as possible, unless the burn is obviously trivial. Severe burns are best treated in a specialized burns unit from the outset. Hypovolaemia takes time to become manifest and it is easy to misjudge the severity of injury, thereby missing the opportunity for uncomplicated early transfer. Patients embarking on a journey expected to take more than 30 minutes should be accompanied by a trained person. An intravenous infusion should be commenced if the burn is extensive. Transfer of patients with large burns between hospitals should be avoided between 8 and 24 hours after injury.

Full-thickness burns are often relatively painless. Partial-thickness injuries can be excruciating and opiates are usually needed. Analgesics must be given intravenously and the dose and route of administration noted.

Adequate ventilation

On arrival at hospital, the maintenance of an adequate airway remains the first priority. Lack of respiratory symptoms on admission is no guarantee that the patient will remain free from airway problems. Every patient who has been exposed to smoke in a closed room should be admitted for observation. Respiratory tract injury is suggested by dyspnoea, cough, hoarseness, cyanosis, coarse crepitations on auscultation, and the presence of soot particles around the nostrils, in the mouth or in the sputum. Endotracheal intubation is advisable if there is anxiety about airway patency, and assisted ventilation may be needed. Tracheostomy is never undertaken lightly in view of the danger of infection of burned tissues around the stoma.

Initial assessment and management

Once airway patency is assured, the time of injury, the type of burn, its previous treatment, and its extent and depth are established (Fig. 18.12). If the burn is over 15% in extent (10% in children), establishing an intravenous infusion takes priority over a detailed history and physical examination. Intravenous therapy may be needed for many days, but there may be few veins available and they must be treated with great respect. It is best to start with the most peripheral vein available in the upper limb, but in shocked patients with vasoconstriction, cannulation of the internal jugular or subclavian vein may be needed. Blood is withdrawn for cross-matching and for determination of haematocrit and urea and electrolyte concentrations. Arterial blood gas analyses are performed and carboxyhaemoglobin levels measured if there is concern about the airway and smoke inhalation. Once an infusion has been established, the pulse rate, blood pressure and core/peripheral temperature difference are monitored. In patients with burns of more than 20%, a catheter is inserted to measure hourly urine output. Severe pain is relieved by intravenous opiates. Tetanus can complicate burns, and tetanus toxoid is given if the patient has not received it recently. In general, patients with burns involving more than 5% of body surface should be admitted to hospital, as should all those with significant full-thickness injury or burns in sites likely to pose particular management problems.

Prevention and treatment of burn shock

The aim of management is to prevent hypovolaemic shock by prompt and adequate fluid replacement (Table 18.4). Opinions vary as to the relative amounts of colloid and crystalloid that should be used. Various formulae are available to help calculate replacement needs, but all are merely guides and the amounts of fluid given must be adjusted in the light of the patient's response to resuscitation.

The Parkland formula, which uses crystalloids, is now widely used in the United Kingdom. The fluid volume in millilitres over the first 24 hours is:

$$4 \times \text{weight (kg)} \times \%\text{BSA}$$

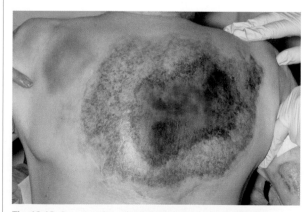

Fig. 18.12 An extensive mixed-depth burn of back with full thickness burn evident centrally.

Table 18.4 **Hypovolaemic shock and burns**
• Anticipate if burn more extensive than 15% (10% in children)
• Prevent by early intravenous resuscitation
• Control pain by adequate intravenous administration of opiates
• Fluid requirements assessed from patient's response
'Formulae' for fluid replacement provide rough guides only

Half of that volume is given in the first 8 hours, the remainder over the next 16 hours. There is debate about introducing colloid, as purified protein solution (PPS) in the second 24 hours. The need for fluid is greatest in the early hours, but excessive losses may persist for 36–48 hours.

Despite renal retention of sodium after injury, there is a tendency to hyponatraemia in the first 2–3 days owing to the secretion of antidiuretic hormone and the sequestration of sodium in oedema. As inflammatory oedema is reabsorbed, the serum sodium concentration returns to normal, and unless water intake is maintained, there is now a danger of hypernatraemia. Tissue destruction releases large amounts of potassium into the extracellular fluid (ECF), but hyperkalaemia is largely prevented by increased renal excretion as part of the metabolic response to injury. Once the first few days have passed, continuing potassium losses can produce hypokalaemia in a patient unable to eat and drink normally.

Water replacement

Daily water losses are replaced using 5% dextrose solution, taking care to avoid water intoxication, especially in young children, in the first few days following injury. Excessive evaporation continues until the burn has re-epithelialized, and a high water intake must be maintained. Although most patients are thirsty, paralytic ileus may occur during the first 48 hours in those with very large burns, so that giving oral fluids too soon can cause gastric distension, vomiting and aspiration. Most patients are able to drink normally after 48 hours and should be encouraged to do so.

Blood transfusion

Blood should not be given in the first 24 hours but may be needed thereafter in patients with large full-thickness burns. Continuing red cell destruction in deep burns with bone marrow suppression can necessitate repeated transfusion. Haemoglobin concentration and haematocrit should be monitored regularly.

Organ failure and burn shock

Organ failure and shock are discussed in detail in Chapter 1.

Respiratory complications

Inhalation of smoke and fumes can cause direct heat damage, carbon monoxide poisoning and damage from other chemicals, all of which predispose to infection. Patients with head and neck burns are best nursed sitting up to encourage the dispersal of oedema. Continued observation is mandatory and physiotherapy is essential to clear bronchial secretions. Chest X-rays and blood gas analyses are repeated regularly in patients with ventilation problems. Arterial hypoxaemia and carbon monoxide poisoning require oxygen therapy, and may necessitate early endotracheal intubation and assisted ventilation. Antibiotics should be prescribed. Tracheostomy is occasionally unavoidable despite the problems associated with its management. Encircling eschar impairing chest or abdominal expansion must be incised (escharotomy) or excised.

Renal failure

Acute tubular necrosis may complicate extensive burns, especially in the elderly, those with pre-existing renal disease and those who develop haemoglobinaemia or myoglobinuria. These pigments appear in the urine after massive red cell destruction or extensive muscle damage (particularly after electrical injury), and can damage the tubules and obstruct urine flow by forming casts. Hourly urine output should be maintained at 30–50 ml in adults. Falling output reflects inadequate resuscitation or impending renal failure (acute tubular necrosis). Measurement of urine osmolality and the response to a test infusion will distinguish between them. Diuretics are used only if oliguria persists despite adequate fluid replacement, when 20% mannitol (1 g/kg) may be infused over 30 minutes.

Nutritional management

The increased energy expenditure following a severe burn can be reduced by nursing in an environmental temperature of 30–32°C. A high-calorie intake is impractical during the period of hypovolaemic shock, but is encouraged as soon as the patient can drink. The daily caloric intake in adults can be calculated as 20 kcal/kg body weight plus 70 kcal/per cent burn. It is particularly important to provide sufficient protein intake (1 g/kg body weight plus 3 g/% burn). In large burns oral intake can usually be supplemented at 48 hours by enteral feeding using a fine-bore nasogastric tube and weight loss can be limited. Vitamin supplements and iron must also be provided. It is considered undesirable to use parenteral nutrition in burned patients.

Sepsis

Septicaemia is a constant threat until skin cover has been fully restored, as resistance to infection is low. The wound provides a reservoir of infecting organisms. Catheters, cannulae and tracheostomy wounds are all potential sources of infection. The incidence of septicaemia has been reduced by topical antibacterial agents and early excision and grafting. However, in large burns the risk remains high. Regular monitoring by means of blood cultures is advisable. Systemic antibiotics are not prescribed routinely for fear of producing superinfection with resistant organisms. Their use is reserved for invasive infection and for patients with positive blood cultures.

Curling's ulcer and gastric erosions

Acute duodenal ulceration (Curling's ulcer) and multiple gastric erosions may follow major burns. Early resumption of feeding reduces their incidence, and H_2-receptor antagonists such as ranitidine are prescribed prophylactically.

Local management of burns

Care of the burn wound commences at the time of injury and continues until epithelial cover has been restored. Infection poses the main threat to life once the first 48 hours have passed.

Initial cleansing and debridement

The wound is cleaned with a mild detergent containing antiseptic and saline in an operating theatre or clean dressing room using aseptic technique. Adherent clothing and loose devitalized tissues are removed. Blisters are punctured and serum expressed. Broken blisters are completely deroofed. General anaesthesia may be necessary, but in most cases pain can be relieved by intravenous opiates. In shocked patients, the wound is covered with a sterile drape and further local care is postponed until the circulatory state has stabilized.

Prevention of contamination

In full-thickness injury, thrombosis of cutaneous vessels impairs the normal response to infection. In large burns, cellular and humoral immune mechanisms are depressed. Organisms readily colonize the burn wound and will multiply and invade surrounding tissues if dead tissue is present. Staphylococci remain the most common infecting organism. *Pseudomonas aeruginosa* remains troublesome in most burn units. Haemolytic streptococci are feared because they can convert superficial into deep burns, and can cause a severe systemic illness.

18

Once contaminating organisms have been cleared, further contamination can be prevented in a number of way as dictated by the patient's needs.

Exposure

After cleansing and debridement, burns to a single surface such as to the face and neck, may be exposed to the air. Evaporation of the protein-rich exudate leaves a dry, adherent crust that is an effective barrier to bacteria as long as it remains intact.

Evaporative dressings

These dressings prevent contamination, allow exudate to evaporate and provide comfortable support. After initial cleansing, the wound is covered by a layer of sterile non-adherent dressing, e.g. paraffin gauze or Mepotil, a layer of cotton gauze swabs, a bulky layer of cotton wool or Gamgee, and an outer retaining crepe bandage. The dressing is reviewed daily but left in place for 8–10 days, unless exudate soaks through to the outside.

Semi-occlusive and occlusive dressings

Clingfilm is useful in first aid, but leaks and is too messy for use as a definitive dressing. OpSite is an adhesive film that is effective for small burns; it may also leak initially, and should be covered with a well-padded dressing for 48 hours, after which time it can be patched or replaced as necessary. Hydrogel and hydrocolloid dressings absorb exudates but offer no particular advantages in acute management. Commercial polythene bags are cheap, sterile when taken from the roll, and useful for treating superficial hand burns. The hands are smeared with liquid paraffin for the first 24–48 hours until a decision as to depth is made. If the decision is made to continue with a conservative regimen, then silver sulfadiazine cream (Flamazine) is applied. The bags are kept in place with a bandage at the wrist. They must be changed at least daily after washing the hand and reapplying the antibacterial cream. Such 'hand bags' allow the patient to continue to use the hand and so prevent stiffness.

Topical antibacterial agents

Silver sulfadiazine cream and povidone-iodine (Betadine) are valuable local antibacterial agents for large burns if reapplied daily. They are not necessary or cost-effective for minor burns.

'Biological' dressings

Freeze-dried xenografts such as porcine skin can be reconstituted for use as temporary occlusive 'biological' dressings, but are expensive. Amnion or stored homograft skin is used rarely because of the danger of infection with human immunodeficiency virus (HIV). Sheets of keratinocytes grown in tissue culture are fragile and easily destroyed by infection – limitations which may be overcome in the future by growing the cells on sheets of collagen or synthetic 'dermis'.

Relief of constriction (escharotomy)

The danger of progressive respiratory embarrassment from encircling eschar has been mentioned. Increasing oedema beneath encircling eschar in the limbs may also imperil the circulation. Relieving incisions (escharotomy), which run from the top to the bottom of circumferential deep burns, may be needed in the first few hours after injury. As these wounds can bleed profusely, it is important to have available methods for controlling haemorrhage.

Restoration of epidermal cover

Full-thickness and deep-dermal burns of less than 10% are suitable for primary excision of eschar and grafting under general anaesthesia within 48–72 hours of injury. Tangential excision is used for deep-dermal burns. The dead outer layers of skin are shaved away down to the deep-dermal layer and a split-skin graft is applied immediately. More extensive burns can be partially excised and grafted soon after injury, and the remaining areas of skin destruction treated by delayed grafting. After some 2 weeks, eschar begins to separate spontaneously but is accelerated by infection and delayed by topical antibacterial agents. As the slough separates, healthy granulation tissue should be revealed, and when all the slough has gone or has been excised, the burn should be ready for grafting. Haemolytic streptococci are a troublesome cause of graft loss, and when such infection is present, grafting should be deferred until the patient has been treated with intravenous penicillin and barrier nursed until three successive wound swabs are negative.

Only split-skin grafts are used to cover acute burns and medium-thickness grafts are most commonly used. The donor site forms a new epidermis from residual islands of epithelium, and more skin can be harvested after 14 days. Excess skin can be stored at 4°C for up to 3 weeks.

Full-thickness grafts are used for secondary reconstruction in cosmetically important areas where contraction has to be avoided, or in areas such as the palm of the hands that are subject to repeated trauma.

Functional and cosmetic result

With energetic treatment, it is usually possible to restore skin cover to even the most extensive injury within 3 months, but wound closure is not the end-point. Skin grafts and donor sites must be kept soft and supple by applying moisturizing cream several times a day for many months. Splints may be needed to prevent contractures, and physiotherapy is essential to mobilize joints. Elastic pressure garments help to prevent the build-up of hypertrophic scars. In spite of all this care, reconstructive procedures may be required for many years to correct contractures or rebuild missing or distorted features. Severely burned patients often have difficulty coming to terms with their disfigurement and limitations to their way of life. Long-term support, with counseling from surgeon and supporting staff, is invaluable.

SKIN AND SOFT TISSUE LESIONS

Diagnosis of skin swellings

In addition to describing the site and size of the lesion, it is necessary to determine whether it arises from the skin or is deep to it. Surface changes indicate an epidermal origin, whereas the surface is stretched over dermal lesions but remains normal. Ulceration may occur as a result of pressure necrosis. The colour of a skin lesion is also an important feature in its diagnosis.

 SUMMARY BOX 18.5

Key questions when examining skin swellings

- Is the swelling located in the skin or in the subcutaneous tissues, i.e. can the overlying skin be pinched up and moved independently of the swelling?
- Is the swelling epidermal or dermal? Epithelial swellings create irregularity of skin surface, whereas dermal swellings do not
- Is the swelling pigmented? Pigmentation most often (although not always) indicates melanocytic activity.

Cysts

Sebaceous cysts

Sebaceous (or epidermoid) cysts are dermal swellings covered by epidermis (Fig. 18.13). They have a thin wall of flattened epidermal cells and contain cheesy white epithelial debris and sebum. They form soft smooth hemispherical swellings over which the skin cannot be moved. A small surface punctum is often visible. If infection supervenes, the cyst becomes hot, red and painful. Infected cysts are incised to allow the infected material to escape. Excision is deferred until the inflammation has settled. In some cases, the inflammation destroys the cyst lining so that excision is not necessary.

Dermoid cysts

Dermoid cysts arise from nests of epidermal cells that have been sequestered in the dermis during development or implanted as a result of trauma. Congenital dermoid cysts are found at sites of embryonic fusion, notably on the face, the base of the nose, the forehead and the occiput. External angular dermoid is the most common congenital dermoid cyst and lies at the junction of the outer and upper margins of the orbit, in the line of fusion of the maxilla and frontal bones. Implantation dermoid cysts are found at sites of injury, notably the palmar surfaces of the hands and fingers. They are lined by squamous epithelium and contain sebum, degenerate cells and, in some cases, hair. A soft rubbery swelling forms deep to the skin. The cyst may be fixed deeply, particularly when situated on the face. Implantation dermoids can be removed under local anaesthesia. Congenital dermoids usually require formal dissection under general anaesthesia, as they may extend deeply.

Tumours of the skin

Epidermal tumours are common and can arise from basal germinal cells or melanocytes, whereas dermal tumours arising from connective tissue elements are rare (Table 18.5).

Table 18.5 Classification of skin tumours	
Epidermal neoplasms (common)	
From basal germinal cells:	**From melanocytes:**
Papilloma	Benign pigmented mole
Infective wart	Common mole
Senile wart	Giant hairy mole
Pedunculated papilloma	Blue naevus
Keratoacanthoma	Halo naevus
Premalignant keratosis	Malignant melanoma
Carcinoma in situ	Melanotic freckle (lentigo maligna)
Epidermoid cancer	Superficial spreading melanoma
Basal cell cancer (rodent ulcer)	Nodular melanoma
Squamous cell cancer	Other forms of melanoma
Dermal neoplasms (rare)	
Fibroma	
Lipoma	
Neurofibroma	

Epidermal neoplasms arising from basal germinal cells

Papillomas

Papillomas (or warts) are common benign skin neoplasms.

Infective warts

These are caused by viral infection. and are found most commonly on the hands and fingers of young children and adults. They spread by direct inoculation and are often multiple. They form greyish-brown, round or oval elevated lesions with a filiform surface and keratinized projections (Fig. 18.14), and may be studded with spots of blood. They often regress spontaneously but can be removed by caustics (acetic acid) or freezing (liquid nitrogen or CO_2 snow). Plantar warts (verruca plantaris) are particularly troublesome infective warts acquired in swimming pools and showers. They are found under the heel and metatarsal heads. They are flush with the surface (Fig. 18.15) and may be intensely painful. If persistent, they are treated by curettage or freezing. Infective warts in the perineum and

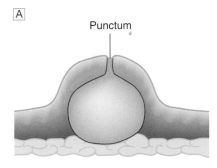

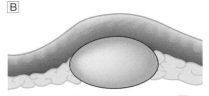

Fig 18.13 Types of cyst. [A] Sebaceous (epidermoid). [B] Dermoid.

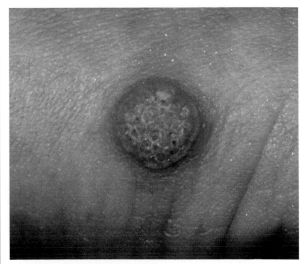

Fig. 18.14 Verruca vulgaris. Infective warts affecting the hands.

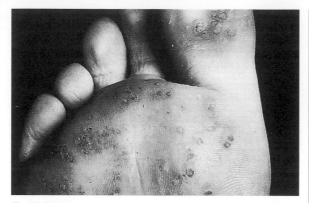

Fig. 18.15 Verruca plantaris (plantar warts). A plaque of closely grouped warts on the sole of the foot.

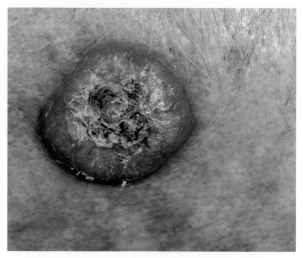

Fig. 18.17 Keratoacanthoma affecting the temple of an elderly man.

on the penis may be of venereal origin and are associated with gonorrhoea, syphilis, HIV infection and lymphogranuloma. Infective warts are also common in immunosuppressed patients.

Senile warts

These are basal cell papillomas and are common in the elderly (Fig. 18.16). They form a yellowish-brown or black greasy plaque (synonym: seborrhoeic keratosis) with a cracked surface that falls off in pieces. Senile warts are often multiple, commonly affect the upper back and trunk, and are best treated by curettage.

Pedunculated papillomas

These simple non-infective papillomas form a flesh-coloured spherical warty mass on a stalk of normal epithelium. If small, they can be dealt with by grasping with fine forceps, pulling out from the skin surface and cutting off with scissors; a stitch is rarely required. If they are large, the papilloma and its pedicle are removed formally with an ellipse of normal skin.

Keratoacanthoma (molluscum sebaceum)

This lesion can be confused with squamous cancer because of its clinical appearance. It grows rapidly over 4–6 weeks and then involutes. Histologically, it has a well-defined

'shoulder', but even under the microscope it may resemble a squamous carcinoma. The distinction between the two is the history. Keratoacanthoma occurs most commonly on the face as a hemispherical nodule with a friable red centre crusted with keratin (Fig. 18.17). It is found mainly in those over 50 years of age. It heals after shedding its central core, but can also be eradicated by curettage.

Actinic (solar) keratosis

This is a premalignant keratosis and is characterized by small, single or multiple, firm warty spots on the face, back of the neck and hands (Fig. 18.18). Such keratoses are particularly common in older, fair-skinned people who have been exposed to excessive sunlight. The scaly lesions drop off periodically to leave a shallow premalignant ulcer. The keratoses should be biopsied to exclude frank malignancy, and then treated by freezing.

Intraepidermal cancer (carcinoma in situ)

This non-invasive form of skin cancer forms a discrete, often solitary, raised brown or red fissured plaque which is keratinized. Histologically, the plaques are composed

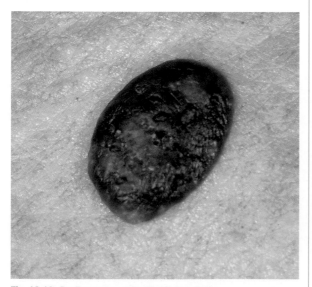

Fig. 18.16 Senile wart or seborrhoeic keratosis.

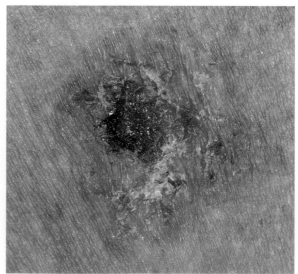

Fig. 18.18 Actinic keratosis.

of hyperplastic atypical epithelial cells, but there is no evidence of invasion through the basement membrane. Intraepidermal skin cancer is also known as Bowen's disease and, when it affects the penis or vulva, as erythroplasia of de Queyrat.

Cancer of the epidermis

Epidermal cancer occurs primarily on exposed areas and in those with poor natural protection against sunlight. Albinos and patients with xeroderma pigmentosa (a congenital defect leading to undue sensitivity to sunlight) are at particularly high risk, whereas skin cancer is rare in black-, brown- and yellow-skinned races. Chronic skin irritation by chemicals (e.g. arsenic, tar and soot), chronic ulceration (e.g. old burns or varicose ulcers) and exposure to other forms of radiation are also established causes. Epidermoid cancer is particularly common in those over 50 years of age. There are two distinct pathological forms.

Basal cell carcinoma (rodent ulcer)

Rodent ulcers are slow-growing, locally invasive and never metastasize. They commonly arise in the skin of the middle third of the face, typically on the nose, inner canthus of the eye, forehead and eyelids (Fig. 18.19). The earliest lesion is a hard pearly nodule, dimpled in its centre and covered by thin telangiectatic skin. Cystic degeneration may make the lesion raised and translucent. Clinical types are described as cystic, nodular, sclerosing, morphoeic, centrally healing and 'field fire'. Over a period of years, the rodent ulcer repeatedly scales over and breaks down. Growth is extremely slow. Occasionally, the tumour is highly invasive and can burrow deeply, despite little apparent surface activity. All suspicious lesions must be biopsied. Surgical excision or radiotherapy can be used for definitive treatment, but the latter is contraindicated if the lesion is close to the eye or overlies cartilage. Complex reconstructive surgery may be needed to restore structure and function in patients who present late.

Squamous cell carcinoma

This tumour may affect any area (Fig. 18.20) but is particularly common on exposed parts such as the ear, cheeks, lower lips and backs of the hands. It commonly develops in an area of epithelial hyperplasia or keratosis. In mucosa, such as the lips, the analogous change is leucoplakia. The lesion starts

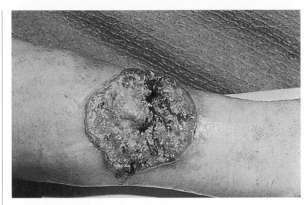

Fig. 18.20 Squamous cell carcinoma. A warty nodule with induration of the adjacent skin.

as a hard erythematous nodule, which proliferates to form a cauliflower-like excrescence or ulcerates to form a malignant ulcer with a raised fixed hard edge. The cancer grows more quickly than a rodent ulcer but more slowly than a keratoacanthoma. The regional nodes can be involved early. The choice of treatment (surgery or radiotherapy) depends on the tumour's size, site and aggressiveness. Palpable lymph nodes require regional lymphadenectomy by block dissection. Adjuvant radiotherapy may be required if histology shows extracapsular spread.

Epidermal neoplasms arising from melanocytes

Benign pigmented moles

The number of melanocytes is relatively fixed (approximately 2000 million), regardless of the colour of the individual, but the amount of pigment produced varies greatly. As a developmental abnormality, conglomerates of melanocytes may migrate to the dermis or epidermis to form a melanocytic naevus or mole. The naevus cells can cause a variety of pigmented spots and swellings (naevi) according to their site and activity (Fig. 18.21). Moles showing melanocyte activity at the junction of epidermis and dermis (junctional change) are common in childhood; all moles on the soles and palms are of this type. Migration of sheets of naevus cells to the dermis produces a dermal naevus; migration to both dermis and epidermis produces a compound naevus.

Common moles

The common mole is a flat or slightly raised brown-black lesion covered by normal epidermis. It has a period of active growth during childhood as a result of junctional activity, but usually becomes quiescent at puberty and may later atrophy. If naevus cells migrate to the dermis, the lesion becomes firm and raised, and there is often aberrant hair growth. The epidermis remains smooth if it remains uninvolved, but can become soft and roughened in a compound naevus. As only 1 in 100 000 moles becomes malignant, they need not normally be removed. Active growth in childhood need not cause concern, but growth after puberty demands removal. An increase in pigmentation, scaliness, itching and bleeding may also give rise to anxiety about malignancy and indicate the need for excision biopsy. Any mole that develops these characteristics should be removed. Further treatment depends on the histological appearances (see below).

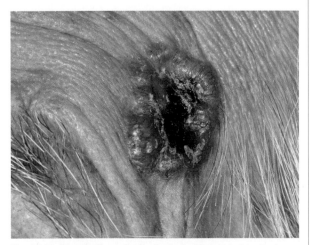

Fig. 18.19 Basal cell carcinoma (rodent ulcer). Note the raised pearly edge.

Normal

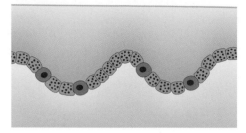

Junctional naevus

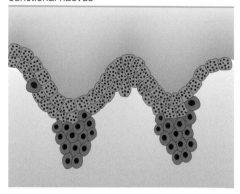

Dermal naevus

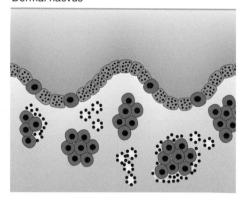

Compound naevus

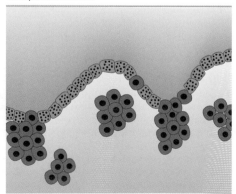

Fig. 18.21 Histopathological types of benign mole.

Giant hairy naevus

Unlike the common mole, this lesion is present at birth. It can cover a large area, which may correspond to a dermatome. Typical sites are the bathing-trunk area and face. The risk of malignant change is small but such moles should be kept under observation, and in some cases there may be cosmetic indications for excision.

Blue naevus

This intradermal naevus can appear blue because the melanin-containing cells are deep in the dermis. It can develop at any time from birth to middle age.

Halo naevus

This pigmented naevus is surrounded by a white circle of depigmentation associated with lymphocytic infiltration.

 SUMMARY BOX **18.6**

Epidermal neoplasms arising from melanocytes

- A mole is due to a conglomeration of melanocytes
- Melanocyte activity at the junction of epidermis and dermis (i.e. junctional activity) is common in childhood
- Migration of melanocytes into the dermis produces a dermal naevus, while migration to both dermis and epidermis produces a compound naevus
- Only 1 in 100 000 moles becomes malignant, so that the presence of a mole is not in itself an indication for removal. Active growth in childhood need not cause concern, but growth thereafter should
- Excision is indicated if a mole shows an increase in pigmentation, scaliness, itching or bleeding. A 3 mm excision margin is adequate in the first instance.

Malignant melanoma

Malignant melanomas predominantly affect fair-skinned people. They are rare in blacks but can occasionally affect the depigmented areas such as the palms, soles and mucosa. Exposure to sunlight is the major precipitating factor. In Scotland, the incidence is 8 per 100 000 individuals per year, compared to 40 per 100 000 in Queensland, Australia. The incidence has increased world-wide, and in Scotland there has been a 100% increase over the last 10 years. Malignant melanomas are more common in females, with a higher incidence on the legs, presumably because of greater exposure. About half of all malignant melanomas are thought to arise in pre-existing naevi. The average individual has 14 melanocytic naevi and the risk of any one of them becoming malignant is very small. However, the greater the number of moles, the greater the risk, particularly in those with a family history of malignant melanoma. The essential feature of malignant melanoma is invasion of the dermis by proliferating melanocytes with large nuclei, prominent nucleoli and frequent mitoses. Three distinct clinicopathological types of malignant melanoma are described.

Hutchison's melanotic freckle (lentigo maligna)

One in 10 malignant melanomas arises in a melanotic or senile freckle. They occur most commonly on the face of elderly women (Fig. 18.22), beginning as a brown-red patch that grows slowly, advancing and receding over the years. The edge of the lesion appears serrated but its margin with normal skin remains abrupt. Kaleidoscopic pigmentation of the surface is typical. This premalignant phase may last for 10–15 years. The first sign of malignancy is a brownish-red papule that develops eccentrically within the freckle and indicates vertical extension of melanocytes into the dermis in the form of a lentigo maligna melanoma.

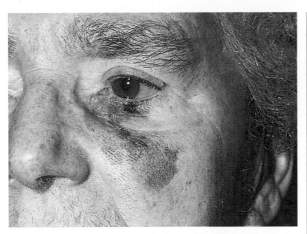

Fig. 18.22 Melanotic freckle on the face of an elderly man.

Superficial spreading melanoma

This is the most common type of malignant melanoma (Fig. 18.23). It occurs on the trunk and exposed parts, and is most common in middle age. During a pre-invasive phase, which lasts for at most 1 or 2 years, malignant cells spread outwards (horizontal growth phase) in the epidermis in all directions. The surface is slightly raised, the outline is indistinct, pigmentation is patchy and there may be a wide range of colours. Invasion of the dermis (vertical growth phase) occurs while the lesion is still relatively small and produces an indurated nodule, which soon ulcerates or bleeds.

Nodular melanoma

This elevated, deeply pigmented melanoma can occur at any site and at any age. Nodular melanomas are particularly common in females on the leg. They may occur at the site of a pre-existing benign naevus. Nodular melanomas are vertically invasive from the start and there is no initial intra-epidermal spread and therefore no surrounding pigmented macule. The nodule enlarges steadily, both centrifugally and on the surface. Surface spread is detected by the destruction of normal skin lines. The lesion darkens progressively and the surface over the area of active growth becomes jet black and glossy. Bleeding may follow trivial injury and is noted as spots of blood on clothes. Crusting, scab formation, itching, irritation and ulceration are typical. Satellite nodules may form around neglected lesions.

Other types of malignant melanoma

Amelanotic melanomas are rare, pale pink lesions that can grow rapidly. Careful histological examination will demonstrate pigment in virtually every case. Acral lentiginous melanoma is seen on the soles and palms (Fig. 18.24). It resembles superficial spreading melanoma in its behaviour,

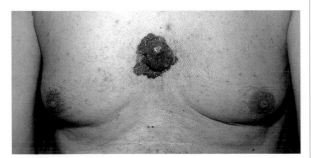

Fig. 18.23 Superficial spreading melanoma.

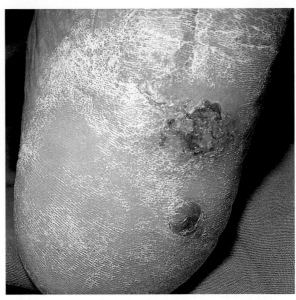

Fig. 18.24 Acral lentiginous melanoma arising on the sole of the foot.

although the thick skin of the affected regions may mask some of the features and cause late presentation, with nodularity and ulceration. Subungual melanomas typically affect the thumb or great toe of the middle-aged and elderly, causing chronic inflammation beneath the nail. Pigmentation is not usually visible in the early stages and the lesion is often misdiagnosed as a paronychia or ingrowing toenail.

Spread of malignant melanoma

Malignant melanomas spread readily via the lymphatics and bloodstream. In transit metastases may develop in the subcutaneous or intracutaneous lymphatics, and form painless discoloured nodules in the line of the lymphatics between the primary and the regional nodes. Lymph node metastases often present as firm enlargement of a node. The disease then spreads to adjacent regional and central nodes. Blood-borne metastases can occur at any site but are common in the brain, liver, lungs, skin and subcutaneous tissues. In about 5% of cases, metastases are present in the absence of a recognizable primary site.

SUMMARY BOX 18.7

Malignant melanoma

- Malignant melanoma is predominantly, but not exclusively, a disease of fair-skinned individuals
- Exposure to sunlight is the key aetiological factor
- The lesion is more common in females, reflecting the higher incidence of malignant melanomas of the lower leg
- 50% of all malignant melanomas arise in a pre-existing naevus
- The essential feature of malignancy is invasion of the dermis by proliferating melanocytes (which show large nuclei, prominent nucleoli and frequent mitoses)
- Malignant melanoma spreads rapidly by the lymphatic system and the bloodstream. 'In transit' metastases may develop in the lymphatics of the skin and subcutaneous tissues.

18

Clinical and pathological staging

Three clinical stages are recognized and staging has major prognostic implications (Table 18.6). For lesions in clinical stage I, the most reliable prognostic indicator is the depth of the lesion (Fig. 18.25); the more superficial the lesion, the better the prognosis. Depth can be measured by reference to the normal layers of skin (Clark) or by a micrometer gauge (Breslow). As the skin layers may be distorted by the tumour, the Breslow system is usually preferred. Mitotic activity also influences prognosis, and tumours can be graded according to the number of mitotic figures in each field. Lymphocytic response and features of regression can also influence prognosis. Melanotic freckles and superficial spreading melanomas tend to remain superficial and so have a better prognosis than nodular melanomas.

Management of malignant melanoma

A biopsy is essential to confirm the diagnosis. Thereafter, the depth and stage of the disease are assessed to define the most appropriate form of treatment. Small pigmented lesions are excised with a margin of 3 mm of normal skin, usually under local anaesthesia. Surgical excision is used to treat stage I lesions. Wide excision with a margin of normal skin of at least 5 cm was once routine but has been shown to be unnecessary, particularly for the more superficial melanomas. Breslow depth is now used as the determinant of clearance margin, using a formula of 1 cm clearance for every millimetre of depth up to 3 cm. A smaller margin may be acceptable to avoid mutilation: for example, on the face. The tumour and surrounding skin are excised down to the deep fascia so that the entire depth of subcutaneous fat can be removed. Smaller defects can usually be closed primarily. Large defects have to be covered with a split-skin graft or flap. A block dissection of regional lymph nodes carries significant morbidity and is no longer carried out routinely. However, if the nodes are involved (clinical stage II), or if the primary tumour overlies the nodes, block dissection can be performed at the time of primary surgery. Isolated limb perfusion with cytotoxic drugs can be used in patients with recurrent disease in a single limb. The treatment of metastatic melanoma remains unsatisfactory. The key to the successful management of malignant melanoma is early diagnosis and appropriate surgical excision (EBM 18.2), with reconstruction as appropriate.

Sentinel lymph node biopsy

This technique is becoming increasingly used in the staging of melanoma. The sentinel lymph node is defined as the first node in the lymphatic basin that drains the lesion and is the node at greatest risk of the development of metastases. Biopsy of this node can assist in staging patients at risk of metastatic disease. Current practice is for patients with a positive sentinel node to proceed to radical node dissection.

Table 18.6 Prognosis in relation to the stage and depth of malignant melanoma

Clinical stage	5-year survival rate (%)
I Primary lesion only	
Breslow depth (mm)	70
< 1.5	93
1.5–3.5	60
> 3.5	48
II Primary lesion + regional lymph node or satellite deposit	30
III Metastatic disease	0

EBM 18.2 Melanoma

'Health-care professionals and members of the public should be aware of the risk factors for melanoma.

'A superficial shave biopsy should not be carried out on suspicious pigmented lesions.

Excision margins for primary melanoma:

< 1 mm	↓ 1 cm
1–2 mm	↓ 1–2 cm
2–4 mm	↓ 2 cm
> 4 mm	↓ 2 cm

Elective lymph node dissection should not be carried out routinely in patients with primary melanoma.

Sentinel lymph node biopsy should be considered as a staging technique in appropriate patients, i.e. primary ≥ 1 mm or < 1 mm but Clark level 4.'

From SIGN Guideline no 72, July 2003 (since writing, Sentinel lymph node biopsy is now considered also in thin (< 1 mm) melanomas with a mitotic rate of 1 per mm^2).

Vascular neoplasms (haemangiomas)

The histological classification of haemangiomas is complex and they are best differentiated by their clinical behaviour: that is, whether they regress or persist.

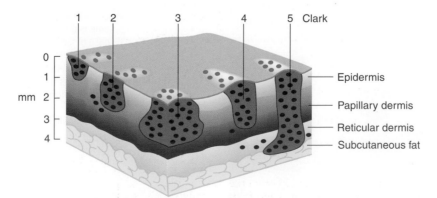

Fig. 18.25 Methods of grading malignant melanoma according to depth of invasion.

Management of malignant melanoma

- The depth of the lesion is a key prognostic factor and can be assessed by micrometer (Breslow) or by reference to normal layers of the skin (Clark). Superficial spreading melanomas and melanotic freckles have a better prognosis than nodular melanomas
- Excision biopsy is essential to confirm malignancy, assess depth and stage, and define the optimal method of treatment
- Once malignancy is confirmed, an excision margin of 1 cm, up to 3cms, for every 1 mm of Breslow depth is advised. The lesion is excised down to the deep fascia to remove all subcutaneous fat. Skin grafting may be required to close the defect
- Lymph node or satellite deposits reduce 5-year survival rates from 70% to 30%, but patients with distant metastases are not expected to survive for 5 years
- Block dissection of regional lymph nodes is no longer practised routinely but is indicated if the nodes are obviously involved or there is a positive sentinel lymph node biopsy.

Involuting haemangiomas

These true neoplasms arise from endothelial cells. They appear at or within weeks of birth, and predominantly affect the head and neck. Superficial involuting haemangiomas form a bright-red raised mass with an irregular bosselated surface (strawberry naevus); deeper lesions form a soft, blue-black tumour covered by normal skin. Active growth continues for about 6 months. The tumour then remains static until the child is 2 or 3 years of age, when it shrinks and loses its colour. The lesion usually disappears before the child is 7 years of age and should be left alone unless it involves the periorbital skin.

Non-involuting haemangiomas

These hamartomas are due to abnormal blood vessel formation, and are of two main types.

Port-wine stain

This bright-red patchy lesion often overlies the area of distribution of a peripheral nerve. The lesion neither grows nor involutes, and good cosmetic results can be achieved by laser therapy.

Cavernous haemangioma

This bluish-purple elevated mass appears in early childhood. It empties on pressure and refills, and histologically consists of mature vein-like structures. It is treated by excision. Cirsoid aneurysm is a rare variant in which the lesion is fed directly by arterial blood and becomes tortuous, dilated and pulsating. Penetrating channels may connect a scalp lesion with a similar malformation in the extradural space. Angiographic embolization may be useful prior to ligation of the feeding vessels and excision of such a lesion.

Tumours of nerves

Neurilemmoma

This is an encapsulated solitary benign tumour that originates from the Schwann cells of a nerve sheath and forms a subcutaneous swelling in the course of the nerve. It is laterally mobile but fixed in the direction of the nerve. It may cause radiating pain in the distribution of the involved nerve. Most neurilemmomas occur superficially in the neck or limbs. They grow slowly, have no malignant potential, and are readily treated by excision. Excision can result in loss of nerve function.

Neurofibroma

This is regarded as a hamartoma of nerve tissue. Such lesions may be solitary, but more commonly they are multiple in von Recklinghausen's disease (neurofibromatosis). This autosomal disorder is present at birth or becomes apparent in early childhood. Multiple dermal and subcutaneous nodules arise from peripheral nerves in association with patches of dermal pigmentation ('café au lait' spots). The tumours can cause bony deformities, particularly of the spine. They are potentially malignant, transforming to neurofibrosarcoma. An increase in size of existing swellings, or the appearance of new swellings suggests malignant change.

Tumours of muscle and connective tissues

Lipoma

A lipoma is a slow-growing benign tumour of fatty tissue that forms a lobulated soft mass enclosed by a thin fibrous capsule. Large lipomas rarely undergo sarcomatous change. Although lipomas can occur in the dermis, most arise from the fatty tissue between the skin and deep fascia. Typical features are their soft fluctuant feel, their lobulation, and the free mobility of overlying skin. Lipomas may also arise from fat in the intermuscular septa, where they form a diffuse firm swelling under the deep fascia, which is more prominent when the related muscle is contracted. Unless it is small and asymptomatic, a lipoma should be removed, either by surgical excision or by liposuction.

Liposarcoma

Liposarcoma is the most common sarcoma of middle age. It may occur in any fatty tissue but is most common in the retroperitoneum and legs. Wide surgical excision is recommended but can be difficult for retroperitoneal tumours; postoperative radiotherapy and chemotherapy are advised but are of doubtful worth. Most liposarcomas grow slowly and recurrence may take a long time to develop.

Fibrosarcoma

This tumour arises from fibrous tissue at any site but is most common in the lower limbs or buttocks. It forms a large, deep firm mass. Wide excision is the initial treatment of choice; radiation therapy may be indicated in the palliation of recurrence.

Rhabdomyosarcoma

This greyish-pink, soft, fleshy lobulated or well-circumscribed tumour arises from striated muscle. It is more common in children, is highly malignant, and requires treatment by radical excision and/or radiotherapy. Amputation of a limb may be unavoidable.

The breast

J.M. Dixon

CHAPTER CONTENTS

ANATOMY AND PHYSIOLOGY

Overview

The breast is an appendage of skin and is a modified sweat gland. It is composed of glandular tissue, fibrous or supporting tissue, and fat. The functional unit of the breast is the terminal duct lobular unit, and any secretions produced in the terminal duct lobular unit drain towards the nipple into 12–15 major subareolar ducts. Although often described as being segmental, the glandular and ductal structures of the breast interweave to form a composite mass. In the resting state, the terminal duct lobular unit secretes watery fluid that is reabsorbed as it passes through the ductules and ducts. This rarely reaches the surface of the nipple because the nipple ducts are blocked or plugged by keratin. If the keratin becomes dislodged, then this physiological secretion can be seen on the surface of the nipple. It varies in colour from white to yellow to green to blue/black, and can be produced in up to two-thirds of non-pregnant women by gentle cleaning of the nipple and massage of the breast.

Anatomy

The breast lies between the skin and the pectoral fascia, to which it is loosely attached. It extends from the clavicle superiorly down on to the abdominal wall, where it extends over the rectus abdominis, external oblique and serratus anterior muscles. The axillary tail of the breast runs between the pectoral muscles and latissimus dorsi to blend with the axillary fat. The breast is supplied by the lateral thoracic artery or the lateral thoracic branch of the axillary artery superolaterally, and by perforating branches of the internal mammary artery superomedially. The functioning unit of the breast, the terminal duct lobular unit, is lined, as are the draining ducts, by a single layer of columnar epithelial cells surrounded by myoepithelial cells. The major subareolar ducts in their terminal portion are lined by stratified squamous epithelium.

The main route of lymphatic spread of breast cancer is to the axillary nodes, which are situated below the axillary vein. On average, there are 20 nodes in the axilla below the axillary vein (Fig. 19.1). These are separated into three levels by their relation to the pectoralis minor muscle. Nodes lateral to the pectoralis minor are considered level I, those beneath are classified as level II, and the nodes medial to pectoralis minor are level III. Level I nodes, which are nearest the breast, are usually affected first by breast cancer. In less than 5% of patients, levels II or III nodes are involved without level I nodes being affected. Lymph also drains to the internal mammary nodes. Occasionally, the main route of lymph drainage of a cancer is to the interpectoral nodes situated between the pectoralis major and minor muscles.

Congenital abnormalities

These are most commonly the result of persistent extramammary portions of the breast ridge. In the sixth week of embryonal development, a bilateral ridge called the 'milk line' develops and extends from the axilla to the groin. Segments coalesce into nests of cells and, in humans, all but one of these nests opposite the fifth intercostal space disappear. In 1–5% of people, one or more of the other nests persists as supernumerary or accessory nipples or, less frequently, as breasts. The most common site for an accessory nipple is in the milk line between the normal breast and the umbilicus; the most common site for an accessory breast is the lower axilla. Supernumerary nipples or breasts rarely require treatment unless they are unsightly. Accessory breast tissue is subject to the same diseases found in normally placed breasts.

Some degree of breast asymmetry is normal, the left usually being the larger of the two. One breast can be absent or hypoplastic, and this is often associated with pectoral

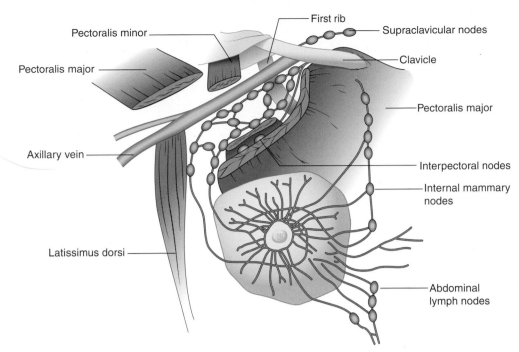

Pectoralis minor

Pectoralis major

Axillary vein

Latissimus dorsi

First rib

Supraclavicular nodes

Clavicle

Pectoralis major

Interpectoral nodes

Internal mammary nodes

Abdominal lymph nodes

Fig. 19.1 Lymph node drainage of the breast.

19

muscle defects. Some patients have abnormalities of the pectoralis muscle and absence or hypoplasia of the breast, associated with a characteristic deformity of the upper limb; this cluster of anomalies is called Poland's syndrome. Abnormalities of the chest wall, such as pectus excavatum and scoliosis of the thoracic spine, can make normal breasts look asymmetric. True asymmetry can be treated by augmentation of the smaller breast, reduction or elevation of the larger breast, or a combination of the two.

Hormonal control of breast development and function

Enlargement of the breast bud in the first week or two of life occurs in approximately 60% of newborn babies; the gland may reach several centimetres in size before regressing. This is because circulating maternal oestrogens cause one or both breasts to enlarge and secrete a colostrum-like fluid (witch's milk) from the nipple. The swelling usually subsides within a few weeks and the breasts then normally remain dormant until puberty, when the onset of cyclical hormonal activity stimulates growth.

The life cycle of the breast consists of three main periods: development (and early reproductive life), mature reproductive life and involution. Development occurs at puberty and involves proliferation of ducts and ductules associated with very rudimentary lobule formation. The breast then undergoes regular changes in relation to the menstrual cycle. During pregnancy, the breast approximately doubles in weight, and lobules and ducts proliferate in preparation for milk production. Lobular development only becomes marked during pregnancy. Milk production during pregnancy is inhibited by ovarian and placental steroids. Delivery reduces the amount of circulating oestrogen and increases the sensitivity of the breast epithelium to prolactin. Suckling stimulates the release of prolactin and oxytocin, with oxytocin stimulating the myoepithelial cells to eject milk into the terminal ducts. By the age of 30, ageing or involution is evident and continues to the menopause and

beyond. During involution, glandular tissue and fibrous tissue atrophy and the shape of the breasts changes and they become more ptotic or droopy. Microscopic changes in the glandular tissue that occur during involution include fibrosis, the formation of small cysts (microcysts) and a focal increase in the number of glandular elements (adenosis). These changes were previously considered abnormal and were called fibrocystic disease or fibroadenosis. However, they occur as part of normal breast ageing or involution and should not be considered as disease.

EVALUATION OF THE PATIENT WITH BREAST DISEASE

Clinical features

Approximately 25% of all surgical referrals relate to breast problems. In the UK, 1 in 4 women will attend a breast clinic, and 1 in 9 will develop breast cancer at some point in their lives. The most common symptoms are a breast lump, which may or may not be painful; an area of lumpiness; pain alone; nipple discharge; nipple retraction; a strong family history of breast cancer; breast distortion; swelling or inflammation; or a scaling nipple or eczema. The most important pointer to the diagnosis is the age of the patient. Although malignant disease can occur in young women, benign conditions are much more common. The duration of any symptom is important; breast cancers usually grow slowly, but cysts may appear overnight. Details of risk factors, including family history and current medication, should be obtained and recorded.

Clinical examination

The patient is asked to undress to the waist and sit facing the examiner. Inspection should take place in good light with the patient's arms by her side, above her head, and then pressing on her hips (Fig. 19.2). Skin dimpling or a change of contour is present in a high percentage of patients

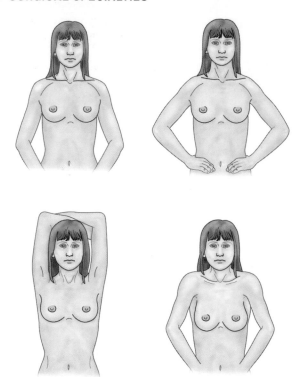

Fig. 19.2 Clinical inspection of the breast.

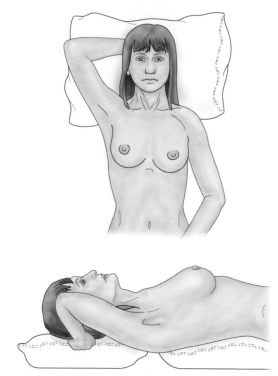

Fig. 19.4 Clinical examination of the breast.

with breast cancer (Fig. 19.3). Breast palpation is performed with the patient lying flat with her arms above or under her head. All the breast tissue is examined, using the fingertips to detect any abnormality (Fig. 19.4). Any abnormal area is then examined in more detail, to determine the texture and outline of the mass. Deep fixation is assessed by asking the patient to tense the pectoralis major muscle; this is accomplished by asking her to press her hands on her hips. All palpable lesions should be measured with callipers and the size and site (using the clock) recorded in the hospital notes.

If the patient complains of nipple discharge, an attempt should be made to reproduce the discharge and to determine

whether it arises from a single or multiple ducts. Any discharge should be tested for haemoglobin. Only marked or moderate amounts of haemoglobin in a nipple discharge are significant.

Assessment of regional nodes

Once the breast has been palpated, the nodal areas are checked (Fig. 19.5). Clinical assessment of axillary nodes is not always accurate. Palpable nodes can be identified in up to 30% of patients with no clinically significant breast disease, while up to 25% of patients with breast cancer who have no palpable nodes on examination will be found histologically to have metastatic disease in the axillary nodes. Ultrasound is better at assessing axillary nodes than clinical examination. The supraclavicular nodes are best examined from behind.

Imaging

Mammography

This requires compression of the breast between two plates and is uncomfortable. By using high-resolution X-rays of low penetrating power, the radiation dose is kept as low as possible (0.5–1.5 mGy per film). Two views, an oblique and a craniocaudal, are usually obtained. Mammography allows the detection of mass lesions, areas of parenchymal distortion and microcalcification. Because the breasts are relatively radiodense in women under 35 years of age, mammography is rarely of value in this group.

Ultrasonography

High-frequency waves are beamed through the breast and reflections are detected and turned into images. Cysts show up as transparent objects (Fig. 19.6) and other benign lesions tend to have well-demarcated edges (Fig. 19.7), whereas

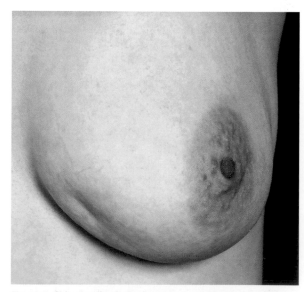

Fig. 19.3 Skin dimpling in the lower inner quadrant of the left breast associated with breast cancer.

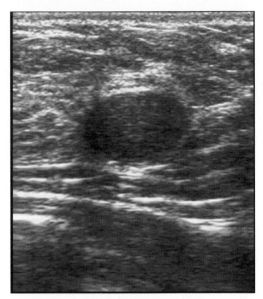

Fig. 19.7 Ultrasound of a fibroadenoma.

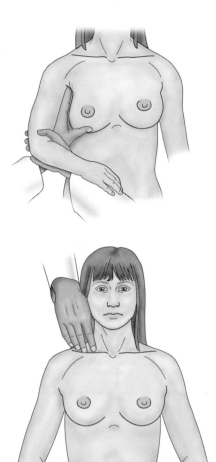

Fig. 19.5 Examination of the regional nodes.

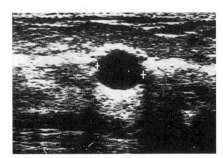

Fig. 19.6 Ultrasound of a cyst.

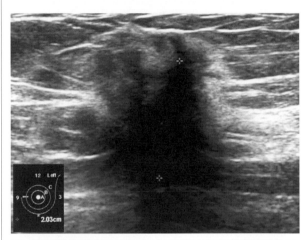

Fig. 19.8 Ultrasound of a cancer.

cancers usually have an indistinct outline and absorb sound, resulting in a posterior acoustic shadow (Fig. 19.8). Ultrasound is also used to assess axillary nodes in patients with breast cancer. Where nodes are enlarged or the cortex of the node thickened, fine needle aspiration cytology or core biopsy should be performed to establish whether nodal metastases are present.

Magnetic resonance imaging (MRI)

This is an accurate way of imaging the breast. It has a high sensitivity for breast cancer and may be of value in demonstrating the extent of both invasive and non-invasive disease. It is particularly useful in the conserved breast to determine whether a mammographic lesion at the site of previous surgery is due to scar or to recurrence. It is currently used as a screening tool for high-risk women between the ages of 35 and 50 (EBM 19.1). MRI is the optimum method of imaging breast implants and detecting implant leakage or rupture.

Ductoscopy, ductography and nipple cytology

None of these investigations have a role in the routine assessment of breast symptoms. Ductoscopy and ductography have a role in determining where in the duct an abnormality is present and can be valuable if surgery to remove an abnormal duct is planned.

EBM 19.1 Screening for breast cancer by MRI

'MRI is more effective than mammography at screening women < 50 years who are at very high risk of breast cancer either because they carry a BRCA1 or BRCA2 mutation or because of their family history.'

MARIBS Study Group. Lancet 2005; 365:1769–1778.

19

Fine needle cytology and biopsy

Core biopsy

Several cores are removed from a mass or an area of microcalcification by means of a cutting needle technique after injection of local anaesthetic (Fig. 19.9). A 14-gauge needle combined with a mechanical gun produces satisfactory samples and allows the procedure to be performed single-handed. Core biopsy can be performed using palpation to guide biopsy but is most successful when image guidance is employed (ultrasound for mass lesions, stereotactic biopsy for calcifications which are usually impalpable). Vacuum-assisted core biopsy devices allow several large cores to be removed without withdrawing the needle from the breast, and have some advantages when biopsying areas of indeterminate microcalcification detected on screening.

Fine-needle aspiration cytology

Needle aspiration can differentiate between solid and cystic lesions. If the lesion is cystic, the fluid is aspirated and, providing it is not blood-stained, discarded. Aspiration of solid lesions requires skill to obtain sufficient cells for cytological analysis and expertise is needed to interpret the smears. Aspiration is usually performed with a 21- or 23-gauge needle attached to a syringe. The needle is introduced into the lesion and suction applied by withdrawing the plunger; multiple passes are then made through the lesion. The plunger is then released and the material spread on to microscope slides. These are then either air-dried or fixed in alcohol and later stained. In some units, a report is available within 30 minutes. Fine-needle aspiration is rarely used now to evaluate solid breast masses because it cannot differentiate invasive from

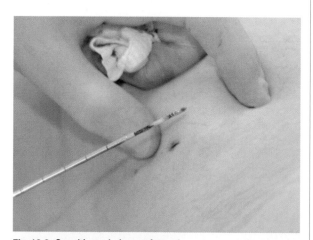

Fig. 19.9 Core biopsy being performed.

in situ cancer. It remains of value in assessing the presence of metastases in axillary lymph nodes. It is best performed under image guidance with use of local anaesthesia.

Open biopsy

An open biopsy should only be performed in patients who have been appropriately investigated by imaging, fine-needle aspiration cytology and/or core biopsy. Removal of a lesion is only indicated if the lesion is benign and the patient requests removal or if core biopsy had not excluded malignancy. Biopsy can be performed under local or general anaesthesia. The removal of impalpable lesions requires localization by a hooked wire. Following excision, the specimen is X-rayed to confirm that the appropriate area has been removed.

Frozen section

The routine use of frozen sections to diagnose breast cancer is no longer practised. Frozen sections can be used to assess lymph nodes, but in this situation the sensitivity (the ability to detect cancer in the lymph nodes) is only 80%.

One-stop clinics

The combination of clinical examination, imaging (mammography with or without ultrasonography for women over 35 years, and ultrasonography for women under 35 years) and core biopsy with or without cytology is known as triple assessment. Patients presenting with a breast lump or suspicious lesion on imaging should have triple assessment performed during a single clinic visit. This allows the majority of patients seen at a breast clinic who have normal breasts to be reassured and discharged after one visit.

Accuracy of investigations

False-positive results occur with all diagnostic techniques. The sensitivity of clinical examination and mammography varies with age, and only two-thirds of cancers in women under 50 years of age are considered suspicious or definitely malignant on clinical examination or mammography (Table 19.1). Image-guided core biopsy is the most accurate and efficient of the various techniques used to diagnose breast masses.

DISORDERS OF DEVELOPMENT

Most benign breast conditions occur during development, cyclical activity or involution, and are so common that they are best considered as aberrations rather than true disease (Table 19.2).

Table 19.1 Accuracy of investigations in the diagnosis of symptomatic breast disease in specialist clinics

	Clinical examination	Mammography	Ultrasonography	Core biopsy	Fine needle aspiration cytology
Sensitivity for cancers[1]	86 %	86 %	90 %	98 %[4]	95 %
Specificity for benign disease[2]	90 %	90 %	92 %	95 %	95 %
Positive predictive value for cancers[3]	95 %	95 %	95 %	100 %	100 %

[1]% of cancers detected by test as malignant or probably malignant (that is, complete sensitivity).
[2]% of benign disease detected by test as benign.
[3]% of lesions diagnosed as malignant by test that are cancers (that is, absolute positive predictive value).
[4]Sensitivity increases if core biopsy is image-guided.

Table 19.2 **Aberrations of normal breast development and involution**

Age (years)	Normal process	Aberration
< 25	Breast development	
	Stromal	Juvenile hypertrophy
	Lobular	Fibroadenoma
25–40	Cyclical activity	Cyclical mastalgia
		Cyclical nodularity
		(diffuse or focal)
30–55	Involution	
	Lobular	Palpable cysts
	Stromal	Sclerosing lesions
	Ductal	Duct ectasia

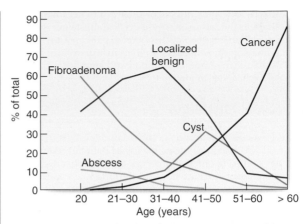

Fig. 19.11 Percentage of patients in 10-year age groups with a discrete breast lump who have common benign conditions and breast cancer.

Juvenile hypertrophy

Uncontrolled overgrowth of breast tissue occurs occasionally in adolescent girls, whose breast development initially begins normally at puberty and is followed by rapid breast growth. These changes are usually bilateral, but may be limited to one breast or part of one breast. This process is often referred to as virginal or juvenile hypertrophy (Fig. 19.10). However, it is not hypertrophy, as there is an increase in the amount of stromal tissue rather than in the number of lobules or ducts. This excessive growth is an aberration rather than a true disease, and presenting symptoms are large breasts and pain in the shoulders, neck and back or under the bra straps. Treatment is by reduction mammaplasty.

Fibroadenoma

Fibroadenomas are classified in most texts as benign tumours, but are best considered as aberrations of development rather than true neoplasms. The reasons are that fibroadenomas develop from a whole lobule rather than from a single cell, and show hormonal dependence similar to that of normal breast tissue, lactating during pregnancy and involuting in the perimenopausal period. Fibroadenomas are most commonly seen immediately following the period of breast development and growth in the 15–25-year age

group (Fig. 19.11). They are usually well-circumscribed, firm, smooth, mobile lumps, and may be multiple or bilateral. Although a small number of fibroadenomas increase in size, most do not and over one-third become smaller or disappear within 2 years. Fibroadenomas have a characteristic appearance with easily visualized margins on ultrasound (Fig. 19.7). Large or giant fibroadenomas (> 5 cm) are infrequent but are more commonly seen in women from certain African countries. Occasionally, a fibroadenoma in an adolescent girl undergoes rapid growth, a condition called juvenile fibroadenoma (Fig. 19.12). Once a diagnosis of fibroadenoma has been established on core biopsy, options for management in lesions measuring less than 4 cm include reassurance with no follow up needed or excision; fibroadenomas over 4 cm in diameter should be excised to ensure that phyllodes tumours are not missed (see below). A carcinoma arising in a fibroadenoma is extremely rare. Patients with simple fibroadenomas are not at significantly increased risk of developing breast cancer.

DISORDERS OF CYCLICAL CHANGE

Premenstrual nodularity and breast discomfort are so common that they are considered part of normal cyclical changes. When premenstrual pain is severe, interferes with

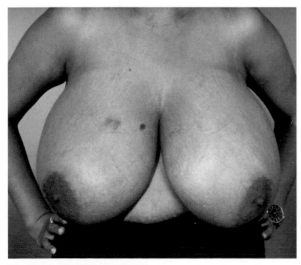

Fig. 19.10 Juvenile hypertrophy.

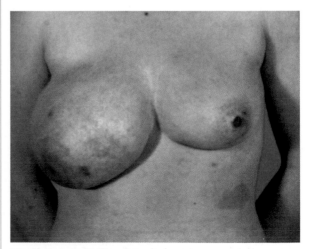

Fig. 19.12 Juvenile fibroadenoma.

19

19

daily activities and influences quality of life, then this is classified as moderate or severe cyclical mastalgia. There is no association between cyclical breast pain and any underlying histological abnormality. The cause of cyclical mastalgia is unknown. Another common and significant problem is non-cyclical mastalgia.

Cyclical mastalgia

Most patients require no specific treatment. Evening primrose oil was previously used for breast pain but recent studies have failed to show any benefit and it is no longer used. Effective agents include danazol (100 mg/day) and tamoxifen (10 mg/day). Tamoxifen does not have a product licence for this condition but it improves pain in 80% of patients. Agnus castis, a fruit extract, has been shown in randomized studies to be somewhat effective in reducing breast pain.

Nodularity

Lumpiness and nodularity in the breast can be diffuse or focal. Diffuse nodularity is normal, particularly premenstrually. In the past, women with lumpy breasts were regarded as having fibroadenosis or fibrocystic disease, but this diffuse nodularity is not associated with any underlying pathological abnormality and so these terms are inappropriate. Focal nodularity is a common cause for women seeking medical advice and is seen in women of all ages (Fig. 19.11). Patients with benign focal nodularity often report that the lump fluctuates in size in relation to the menstrual cycle. Breast cancer should be excluded by imaging +/- core biopsy in women with persistent localized asymmetric areas of nodularity, as breast cancer in younger women often presents as nodularity rather than a discrete mass.

Non-cyclical breast pain

Localized pain in the chest wall is a common reason for patients to be referred for advice. The pain may appear to be in the breast but examining a patient on her side to move the breast away from the chest wall demonstrates that the ribs or chest wall muscle are the site of origin of the pain. Oral nonsteroidal anti-inflammatory agents (NSAIDs) are usually effective in improving chest-wall pain. Up to 60% of patients with a persistent localized painful area in the chest wall can be effectively treated by infiltration of local anaesthetic and steroid (2-5 ml 0.5% bupivacaine added to 40 mg of methylprednisolone).

DISORDERS OF INVOLUTION

Aberrations of the normal ageing process include cyst formation, areas of scarring (sclerosis), duct ectasia and epithelial hyperplasia.

Palpable breast cysts

Approximately 7% of women in developed countries develop a palpable breast cyst at some time in their life. Cysts constitute 15% of all discrete breast masses. They are distended, involuted lobules and are most frequently seen in the perimenopausal period (Fig. 19.11). Clinically, they are smooth discrete lumps that can be painful and are sometimes visible. Mammographically, they have characteristic haloes and are easily diagnosed by ultrasonography (see Fig. 19.6). Symptomatic palpable cysts are treated by aspi-

ration and, provided the fluid is not blood-stained, it is discarded. Cysts that contain blood-stained fluid require excision to exclude an associated intracystic cancer. Such cancers are rare and are usually evident on ultrasound. Most cysts are asymptomatic and, following ultrasound assessment, do not need aspiration. All patients with cysts should have mammography, preferably before cyst aspiration, as between 1 and 3% will have a cancer, usually remote from the cyst, visible on mammography (Fig. 19.13). Patients with cysts have a slightly increased risk of developing breast cancer, but the magnitude of this risk is not considered of clinical significance.

Sclerosis

Areas of excessive fibrosis or sclerosis can occur as part of stromal involution. Sclerosing lesions include radial scars, complex sclerosing lesions and sclerosing adenosis and can produce stellate lesions or localized calcification that mimic breast cancer mammographically, and so can cause diagnostic problems during screening. Radial scars are difficult to differentiate on imaging from small cancers and sometimes have small areas of pre cancer (DCIS see page 312) down one of the legs of the scar so most are removed.

Duct ectasia

The major subareolar ducts dilate and shorten with age; when symptomatic, this is known as duct ectasia. By the age of 70, 40% of women have dilated ducts, some of whom present with nipple discharge or retraction. The discharge is usually cheesy and the retraction is classically slit-like (Fig. 19.14), which contrasts with breast cancer, in which the whole nipple is pulled in (Fig. 19.15). Surgery is indicated if the discharge is troublesome or if the patient wishes the nipple to be everted.

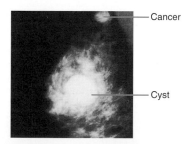

Fig. 19.13 Mammogram of a cyst and a cancer.

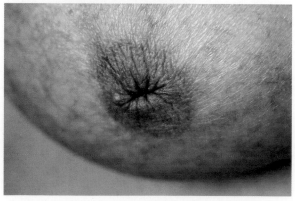

Fig. 19.14 Duct ectasia showing slit-like nipple retraction.

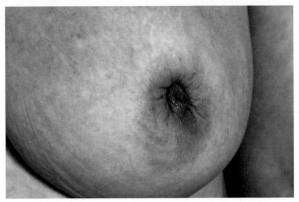

Fig. 19.15 Asymmetric nipple inversion in a patient with breast cancer.

Epithelial hyperplasia

An increase in the number of cells lining the terminal duct lobular unit is known as epithelial hyperplasia, the degree of which is graded as mild, moderate or florid. If the hyperplastic cells show cellular atypia, the condition is called atypical hyperplasia. Women with atypical hyperplasia have a significant increase in their risk of breast cancer. The absolute risk of developing breast cancer for a woman with atypical hyperplasia without a first-degree relative with breast cancer is 8% at 10 years; for women with a first-degree relative with breast cancer the risk is 20–25% at 15 years.

BENIGN NEOPLASMS

Duct papillomas

These can be single or multiple. They are very common, and should be considered as aberrations rather than true neoplasms as they show minimal malignant potential. They can cause persistent and troublesome nipple discharge, which can be either frankly blood-stained (Fig. 19.16), or serous. Treatment comprises removal of the discharging duct (microdochectomy), which removes the papilloma (if this is the cause) and allows exclusion of an underlying neoplasm, seen in approximately 5% of women who present with a blood-stained nipple discharge.

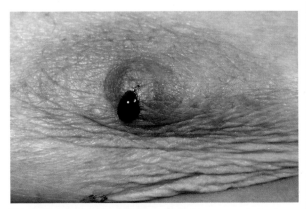

Fig. 19.16 Blood-stained nipple discharge.

Lipomas

These are soft, lobulated, radiolucent lesions and are common. Interest lies in their confusion with pseudolipoma (a soft mass that can be felt around a cancer, caused by indrawing of surrounding fat).

Phyllodes tumours

These rare fibro-epithelial neoplasms may be malignant in their behaviour, although most are benign. They present as localized discrete masses that clinically feel like fibroadenomas, although they tend to be larger (> 4 cm). Up to 20% of benign phyllodes tumours recur locally following simple excision. In more malignant lesions it is the sarcomatous element that recurs; approximately one-quarter of lesions reported as malignant metastasize. Treatment of phyllodes tumours, whether malignant or benign, is wide excision. If the lesion is large, mastectomy may be needed to ensure complete removal.

Other benign tumours that occur in the breast include granular cell tumours, neurofibromas and leiomyomas.

 SUMMARY BOX **19.1**

Benign breast disease

- Is more common than breast cancer
- Can be difficult to differentiate from breast cancer
- Inappropriate treatment of benign conditions is associated with significant morbidity
- Occurs against the background of breast development (age < 25), cyclical activity (up to menopause) and involution (following the menopause)
- The only benign condition associated with a significant increased risk of subsequent breast cancer is atypical hyperplasia.

BREAST INFECTION

Breast infection is less common than it used to be. It is seen occasionally in neonates but most commonly affects women between the ages of 18 and 50. In this age group, infection can be divided into lactational and non-lactational. Infection can also affect the skin overlying the breast, when it can be a primary event or secondary to a lesion in the skin (such as a sebaceous cyst or an underlying condition such as hidradenitis suppurativa).

The principles of treating breast infection are:

- Give appropriate antibiotics early to reduce the incidence of abscess formation (Table 19.3)
- If an abscess is suspected, confirm pus is present by ultrasound or aspiration before embarking on surgical drainage
- Exclude breast cancer using imaging and core biopsy in an inflammatory lesion that is solid and that does not settle despite adequate antibiotic treatment.

Most breast abscesses can be managed by repeated aspiration (preferably guided by ultrasound), combined with oral antibiotics or incision and drainage under local anaesthetic. Few abscesses, except those in children, require drainage under general anaesthesia. Placement of a drain or packing the abscess cavity after incision and drainage is unnecessary.

19

Table 19.3 Antibiotics most appropriate for treating breast infections*		
Type of infection	**No allergy to penicillin**	**Allergy to penicillin**
Lactating and skin-associated Non-lactating	Flucloxacillin (500 mg 6-hourly) Co-amoxiclav (375 mg 8-hourly)	Clarithromycin (500 mg 12-hourly) Combination of clarithromycin (500 mg 12-hourly) with metronidazole (200 mg 8-hourly)

*Doses are for adults.

Lactating infection

Improvements in maternal and infant hygiene have reduced considerably the incidence of infection associated with breastfeeding. When infection does occur, it usually develops within the first 6 weeks of breastfeeding. Presenting features are pain, swelling, tenderness and a cracked nipple or skin abrasion. *Staphylococcus aureus* is the most common organism, although *Staph. epidermidis* and streptococci are occasionally implicated. Drainage of milk from the affected segment is reduced, with the resultant stagnant milk becoming infected. Early infection is treated with flucloxacillin or co-amoxiclav. An established abscess should be treated by recurrent aspiration, or by incision and drainage (Fig. 19.17). Women should be encouraged to breastfeed, as this promotes milk drainage from the affected segment. Rarely, milk flow needs to be stopped using cabergoline, a prolactin antagonist.

Non-lactating infection

This can be separated into infections that occur centrally in the periareolar region and those affecting the periphery of the breast.

Central (periareolar) infection

This is most commonly seen in young women (mean age 32 years). The underlying cause is periductal mastitis. Current evidence suggests that smoking is important in the aetiology of non-lactational infection, 90% of women who present with periductal mastitis or its complications being smokers. Substances in cigarette smoke either directly or indirectly damage the subareolar breast ducts, and the damaged tissue then becomes infected by either aerobic or anaerobic organisms. Initial presentation is with periareolar inflammation, with or without an associated mass, or with an established abscess. Clinical features include breast pain, erythema, periareolar swelling and tenderness, and/or nipple retraction; these occur in relation to the affected duct.

Treatment of periductal mastitis is with appropriate antibiotics (Table 19.3). Abscesses are managed by aspiration or incision and drainage. Infection is commonly recurrent because treatment does not remove the damaged subareolar duct(s). Following drainage of a non-lactating abscess, up to one-third of patients develop a mammary duct fistula. Recurrent episodes of peri-areolar infection require excision of the diseased duct(s) (total duct excision).

Mammary duct fistula

This is a communication between the skin – usually at the areolar margin – and a major subareolar duct (Fig. 19.18). Treatment is by excision of the fistula and diseased duct(s) under antibiotic cover.

Peripheral non-lactating abscesses

These are less common than periareolar abscesses and are sometimes associated with an underlying condition, such as diabetes, rheumatoid arthritis, steroid treatment, granulomatous lobular mastitis or trauma. Infection associated with granulomatous lobular mastitis can be a particular problem, as there is a strong tendency for this condition to persist and recur despite surgery. Peripheral abscesses should be treated by recurrent aspiration with antibiotics (Table 19.3), or incision and drainage under local anaesthesia.

SUMMARY BOX 19.2

Breast infection

- Antibiotics should be given early to reduce abscess formation
- Hospital referral is indicated if infection does not settle rapidly on antibiotics
- If an abscess is suspected, this should be confirmed by ultrasound or aspiration
- If the lesion is solid on ultrasound or aspiration a core biopsy should be performed to exclude an underlying inflammatory carcinoma.

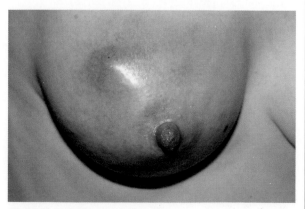

Fig. 19.17 Lactating breast abscess.

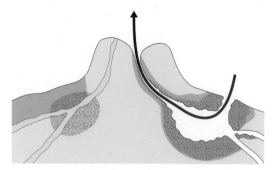

Fig. 19.18 Mammary duct fistula and periductal mastitis.

Skin-associated infection

Primary infection of the skin most commonly affects the lower half of the breast and can be recurrent in women who either are overweight or have large breasts. It is more common after previous surgery or radiotherapy. Treatment is with antibiotics (Table 19.3) and drainage or aspiration of abscesses. Women with recurrent infection should be advised about weight reduction and keeping the area as clean and dry as possible.

Sebaceous cysts are common in the skin of the breast and may become infected. Some recurrent infections in the skin of the lower part of the breast are due to hidradenitis suppurativa, which is more common in smokers. This condition, which affects the apocrine glands of the breast, is difficult to treat. Excision of the affected skin is effective at stopping further infection in about half of patients.

BREAST CANCER

Epidemiology

Over 1 million new cases of breast cancer are diagnosed each year world-wide. It is the most common malignancy in women comprising 18% of all female cancers. In the UK, approximately 1 in 9 women will develop breast cancer. Known risk factors are shown in Table 19.4.

The incidence of breast cancer increases with age, doubling every 10 years until the menopause, when the rate of increase slows dramatically (Fig. 19.19). Compared with lung cancer, the incidence of breast cancer is higher at young ages. There is a variation in incidence by up to a factor of 5 between different countries. Studies of migrants from Japan, a low-risk area, to Hawaii show that the rate of breast cancer in migrants becomes the same as the rate in the host country within one or two generations. This suggests that environmental rather than genetic factors are important in the

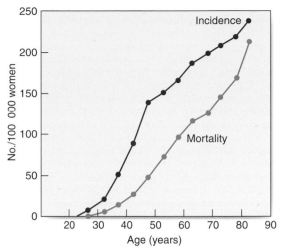

Fig. 19.19 Percentage of all deaths in women attributable to breast cancer.

aetiology. Women who start menstruating early in life, or who have a late menopause, have a slightly increased risk of developing breast cancer. Young age at first delivery protects against breast cancer. The risk of breast cancer in women who have their first child after the age of 30 is twice that of women who have their first child before the age of 20. Breast cancer is also increased in nulliparous women, who have a risk approximately 2.4 times that of women having their first child before the age of 20. The highest risk is in women who have a first pregnancy over the age of 40 years. Breastfeeding has a small protective effect and women who have breastfed have a slightly reduced incidence of breast cancer.

Severe atypical hyperplasia carries a four- to five-fold higher risk of breast cancer than when no proliferative changes are evident. A doubling of breast cancer was observed among teenage girls exposed to radiation during the Second World War. Women treated by radiation therapy for lymphoma during adolescence and teenage years are also at significant risk of developing early-onset breast cancer. Although there is a close correlation between the incidence of breast cancer and dietary fat intake in populations, the relationship is neither particularly strong or consistent. A high alcohol intake does appear to increase breast cancer risk. Patients taking the oral contraceptive pill have a 1.24 times increased relative risk of breast cancer compared to that of the general population. This rapidly falls to normal after stopping the pill. Hormone replacement therapy (HRT) increases breast cancer risk. Combined oestrogen and progestogen HRT is associated with a greater risk than preparations containing oestrogen alone (Table 19.5).

Table 19.4 Established and probable risk factors for breast cancer

Factor	Relative risk	High-risk group
Age	> 10	Elderly
Geographical location	5	Developed country
Age at first full pregnancy	3	First child in early 40s
Previous benign disease	4–5	Atypical hyperplasia
Cancer in other breast	> 4	Women treated for breast cancer
Socioeconomic group	2	Social classes I and II
Diet	1.5	High intake of saturated fat
Exposure to ionizing radiation	3	Abnormal exposure in young females after age 10
Taking exogenous hormones		
Oral contraceptives	1.24	Current use
Combined hormone replacement therapy	2.3	Use for ≥ 10 years
Family history	≥ 2	Breast cancer in first-degree relative

Table 19.5 Relationship of HRT to breast cancer development: relative risk of breast cancer related to type and recency of HRT use*

Patient group	Relative risk (95% confidence intervals)
Never used HRT	1.0 (0.96–1.04)
All previous users	1.01 (0.95–1.08)
Current users of:	
Oestrogen only+	1.3 (1.22–1.38)
Oestrogen/progestogen combinations	2.0 (1.91–2.09)

*Lancet 2003; 362:419–427.
+Data from WH1 study suggest risk is lower from oestrogen only than combined HRT and may not exceed 1.

19

Up to 10% of breast cancers in developed countries are due to genetic predisposition. This is mainly through single genes inherited as autosomal dominants but with limited penetrance. Not all gene carriers develop breast cancer. Human breast cancer genes that have been identified and that affect different families include *BRCA1* on chromosome 17, *BRCA2* on chromosome 13, *p53* on chromosome 17 and *PTEN* on chromosome 10. Throughout the USA and most of Europe, germline mutations in *BRCA1* and *BRCA2* are believed to occur in just over 1 in 1000 of the population.

In some populations, e.g. Ashkenazi Jews and Icelanders, particular mutations in *BRCA1* and *BRCA2* may be relatively common. In 'breast cancer families', there is also an increased risk of other tumours, notably ovarian cancer. Most *BRCA1* and *BRCA2* mutations confer a 50–60% lifetime risk of breast cancer. Environmental factors probably modify inherited breast cancer risk, and other genes probably interact with *BRCA1* and *BRCA2* to modify risk. Pointers to an inherited disposition are a first-degree relative who developed breast cancer, particularly bilateral cancer, under the age of 40 years, numerous female relatives with breast cancer on the same side of the family, or a close female relative who has had ovarian cancer. Options for high-risk women include regular screening, prevention using hormonal agents such as tamoxifen, raloxifene and aromatase inhibitors, or prophylactic bilateral mastectomy. Tamoxifen and raloxifene appear to reduce the risk of developing breast cancer by 40–50%, whereas surgery reduces the risk by over 90%.

Types of breast cancer

Breast cancers are derived from the epithelial cells that line the terminal duct lobular unit. Cancer cells that remain within the basement membrane of the lobule and the draining ducts are classified as in situ or non-invasive. An invasive cancer is one in which cells have moved outside the basement membrane of the ducts and lobules into the surrounding adjacent normal tissue. Both in situ and invasive cancers have characteristic patterns by which they are classified.

Non-invasive

Two main types of non-invasive cancer can be recognized on the basis of cell type. Ductal carcinoma in situ (DCIS) is the most common form (Fig. 19.20), making up to 3–4% of symptomatic and 17–25% of screen-detected cancers. Screen-detected DCIS is most commonly associated with

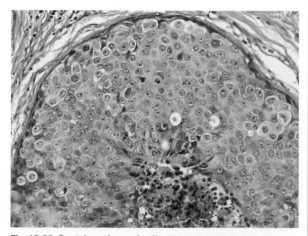

Fig. 19.20 Ductal carcinoma in situ. This is characterized by cells with irregularly shaped and often angular nuclei with variable amounts of chromatin. The cells themselves are variable in size and the necrosis seen in the lumen is a frequent finding.

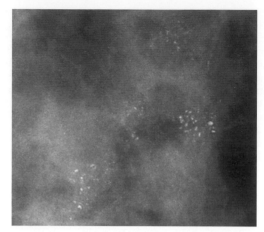

Fig. 19.21 Diffuse microcalcification in the breast affected by ductal carcinoma in situ.

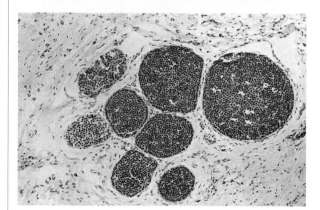

Fig. 19.22 Lobular carcinoma in situ (now called LIN). This is characterized by regular cells with regular round or oval nuclei. (Compare this with DCIS.)

microcalcifications on mammograms (Fig. 19.21), which can be either localized or widespread. Lobular carcinoma in situ (LCIS) (Fig. 19.22) and atypical lobular hyperplasia (ALH) have been combined into a single diagnostic condition called lobular intraepithelial neoplasia (LIN). This is usually an incidental finding and is generally treated by regular follow-up, as these women are at significant risk of developing invasive cancer in either breast.

Invasive

The most commonly used classification of invasive cancers divides them into ductal and lobular types and is based on the belief that ductal carcinomas arise in ducts and lobular carcinomas in lobules. This is now known to be incorrect, as almost all cancers arise in the terminal duct lobular unit. The two types behave differently, however, so the classification remains in use. Certain invasive ductal carcinomas show distinct patterns of growth and are classified separately as tumours of 'special type'; this includes tubular, cribriform, papillary, mucinous and medullary cancers. Tubular, cribriform and mucinous cancers are well differentiated and have a better than average prognosis. Mucinous cancers are rare circumscribed tumours characterized by tumour cells that produce mucin; these also have a good prognosis. Medullary cancers are circumscribed and soft, and consist of aggregates of high-grade pleomorphic cells surrounded by lymphoid cells. Invasive lobular cancer accounts for up to 10% of invasive cancers and is characterized by a diffuse pattern of spread that causes problems with clinical and mammographic detection. These tumours are often large at diagnosis.

Breast cancers are graded on the presence or absence of glands, the extent of nuclear pleomorphism and the mitotic rate of the tumour. Grade I are the best differentiated and have the best prognosis, grade II have an intermediate prognosis, and grade III or high-grade cancers have a poor prognosis. The presence of tumour cells in lymphatics or blood vessels is a marker of more aggressive disease and is associated with an increased rate of both local and systemic recurrence.

Hormone and growth factors receptors

The hormones oestrogen and progesterone play important roles in breast cancer. Oestrogen receptors, called ERs after the American spelling (estrogen) are present in approximately 75% of breast. ER is expressed in much greater amounts in cancer cells than in normal breast tissue. ER is thus an important target for treatment, and depriving cancer cells of oestrogen causes the cancer cells to stop growing and the tumour to eventually shrink. The majority of cancers that express ER also have receptors for progesterone and these are called PgRs. The presence of ER and PgR indicates the cancer is likely to benefit from removing oestrogen compared to a cancer which has no ER or PgR (ER and PgR negative) where there is no benefit from hormone treatment.

Growth factors in cancer cells control the rate of growth of the cancer. The most important group of growth factors are the human epidermal growth factor receptors, also known as the HER group. There are four HER receptors, the most important of which is HER2. Around 15–20% of all cancers are HER2 receptor rich and rely on HER2 which can be blocked with a new type of drug called trastuzumab, also known as herceptin®. This reduces growth and leads to cancers shrinking, and in some patients results in eradication of the cancer. Treatments that block HER1 have been developed. A new oral drug, lapatanib, blocks both HER1 and HER2 and pertuzumab (see p. 319) blocks HER1, HER2 and HER3.

Currently all breast cancers are checked for ER and HER2. Some units check routinely for PgR but others only check PgR in ER negative cancers to make sure they are not likely to benefit from hormone treatment. The amount of ER is reported as ER positive (+ve) or ER negative (−ve) and a commonly used scale classifies the amount of ER and PgR between 0 and 8. Zero is negative. There is no score of 1, and score 2 indicates a very low level of receptors. Most cancers have high levels of ER or PgR with scores of 6, 7 or 8 (ER rich).

HER2 is reported as positive or negative but sometimes two tests are needed in borderline cases and it may take 10–14 days to get a HER2 result.

Cancers may be classified as hormone sensitive, (ER+, PgR+); there are few if any ER-, PgR+. About 20–25% of cancers are hormone resistant (ER− PgR−). Cancers are considered triple negative (ER−, PgR−, HER2−) if all three markers are negative on testing. Triple negative cancers, which are often seen in women carrying an abnormal BRCA1 gene (see p. 312), tend to have a worse outcome, although about half do respond very well to chemotherapy. HER2 positive cancers used to have a worse outlook to HER2 negative cancers before the widespread use of trastuzumab. This drug dramatically improves outcome in HER2 positive disease so that the prognosis for patients with HER2+ and HER2− cancers is similar.

Screening for breast cancer

Randomized controlled trials have shown that screening by mammography can significantly reduce mortality from breast cancer (EBM 19.2). Mortality is reduced by up to 40%

EBM 19.2 **Breast screening by mammography**

'Mammography is at present the best screening tool available. Randomized controlled trials have shown screening by mammography reduces mortality from breast cancer by 40% in those who attend. Benefit is greatest in women aged 50–70 years. Two-view mammography should be performed at each screening visit.'

Nystrom L, et al. Lancet 1993; 341(8851):973–978.

in women who attend for screening, with the greatest benefit being seen in women aged over 50. To be effective, attendance at screening programmes has to be greater than 70%. The UK programme screens the 50–70-year age group but may extend from 47–73 over the next decade.

The most appropriate interval between mammographic screens is yet to be determined. In the UK, screening takes place every 3 years but the rate of cancers diagnosed between the second and third years after the initial screen climbs rapidly, suggesting that this interval may be too long, at least for women aged 50–60. Patients are currently screened by two-view mammography.

About two-thirds of screen-detected abnormalities are shown to be benign or normal on further mammographic or ultrasound imaging. Among women aged 50–70, approximately 75 cancers (invasive and non-invasive) are detected for every 10 000 attending for their initial screen. At subsequent screens, approximately 50 cancers should be identified for every 10 000 attenders. Up to 70% of important abnormalities are impalpable, and for these, image-guided (ultrasound or stereotactic radiography) core biopsy is necessary to establish a diagnosis. Compared with symptomatic cancers, screen-detected cancers are smaller and more likely to be non-invasive. The ability of screening to influence mortality from breast cancer (EBM 19.3) indicates that early diagnosis identifies cancers at an earlier stage of evolution, when metastasis is less likely to have occurred.

EBM 19.3 **Mortality rates in breast cancer**

'Mortality from breast cancer has reduced by 15% over the last decade despite a rising incidence. The fall in mortality is a consequence of screening and better treatment.'

Breast Cancer UK. In: Toms JR (ed). Cancer Stats Monograph. Cancer Research UK; 2004:21–30.

Mammographic features of breast cancer

Mammographically, a cancer most commonly appears as a dense opacity with an irregular outline from which spicules pass into the surrounding tissue (Fig. 19.23). Associated features include microcalcifications, which can occur within or outside the lesion, skin tethering or thickening, distortion of the shape of the breast or overlying skin, and tenting or direct involvement of underlying muscle. Involved lymph nodes can also sometimes be seen (Fig. 19.24). Microcalcification alone is a feature of DCIS.

Staging

When invasive cancer is diagnosed, the extent of the disease should be assessed. The currently used TNM (tumour, nodes and metastases) system depends on clinical measurements

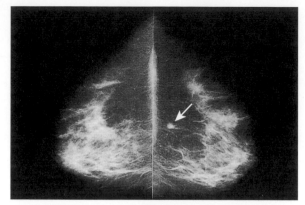

Fig. 19.23 Mammogram of a cancer detected at breast screening.
A small lesion at the back of the left breast (arrow).

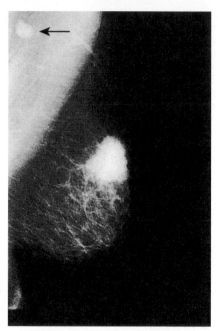

Fig. 19.24 Mammogram of a cancer (irregular dense mass) and involved axillary nodes (localized density in the axillary tail).

Table 19.6 TNM Staging for breast cancer
T (Primary tumour)
• T_x — Primary tumour cannot be assessed
• T_0 — No evidence of primary tumour
• T_{1s} — Carcinoma in situ: intraductal carcinoma, lobular carcinoma in situ, or Paget's disease of the nipple with no associated tumour mass[1]
• T_1 — Tumour 2.0 cm or less in greatest dimension[2]
• T_{1a} — 0.5 cm or less in greatest dimension
• T_{1b} — More than 0.5 cm but not more than 1.0 cm in greatest dimension
• T_{1c} — More than 1.0 cm but not more than 2.0 cm in greatest dimension
• T_2 — Tumour more than 2.0 cm but not more than 5.0 cm in greatest dimension[2]
• T_3 — Tumour more than 5.0 cm in greatest dimension[2]
• T_4 — Tumour of any size with direct extension to chest wall or skin
• T_{4a} — Extension to chest wall
• T_{4b} — Oedema (including peau d'orange), ulceration of the skin of the breast or satellite nodules confined to the same breast
• T_{4c} — Both of the above (T_{4a} and T_{4b})
• T_{4d} — Inflammatory carcinoma
N (Regional lymph nodes)
• N_x — Cannot be assessed (e.g. previously removed)
• N_0 — No regional lymph node metastasis
• N_1 — Movable ipsilateral axillary lymph node(s)
• N_2 — Ipsilateral lymph node(s) fixed to one another or to other structures
• N_3 — Ipsilateral internal mammary lymph node(s)
M (Distant metastases)
• M_x — Cannot be assessed
• M_0 — No distant metastasis
• M_1 — Distant metastasis present (includes metastasis to ipsilateral supraclavicular lymph nodes)

Note: Chest wall includes ribs, intercostal muscles and serratus anterior muscle, but not pectoral muscle.
[1]Paget's disease associated with tumour mass is classified according to the size of the tumour.
[2]Dimpling of the skin, nipple retraction or other skin changes may occur in T_1, T_2 or T_3 without changing the classification.

and clinical assessment of lymph node status, both of which are inaccurate (Table 19.6). To improve the TNM system, a separate pathological classification has been added. Patients with small breast cancers (< 4 cm) have a low incidence of detectable metastatic disease and, unless they have specific symptoms, should not undergo investigations to search for metastases other than in the axilla which can be assessed by ultrasound and/or FNAC or core biopsy. Patients with larger or more locally advanced breast cancers are more likely to have metastases and should be considered for bone scan and liver ultrasound. A simpler classification of breast cancer separates patients into three groups: operable, locally advanced and metastatic.

The curability of breast cancer

Almost half the women with operable breast cancer treated by the local treatments of surgery, with or without radiotherapy, die from metastatic disease. This indicates that in most cases the cancer has already spread at the time of presentation. Invasive breast cancers spread via lymphatics and the bloodstream. The first lymph node that drains the tumour is called the sentinel node and is most commonly a level I axillary node. However, in 5% of women the sentinel node is in the internal mammary chain. In most patients with internal mammary node metastases, axillary nodes are also involved. Rarely (usually in medial tumours), the internal mammary nodes are the only regional nodes involved. It was believed that haematogenous spread took place after lymph node involvement, but it is now appreciated that lymph nodes do not act as a filter and that the presence of nodal metastases usually means that the cancer has spread systemically. Metastasis can occur at any site, but the most commonly affected organs are the bony skeleton, lungs, liver, brain, ovaries and peritoneal cavity.

Prognostic factors

Factors related to prognosis include:

- the stage of the tumour at diagnosis: principally, its size and the involvement of the axillary lymph nodes or the presence of clinically evident metastases
- biological factors that relate to tumour aggressiveness: these include histological grade, histological type, the presence of lymphatic or vascular invasion, hormone receptor content and HER2 status (see above).

The single most important prognostic factor is the number of axillary lymph nodes involved (Fig. 19.25). It is possible to combine prognostic factors to form an index that allows the identification of groups with different prognoses. The Nottingham Prognostic Index (Table 19.7) is the most widely used and incorporates three factors: tumour size, node status and histological grade.

- Tumour size (pathological size of lesion in centimeters)
- Node status (scored 1 if no nodes involved, 2 if 1–3 nodes positive, 3 if ≥ 4 nodes involved)
- Grade I tumours (scored as 1) grade II (scored as 2) grade III (scored as 3).

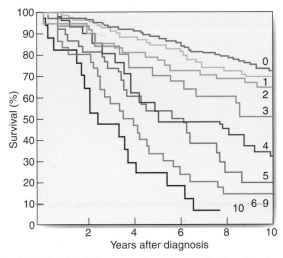

Fig. 19.25 Relation between number of involved axillary lymph nodes (numbered 0–10) and survival after breast cancer.

Table 19.7 Nottingham prognostic index (NPI) and survival

NPI = (0.2 × size in cm)
+ lymph node stage (score 1 for no nodes, 2 for 1-3 nodes, 3 for ± 4 nodes)
+ grade (score 1 for grade I, 2 for grade II, 3 for grade III)

Originally, the NPI was used to divide women into good, intermediate or poor prognostic groups; several confirmatory studies have led to a refined NPI with five categories

Group	Index value	10-year survival (%)
Excellent (EPG)	≤ 2.4	98
Good (GPG)	≤ 3.4	90
Moderate I (MPGI)	≤ 4.4	83
Moderate II (MPGII)	< 5.4	75
Poor (PPG)	> 5.4	47

Adjuvant! Online® provides an online tool for evaluating prognosis and the potential benefits from hormonal and chemotherapy and incorporates the tumour size, node status, grade, patient age, their general health status and the hormonal receptor status of the cancer.

Presentation of breast cancer

The most common presentation is with a breast lump or lumpiness, which is usually painless. Any discrete lump, no matter how small or mobile, can be a cancer. The investigation of a breast lump is shown in Figure 19.26. Malignant lesions may be firm and irregular and produce visible signs of breast

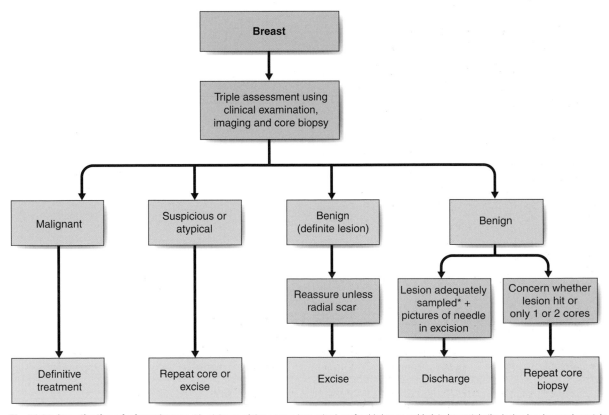

Fig. 19.26 Investigation of a breast mass. *A minimum of three cores is required, preferably image-guided, to be certain the lesion has been adequately sampled.

asymmetry, such as flattening, dimpling or puckering of the overlying skin, or retraction or alteration in nipple contour. Approximately 50% of breast cancers are located in the upper outer quadrant of the breast. Diagnosis of breast lumps is a particular problem in young women, in whom the breasts are dense and lumpier and cancer is rare. Some patients present with features of locally advanced breast cancer such as skin ulceration, with direct infiltration of the skin by tumour or with oedema (Fig. 19.27) of the overlying skin.

Breast pain alone is a rare presenting feature of breast cancer; 2.7% of patients with breast pain have cancer, whereas 4.6% of patients presenting with breast cancer have pain as their only symptom. Nipple discharge, which is either blood-stained or contains moderate or large amounts of blood on testing, can be a presenting feature of breast cancer. However, only 5–10% of patients with this symptom will have underlying malignancy. Investigation of patients who present with nipple discharge is shown in Figure 19.28. Patients with breast cancer occasionally present with a dry scaling or red weeping appearance of the nipple known as Paget's disease; this signifies an underlying invasive or non-invasive cancer (Fig. 19.29) and should be differentiated from eczema (Fig. 19.30). Paget's disease always affects the nipple and only involves the areola as a secondary event, whereas eczema primarily involves the areola and only secondarily affects the nipple. Approximately 1–2% of

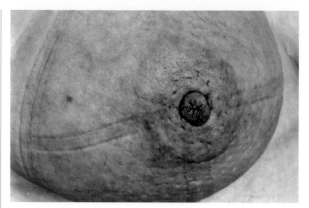

Fig. 19.27 Peau d'orange of the skin around the nipple in a patient with inflammatory carcinoma.

patients with breast cancer present with Paget's disease. In half of these, it is associated with an underlying mass lesion, and 90% of such patients will have an invasive cancer. Of the patients without a mass lesion, 30% have an invasive cancer and the rest have in situ disease alone.

Patients can also present initially with palpable axillary nodes or signs and symptoms of distant metastatic disease:

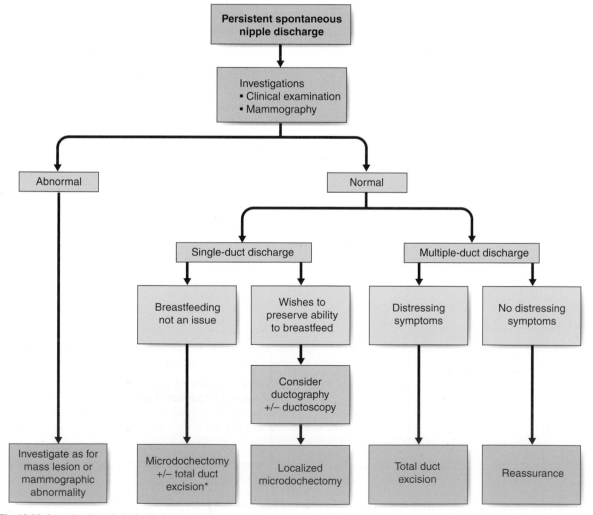

Fig. 19.28 Investigation of nipple discharge. *Some surgeons prefer total duct excision in women > 45 to reduce the incidence of further discharge from ducts - microdochectomy: removal of diseased duct.

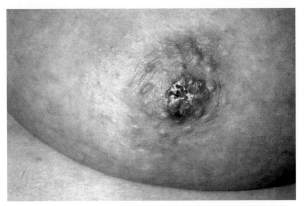

Fig. 19.29 Paget's disease.

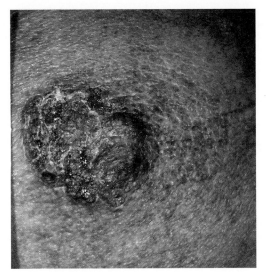

Fig. 19.30 Eczema of the nipple.

for example, palpable supraclavicular nodes, bone pain, a cough or breathlessness, lethargy and tiredness, jaundice and headaches, or a sudden onset of grand mal seizures. Fewer than 1 in 300 patients with breast cancer present with nodal metastases and an occult primary cancer. Up to 70% of women shown histologically to have metastatic adenocarcinoma in the axillary nodes without an obvious breast cancer will have an occult breast cancer. Most of these cancers will be visible on mammography or, if not, can be visualized by MRI of the breast.

Management of operable breast cancer

In situ breast cancer

Localized DCIS (usually considered as less than 4 cm in maximum dimension) should be treated by complete wide excision, ensuring that surrounding normal tissue is present at all lateral margins. Following wide excision alone, approximately 2% per year will recur; half of these will be further in situ disease, the other half being invasive. For this reason, following wide excision, patients should be considered for postoperative radiotherapy particularly if the DCIS is high grade. Patients with small areas of DCIS or who have low or intermediate grade DCIS that have been completely excised may not require radiotherapy. Tamoxifen appears to reduce both the risk of recurrence and the rate of development of

contralateral cancer in those women with oestrogen receptor-positive disease. It is not without side effects and its use for DCIS is not widespread. Current studies are evaluating the role of aromatase inhibitors in reducing recurrence. DCIS that is incompletely excised requires re-excision or mastectomy. Widespread (≥ 4 cm) DCIS is usually treated by mastectomy, with or without immediate breast reconstruction but can be treated by breast conservation providing a satisfactory cosmetic outcome can be obtained.

 SUMMARY BOX 19.3

Ductal carcinoma in situ (DCIS)

- Localized disease is treated by wide local excision to clear margins
- All patients other than those at low risk of recurrence should be considered for adjuvant radiotherapy to the breast following wide local excision
- Tamoxifen reduces all breast cancer events following wide excision, but its exact role in reducing local recurrence following conservative treatment is not clear
- The value of aromatase inhibitors is being investigated
- Large areas of DCIS are usually treated by mastectomy ± reconstruction.

Operable breast tumours

Operable breast tumours are those restricted to the breast or associated with mobile axillary lymph nodes on the same side: T_1, T_2, T_3, N_0, N_1, M_0. As only a minority of patients are cured by locoregional treatments alone, all should be considered for systemic therapy after local therapy (EBMs 19.4 and 19.5M).

EBM 19.4 Breast conservation in operable cancers

'Breast-conserving surgery followed by radiotherapy is as effective as mastectomy for small operable breast cancer.'

Fisher B, et al. N Engl J Med 2002; 347(16):1270–1271.

EBM 19.5 Radiotherapy after surgery for breast cancer

'Radiotherapy reduces local recurrence after surgery and reduces deaths from breast cancer.'

Early Breast Cancer Trialists' Collaborative Group. Lancet 2005; 366:2087-2106.

Local therapy

There are currently two accepted methods of local therapy for operable breast cancer.

Breast-conserving treatment (wide local excision and radiotherapy)

This involves excising the tumour with a 1 cm margin of macroscopically normal tissue. Breast conservation is usually only suitable for single cancers measuring less than 4 cm in diameter. Complete excision of all invasive and non-invasive cancer is necessary. Wide excision should be combined with an axillary node staging procedure. This involves either removing the first node or nodes draining the tumour (sentinel node biopsy), or axillary clearance (removing all nodes at levels I, II and III). To identify the sentinel node(s), blue dye usually combined with radioisotope is injected either under the nipple into the skin over the cancer or around the cancer. Sentinel nodes can be seen on scintigraphy or can be identified with a hand-held probe, or are stained blue. There is rarely a single sentinel node and the average number of sentinel nodes removed at surgery is 3. When blue dye and radioactively labelled sulphur colloid or albumin techniques are combined, one or more sentinel nodes will be identified in approximately 97% of patients, and this sentinel node is accurate in determining the presence of any involved nodes in the axilla in approximately 98% of patients.

The cosmetic outcome following breast conservation relates to psychological well-being. Patients who have a good cosmetic result have low levels of anxiety and depression and improved body image and self-esteem. The larger the volume of tissue excised, the poorer the cosmetic result. The aim of breast-conserving surgery is to remove the cancer completely in as small a volume of tissue as possible.

Wide excision should be followed by radical radiotherapy using megavoltage equipment to deliver 45–50 Gy to the whole breast. An additional boost of 10–15 Gy by electrons of appropriate energy, or an iridium-192 (^{192}Ir) implant, is given to the tumour bed in women under 50 years of age or those with close margins. For patients with involved nodes identified by a sentinel node biopsy or an axillary node sampling procedure, the remaining axillary nodes should be removed or treated by radiotherapy to the axilla and/or the medial supraclavicular fossa. Studies of local radiotherapy to the tumour bed given intraoperatively or after operation using external beam or an intracavity balloon device have been reported and seem to show satisfactory rates of local control in patients at low risk of local recurrence after breast conserving surgery.

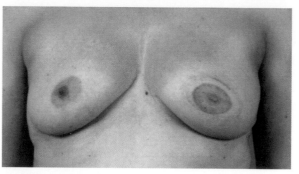

Fig. 19.31 A patient who had a left mastectomy and breast reconstruction with a latissimus dorsi reconstruction. The patient also had a nipple reconstruction with tattooing.

Mastectomy removes all breast tissue with some overlying skin (usually including the nipple), but leaves the chest wall muscles intact. If reconstruction is being performed, minimal skin around the tumour can be excised. Mastectomy should be combined with some form of axillary surgery. Radiotherapy is given after mastectomy to patients who are at high risk of local recurrence. Risk factors for local recurrence after mastectomy include axillary lymph node involvement, lymphatic or vascular invasion by tumour, a grade III cancer, a cancer more than 4 cm in diameter (pathological measurement), or a tumour that involves the pectoral fascia or pectoral muscle.

 SUMMARY BOX 19.4

Breast conservation

- Suitable for localized, operable breast cancers in which there is no evidence of metastatic disease beyond regional nodes; excision must leave a reasonable cosmetic result to produce benefits compared with mastectomy
- Includes wide local excision of the cancer to clear histological margins, axillary surgery (sentinel node biopsy, or clearance of the axillary nodes) and whole-breast radiotherapy consisting of a 45–50 Gy dose of radiotherapy applied to the whole breast, with an optional 10–15 Gy boost to the tumour bed.

 SUMMARY BOX 19.5

Mastectomy

- Is appropriate for large operable breast cancers or in patients with extensive non-invasive disease, an incomplete excision after attempted breast-conserving surgery or some women with central tumour
- Consists of total removal of the breast together with sentinel node biopsy, axillary node sampling or axillary clearance
- Should be followed by chest-wall radiotherapy in those women identified to be at significantly increased risk of local recurrence.

Systemic therapy

Systemic treatment may be given as adjuvant therapy after surgery and/or radiotherapy, or as primary or neoadjuvant treatment before surgery and/or radiotherapy. The effectiveness of adjuvant treatment has been shown in clinical trials (EBM 19.6). Randomized studies comparing primary systemic treatment with adjuvant treatment have shown similar survivals, with a higher rate of breast-conserving surgery in patients having initial medical treatment. Adjuvant treatments consist of chemotherapy or hormonal therapy.

Adjuvant chemotherapy

A combination of drugs is more effective than a single agent and the optimal benefit seems to come from at least four cycles of postoperative chemotherapy. The benefits of chemotherapy are greatest in women under the age of 50 (Table 19.8); a smaller but still significant benefit is seen in older women. Regimens that include anthracyclines are more effective than non-anthracycline containing regimens. Commonly used regimens include AC (adriamycin, cyclo-

Mastectomy

This is an alternative method of local treatment. It is indicated in patients:

- for whom radiotherapy is not available or when there is a wish to avoid radiotherapy
- who elect to have a mastectomy
- who have more than one focus of cancer in their breast and where removal of all the cancers would produce an unacceptable cosmetic result
- who have a localized invasive cancer but a large area of surrounding non-invasive disease
- when breast conservation would produce an unacceptable cosmetic result. (This includes some central lesions directly underneath the nipple, and most cancers measuring more than 4 cm in diameter.) Breast-conserving surgery is possible in these women if they have shrinkage following initial systemic therapy, or if the breast defect is filled with a latissimus dorsi flap (Fig. 19.31).

Table 19.8 Reduction in recurrence and mortality in polychemotherapy trials

Age	Reduction in annual odds of recurrence (% ± SD)	Reduction in annual odds of death (% ± SD)
< 40	37 ± 7	27 ± 8
40-49	34 ± 5	27 ± 5
50–59	22 ± 4	14 ± 4
60–69	18 ± 4	8 ± 4
All ages	23 ± 8	15 ± 2

phosphamide) or FEC (5-fluorouracil, epirubicin and cyclophosphamide) alone, or four courses of epirubicin alone, or FEC followed by four courses of CMF (cyclophosphamide, methotrexate and 5-fluorouracil). The taxanes (taxol and taxotere) combined with an anthracycline such as AT (adriamycin, taxotere/taxol) or ET (epirubicin and taxotere/taxol) appear more effective than anthracyclines alone.

Adjuvant hormone therapy

Adjuvant hormonal treatments consist of oophorectomy, tamoxifen and the aromatase inhibitors letrozole, anastrozole and exemestane. Oophorectomy is only of benefit in women under 50 years of age with ER positive cancers and produces survival benefits of similar magnitude to those obtained by polychemotherapy in younger women. It can be achieved surgically, by radiation or by the administration of gonadotrophin-releasing hormone (GnRh) analogues such as goserelin. Tamoxifen is a par-

tial oestrogen agonist that is given in a dose of 20 mg once daily. At least 5 years of tamoxifen should be given. It reduces the risk of contralateral breast cancer by between 40 and 50%. The benefits of tamoxifen and oophorectomy are greatest in patients with tumours that are rich in oestrogen receptors. Tamoxifen is effective in both pre- and postmenopausal women. The aromatase inhibitors, which block the conversion of androgens to oestrogen in postmenopausal women, appear more effective than tamoxifen. They can be given immediately after surgery, after 2 years of tamoxifen or after 5 years of tamoxifen to reduce recurrence rate and improve survival. The current view is that aromatase inhibitors should be included as part of the adjuvant therapy programme of most postmenopausal women with hormone receptor-positive breast cancer.

Adjuvant anti-HER2 *therapy*

Overall, 15–20% of cancers over-express the oncogene *HER2* and these cancers have a worse prognosis than those that are *HER2*-negative. A humanized monoclonal antibody (trastuzumab) has been shown to reduce the risk of cancer recurrence by up to 50% in women whose cancers over-express *HER2* (EBM 19.7).

Studies with lapatanib, an oral agent which targets HER1 and HER2 are in progress. Adjuvant systemic therapy is effective in patients at both low and high risk of recurrence, but the absolute gains in survival are greatest in the latter. Risk of recurrence can be calculated using the Nottingham Prognostic Index (see Table 19.7) or can be based on individual factors. *Adjuvantonline.com®* presents absolute benefits in individual patients from different endocrine and chemotherapy regimens. An outline of the use of adjuvant treatment in different groups and factors which should be taken into consideration are presented in Tables 19.9 and 19.10.

Table 19.9 Indications and factors helpful in deciding whether ER-positive HER2-negative breast cancer should be treated with chemo and endocrine therapy combined, or endocrine therapy alone

Clinicopathological features	Relative indications for chemoendocrine therapy	Factors not useful for decision	Relative indications for endocrine therapy alone
ER and PgR	Lower ER and PgR level		Higher ER and PgR level
Histological grade	Grade 3	Grade 2	Grade 1
Proliferation	High*	Intermediate*	Low*
Nodes	Node positive (4 or more)	Node positive (1–3 involved nodes)	Node negative
LVI	Presence of extensive LVI		Absence of extensive LVI
pT size	> 5 cm	2.1–5 cm	≤ 2 cm
Patient preference	Happy to have all treatments		Wants to avoid chemorelated side effects

ER = oestrogen receptor; PgR = progesterone receptor; *proliferation can be measured using a variety of different methods by immunohistochemistry or by genetic signature; LVI = lymphatic vascular invasion

19

Table 19.10 **Suggested adjuvant treatment for patients with breast cancer[1]**

Risk group	Premenopausal	Postmenopausal
Very low-risk	Nil or tamoxifen	Nil or tamoxifen
Low-risk ER+	Tamoxifen ± OS[2]	Tamoxifen
Low-risk ER−	Chemotherapy	Chemotherapy
Moderate-risk ER+	Chemotherapy + tamoxifen ± OS	Chemotherapy + AI/tam[3]
Moderate-risk ER−	Chemotherapy	Chemotherapy
High-risk	Chemotherapy + tamoxifen + OS (if ER+)	Chemotherapy + AI/tam[3]

(ER = oestrogen receptor)

[1]Patients whose tumours over-express *HER2* should also be considered for adjuvant trastuzumab.

[2]Ovarian suppression (OS): either luteinizing hormone releasing hormone (LHRH) analogue or surgical oophorectomy.

[3]With the data showing superiority of aromatase inhibitors (AIs) over tamoxifen, the former are being increasingly used either as first-line treatments in high-risk women or in sequence with tamoxifen.

 SUMMARY BOX 19.6

Adjuvant therapy

Following surgery and/or radiotherapy for operable breast cancer, patients should receive adjuvant systemic therapy, which can be either hormonal therapy or chemotherapy.

Examples of hormonal therapy
- Premenopausal women: tamoxifen, goserelin, or both together
- Postmenopausal women: tamoxifen or aromatase inhibitors, or tamoxifen followed by an aromatase inhibitor.

Chemotherapy
- Commonly used regimens are AC, FEC, Epi CMF, AT, ET*.

Positive factors influencing the use of chemotherapy
- Young age (especially < 50 years)
- Axillary node involvement
- Large tumour size
- Histological features
  grade III
  lymphatic/vascular invasion
- Negative oestrogen receptor.

*Defined in text.

Primary systemic therapy

The use of primary medical (neoadjuvant) or preoperative treatment for operable breast cancer allows large tumours that would otherwise require a mastectomy to become suitable for breast-conserving surgery. Both the primary tumour and lymph node metastases can be shown to respond. With conventional chemotherapy regimens, approximately 70% of patients will demonstrate tumour shrinkage of over 50%. Although chemotherapy is most commonly used as preoperative treatment, particularly in premenopausal women, primary hormonal therapy is being increasingly used in post-menopausal women with strongly oestrogen receptor-positive breast cancers. Response rates of over 75% are reported. Randomized studies have suggested that the aromatase inhibitor, letrozole, produces significantly better responses in postmenopausal women with ER rich cancers in the neoadjuvant setting than tamoxifen, and this is currently the first-line agent of choice in this setting.

Complications of treatment

Haematoma and infection are uncommon (less than 5%) after breast surgery. Removal of all the axillary nodes often damages the intercostobrachial nerve, which results in numbness and paraesthesia down the upper inner aspect of the arm. Other nerves that can potentially be damaged during axillary surgery are the long thoracic nerve, damage to which causes winging of the scapula, and the thoracodorsal nerve, which can lead to atrophy of the latissimus dorsi muscle and prominence of the scapula. Axillary surgery is associated with some short-term reduction in shoulder movement and about 5% of women develop a frozen shoulder. Approximately 5–10% of patients treated by a full axillary dissection develop lymphoedema. The treatment of lymphoedema is unsatisfactory and is best managed by bandaging and a supportive elastic arm stocking.

Radiotherapy

Following radiotherapy, the skin develops an erythematous reaction, which often lasts for 3–4 weeks. Patients should avoid exposing the area to direct sunlight for several months. Subsequent exposure is possible with an appropriate sunscreen. Following radiotherapy to the axilla, some patients develop fibrosis around the shoulder, which can lead to some restriction in their range of movement.

Chemotherapy

Although hair loss is the most common concern of patients before starting chemotherapy, 80% report fatigue and lethargy as the most troublesome side effects. The occurrence of alopecia with some chemotherapy regimens may be reduced by scalp cooling. Nausea and vomiting are unpleasant side effects but in most patients can be controlled with appropriate antiemetic drugs. Trastuzumab, when combined with anthracycline-containing chemotherapy, can result in cardiac failure in a small but significant number of patients.

Hormonal treatments

The side effects of hormonal treatments are greatest in premenopausal patients. Less than 10% of patients stop taking tamoxifen because of side effects, but vaginal dryness or vaginal discharge, loss of libido and hot flushes all have a considerable impact on quality of life. Aromatase inhibitors in post-menopausal women cause fewer hot flushes than tamoxifen and fewer vaginal problems, but more muscular aches and pains and fractures with up to a quarter of patients having to stop them early due to side effects.

Psychological aspects

Most women who present with breast lumps are emotionally distressed. When breaking bad news, the first step should be to check the patient's perception of what is wrong. Almost two-thirds of patients with breast cancer already suspect that their lump is malignant. In patients with proven malignancy, the doctor's role is to confirm that their diagnosis is correct, pause to let this sink in, acknowledge their distress and establish what concerns are contributing to this distress. When a patient is unaware that she has cancer, the doctor should break the news more slowly. Most specialist units employ nurse counsellors who ensure that the patient is fully informed about the nature of the disease and its treatment. They provide advice on prostheses after surgery, and help recognize and support patients with significant psychiatric problems.

Up to 30% of women with breast cancer develop an anxiety state or depressive illness within a year of diagnosis, 3–4 times the expected rate. After mastectomy, 20–30% of patients develop persisting problems with body image and sexual difficulties. Breast-conserving surgery reduces problems with body image. Psychiatric morbidity is increased when radiotherapy or chemotherapy is used. Few patients mention psychological problems to their doctor because they think it is unacceptable to do so. Doctors can promote the disclosure of such problems by being empathetic, making educated guesses about how patients are feeling, and summarizing what they have disclosed.

There is evidence that patients benefit psychologically from immediate breast reconstruction. Options for reconstruction include the placement of an implant behind the chest wall muscles at the time of mastectomy. The problem with this approach is that the size of implant that can be inserted is limited and symmetry is difficult to obtain. Another option is to place a tissue expander behind the pectoral muscles. The use of implants has increased because larger pockets can now be created by the use of decellularized human or pig skin sutured from the pectoralis major to the chest wall to create a larger pocket into which an implant or expander can be placed. Small amounts of fluid are injected regularly into an expander over a period of months before replacing it, at a second operation, with a permanent prosthesis. Alternative options include using myocutaneous flaps; the most commonly used are the latissimus dorsi myocutaneous flap with or without an implant (Fig. 19.31), and the rectus abdominis myocutaneous flap alone.

Follow-up

Patients treated by wide local excision and radiotherapy have between a 0.4 and 1% per year rate of local recurrence in the treated breast. Those with cancer in one breast are also at risk of cancer in the other breast (0.4–0.6% per year). The majority of local recurrences after mastectomy occur within the first few years. The aim of follow-up is to detect local recurrence at a stage when it is treatable, to support the patient psychologically and to discuss problems associated with adjuvant therapy. Patients should have an annual mammogram of one or both breasts every 1–2 years for life. No investigations should be performed to detect asymptomatic metastases, as there is no evidence that this influences survival.

Management of locally advanced breast cancer

Locally advanced breast cancer (LABC) is characterized by features suggesting infiltration of the skin or chest wall by tumour or matted involved axillary nodes (Table 19.11).

Table 19.11 Clinical features of locally advanced breast cancer

Skin
- Ulceration
- Satellite nodules
- Dermal infiltration
- Peau d'orange
- Erythema over tumour

Chest wall
- Tumour fixation to:
  ribs
  intercostal muscles
  serratus anterior

Axillary nodes
- Nodes fixed to one another or to other structures

It has a variable natural history, with reported 5-year survivals of between 1 and 30%. The median survival was previously about 2–2.5 years but this has improved with better systemic therapy. LABC can arise because of its position in the breast (for example, peripheral), neglect (some patients do not present to hospital for months or years after they notice a mass) or biological aggressiveness. The latter includes inflammatory cancers that present with erythema and/or widespread peau d'orange affecting the breast skin. The peau d'orange is because of lymphatic obstruction by cancer cells in lymphatics or in lymph nodes (see Fig. 19.27). Inflammatory carcinomas are uncommon and are characterized by brawny, oedematous, indurated and erythematous skin changes (Fig. 19.32). They have the worst prognosis of all LABCs.

Local and regional relapse was formerly a major problem in LABC and affected more than half of patients. By treating patients initially with systemic therapy, followed by surgery and radiotherapy or radiotherapy alone, improvements in local control have been achieved. Systemic treatment consists of either chemotherapy (inflammatory cancers, oestrogen receptor-negative tumours and rapidly progressive disease) or hormonal treatment (slow or indolent disease, oestrogen receptor-positive cancers, or women who are elderly or unfit). Following systemic therapy, the disease may become operable, at which point surgery, usually mastectomy, is followed by radiotherapy. In women whose disease remains inoperable following systemic treatment, radiotherapy is given. This is followed by surgery in some women in whom viable resectable cancer remains following radiotherapy (Fig. 19.32). Systemic therapy, either chemotherapy (for 3–4 months) or hormone treatment (usually for 5 years), is often given after surgery.

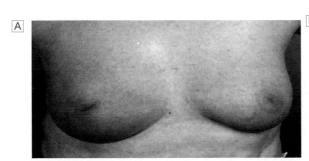
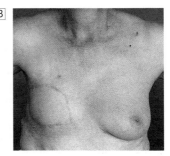

Fig. 19.32 Inflammatory breast cancer. [A] Inflammatory breast cancer at diagnosis. [B] Following chemotherapy and radiotherapy, then surgery to excise residual disease using myocutaneous flap for skin closure.

SUMMARY BOX **19.7**

Locally advanced breast cancer

- For the majority, consider systemic chemotherapy or, in the elderly or those who have indolent hormone-sensitive cancers, prescribe hormonal therapy
- Radiotherapy can be used following primary chemotherapy, or can be given concurrently with hormonal therapy
- Consider surgery if the disease becomes operable following primary systemic therapy, or in patients with locally advanced breast cancers that have occurred because of either a delay in diagnosis or their position in the breast, e.g. superficial or at the breast margin. Surgery is also possible in those with locally advanced disease following radiotherapy.

Breast cancer in pregnancy

Overall, 1–2% of breast cancer occurs during pregnancy. It affects 1–3 of every 10 000 pregnancies. Although there is no evidence that breast cancer occurring during pregnancy is more aggressive, up to 65% of patients have involved axillary nodes because the diagnosis is often delayed. Treatment during the first two trimesters is with mastectomy. Radiotherapy should not be delivered during pregnancy. Chemotherapy can be given but is associated with a small risk of fetal damage. Breast cancer during the third trimester can be managed either by immediate surgery or by monitoring the tumour and delivering the baby early at 32 weeks, and then instituting treatment after delivery.

Pregnancy after treatment for breast cancer

There is only limited information on the effect of pregnancy on the outcome of patients with breast cancer, but the available data show no detrimental effect.

Management of metastatic or advanced breast cancer

The average period of survival after a diagnosis of metastatic disease is 20–30 months, but this varies widely between patients. A patient may present with metastatic breast carcinoma or can develop metastases following treatment of an apparently localized breast cancer. The aim of treatment is to produce effective symptom control with minimal side effects. This ideal is only achieved in the 40–50% of patients whose cancers respond to hormonal therapy or chemotherapy. There is no evidence that treating asymptomatic metastases improves overall survival, and chemotherapy is normally given only to symptomatic patients. Even in patients with metastatic breast cancer, surgery to control local disease has an important role and may improve long-term outcome.

Chemotherapy

With chemotherapy, a balance must be achieved between a high response rate and limiting side effects. The best palliation is obtained with regimens that produce the highest response rates. The most frequently used drugs in metastatic breast cancer are the anthracyclines, adriamycin and epirubicin. Taxanes (taxol and taxotere) are also commonly used. Overall rates of response to chemotherapy are approximately 40–60%, with a median time to relapse of 6–10 months. Subsequent courses have response rates of less than 25%.

Hormonal treatment

A variety of hormonal interventions are available for use in metastatic breast cancer (Table 19.12). In premenopausal women these include oophorectomy (surgical, radiation- or drug-induced by GnRh analogues) combined with tamoxifen. Options in postmenopausal women include the new aromatase inhibitors (anastrozole, letrozole and exemestane) and the progestogens (such as medroxyprogesterone acetate or megestrol acetate). First-line treatment is with letrozole or anastrozole. Objective responses to hormonal treatments are seen in 30% of all patients and in 50–60% of those with oestrogen receptor-positive tumours. Response rates of 25% are seen when using second-line hormonal agents, although fewer than 15% of patients who show no response to first-line treatment will have a response to second-line agents. Approximately 10–15% of patients respond to third-line endocrine agents.

Anti-*HER2* therapy

The humanized monoclonal antibody trastuzumab, raised against *HER2*, increases both the rate and duration of response of patients with metastatic disease when combined with chemotherapy in patients with tumours over-expressing *HER2*. The oral agent lapatanib which targets HER1 and HER2 is in clinical trials.

SUMMARY BOX **19.8**

Metastatic breast cancer

- The primary aim is to improve symptoms as well as improving the quantity and quality of life
- Consider hormone therapy if there is a long disease-free interval and the tumour is hormone receptor-positive
- Consider chemotherapy if there is a short disease-free interval, vital organs are affected and/or the tumour is oestrogen receptor-negative.

Table 19.12 Hormonal treatment of metastatic breast cancer

Premenopausal

- Ovarian suppression
- Gonadotrophin-releasing hormone analogues
- Oophorectomy
- Radiation menopause
- Tamoxifen
- Ovarian suppression + tamoxifen[1]
- Ovarian suppression + an aromatase inhibitor

Postmenopausal

- Aromatase inhibitor[2,3]
- Tamoxifen
- Progestins, e.g. megestrol or medroxyprogesterone acetate
- Fulvestrant[4]

Note These agents can be used in any order.
[1]There is evidence that combined ovarian suppression plus an anti-oestrogen is superior to single-agent treatment in premenopausal women.
[2]Letrozole or anastrozole are first-line agents in postmenopausal women. Data for letrozole is more impressive than for anastrozole.
[3]A steroidal aromatase inhibitor (e.g. exemestane) can have efficacy even if a tumour is resistant to the non-steroidal aromatase inhibitors letrozole and anastrozole.
[4]Licensed in England, Wales and Northern Ireland, but not Scotland; continues to be evaluated in trials.

Specific problems

Bone disease

Three-quarters of patients who develop secondary breast cancer have disease involving the bony skeleton. Widespread bony disease responds well to hormonal treatment, but in young patients cytotoxic agents may be required. Treatment of localized pain includes external beam radiotherapy and analgesics, including NSAIDs and opiates. Pathological fractures due to bone disease should be avoided and can be predicted by a sharp increase in pain over a few days or weeks. When X-rays show that fracture is likely, a combination of internal fixation and radiotherapy should be used. Options for widespread bony pain include the use of bisphosphonates (which reduce osteoclast activity) and sequential upper and lower body hemiradiotherapy or radioactive strontium. Bisphosphonates are also showing promise as adjuvant treatments in early breast cancer.

Hypercalcaemia

Seen in up to 40% of patients with bony metastases, symptoms include nausea, constipation, thirst, polyuria, personality change, muscle weakness and bone pain. Treatment consists of hydration with saline (about 3 litres given over 24 hours) and the administration of intravenous bisphosphonates, followed by a change in systemic anticancer therapy.

Marrow infiltration

A leucoerythroblastic blood picture (immature cells in the peripheral blood) suggests extensive marrow infiltration. Chemotherapy is generally required, although hormones can be effective in oestrogen receptor-rich disease. Chemotherapy should be given initially in reduced doses with careful monitoring and adequate supportive care.

Spinal cord compression

This is most often seen in patients with thoracic spinal metastases. It must be recognized early and treated promptly. Patients with isolated metastases causing cord compression, and who are fit, should be treated by surgery followed by postoperative radiotherapy and appropriate systemic therapy. In the remaining patients, treatment consists of steroids and fractionated radiotherapy.

Pleural effusion

Up to half of patients with metastatic breast cancer will develop a malignant pleural effusion. Cytological examination of aspirated fluid reveals malignant cells in only 85% of patients. Aspiration alone of pleural effusions is ineffective treatment, as between 97 and 100% of patients will re-accumulate fluid. In contrast, tube drainage alone is effective in controlling effusions in over one-third of patients. The instillation of bleomycin, tetracycline or talc to cause pleurodesis reduces recurrence.

Liver metastases

Right upper quadrant pain, general debility, tiredness, a feeling of nausea and lack of appetite, and the onset of jaundice are all symptoms suggestive of liver metastases. Chemotherapy is usually indicated, except in postmenopausal patients with oestrogen receptor-rich tumours in whom the new aromatase inhibitors can be effective. Where jaundice is due to nodal disease at the porta hepatis, a stent inserted in the common bile duct using endoscopic retrograde pancreatography (ERCP) should be considered.

Brain metastases

These should be suspected in any patient with breast cancer who presents with focal neurological symptoms particularly if the cancer is HER2 positive. CT or MRI can detect even small volumes of disease. Treatment consists of high-dose corticosteroids (16 mg dexamethasone daily), followed by radiotherapy. The greatest benefits of radiotherapy are seen in patients whose neurological symptoms improve following steroid treatment, but the long-term results of treatment are disappointing. A small group of patients with solitary brain metastases, and without evidence of involvement at other sites, are suitable for local excision followed by postoperative radiotherapy and appropriate systemic treatment. A few patients remain well without other evidence of disease for many years.

 SUMMARY BOX **19.9**

Metastatic disease: specific problems

- Bone metastases may require local radiotherapy, bisphosphonates or orthopaedic intervention, combined with systemic hormonal therapy or chemotherapy
- Hypercalcaemia causes nausea, constipation, thirst, polyuria, weakness, pain and personality change, and is treated by rehydration followed by bisphosphonates
- Spinal cord compression should be treated by surgical decompression if appropriate, or by steroids and radiotherapy
- Pleural effusions should be treated by tube drainage, followed by instillation of bleomycin, tetracycline or talc
- Discrete lung metastases may not cause acute symptoms but lymphangitis carcinomatosa can cause severe bronchospasm and dyspnoea, which may be relieved by steroids, bronchodilators and chemotherapy
- Liver metastases present most commonly with general debility, nausea and lack of appetite; they are usually treated by chemotherapy but hormone therapy with aromatase inhibitors is an option in postmenopausal women with ER+ rich cancers
- Brain metastases are treated initially with steroids, followed by radiation. Surgery can be used for isolated single metastases

Miscellaneous tumours of the breast

Lymphoma

This is rare in the breast. Staging investigations are necessary because patients will usually have disease elsewhere. Characteristically, lymphoma presents as a discrete smooth rubbery mass.

Sarcomas

Sarcomas can develop in breast tissue and can affect the skin overlying the breast. Rarely, they are induced by radiotherapy to the chest wall. Sarcomas are treated by excision. These tumours are usually large at diagnosis, so mastectomy is generally necessary. Radiotherapy should be given to the chest wall after excisional surgery, but there is no evidence that adjuvant chemotherapy is of benefit.

19

19

Malignant phyllodes tumours

Previously called cystosarcoma phyllodes, these present as large lobulated lesions that can involve the overlying skin. Initial treatment is by wide excision or mastectomy. The roles of radiotherapy and chemotherapy in these lesions are unclear.

Secondary tumours

Metastases from tumours elsewhere, e.g. bronchus, thyroid, melanoma or the opposite breast, produce a well-defined mass both clinically and mammographically.

MALE BREAST

Gynaecomastia

Gynaecomastia (the growth of breast tissue in males to any extent in all ages) is entirely benign and usually reversible. It commonly occurs at puberty and in old age and is seen in 30–60% of boys aged 10–16. In this age group it usually requires no treatment, as 80% resolve spontaneously within 2 years (Fig. 19.33). Embarrassment or persistent enlargement is an indication for surgery. Senescent gynaecomastia usually affects men between 50 and 80, and in most cases does not appear to be associated with any endocrine abnormality. Causes include excess alcohol intake and drugs including cannabis, cirrhosis, hypogonadism and, rarely, testicular tumours. Rapidly progressive gynaecomastia is an indication for an assessment of hormonal profile. A history of recent progressive breast enlargement without pain and tenderness, or an easily identifiable cause, should raise the suspicion of breast cancer. If there is a localized mass, then further investigations should be performed. Surgery consists of excision of glandular tissue combined with liposuction or liposuction alone and is reserved for patients with significant social embarrassment.

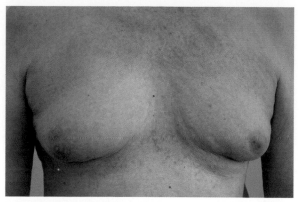

Fig. 19.33 Gynaecomastia in a male.

Male breast cancer

Fewer than 0.5% of all breast cancers occur in men, and breast cancer comprises 0.7% of all male cancers. The peak incidence in males is 5–10 years later than in women. Klinefelter's syndrome and a strong family history are the only known risk factors. Male breast cancers can be associated with *BRCA2* gene mutations. Cancer usually presents with an eccentric breast mass or retraction of the overlying skin. Direct involvement of the skin occurs more often in male breast cancer because of the smaller breast volume compared to the female breast, and so the disease is more likely to be advanced at diagnosis. Mammography and core biopsy will confirm the diagnosis. Treatment for localized breast cancer is by breast conserving surgery or total mastectomy and the removal of the sentinel or all the axillary nodes, usually followed by postoperative radiotherapy to the chest wall. Adjuvant tamoxifen is effective at reducing recurrence. Adjuvant chemotherapy should be considered for fit patients with tumours that have nodal involvement or are oestrogen receptor-negative.

20

Endocrine surgery

CHAPTER CONTENTS

Introduction

In surgical endocrine disease, thyroid disorders are common, adrenal disease is uncommon and parathyroid disease is rare.

THYROID GLAND

Surgical anatomy and development

The thyroid gland develops from the thyroglossal duct, which grows downwards from the pharynx through the developing hyoid bone. On the front of the trachea, the duct bifurcates and fuses with elements from the fourth branchial arch, from which the parafollicular (C) cells are derived.

The duct is normally obliterated in early fetal life but can persist in part to produce a thyroglossal cyst. The upper end of the duct is identified in adults as the foramen caecum at the junction of the anterior two-thirds and the posterior third of the tongue. Arrest of descent of the duct may result in an ectopic thyroid (e.g. lingual thyroid).

There are two pairs of parathyroid glands. The upper glands arise from the fourth branchial arch and are usually found at the back of the thyroid above the inferior thyroid artery. The lower glands arise from the third arch (in association with the thymus) and are less constant in position. They are usually found posterior to the lower pole of the thyroid lobes but can lie within the gland, some distance below it, in the upper mediastinum or within the thymus.

The lobes of the thyroid lie on the front and sides of the trachea and larynx at the level of the 5–7th cervical vertebrae (Fig. 20.1). They are connected by a narrow isthmus, which overlies the second and third tracheal rings. The thyroid normally weighs 15–30 g and is invested by the pretracheal fascia, which binds it to the larynx, cricoid cartilage and trachea (Fig. 20.2). The strap muscles (sternohyoid and sternothyroid) lie in front of the pretracheal fascia and must be separated to gain access to the gland. It is difficult to feel the normal thyroid gland except at puberty and during pregnancy, when physiological enlargement occurs.

The superior thyroid artery runs down to the upper pole of the gland as a branch of the external carotid artery, whereas the inferior thyroid artery runs across to the lower pole from the thyrocervical trunk (a branch of the subclavian artery). As it nears the gland, the inferior thyroid artery usually passes in front of the recurrent laryngeal nerve, but may branch around it. Blood drains through superior, middle and inferior thyroid veins into the internal jugular and innominate veins. Lymphatics pass laterally to the deep cervical chain and downwards to pretracheal and mediastinal nodes. The recurrent laryngeal nerve, a branch of the vagus, passes upwards in the groove between the oesophagus and trachea to enter the larynx and supply all of its intrinsic muscles except the cricothyroid. The superior laryngeal nerve (also a branch of the vagus) runs with the superior thyroid vessels and supplies the cricothyroid muscles (external branch), which tense the vocal cords. The recurrent nerve also supplies sensation to the larynx below the vocal cords. The internal branch of the superior laryngeal nerve provides sensation above the cords. Normal sensory and motor function within the larynx is necessary for speech and coughing. Both nerves are at risk of damage during thyroid surgery and the consequences, if permanent, can be disabling.

Thyroid function

Histologically, the gland is made up of follicles containing colloid. The follicles are spheroids lined by cuboidal epithelium (thyrocytes). The parafollicular or C cells may be seen between follicles. The gland has a rich blood supply. The thyrocytes secrete triiodothyronine (T_3) and thyroxine (T_4). T_3 is the active hormone, and T_4 is converted to T_3 in the periphery.

Secretion of T_3 and T_4 is controlled by thyroid-stimulating hormone (TSH), which is secreted by the anterior pituitary. TSH release is in turn controlled by thyrotropin-releasing hormone (TRH) from the hypothalamus. Circulating levels of T_3 and T_4 exert a negative feedback effect on the hypothalamus and anterior pituitary. Calcitonin, which is released by the parafollicular cells following stimulation by ingested food, lowers the serum calcium but it is not an essential hormone and does not require replacement after total thyroidectomy.

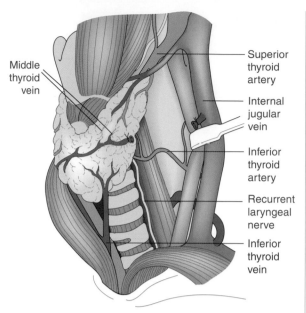

Fig. 20.1 Anatomy of the thyroid gland. The middle thyroid vein has been divided to allow forward rotation of the left lobe of the gland.

Middle thyroid vein

Superior thyroid artery

Internal jugular vein

Inferior thyroid artery

Recurrent laryngeal nerve

Inferior thyroid vein

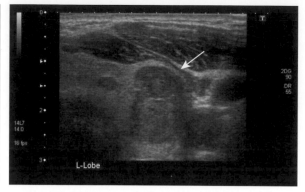

Fig. 20.3 Ultrasound demonstrating thyroid nodule (arrowed).

Enlargement of the thyroid gland (goitre)

Clinical features

Goitre is a visible or palpable enlargement of the thyroid (Fig. 20.4). The swelling appears in the lower part of the neck and retains the shape of the normal gland (*thyreos* – Greek for shield). The swelling characteristically moves upwards on swallowing because of the gland's attachment to the trachea. Patients may have a dry mouth, and when asking them to swallow, water should be provided.

Assessment of thyroid disease

Measurement of T_3, T_4 and TSH gives a biochemical estimation of thyroid function. TSH is totally suppressed in thyrotoxicosis and elevated in hypothyroidism. Pregnancy or oestrogen administration increases the level of thyroid-binding globulin, so that estimation of the ratio of free to bound hormone may be needed. TRH and TSH stimulation tests may be required to determine the site of failure of production of thyroid hormones.

The thyroid can be imaged by ultrasonography (Fig. 20.3) or radioisotope scanning (^{99m}Tc-sodium pertechnetate behaves like iodine and is 'trapped' by the gland). The main value of scanning is to differentiate between 'hot' (actively functioning), 'cool' (normally functioning) and 'cold' (non-functioning) thyroid nodules. Total isotope uptake also reflects thyroid activity.

Magnetic resonance imaging (MRI) and computed tomography (CT) provide excellent means of determining the extent of goitre. Fine-needle aspiration cytology is used to determine the nature of thyroid nodules. Thyroid antibodies detected in significant titre may indicate autoimmune thyroid disease.

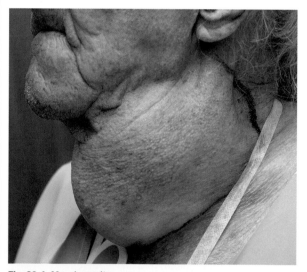

Fig. 20.4 Massive goitre.

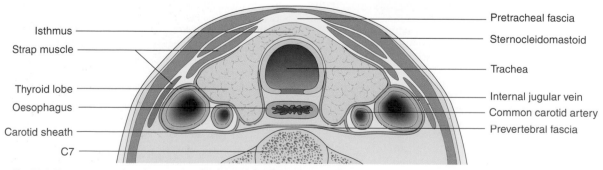

Isthmus

Strap muscle

Thyroid lobe

Oesophagus

Carotid sheath

C7

Pretracheal fascia

Sternocleidomastoid

Trachea

Internal jugular vein

Common carotid artery

Prevertebral fascia

Fig. 20.2 Transverse section of the neck at the level of the 7th cervical vertebra to show the arrangement of the deep cervical fascia.

'Physiological' enlargement

Transient enlargement may occur during puberty or pregnancy.

Non-toxic nodular goitre

Aetiology

This common disease occurs endemically in areas of iodine deficiency, but can be sporadic or a reaction to drugs. It occurs much more commonly in females. In the past, lack of iodine in the diet was a common cause of thyroid enlargement, but 'endemic goitres' in populations where iodine was deficient are now rare because table salt is iodized.

Pathology

In iodine deficiency, the gland initially enlarges diffusely as the follicles fill with colloid. Later, multiple nodules develop, some of which contain abundant colloid; others show degenerative changes, with the formation of cysts, areas of old and new haemorrhage, and even calcification. The goitre varies greatly in size, from little more than normal to weighing several hundred grams. The whole gland may be involved, or the changes may be confined to one lobe.

Clinical features

Most multinodular goitres are asymptomatic. Others cause tracheal compression and dyspnoea, particularly when they extend behind the sternum (retrosternal goitre). Oesophageal compression can cause dysphagia. Very rarely, bleeding into a nodule may cause pain and rapid enlargement and, for retrosternal goitre, respiratory distress. The thyroid is visibly enlarged and multiple nodules are usually palpable. Sometimes only one nodule is palpable, giving the erroneous impression of a solitary nodule.

Investigations

In the case of retrosternal goitre, plain films of the thoracic inlet may reveal tracheal deviation (Fig. 20.5A) and CT may show tracheal compression (Fig. 20.5B) The presence of stridor indicates compromise of the tracheal lumen. T_3, T_4 and TSH are usually normal and that being the case isotope scans are not indicated.

Management

The administration of thyroxine rarely prevents further gland enlargement via the negative feedback loop. Large goitres and those causing symptoms of compression require total or subtotal thyroidectomy. Some patients request surgery for cosmetic reasons. Patients usually choose total thyroidectomy with lifelong replacement therapy in preference to the high chance of recurrence and the need for reoperation with subtotal thyroidectomy.

Thyrotoxic goitre

Diffuse thyroid enlargement can result from stimulation by TSH or TSH-like proteins, resulting in increased production of T_3 and T_4 and thyrotoxicosis.

SUMMARY BOX 20.1

Goitres

- Physiological thyroid enlargement may occur during puberty or pregnancy
- Non-toxic nodular goitre can be associated with iodine deficiency and drug reactions; it is usually asymptomatic but can cause compression symptoms
- Thyrotoxic goitre results from stimulation of the gland by TSH or TSH-like proteins, resulting in excessive production of T_3 and T_4. About 25% of cases of thyrotoxicosis are due to a toxic multinodular goitre (a long-standing non-toxic goitre develops hyperactive nodule(s) that function independently of TSH levels)
- Thyroiditis can produce diffuse painful swelling that may be subacute (de Quervain's disease) or autoimmune (Hashimoto's disease). Riedel's thyroiditis is a very rare cause of painless thyroid swelling and tracheal compression
- A solitary thyroid nodule is often a conspicuous palpable nodule in a multinodular goitre. True solitary nodules may be adenomas, cysts or cancers, conditions that are distinguished by fine-needle aspiration cytology, ultrasonography, isotope scans and function tests
- Thyroid cancers can produce a goitre, particularly in the case of medullary carcinoma of the thyroid and lymphoma.

20

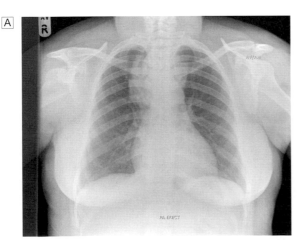

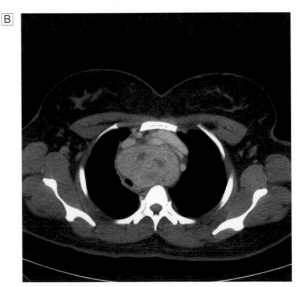

Fig. 20.5 Retrosternal goitre images showing marked tracheal deviation. **A** Plain X-ray. **B** CT.

20

Thyroiditis

Subacute thyroiditis (de Quervain's disease)

This rare condition is associated with an influenza-like illness, during which there is painful diffuse swelling of the gland. Thyroid antibodies may appear in the serum. The disease may be due to a viral infection and usually resolves spontaneously.

Autoimmune thyroiditis (Hashimoto's disease)

Aetiology

This condition is believed to be due to the destruction of thyroid follicles by lymphocytes. Antibodies are detected in the serum against thyroglobulin, thyroid cell cytosol and microsomes. Histologically, there is marked lymphocytic infiltration around destroyed follicles.

Clinical features

The patient is usually euthyroid, but early in the disease thyrotoxicosis can occur. In the long term, the patient becomes hypothyroid as the gland is progressively destroyed. Postmenopausal women are most commonly affected (female:male ratio 10:1). The thyroid is diffusely enlarged and firm. A nodular form may be confused with multinodular goitre. Lymphoma may occur in a thyroid that has been affected by long-standing Hashimoto's disease.

Investigations

The diagnosis is made by demonstrating antithyroid antibodies, particularly to microsomal components of the follicle cells. Biopsy for cytology helps to confirm the diagnosis.

Management

Thyroidectomy is seldom needed and can be difficult because of the firm nature of the gland and inflammation of the surrounding structures. There is a higher than normal risk of damage to the recurrent laryngeal nerves or parathyroid glands.

Riedel's thyroiditis

In this very rare condition the thyroid is replaced by dense fibrous tissue, resulting in a firm painless swelling and tracheal compression. The cause is unknown. Surgery is reliably difficult but decompression of the trachea may be required.

Solitary thyroid nodules

Slow-growing and painless clinically 'solitary' nodules are common, although 50% of them are really part of a multinodular goitre. Of the true solitary nodules, half are benign adenomas and the rest are cysts or differentiated cancers. The pivotal diagnostic test is fine-needle aspiration cytology, complemented by ultrasonography, isotope scans and thyroid function tests (Fig. 20.6). Cysts can be aspirated and, provided that they do not refill and that the cytology is negative for neoplastic cells, they need not be removed. Very rarely, a cyst contains a carcinoma (often papillary) within its wall, and blood-stained aspirate or a residual swelling after aspiration should raise this possibility. A cytopathologist cannot distinguish between a follicular adenoma and follicular carcinoma; this can only be achieved on definitive histopathology by looking for capsular or vascular invasion. Diagnostic surgery is needed if aspiration reveals a follicular neoplasm. Intraoperative frozen section does not always provide a definitive diagnosis, but the demonstration of carcinoma by whatever means indicates that more extensive surgery may be needed (e.g. complete total thyroidectomy).

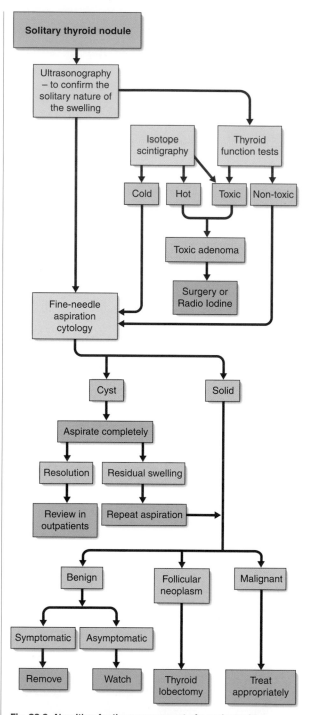

Fig. 20.6 Algorithm for the management of a patient with a suspected solitary thyroid nodule.

Other forms of neoplasia

All forms of thyroid cancer can produce goitre. Lymphoma and anaplastic tumours may cause diffuse thyroid swellings. Medullary and follicular tumours are often solitary swellings.

Hyperthyroidism

Thyrotoxicosis results from the overproduction of T_3 and T_4 and, because of the feedback mechanism, serum TSH levels are reduced or undetectable. The three conditions that may produce thyrotoxicosis are primary thyrotoxicosis (Graves' disease), toxic multinodular goitre and toxic adenoma.

Primary thyrotoxicosis (Graves' disease)

Pathophysiology

This condition accounts for 75% of cases. It is an autoimmune disease in which TSH receptors in the thyroid are stimulated by circulating thyroid receptor antibodies (TRAbs). The gland is uniformly hyperactive, very vascular and usually symmetrically enlarged. Histologically, there is marked epithelial proliferation, with papillary projections into follicles devoid of colloid. TRAbs can cross the placental barrier, so that neonatal thyrotoxicosis can occur.

Clinical features

The patient is usually a young female (male:female ratio 1:8) and the condition can be familial. The thyroid is usually moderately and diffusely enlarged and soft, and because of its vascularity a bruit may be audible. High circulating levels of T_3 and T_4 increase the basal metabolic rate and potentiate the actions of the sympathetic nervous system.

Metabolic effects

The patient feels hot at rest and heat intolerant. The skin is moist and warm because of peripheral vasodilatation and excess sweating. Weight loss is the rule, despite an increased appetite. Cardiac output is increased to meet the metabolic demands.

Sympathetic effects

Tachycardia is present, even during sleep. Palpitations can be troublesome, and cardiac irregularities and arrhythmias (especially atrial fibrillation) are common in older patients. The hands exhibit a fine tremor. The upper eyelids are retracted (the levator palpebrae superioris has some non-striated muscle which is innervated by the sympathetic nervous system) and there is lid lag. Gastrointestinal motility is increased. There is general hyperkinesia; anxiety and psychiatric disturbance may occur.

Other features

Exophthalmos is usual but not invariable (Fig. 20.7). Ophthalmoplegia, pretibial myxoedema, proximal muscle myopathy and finger clubbing are sometimes present. Menstrual irregularity and infertility can occur.

Diagnosis

The diagnosis is usually obvious clinically, although in patients with anxiety, distinction from neurosis can be difficult. Raised T_3 and T_4 levels, coupled with low TSH levels, are confirmatory. The TSH response to intravenous injection of TRH is absent owing to atrophy of the TSH-producing cells of the pituitary.

Management

Antithyroid drugs

These drugs block the incorporation of iodine into tyrosine and so prevent the synthesis of T_3 and T_4. Carbimazole, given in full blocking doses (30–60 mg daily in four divided doses), can render the patient euthyroid within 4–6 weeks. However, up to 60% of patients will relapse within 2 years of stopping treatment.

Radioactive iodine

Many consider this to be the treatment of choice. As long as it is not used in pregnancy, the risks of genetic damage are minimal in both patients and their offspring. If ablative doses of iodine are used, patients require thyroxine replacement, but can lead an otherwise normal life with little risk of recurrence.

Surgery

Thyroidectomy is a highly successful form of treatment for many patients, especially younger ones. In experienced hands, operative mortality and morbidity are low. Patients are cured by surgery, total thyroidectomy being the operation of choice.

Before surgery, patients must be rendered euthyroid with antithyroid drugs. Iodine has historically been given orally for 10 days before surgery to reduce vascularity, but the evidence base to support this is weak. β-Adrenergic blocking drugs can be used as an alternative means of countering the effects of thyrotoxicosis before operation. They block sympathetic over-activity and make the gland less vascular. Cardiac failure, obstructive airways disease and diabetes (where they may mask hypoglycaemic symptoms) are contraindications to the use of β-blockers. Propranolol is given in a dose of 40–80 mg 6-hourly, the aim being to reduce the pulse rate to below 80 beats per minute. Long-acting preparations may be preferred. The drug is continued on the morning of operation and for 7 days thereafter to avoid 'thyroid storm' or 'thyrotoxic crisis'. Excessive sweating or tachycardia after operation is an indication to increase the dose.

Toxic multinodular goitre and toxic adenoma

Pathophysiology

A toxic multinodular goitre is responsible for thyrotoxicosis in about 25% of patients. There is usually a long-standing non-toxic goitre in which one or more nodules become hyperactive and begin to hyperfunction independently of TSH levels. A single hyperfunctioning adenoma is a rare cause of thyrotoxicosis (1–2% of patients). The adenoma secretes thyroid hormones autonomously; TSH secretion and the remainder of the gland are suppressed.

Clinical features

Toxic multinodular goitre is more common in older women, and cardiac complications such as arrhythmias are particularly frequent. Eye signs are rare in these patients.

Diagnosis

In a toxic multinodular goitre, the isotope scan demonstrates one or more areas of increased uptake. In toxic adenoma, the nodule is 'hot' and the remainder of the gland is 'cold'.

Management

Treatment consists of removal of the hyperfunctioning glandular tissue by total thyroidectomy (multinodular goitre) or lobectomy (toxic adenoma), or if surgery is contraindicated, radioiodine.

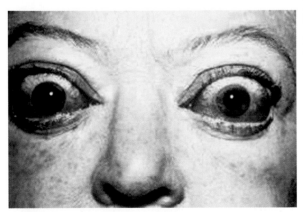

Fig. 20.7 Thyroid-associated ophthalmopathy. (Courtesy of Prof Michael Sheppard, University of Birmingham Medical School.)

20

20

Malignant tumours of the thyroid

Thyroid cancer accounts for less than 1% of all forms of malignancy. As with all thyroid disease, females are more often affected (male:female ratio 1:3). The two main types of thyroid carcinoma are papillary (50%) and follicular (30%), with the remainder comprising medullary carcinoma, anaplastic carcinoma and lymphoma (EBM 20.1). The incidence of thyroid cancer is increased by exposure to ionizing radiation: for example, following the Chernobyl disaster.

EBM	20.1 Relevant websites and publications for the management of thyroid cancer are:

- www.aace.com/pub/guidelines/index.php American Association of Endocrine Surgeons, thyroid_carcinoma guidelines.
- www.baets.org.uk/Pages/guidelines/.php British Association of Endocrine and Thyroid Surgeons.
- www.british-thyroid-association.org National thyroid cancer guidelines group of the British Thyroid Association.
- Northern Cancer Network. Guidelines for management of thyroid cancer. Clinical Oncology 2000; 12:373–391.

Papillary carcinoma

Clinical features

This tumour is most prevalent before the age of 40 years and presents as a slow-growing solitary thyroid swelling. Enlarged lymph nodes are palpable in one-third of patients and may be the only finding in some patients with a microscopic primary (the so-called 'lateral aberrant thyroid'). Distant metastases are rare. In thyroid glands resected for non-malignant causes, microscopic papillary carcinoma is discovered as an incidental finding in up to 20%. Histologically, complex papillary folds lined by several layers of cuboidal cells project into what appear to be cystic spaces.

Management

The disease is commonly multifocal, so bilateral total lobectomy is commonly indicated. Microscopic disease (< 1cm and unifocal) and tumours with favourable histology and < 2cm in size may be treated by single lobectomy alone.

Involved lymph nodes, usually identified by preoperative ultrasound scanning, are removed according to selective anatomical compartments, but routine radical neck dissection is unnecessary. Thyroid replacement therapy (T_3, 20 μg 6–8-hourly, or thyroxine 150 μg/day) is given with the intention of suppressing TSH. Widespread metastases are rare but may be amenable to radioactive iodine therapy. For this reason an isotope scan should be performed postoperatively to identify any iodine uptake in the neck or elsewhere. The disease has an excellent prognosis, with 10-year survival rates approaching 90%.

Follicular carcinoma

Clinical features

This disease typically presents as a solitary thyroid nodule in patients aged 30–50 years. Lymph node metastases are much less common than haematogenous spread, with deposits in the lungs, bone or liver (Fig. 20.8). Histologically, malignant cells are arranged in solid masses with rudimentary acini. Vascular and capsular invasion characterize this neoplasm and distinguish it from a benign follicular adenoma.

Management

Treatment consists of total thyroidectomy with preservation of the parathyroids. If a postoperative radioisotope scan (challenge scan) reveals increased uptake in the skeleton or neck, therapeutic doses of radioiodine are given. Prior to challenge scanning the short half-life hormone T3 should be given and once all treatment is completed T_4 is administered to suppress TSH secretion. Plasma thyroglobulin levels should be undetectable after surgery and radioiodine therapy. Subsequent detection of thyroglobulin indicates recurrent disease. The disease is more aggressive than papillary carcinoma and the 10-year survival rate is 75%.

Anaplastic carcinoma

Clinical features

These rapidly growing, highly malignant tumours tend to occur in older patients. Local invasion may involve the recurrent laryngeal nerve(s) and cause hoarseness, the trachea causing dyspnoea and stridor, and the oesophagus causing dysphagia. Invasion of the cervical sympathetic nerves may cause Horner's syndrome (contraction of the

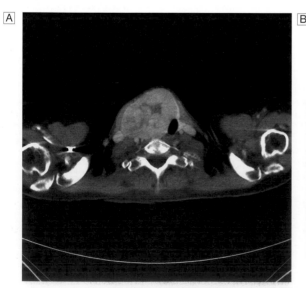

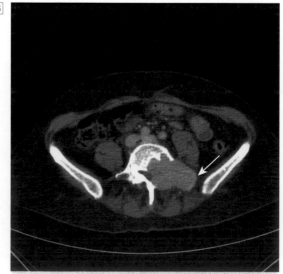

Fig. 20.8 Metastatic follicular cancer. **A** Primary tumour. **B** Bony metastases (arrowed).

pupil, enophthalmos, narrowing of the palpebral fissure and loss of sweating on the face and neck). Pulmonary metastases are common.

Management

Resection is rarely appropriate but surgery can relieve tracheal compression. External beam radiotherapy may be of value but chemotherapy seldom is.

Medullary carcinoma

Clinical features

This tumour arises from the parafollicular C cells. There is hard enlargement of one or both thyroid lobes, and in 50% of patients the cervical lymph nodes are involved. The tumour may occur sporadically or as part of an inherited multiple endocrine neoplasia (MEN) syndrome type II (Sipple's syndrome). Calcitonin levels are elevated, and can be used to monitor progress and screen relatives. The gene causing the inherited form of this tumour is the *Ret* proto-oncogene, and the finding of a mutation allows the diagnosis to be made at any age. Prophylactic thyroidectomy for affected children is recommended at different ages depending on the specific mutation and level of risk associated with that mutation. This varies from age 1 for the 918 mutation through to age 5 for the commonest 634 mutation and in some good prognosis families may be delayed to age 13.

Management

Treatment consists of total thyroidectomy and, if the calcitonin level is raised, dissection of the lymph nodes in the central compartment of the neck (levels 6 and 7). Medullary carcinoma in MEN IIb syndrome (918 mutation) is particularly aggressive, and those affected rarely live beyond 30–40 years of age. Other forms, e.g. pure inherited medullary thyroid cancer occurring without other endocrine tumours, can be very indolent. Preoperative CT of the neck and mediastinum is advised and the exclusion of a phaeochromocytoma before neck surgery is mandatory.

Lymphoma

Primary lymphoma of the thyroid is a rare complication of autoimmune thyroiditis. It can also occur as a primary tumour that originates in an otherwise normal gland. It is amenable to treatment by radiotherapy and chemotherapy, but patients often require core biopsy of the gland to characterize the type of lymphoma. CT is used to stage the disease fully.

Thyroidectomy

Technique

The gland is exposed through a transverse skin-crease incision placed 2–3 cm above the sternal notch. The deep cervical fascia is divided longitudinally in the midline and the strap muscles are separated. Each lobe is mobilized by dividing the vessels supplying the superior pole, the middle and inferior thyroid veins, and the inferior thyroid artery. It is quick, easy and safe to do this using for example the harmonic scalpel in place of ligatures or clips. The recurrent laryngeal nerves should be identified, so that they can be protected from injury. Generally nothing less than a total lobectomy should be performed, to avoid the need for reoperation on that side. Care is taken to preserve the parathyroid glands. Haemostasis must be meticulous and drains are rarely necessary. The layers of the neck are reconstituted with continuous absorbable sutures and the skin with a subcuticular suture. Minimally invasive thyroidectomy is being explored in the minority of very small goiters.

> ### SUMMARY BOX 20.2
>
> **Thyroid cancer**
>
> - Thyroid cancers may arise from the epithelium (papillary 50%, follicular 30%). Remainder comprise anaplastic, parafollicular C cells (medullary carcinoma) or lymphoreticular tissue (lymphoma)
> - Papillary cancers are rare after the age of 40 years, are often multifocal and spread to lymph nodes, but rarely disseminate widely. Total or near-total thyroidectomy with the removal of involved nodes may be followed by radioiodine, and thyroid replacement therapy to suppress TSH. Ten-year survival rates approach 90%
> - Follicular carcinoma occurs in the 30–50-year age group, spreads preferentially via the bloodstream, and is treated by total thyroidectomy. Residual neck or skeletal radioisotope uptake signals the need for radioiodine therapy. T_4 is used routinely to suppress TSH production. The 10-year survival rate is 75%
> - Anaplastic carcinoma occurs in older patients, spreads locally and frequently gives rise to pulmonary metastases. Curative resection is rarely possible, radiotherapy/chemotherapy is of little value, and most patients die within 1 year
> - Medullary carcinomas secrete calcitonin, may involve both lobes, and involve neck nodes. They may be sporadic or part of MEN II. Treatment consists of total thyroidectomy and node dissection.

Complications

Haemorrhage

Early secondary haemorrhage should not occur if meticulous haemostasis is achieved before closure. If bleeding does occur, it can compress structures in the thoracic inlet, leading to venous engorgement, laryngeal oedema, tracheal compression and asphyxia. The wound must be reopened urgently prior to intubation and return to theatre.

Nerve damage

The external branch of the superior laryngeal nerve may be damaged while securing the superior thyroid pedicle causing inability to tense the vocal cord and a weaker voice with noticeable pitch range changes. Anaesthesia of the mucous membrane of the upper larynx allows foreign bodies to enter the larynx more readily.

Damage to the recurrent laryngeal nerve is more serious. Traction or bruising of this nerve causes temporary paralysis of a vocal cord in 1% of patients undergoing thyroidectomy, but recovery within 3 months is the rule. Division of the nerve paralyses the cord in the 'cadaveric' position (i.e. midway between the closed and open positions). The normal cord on the other side compensates by crossing the midline in phonation, but the voice is altered in timbre, hoarse, weak and breathy. Some degree of stridor, especially on exertion, may be noted.

Bilateral nerve injury results in stridor and ineffective coughing when the endotracheal tube is withdrawn at the end of the operation. The tube is reinserted immediately and, if there is no early improvement, tracheostomy may be required. The paralysis is originally flaccid, but fibrosis draws the cords together and, even if tracheostomy has been avoided, increasing dyspnoea on exertion may be troublesome. Laryngoplasty may be needed to reconstitute the cords, but if this fails, permanent tracheostomy may be unavoidable.

20

Hypothyroidism

Thyroid function is monitored after unilateral lobectomy in case replacement therapy is needed. After total thyroidectomy, replacement therapy should commence the following day. A standard dose for adults is 150 mg thyroxine daily, adjusted according to clinical findings and thyroid function tests.

Hypoparathyroidism

Bruising or accidental removal of the parathyroid glands leads to hypoparathyroidism, manifest by hypocalcaemia and symptoms of increased neuromuscular excitability. Early symptoms are tingling or numbness around the mouth and in the fingers. Hypercontractility can be demonstrated in the muscles of facial expression by tapping the facial (VII) nerve over the parotid gland (Chvostek's sign). In extreme cases, tetany may develop. Serum calcium must be checked 24 hours after thyroid surgery. Hypocalcaemic symptoms, or serum calcium less than 2.0 mmol/l, require calcium supplements. Severe hypoparathyroidism may require vitamin D therapy as well. Serum calcium checks are required, with gradual withdrawal of supplements as the parathyroids recover. If supplementation is still necessary at 12 months, then the patient is likely to require lifelong treatment.

Scar complications

The scar can become hypertrophic or keloid, particularly when the incision has been placed low in the neck. Recurrent keloid formation is common after excision of the scar (with or without steroid infiltration), and reoperation is not advised lightly.

Patient information

A forewarned patient is much less aggrieved than one who learns about previously unmentioned complications on the first postoperative day. Full informed consent should be obtained by the surgeon who will carry out the procedure and should describe the potential complications with their own complication rates and information on how these compare with national averages. Explanations should be given in simple language and should be full and honest. Written advice may better inform the patient who may have accessed the Internet which may not provide accurate and appropriate information.

PARATHYROID GLANDS

Surgical anatomy

The parathyroid glands receive a rich blood supply from the inferior thyroid artery, the branches of which are a valuable guide to their position. Histologically, the glands contain chief cells that secrete parathormone (PTH).

Calcium metabolism

Plasma calcium levels are kept constant in the range 2.25–2.6 mmol/l by regulating the amounts absorbed from the intestine, deposited in or withdrawn from bone, and excreted in the urine. PTH and vitamin D are the main regulators, with minimal modulation by calcitonin.

Hypercalcaemia and hypocalcaemia

Hypercalcaemia is a common biochemical abnormality and may be due to many causes other than excess PTH secretion (Table 20.1). Similarly, hypocalcaemia may be due to causes other than parathyroid removal or damage (Table 20.2).

Table 20.1 Causes of hypercalcaemia

Hyperparathyroidism
- Primary
- Secondary
- Tertiary

Increased calcium absorption
- Vitamin D excess
- Sarcoidosis
- Drugs (e.g. diuretics, lithium)

Excessive bone breakdown
- Metastatic disease (particularly breast cancer)
- Myeloma
- Immobilization following multiple fractures

Ectopic secretion of parathyroid-like hormone
- Cancer of bronchus
- Cancer of breast

Table 20.2 Causes of hypocalcaemia

Hypoparathyroidism
- Thyroid surgery
- Parathyroid surgery

Hypoproteinaemia
- Nephrosis (excessive protein loss)
- Malnutrition (inadequate intake)
- Cirrhosis (deficient synthesis)
- Severe inflammation (e.g. burns, acute pancreatitis)

Vitamin D deficiency
- Pseudohypoparathyroidism

Primary hyperparathyroidism

Pathology

In 90% of patients, primary hyperparathyroidism is due to an adenoma, in 10% it results from hyperplasia (usually affecting all four glands), and in less than 1% it results from parathyroid carcinoma. Adenomas are normally small spherical brown nodules but can be 10 times larger than the normal gland. Most are single, but 20% of patients have multiple adenomas. Histologically, chief cells predominate. In hyperplasia, the gland is usually twice the normal weight, i.e. more than 70 mg.

Clinical features

Women are affected twice as often as men. The disease usually presents in middle age and is increasingly being diagnosed in asymptomatic patients found to have hypercalcaemia on routine biochemistry. If clinical manifestations occur, renal and bone effects predominate, including nephrocalcinosis (diffuse calcification) and urinary calculi. Polyuria is an early symptom of hyperparathyroidism.

Bone damage used to be common but is now rarely seen as the disease is diagnosed earlier. Gross demineralization, subperiosteal bone resorption (seen typically in the middle and distal phalanges of the fingers), cysts in the long bones and jaw, and the moth-eaten appearance of the skull gave rise to the descriptive term 'osteitis fibrosa cystica'. Multiple pathological fractures were also once common.

Other manifestations of hyperparathyroidism include peptic ulceration, acute and chronic pancreatitis, lethargy, muscle weakness and psychotic symptoms. The clinical picture of florid hyperparathyroidism is often summarized as one of 'bones, stones and groans'. Rarely, patients present with a hypercalcaemic crisis characterized by marked hypercalcaemia (> 3.5 mmol/l), mental confusion, nausea and vomiting. The vomiting increases pre-existing dehydration, leading to higher levels of serum calcium, more confusion and prostration, more dehydration, and so on. Urgent expert attention is required to reverse this vicious downward spiral. The most pressing need is to correct the dehydration. The calcium may be further reduced by the use of bisphosphonates.

Diagnosis

If hyperparathyroidism is suspected, serum calcium and PTH levels must be measured on more than one occasion. PTH levels may be normal, but the detection of PTH in a patient with hypercalcaemia supports the diagnosis of primary hyperparathyroidism. Other supportive findings include a low serum phosphate, hyperchloraemia (and an abnormal Cl/PO_4 ratio), and a raised 24-hour urinary calcium excretion. A low urinary calcium excretion should alert the clinician to the possibility of familial hypercalcaemic hypocalciuria, a disease of the renal tubules in which the parathyroids are normal. Alkaline phosphatase (skeletal) levels may be raised, even if there is no radiological evidence of bone disease.

Management

The aim of treatment is to identify and remove all overactive parathyroid tissue. Preoperative imaging with ultrasound and MIBI scans will allow selection of patients for a focused approach. Concordant scans permit a direct targeted incision over the suspected adenoma, with or without frozen section confirmation and intraoperative PTH monitoring. The latter two intraoperative tests are not employed by all surgeons and rarely make a difference to the outcome of surgery enough to justify their expense. With discordant imaging or associated multinodular goiter and previous neck surgery, traditional cervicotomy and four-gland exploration will be required. If two or more glands are enlarged, they should be removed. If all four glands are thought to be hyperplastic, then all but a portion of the smallest gland should be removed. If exploration fails to identify an adenoma or hyperplasia, the incision is closed. Reoperation is considered after (re)confirming the diagnosis and attempting to localize the gland using CT, MRI or selective venous catheterization (Fig. 20.9). Recurrent hyper-parathyroidism is approached in the same way but repeating first ultrasound and MIBI scans.

Secondary and tertiary hyperparathyroidism

In secondary hyperparathyroidism, there is over-secretion of PTH in response to low plasma levels of ionized calcium, usually because of renal disease or malabsorption. This is an increasing problem in patients on long-term dialysis for chronic renal failure. It is managed initially by giving 1-α-hydroxyvitamin D_3 (alfacalcidol) to increase calcium absorption and provide negative feedback on the parathyroids.

Excessive PTH secretion in secondary hyperparathyroidism may become autonomous; it is then termed tertiary hyperparathyroidism. This may occur after renal transplantation. Total parathyroidectomy may be needed, with calcium and vitamin D replacement therapy, subtotal parathyroidectomy leaving half equivalent of a normal gland in situ or autotransplantation of parathyroid tissue (equivalent in size to one normal gland) into an arm muscle (where it can be readily located if problems persist). Postoperatively, alfacalcidol and calcium are continued to heal bone disease and reduce the risk of recurrent hyperparathyroidism.

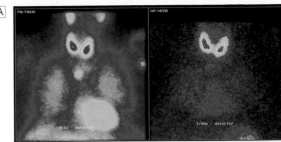
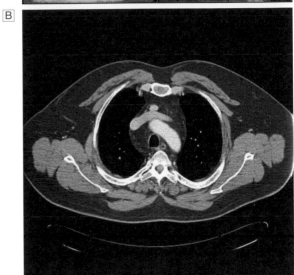

Fig. 20.9 Images of mediastinal parathyroid tissue. MIBI scan. **B** CT.

SUMMARY BOX 20.3

Hyperparathyroidism

- Serum calcium levels are normally controlled by parathormone (mobilizes calcium from bone, and increases renal calcium absorption and phosphate excretion) and vitamin D (promotes absorption from the intestine and augments effect of parathyroid hormone (PTH) on osteoclasts), with an uncertain contribution from calcitonin
- Hyperparathyroidism may be primary (90% adenoma, 10% hyperplasia, 1% carcinoma), secondary to renal disease/malabsorption (low serum Ca^{2+} triggers PTH secretion) or tertiary (development of autonomous secretion in secondary hyperparathyroidism)
- Hyperparathyroidism is now normally diagnosed while asymptomatic, but can produce renal effects (nephrocalcinosis, calculi and failure), skeletal effects (demineralization), gastrointestinal upsets (peptic ulcer, pancreatitis) and psychotic symptoms, i.e. 'stones, bones and groans'
- The diagnosis of primary hyperparathyroidism is supported by detection of circulating PTH in the presence of hypercalcaemia
- Primary hyperparathyroidism is treated surgically by removing an adenoma. If all four glands are involved by hyperplasia, all but a portion of one gland is removed.

20

Hypoparathyroidism

Hypoparathyroidism may occur temporarily after parathyroidectomy until the suppressed residual glands assume normal function. A fall in ionized calcium levels gives rise to paraesthesiae ('pins and needles') in the hands and feet, and muscle cramps and spasms (tetany) that cause bunching and flexion of the fingers and toes. Respiratory obstruction with stridor due to spasm of the laryngeal muscles can prove fatal. Clinical signs include Chvostek's sign (twitching of the facial muscles on tapping of the facial nerve), Trousseau's sign (spasm of hand and forearm muscles after applying a tourniquet to occlude the pulse) and Erb's sign (hyperexcitability of muscles on electrical stimulation). The patient is lethargic and depressed. Blood levels of ionized calcium and PTH are low, and the electrocardiogram (ECG) shows a lengthened Q–T interval. Acute hypoparathyroidism is treated with intravenous calcium gluconate (20 ml of a 10% solution given intravenously diluted in 100 ml of saline) 4-hourly until calcium levels rise. Oral calcium (effervescent calcium gluconate) and if required vitamin D (cholecalciferol) are prescribed according to serial blood calcium levels.

Parathyroidectomy

Patient information

In order to provide informed consent, it is important that patients understand several aspects of the glands and the disease, specifically:

- the variable position of the glands
- the function of the glands
- the results of hyperfunction: renal effects, bone disease and systemic effects
- that only one gland is likely to be diseased and overactive, and that this is very rarely malignant (< 1%)
- that surgery will attempt to remove the abnormal gland but may fail to locate it because it is in an ectopic position
- that there may be a need for calcium and vitamin D supplements after surgery.

PITUITARY GLAND

Surgical anatomy

The pituitary gland is small and weighs about 500 mg. It is enclosed within a bony shell, the sella turcica, which is sealed superiorly by a fold of dura mater, the diaphragma sellae. The pituitary stalk connects the pituitary to the hypothalamus. The pituitary has two parts: the anterior pituitary (adenohypophysis) and the posterior pituitary (neurohypophysis) (Fig. 20.10).

Anterior pituitary

The anterior pituitary develops from an epithelial outgrowth from the pharynx (Rathke's pouch). Some cells are thought to be of neural crest origin and belong to the APUD (amine and precursor uptake and decarboxylation) system. The anterior pituitary contains solid cords of secreting cells that used to be classified as acidophil, basophil or chromophobe on staining with haematoxylin and eosin. On the basis of immunofluorescence and other specific stains, these are now subdivided into cell types that secrete (Fig. 20.11):

- the polypeptides: growth hormone (GH), prolactin (PRL) and adrenocorticotrophic hormone (ACTH)
- the glycoproteins: luteinizing hormone (LH), follicle-stimulating hormone (FSH) and TSH.

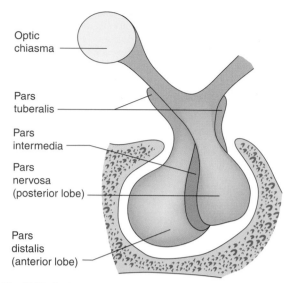

Fig. 20.10 Sagittal section through the pituitary gland.

Optic chiasma

Pars tuberalis

Pars intermedia

Pars nervosa (posterior lobe)

Pars distalis (anterior lobe)

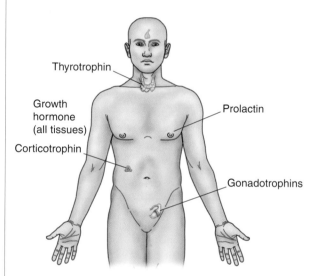

Fig. 20.11 The anterior pituitary hormones and their target organs.

Thyrotrophin

Growth hormone (all tissues)

Corticotrophin

Prolactin

Gonadotrophins

The hypophysial stalk contains a portal venous system that connects capillaries in the median eminence of the hypothalamus with capillaries and sinusoids of the anterior pituitary. This system carries neurosecretory hormones that stimulate or inhibit specific endocrine cells in the pituitary. The most important messengers are GH-releasing and inhibiting factors, corticotrophin-releasing factor (CRF), gonadotrophin-releasing hormone (GnRH), TRH and prolactin-inhibiting factor (PIF). If the portal tract is divided, the secretion of all anterior pituitary hormones is suppressed, with the exception of prolactin, the secretion of which is increased. A number of feedback loops ensure that the secretion of pituitary hormones is adjusted to need.

Tumours of the anterior pituitary

Pathophysiology

Functioning pituitary adenomas may result from over-stimulation by hypothalamic factors. Initially small and confined within the gland (microadenomas), they grow slowly and can ultimately expand the sella turcica. Eccentric enlargement is common. Upward extension of the adenoma may

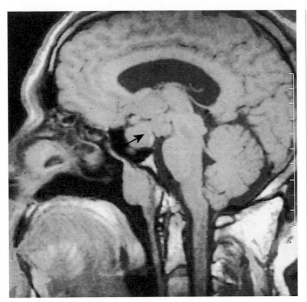

Fig. 20.12 MRI scan showing a pituitary tumour (arrow).

stretch the diaphragm or herniate through it, to compress the optic chiasma and cause visual defects. It is therefore important that pituitary adenomas are detected before they enlarge the fossa or extend above it. CT with contrast enhancement and MRI (Fig. 20.12) are used to image the tumour. Three endocrine syndromes caused by anterior pituitary disorders have surgical relevance.

Acromegaly

Excess secretion of GH occurs most often in early adult life and results in overgrowth of the soft tissues of the hands, feet and face. This gives the patient 'large extremities' and a characteristically coarse face, with bulging supraorbital ridges and a protruding jaw. Endochondral ossification and periosteal new bone formation account for some of these changes. All viscera are enlarged and there is muscle hypertrophy, although muscle weakness and cardiac failure develop later. The skin is coarse and greasy and acne is common. Headaches, sweating and the carpal tunnel syndrome often develop. Glucose tolerance is impaired and galactorrhoea can occur in females. GH and somatomedin levels are increased, and glucose or a meal does not suppress their secretion.

Treatment is directed at restoring GH levels to normal. For small adenomas, transsphenoidal removal is the treatment of choice. Although bromocriptine inhibits GH release, it achieves normal levels in only 20% of patients with acromegaly. Somatostatin analogues offer a more effective way of normalizing GH levels and can be used to reduce the size of macroadenomas or to treat recurrent or residual tumour.

Hyperprolactinaemia

Prolactin is the most common hormone secreted by pituitary tumours. Hypersecretion results in galactorrhoea and amenorrhoea (owing to the suppression of gonadotrophin secretion) in young women, whereas in men gynaecomastia and impotence may occur. Basal levels of prolactin are high, the nocturnal increase is absent, and the response to TRH is diminished. It is important to exclude other causes of hyperprolactinaemia, notably the administration of drugs such as metoclopramide.

To preserve pituitary function in younger patients, small adenomas are enucleated and larger tumours are treated by bromocriptine, with monitoring to ensure that tumour expansion does not threaten visual integrity.

Cushing's disease

This may be due to a functioning adenoma of ACTH-secreting cells. Only 15% of patients show expansion of the pituitary fossa. Removal of the microadenoma or its irradiation will relieve symptoms. Unsuccessful surgery may require bilateral adrenalectomy (removal of end organs) to terminate the syndrome of hypercortisolism, with its widespread destructive systemic effects.

SUMMARY BOX 20.4

Tumours of the anterior pituitary gland

- May be detected while still small (microadenoma) or after it has expanded, often with upward extension to compress the optic chiasma
- The three endocrine syndromes that have surgical importance are acromegaly, hyperprolactinaemia and Cushing's disease
- Acromegaly is due to excessive secretion of growth hormone (GH). Somatostatin analogues (or bromocriptine) can be used to normalize GH levels. Small adenomas are treated by removal; radiotherapy can be used for larger inoperable tumours
- Hyperprolactinaemia causes galactorrhoea and amenorrhoea in females, and impotence and gynaecomastia in men. Small adenomas are usually enucleated, whereas larger tumours are treated by bromocriptine
- Cushing's disease may result from a functioning adenoma of ACTH-secreting cells, which is treated by removal or irradiation.

Surgical hypophysectomy

The transsphenoidal approach is preferred for the removal of a small adenoma. An operating microscope is used to approach the gland through the sphenoidal or ethmoidal sinuses (Fig. 20.13). Diabetes insipidus is rare. By placing a free flap of muscle in the fossa, cerebrospinal fluid (CSF) rhinorrhoea is prevented. The transcranial approach is a major neurosurgical procedure that results in loss of the sense of smell and the development of diabetes insipidus. It is now reserved for the removal of large tumours with suprasellar extension, often in combination with a transsphenoidal approach.

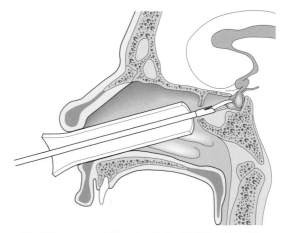

Fig. 20.13 Transsphenoidal removal of a pituitary adenoma.

20

Radiation therapy

The pituitary is comparatively radioresistant and at least 100 Gy are needed to affect the function of a normal gland. Smaller doses (40–50 Gy) are used to treat acromegaly and Cushing's disease. A rotational technique avoids excessive irradiation of surrounding neural tissue. Larger doses can be delivered by the narrow focused beam of heavy particles that are generated by a cyclotron.

Replacement therapy

After total hypophysectomy, replacement therapy is required for life (hydrocortisone 20 mg each morning and 10 mg each evening). All episodes of stress or trauma, including hypophysectomy itself, require additional steroid to cover the stress response. An alert wrist band should be given to patients who are steroid dependant. Aldosterone secretion is unaffected and there is no need for mineralocorticoid replacement. TSH secretion is suppressed and thyroxine must be given. Diabetes insipidus is a common but often transient complication of pituitary surgery or the insertion of radioactive implants. Vasopressin, or an analogue, relieves polyuria.

The posterior pituitary

Pathophysiology

The neurohypophysis is part of a secretory and storage unit that includes the nerve cells of the supraoptic and paraventricular hypothalamic nuclei (Fig. 20.14). Fibres pass from these nuclei via the hypothalamo-hypophysial tract to the median eminence of the hypothalamus and posterior pituitary. The nerve cells secrete arginine vasopressin (antidiuretic hormone, ADH) and oxytocin, both of which pass down the nerve fibres to be stored in vesicles in the pituitary. The close anatomical relationship of the anterior and posterior pituitary has functional significance in that oxytocin release during lactation is paralleled by increased TSH and prolactin production, and the posterior pituitary may influence prolactin secretion by dopamine release.

ADRENAL GLAND

Surgical anatomy and development

Each adrenal gland weighs approximately 4 g and lies immediately above and medial to the kidneys. The right adrenal lies in close contact with the inferior vena cava, into

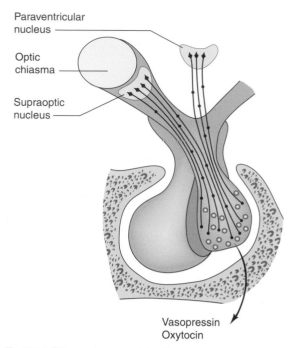

Fig. 20.14 The neurohypophysial system.

which it drains by a short wide vein that can be difficult to ligate at operation. The left adrenal vein drains into the left renal vein (Fig. 20.15). The glands are supplied by small vessels that arise from the aorta and the renal and inferior phrenic arteries.

Each gland has an outer cortex and inner medulla. The cortex, like the gonads, is derived from mesoderm, whereas the medulla is derived from the chromaffin ectodermal cells of the neural crest. The cortex secretes corticosteroids. The medulla is part of the sympathetic nervous system. Its APUD cells secrete the catecholamines, adrenaline (epinephrine), noradrenaline (norepinephrine) and dopamine, and are supplied by preganglionic sympathetic nerves.

Adrenal cortex

Cortical function

Microscopically, the adrenal cortex has three zones (Fig. 20.16). The outer zona glomerulosa secretes the mineralocorticoid, aldosterone. The zona fasciculata and zona

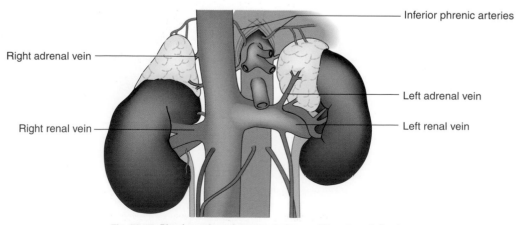

Fig. 20.15 Blood supply and venous drainage of the adrenal glands.

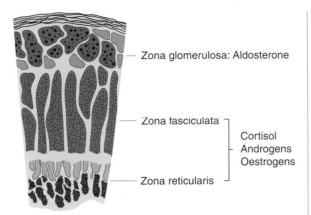

Zona glomerulosa: Aldosterone

Zona fasciculata ⎤
⎟ Cortisol
⎟ Androgens
⎥ Oestrogens
Zona reticularis ⎦

Fig. 20.16 Functional zones of the adrenal cortex.

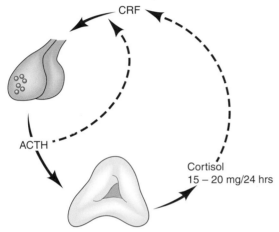

Fig. 20.17 Feedback loop in the control of cortisol secretion.
(ACTH = adrenocorticotrophic hormone; CRF = corticotrophin-releasing factor)

reticularis act as a functional unit and secrete glucocorticoids (cortisol and corticosterone) (Fig. 20.17), androgenic steroids (androstenedione, 11-hydroxy-androstenedione and testosterone) and the inactive androgen and oestrogen precursor, dehydroepiandrosterone sulphate (DHA-S). Precursors of aldosterone (Fig. 20.18) are also synthesized by the fasciculata-reticularis zone, as are small amounts of

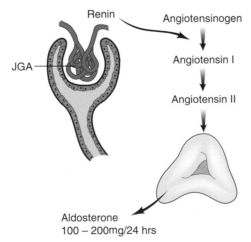

Fig. 20.18 Control of aldosterone secretion by the adrenal cortex.
(JGA = juxtaglomerular apparatus)

progesterone and oestrogen. Only a fraction of the amount of hormone needed daily is stored in the cortex. The hormones are, therefore, secreted 'to order' and circulate either free (5%) or bound to α-globulin.

SUMMARY BOX 20.5

Adrenocortical hormones

- Cortisol secretion is controlled by pituitary adrenocorticotrophic hormone (ACTH). Cortisol protects against stress, maintains blood pressure and aids recovery from injury/shock. Its metabolic activities include protein breakdown, increased gluconeogenesis, reduced glucose utilization and mobilization/redistribution of fat and water
- In excess, cortisol has mineralocorticoid activity, can cause psychosis, and has anti-inflammatory effects (used in transplantation immunosuppression)
- Aldosterone secretion is controlled mainly by angiotensin levels (and thus by renin release from the juxtaglomerular apparatus during decreased renal perfusion)
- Aldosterone conserves sodium (by facilitating its exchange for potassium and hydrogen ions in the kidney) and is a major determinant of extracellular fluid conservation
- Androgenic steroids and dehydroepiandrosterone sulphate (DHA-S) are also secreted by the adrenal cortex. DHA-S is converted to testosterone and oestrogen in fat and liver, and this peripheral aromatization is the main source of oestrogen in postmenopausal women.

Cushing's syndrome

This syndrome was first described by the American neurosurgeon, Harvey Cushing. It results from any prolonged and inappropriate exposure to cortisol and has the following causes (Fig. 20.19):

- *Tumours of the adrenal cortex* (20%). Benign adenoma is the most common adrenal cause of Cushing's syndrome. It is almost invariably unilateral and is

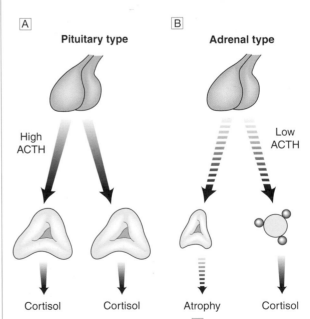

Fig. 20.19 Types of Cushing's syndrome. **A** Overstimulation of the normal adrenal glands by excess ACTH. **B** Oversecretion of cortisol by a functioning tumour of the left adrenal gland, leading to suppression of function in the opposite gland.

more common in females. Histologically, the tumour contains clear cells like those of the zona fasciculata, or compact cells like those of the zona reticularis. Autonomous cortisol secretion inhibits ACTH production, so that the contralateral gland becomes atrophic and ceases to function. Adrenal carcinoma is a rare cause of Cushing's syndrome that occurs more frequently in young adults and children. The tumour grows to a large size and has frequently metastasized by the time of presentation.

- *Pituitary disease* (80%). Pituitary tumours causing Cushing's syndrome are usually basophil or sometimes chromophobe adenomas of ACTH-secreting cells. They range from tiny 'microadenomas' to large and even invasive tumours. Because of the continued ACTH secretion, both adrenals become hyperplastic. When Cushing's syndrome is caused by a pituitary tumour, it is referred to as Cushing's disease.
- *Ectopic ACTH production*. Inappropriate secretion of ACTH-like peptide by tumours of non-pituitary origin (e.g. pancreas, bronchus, thymus) is a rare cause.
- *Iatrogenic*. Cushing's syndrome can be a major side effect of therapeutic steroid use. Adrenal atrophy occurs if the steroid dosage is supraphysiological (> 20 mg equivalent of prednisone per day) and prolonged in duration.

Clinical features

Cushing's syndrome occurs most frequently in young women. The most striking feature is truncal obesity, a 'buffalo hump' (due to redistribution of water and fat) and 'mooning' of the face (Fig. 20.20). Cushing's original description was a 'tomato head, potato body and four matches as limbs'. As a result of protein loss, the skin becomes thin, with purple striae, dusky cyanosis and visible dermal vessels. Proximal muscle weakness is prominent. Other features include increased capillary fragility, purpura, osteoporosis, acne, loss of libido, hirsutism, diabetes, hypertension and amenorrhoea. The clinical signs develop insidiously over years and sometimes are only fully appreciated when the patients and their family review old photographs. In some cases, the disease runs a fulminant course, particularly when due to an adrenal carcinoma or ectopic ACTH secretion. Electrolyte disturbances, cachexia, pigmentation, severe diabetes and psychosis are common in these patients.

Investigations

Before proceeding to adrenalectomy, the surgeon must be convinced that:

- Cortisol secretion is beyond normal control. In Cushing's syndrome plasma cortisol levels are high, diurnal variation is lost and secretion is not suppressed by low-dose dexamethasone
- The primary problem is in the adrenal. In patients with a functioning adrenal tumour, ACTH cannot be detected in the plasma, and urinary excretion of cortisol is not suppressed by high-dose dexamethasone (Fig. 20.21)
- Pituitary and ectopic sources of excessive ACTH production have been excluded. In Cushing's disease due to a pituitary adenoma, plasma ACTH levels are inappropriately high and urinary cortisol excretion is suppressed by dexamethasone. In ectopic ACTH

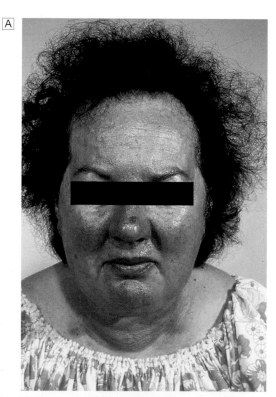

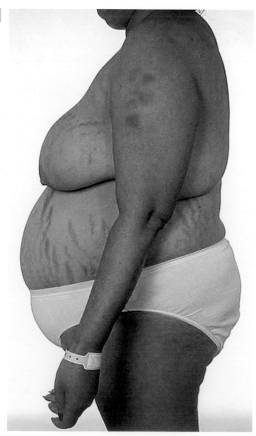

Fig. 20.20 Features of Cushing's syndrome. ☐A☐ Moon face and puffy eyes. ☐B☐ Papery skin with striae and a propensity to bruising, muscle wasting of limbs and centripetal obesity. (Courtesy of Prof Michael Sheppard, University of Birmingham Medical School.)

Pituitary-dependent   **Autonomous adrenal tumour**

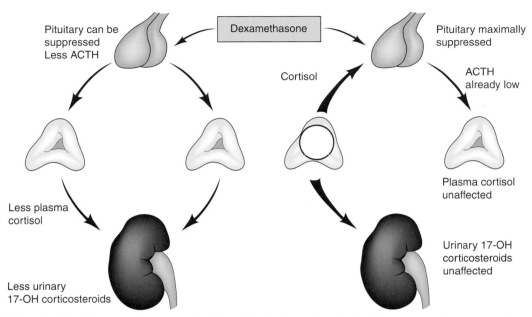

Pituitary can be suppressed
Less ACTH

Dexamethasone

Pituitary maximally suppressed

Cortisol

ACTH already low

Less plasma cortisol

Plasma cortisol unaffected

Less urinary 17-OH corticosteroids

Urinary 17-OH corticosteroids unaffected

Fig. 20.21 The principle of the dexamethasone test in differentiating between adrenal and pituitary causes of excess cortisol secretion.

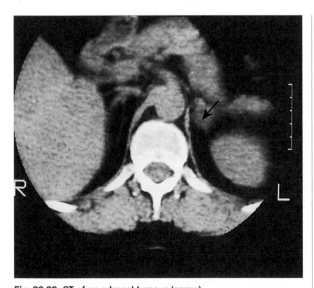

Fig. 20.22 CT of an adrenal tumour (arrow).

syndrome, the ACTH levels are often exceedingly high and there is an associated electrolyte disturbance. These patients may also have cancer cachexia
• Attempts have been made to localize the lesion by techniques such as CT (Fig. 20.22) or MRI.

Management

Adrenal adenoma
Adrenal adenomas are rarely bilateral and unilateral adrenalectomy is most commonly indicated. As the other adrenal is suppressed and atrophic, cortisone replacement is needed until the pituitary–adrenal axis recovers. This may take up to 2 years, and steroids must not be reduced or discontinued until a low-dose dexamethasone test shows normal function in the remaining gland.

Adrenal carcinoma
Adrenal carcinomas should be completely removed whenever possible; debulking may be helpful if chemotherapy is to be used. Patients often present late, with large tumours and lung metastases. Chemotherapy with mitotane or p-p-DDD may be tried, but this is a toxic drug and is often poorly tolerated. The therapeutic gain may be small.

Pituitary disease
The symptoms of bilateral adrenal hyperplasia due to pituitary hyperfunction can be relieved by bilateral adrenalectomy, but at the price of lifelong steroid therapy. Furthermore,

---

⟳ SUMMARY BOX 20.6

Cushing's syndrome

• Cushing's syndrome results from inappropriate secretion of cortisol
• May be caused by tumours of the adrenal cortex (20%), tumours of the anterior pituitary (80%), ectopic ACTH production (rare), or may be a side effect of steroid therapy
• The main clinical features are truncal obesity, buffalo hump, mooning of the face ('tomato head, potato body, four matchsticks as limbs'), thinning of the skin, livid striae and proximal muscle weakness
• An adrenal tumour is usually treated by unilateral adrenalectomy, but cortisone replacement is needed until the suppressed contralateral adrenal recovers
• Before proceeding to adrenalectomy, the surgeon should confirm that cortisol secretion is beyond normal control, that the primary problem is not pituitary or ectopic ACTH production. CT scan is the optimal method of localization.
• Pituitary disease is best treated by pituitary surgery (or irradiation) rather than by bilateral adrenalectomy. This avoids continued growth of the pituitary tumour, problems due to ACTH and MSH production (pigmentation, Nelson's syndrome), and the risks of adrenalectomy.

20

adrenalectomy removes all feedback control, so that over-production of ACTH and melanocyte-stimulating hormone (MSH) produces characteristic skin pigmentation, and continued growth of the adenoma may compress the optic chiasma (Nelson's syndrome). Pituitary irradiation or surgery avoids the side-effects of adrenalectomy, and microsurgical removal of the adenoma is now the treatment of choice.

Hyperaldosteronism

Primary hyperaldosteronism (Conn's syndrome)

This is usually due to a benign adenoma and is most common in young or middle-aged women. The adenoma is small, single, canary yellow on bisection and composed of cells of the glomerulosa type. Only rarely is the syndrome due to bilateral adrenal hyperplasia or multiple microadenomas. The high circulating levels of aldosterone suppress renin secretion – a helpful biochemical diagnostic observation.

Clinical features
Retention of sodium increases plasma volume and produces hypertension, often in association with headaches and visual disturbance (although serious retinopathy is uncommon). Potassium loss leads to worsening hypokalaemia, episodes of muscle weakness and nocturnal polyuria. Unrecognized, the syndrome progresses to severe hypokalaemic alkalosis, with periodic muscle paralysis, paraesthesia and tetany.

Diagnosis
Low serum potassium in a hypertensive patient should signal the possibility of hyperaldosteronism. Diagnosis then rests on the following:

- *Confirm hypokalaemia.* This may require repeated blood sampling without an occluding cuff; 24-hour urine collections usually show increased potassium excretion.
- *Demonstrate hypersecretion of aldosterone.* Plasma and/or urinary aldosterone levels are measured at 4-hourly intervals to allow for diurnal variations. Giving the aldosterone antagonist, spironolactone, should reduce blood pressure and reverse hypokalaemia.
- *Exclude secondary hyperaldosteronism.* Measurement of plasma renin is the critical investigation; renin levels are increased in secondary hyperaldosteronism but undetectable in the primary disease. Spironolactone causes further increases in renin levels in secondary hyperaldosteronism.
- *Localize the adenoma.* If primary hyperaldosteronism is confirmed biochemically, attempts should then be made to localize the adenoma by CT or MRI. Failure to 'see' an adenoma may mean that there is no discrete tumour and that the patient has bilateral cortical hyperplasia. Plasma cortisol levels should always be measured to exclude Cushing's syndrome. Selective adrenal vein samplingto determine aldosterone levels is required to help localize small adenomas to one or other gland, and confirm which gland is hyperfunctioning.

Management
Primary hyperaldosteronism due to an adenoma is treated by removal of the affected gland *after* correcting the hypokalaemia with oral potassium and spironolactone. Hyperaldosteronism due to adrenal hyperplasia can be cured by bilateral adrenalectomy, but at such a high price that long-term drug treatment is preferable.

Secondary hyperaldosteronism

Hyperaldosteronism is most commonly secondary to excessive renin secretion (and stimulation of the zona glomerulosa by angiotensin) in chronic liver, renal or cardiac disease.

Adrenogenital syndrome (adrenal virilism)

Pathophysiology
This syndrome is due to one of a number of genetically determined enzyme defects that impair cortisol synthesis. The resultant increase in pituitary ACTH production causes adrenal hyperplasia and inappropriate adrenal androgen secretion.

Clinical features
The effects depend on the patient's sex and age. Female infants show enlargement of the clitoris and varying fusion of the labial folds. Later, other signs of virilism appear, leading to precocious heterosexual puberty. Young boys have precocious isosexual puberty. In both sexes, growth is at first rapid, but the epiphyses fuse early so that the final height is stunted. Excess muscle growth produces an 'infant Hercules' appearance. Milder forms of the disease may affect older girls and cause hirsutism and acne.

Management
The patient is given cortisol for replacement purposes and to suppress ACTH production. Surgical correction of the genital abnormality may be needed. Rarely, virilism is due to an adrenal tumour, which is usually large and malignant.

Adrenal feminization

Exceptionally, a tumour of the adrenal cortex may secrete oestrogens. Such tumours are usually large and malignant. In the female, there is sexual precocity; in the male, there is feminization, with gynaecomastia, decreased libido and testicular atrophy. Treatment consists of removing the tumour, although recurrence and metastatic spread are common.

SUMMARY BOX 20.7

Management of pituitary disease

- Secreting macroadenomas are usually resected surgically
- Secreting microadenomas can be treated by specific drugs targeting the relevant hormone (e.g. bromocriptine for prolactin, somatostatin for growth hormone)
- Failed pituitary surgery for Cushing's disease may require bilateral adrenalectomy to control hypercorticolism
- Following pituitary surgery careful monitoring of all pituitary hormones is required, as collateral damage can occur leading to occult deficiencies (e.g. TSH, ACTH, LH and FSH).

Adrenal medulla

Pathophysiology
The adrenal medulla is not essential for life. There are other collections of chromaffin cells in paraganglia in the retroperitoneum, mediastinum and neck that release noradrenaline (norepinephrine). The normal adrenal medulla secretes catecholamines in the ratio 80% adrenaline to 20% noradrenaline. It also secretes the noradrenaline precursor, dopamine. Small amounts of catecholamines are excreted in the urine in free and conjugated form. Larger amounts are excreted as metnoradrenaline and 3-methoxy-4-hydroxymandelic acid (VMA).

Phaeochromocytoma
Pathology
Phaeochromocytomas are tumours either of the adrenal medulla (80%) that secrete large amounts of adrenaline (epinephrine) and noradrenaline (norepinephrine), or of

the extra-adrenal paraganglionic tissue (20%) that secrete only noradrenaline. Virtually all (99%) arise within the abdomen, 10% are multiple and 10% are malignant. Benign tumours are usually chocolate-brown and highly vascular. Associated conditions are neurofibromatosis, medullary carcinoma of the thyroid (as part of MEN type II), duodenal ulcer and renal artery stenosis. If it presents in pregnancy, phaeochromocytoma can be mistaken for hypertension of pregnancy and may cause maternal and fetal mortality. Genetic testing for predisposition syndromes such as SDHB, C and D should be done in all patients under 50.

Clinical features

The median age for presentation of phaeochromocytomas is 40 years. Excess noradrenaline secretion causes hypertension; adrenaline excess has metabolic effects (e.g. diabetes and thyrotoxicosis). Paroxysmal hypertension is a very characteristic symptom; due to the sudden release of catecholamines. It may be precipitated by abdominal pressure, exercise stress or postural change. During a paroxysm the blood pressure may rise to 200/100 mmHg and there is headache, palpitation, sweating, extreme anxiety, chest and abdominal pain. Pallor, dilated pupils and tachycardia are prominent features. In some patients, persistent and severe hypertension develops at the age of 30–40 years, often in association with severe retinopathy, which can cause optic atrophy and blindness. Glycosuria is common. The skin may be mottled, with tingling of the extremities. Extra-adrenal phaeochromocytomas are also associated with persistent hypertension. On rare occasions, the tumour is in the bladder, and micturition may precipitate a syncopal attack. A few patients present with predominantly metabolic effects, such as those found in thyrotoxicosis. Occasionally, a phaeochromocytoma may cause sudden and unexplained death after trauma or during surgery, owing to severe hypertension causing a cerebrovascular accident or by precipitating a fatal arrhythmia.

Investigations

All young hypertensive patients (age < 40 years) should be screened for a catecholamine-secreting tumour. Twenty-four hour or overnight collections of urine should be analysed for metadrenaline and normetadrenaline levels. A CT or MRI may show the tumour. It may also be demonstrated by scintigraphy after giving radio-iodine-labelled metaiodobenzylguanidine (MIBG), a catecholamine precursor taken up by sites of synthesis (Fig. 20.23).

Management

Surgical removal of the tumour is the treatment of choice. The use of α- and β-blocking drugs has greatly reduced the risk of hypertensive crisis, tachycardia and arrhythmias during induction of anaesthesia or tumour handling. The patient should come to operation with blood pressure and pulse rate controlled. Adrenergic blockade also allows restoration of blood volume, so that sudden hypotension after removal of the tumour is unusual. To achieve blockade, an α-adrenergic receptor blocker such as phenoxybenzamine or doxazosin should be used, with incremental dose escalation according to response A typical starting dose for doxazocin would be 1 mg 12-hourly, building up to 6 or 8 mg a day until hypertension is controlled and postural symptoms occur.

Once and only once α-blockade has been established, unopposed β effects, such as tachycardia, may become evident and are treated with a β-blocker such as propranolol. β-blockade should not be instituted first, as this may allow unopposed α-agonist effects, which may make hypertension worse and precipitate heart failure.

Peroperatively, short-acting α- and β-blocking agents and sodium nitroprusside (which acts directly on vessels independent of adrenergic receptors and gives additional control of hypertension) should be available.

20

SUMMARY BOX 20.8

Phaeochromocytoma

- Usually benign tumour of the adrenal medulla (80%) but 20% arise in extra-adrenal paraganglionic tissue. 10% are multiple and 10% are malignant
- May be associated with neurofibromatosis, medullary carcinoma of the thyroid (MEN II), Von Hipple–Lindau disease, duodenal ulcer and renal artery stenosis
- Usually presents clinically with hypertension, which is often paroxysmal, and with metabolic effects such as diabetes mellitus
- All hypertensive patients < 40 years old should be screened for phaeochromocytoma; Overnight or 24 hour urinary and plasma metadrenaline and normetadrenaline levels are reliable methods of diagnosis
- Location is best defined by CT and radiolabelled metaiodobenzylguanidine (MIBG) scanning
- Treatment consists of adrenalectomy after careful preparation to control blood pressure and heart rate and to re-expand blood volume (by α-adrenergic blockade with β-blockade)

Non-endocrine adrenal medullary tumours

Ganglioneuromas

These are benign, firm, well-encapsulated tumours of ganglion cells. They grow slowly, may become large and can cause diarrhoea. Surgical excision gives excellent results.

Neuroblastomas

These are highly malignant tumours arising from sympathetic nervous tissue. They are one of the most common malignant tumours of infancy and childhood, and metastasize widely. About 75% secrete catecholamines. Treatment by radical excision, radiotherapy and chemotherapy offers the only hope of cure, although spontaneous regression has been reported.

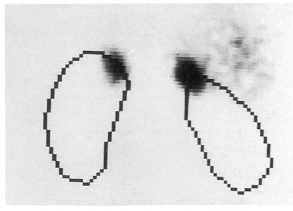

Fig. 20.23 Extra-adrenal phaeochromocytoma. **A** MIBI scan. **B** CT scan.

Adrenal 'incidentaloma'

The increasing use of imaging modalities such as CT or MRI has led to adrenal tumours being discovered incidentally in patients being investigated for other reasons. In such cases, it is important to determine whether there is cortical or medullary hyperfunction, by the use of appropriate biochemical tests as detailed above. If there is no hyperfunction and the swelling is < 3.5 cm in diameter, further investigation and exploration are unwarranted. The lesion is likely to be a benign non-functioning cortical adenoma. Endocrine hyperfunction, a swelling > 3.5 cm or the suspicion of malignancy is an indication for further assessment and exploration.

Adrenalectomy

Indications

Indications for adrenalectomy include adrenal adenomas producing Cushing's syndrome, Conn's syndrome or excess catecholamines (phaeochromocytoma). Bilateral adrenalectomy may be needed for bilateral tumours, nodular hyperplasia producing Conn's or Cushing's syndrome, and if pituitary surgery fails to cure Cushing's disease.

Technique

The approach of choice is laparoscopically by the transperitoneal or posterior route. The exception to this is the known or suspected adrenal malignancy. If an open approach is required then the anterior transperitoneal route requires a large incision, inevitably causes ileus, and has a high incidence of wound and respiratory complications (especially in patients with Cushing's syndrome).

Large tumours which may be malignant are best approached through a flank incision, after removing a rib to allow access; if possible, the diaphragm, pleura and peritoneum are left intact.

The open posterior approach through the bed of the 11th or 12th rib is technically more difficult, but has low morbidity and patients return to normal activity more quickly. If the pleura is breached in the course of adrenalectomy, it can be repaired on closing the wound, ensuring that the lung is fully inflated. There is no need for pleural or wound drains.

Adrenalectomy, however, is best carried out using minimally invasive techniques. The usual route is anteriorly, beneath the costal margins, transperitoneally with reflection of liver on the right and spleen, pancreas and colon on the left. The adrenal vein can often be divided early in laparoscopic surgery which, in phaeochromocytomas, prevents catecholamines from circulating, thereby reducing blood pressure swings following manipulation of the tumour. It is occasionally necessary to convert to an open procedure if bleeding is encountered or there are other technical or access problems. The posterior extra peritoneal approach is gaining popularity.

Replacement therapy

Corticosteroid replacement is needed for life after bilateral total adrenalectomy, but may not be needed permanently after unilateral adrenalectomy. Replacement is best achieved by a combination of oral hydrocortisone (30 mg daily in divided doses) and the mineralocorticoid fludrocortisone acetate (0.1 mg daily). If both adrenals are removed or the remaining adrenal is non-functional, the operation must be covered by commencing steroid replacement at the time of surgery. Adequacy of replacement is assessed by serum levels and response to the dexamethasone test.

Doses of hydrocortisone are given intravenously until the patient can take oral steroid. It cannot be overemphasized that blood pressure is the best early guide to adequacy of therapy. If hypotension occurs, 100 mg hydrocortisone is given immediately by intravenous injection, followed by 100 mg every 6–8 hours All adrenalectomized patients must be warned to increase the dose of steroid if stress or infection occurs. Failure to anticipate the need for added steroid may precipitate an 'adrenal crisis', with acute hypotension and collapse. Such patients should carry a 'steroid card' giving details of dosage and possible complications, and should be able to recognize the symptoms of adrenal insufficiency (i.e. loss of appetite, nausea, cramps, muscle pains and malaise). If such symptoms occur, the patient should take an extra two tablets of hydrocortisone and seek urgent medical help.

Patient information

Although adrenal cortical function is vital for life, patients are unlikely to have heard of the adrenal glands. Adrenal tumours occur at a rate of about 1 per million population per annum, so patients may not have an awareness of cortisone or adrenaline. It is necessary to discuss the technicalities of surgery and the approach to be used, and to forewarn patients that a laparoscopic procedure may have to be converted to an open one. Complications should be minimal, but it is essential to mention blood loss and common complications as well as ones which though rare have a major impact on quality of life.

One of the most important features to describe will be any requirement for steroid replacement therapy (necessary after bilateral adrenalectomy, unilateral adrenalectomy

---

 SUMMARY BOX 20.9

Management of adrenal pathologies

- Hyperfunctioning benign adrenal masses should be removed surgically (phaeochromocytoma, cortisol secreting adenomas and Conn's syndrome). The laparoscopic approach is the preferred one
- Careful preoperative assessment to exclude multiple hormone secretions from a single or bilateral adrenal masses must be undertaken (e.g. a phaeochromocytoma that is also secreting cortisol)
- In primary hyperaldosteronism (Conn's syndrome) preoperative selective venous sampling from both adrenals should be considered to confirm the site of maximal secretion. It can be misleading to assume this will be the side with the mass lesion in it
- Incidentally found adrenal masses must be investigated for possible hypersecretion of all adrenal hormones prior to their removal or a decision to leave them in situ and follow up.
- Have a low threshold to remove non-functioning incidentalomas > 3.5 cm in size, as the incidence of adrenocortical carcinomas increases significantly above this size
- Only biopsy an adrenal mass if you think it is due to a metastasis from a previous known malignancy. Always exclude a phaeochromocytoma before biopsy of any adrenal mass.

British Association of Endocrine and Thyroid Surgeons' Guidelines at www.BAETS.ORG.UK

for an adenoma producing Cushing's syndrome, and after pituitary surgery) and the need for dosage increase at times of stress (e.g. other surgery) or intercurrent illness (e.g. pneumonia).

OTHER SURGICAL ENDOCRINE SYNDROMES

Apudomas and multiple endocrine neoplasia

The APUD cell series

Distributed throughout the body (anterior pituitary, adrenal medulla, thyroid gland and intestine) are *a*mine *p*recursor *u*ptake and *d*ecarboxylation (APUD) cells that have in common the capacity to synthesize and store amines (e.g. ACTH, catecholamines, calcitonin, secretin, gastrin, cholecystokinin, enteroglucagon, somatostatin, vasoactive intestinal peptide). Hyperplasia and tumour of any APUD cell can produce specific endocrine syndromes.

Multiple endocrine neoplasia (MEN) syndromes

In MEN syndromes, which are inherited as autosomal dominant traits of variable penetrance and expression, patients develop benign or malignant tumours in more than one endocrine gland.

MEN type I

This is characterized by hyperplasia and/or adenomas of the parathyroid, pancreatic islets and anterior pituitary. There may also be non-functioning tumours of the thyroid, pituitary, adrenal cortex and soft tissues (lipomas), and functioning carcinoid tumours of the gut or lungs. The earliest biochemical sign in affected individuals is usually hypercalcaemia from hyperparathyroidism or hyperprolactinaemia from an asymptomatic pituitary tumour. Families are often uncovered when an index patient presents dramatically with small bowel perforation or bleeding due to the Zollinger–Ellison syndrome, or with hypoglycaemia due to an insulinoma of the pancreas. Family members should be screened by measurement of fasting serum calcium and other hormonal markers such as prolactin. Mutations in the MENIN gene on chromosome 11 can be detected. A bracelet may be worn to alert medical attendants to the condition. Treatment is directed at the dominant clinical or biochemical feature. For example, pancreatic endocrine tumours are localized by endoscopic ultrasonography or CT and removed as necessary. Hypercalcaemia is treated by parathyroid surgery, where either all diseased glands are excised, followed by calcium replacement therapy, or by subtotal (three and half glands) parathyroidectomy, when replacement therapy can be avoided, but recurrence of the remnant to a hyperfunctioning state at some later date is inevitable.

MEN type II

This is characterized by medullary carcinoma of the thyroid, phaeochromocytoma and parathyroid hyperplasia. Genetic diagnosis, based on a mutation in *Ret* proto-oncogene chromosome 10, obviates the need for biochemical testing in family members. Unlike in MEN I, there is advantage in prophylactic surgery with affected individuals undergoing total thyroidectomy at an age dictated by the mutation identified and the level of risk associated with that mutation. Kindred members not showing the mutation can be dismissed from follow-up and can be reassured that they will not pass on the genetic abnormality to their offspring. Phaeochromocytomas are diagnosed by annual screening using urinary and or plasma metadrenaline and normetadrenaline levels, and localized by CT and MIBG scanning. Surgical treatment of the phaeochromocytoma must take precedence over the thyroid and parathyroid disease, as anaesthesia and surgery in patients with undiagnosed or untreated phaeochromocytoma can be life-threatening.

Carcinoid tumours and the carcinoid syndrome

20

Carcinoid tumours are most frequently found incidentally in the appendix of a patient undergoing appendicectomy for acute appendicitis, and account for 85% of all appendiceal tumours. They are usually less than 1 cm in diameter and are cured by appendicectomy, as metastases are exceptional in this situation. Carcinoid tumours larger than 2 cm in diameter are rare, but may have spread to lymph nodes and are best treated by right hemicolectomy. Liver metastases are extremely rare in patients with appendiceal carcinoids. Carcinoids occurring in the small intestine frequently spread to lymph nodes, and in 10% of cases there are liver metastases by the time the patient presents with obstructive symptoms or bleeding. Carcinoids in any site produce 5-hydroxytryptamine (5-HT) and other biologically active amines and peptides. In the case of gut carcinoids, these products are normally inactivated by the liver, but liver secondaries secrete these substances directly into the systemic circulation, giving rise to the carcinoid syndrome: periodic flushing, diarrhoea, bronchoconstriction, wheezing and distinctive red-purple discoloration of the face. Right-sided heart disease, notably pulmonary stenosis, may result and can prove fatal.

The diagnosis of carcinoid syndrome is confirmed by detecting 5-hydroxyindoleacetic acid (a breakdown product of 5-HT) in the urine. If the primary tumour is causing symptoms, it should be removed surgically if possible (e.g. right hemicolectomy, small bowel resection, lung resection). Hepatic metastases can be dealt with by resection, radiofrequency ablation or angiographic embolization.

Somatostatin analogues or α-adrenergic antagonists may be useful in controlling symptoms. Chemotherapy (e.g. 5-fluorouracil) is sometimes effective, as is interferon but side effects can be troublesome.

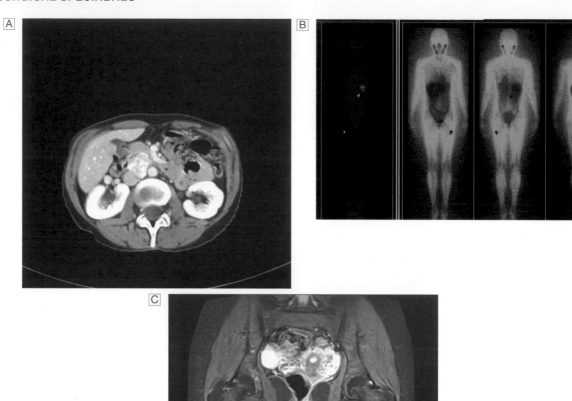

Fig. 20.24 Malignant paraganglioma A CT scan abdomen showing primary. B MIBG showing femoral metastases. C MRI showing femoral deposit.

A.W. Bradbury
T.J. Cleveland

21

Vascular and endovascular surgery

CHAPTER CONTENTS

INTRODUCTION

The management of patients with vascular disease requires a multidisciplinary approach involving vascular surgeons and interventional radiologists, anaesthetists, physicians (angiologists), nursing and rehabilitation specialists, physiotherapists, occupational therapists and orthotists. Many open surgical procedures have been complemented or replaced by less invasive, percutaneous interventions. Despite recent reductions in smoking in many developed countries, the socioeconomic burden of arterial and venous disease is likely to grow as the population ages and the prevalence of diabetes and obesity increases. In the so-called emerging economies and developing world, the prevalence of vascular disease is increasing rapidly.

PATHOPHYSIOLOGY OF ARTERIAL DISEASE

Pathology

Most patients presenting to vascular specialists in developed countries have atherosclerosis which is characterized histopathologically by endothelial cell injury; sub-endothelial deposition of lipids and inflammatory cells; and smooth muscle cell migration and proliferation, all of which lead to plaque haemorrhage and rupture resulting in thrombosis and embolism (Fig. 21.1).

Endothelial injury

Chemical injury

The main risk factor for the development of atherosclerosis is smoking. Hypercholesterolaemia and hypertriglyceridaemia are also important risk factors. Arterial disease is commoner in diabetics, who have disordered glucose and lipid metabolism.

Physical injury

Atheroma often appears first where blood flow exerts high levels of shear stress on the arterial wall: for example, at bifurcations. Hypertension, which increases this stress, is an important predisposing factor for arterial disease.

Lipid deposition

Injury increases the permeability of the endothelium to lipids and inflammatory cells, which become deposited in the subendothelial layer. At this point, atheroma forms a discolored but flat yellow patch (fatty streak). In developed countries, many young adults will have such lesions, which may progress to atherosclerosis.

Inflammatory cell infiltrate

Leucocytes adhere to the overlying damaged endothelium, migrate into the subendothelial space, digest lipid to become 'foam' cells, and liberate free radicals and proteases that destroy the arterial wall. They also liberate cytokines, which attract further leucocytes and smooth muscle cells from the media. The overlying endothelium becomes increasingly 'sticky', leading to platelet deposition and thrombosis.

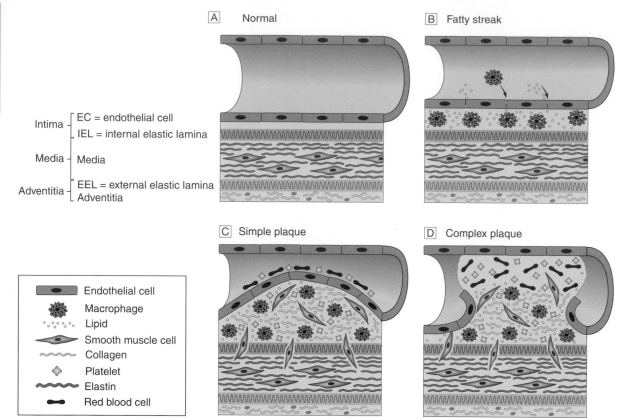

Fig. 21.1 Pathophysiology of atherosclerosis. **A** Normal arterial wall. The intima, comprising a single layer of endothelial cells, rests upon a basement membrane and the internal elastic lamina. The media comprises smooth muscle cells and elastin, and the adventitia consists of collagenous tissue and vasa vasorum. **B** Fatty streak. Injured endothelial cells permit the sequestration of lipids and macrophages in the subendothelial space. **C** Simple plaque. Through the internal elastic lamina, smooth muscle cells enter the media, where they proliferate, take on the characteristics of fibroblasts and produce collagen. **D** Complex plaque. The endothelial cap has ruptured, leading to acute thrombosis and distal embolization.

Smooth muscle cells

Smooth muscle cells migrate from the media into the subendothelial space and begin to proliferate. They take on the properties of fibroblasts and lay down collagen. At this stage, the atheroma is raised and encroaches upon the lumen of the artery.

Plaque rupture

At this point, the plaque comprises a thin 'cap' of endothelium stretched over a mass of lipid and inflammatory and smooth muscle cells. Intra-plaque haemorrhage from immature new blood vessels that infiltrate the lesion (angiogenesis) weakens the plaque. Further chemical and/or physical injury can lead to rupture and the exposure of highly thrombotic plaque contents to the flowing blood. This results in acute thrombotic occlusion of the vessel and/or distal embolization. It is this sudden decompensation that leads to the most serious and dramatic clinical presentations of arterial disease. Rupture can also occur in a plaque that has hitherto been completely asymptomatic.

Clinical features

The clinical manifestations of arterial disease depend upon:
- The site of the disease
- Whether the artery is an end-artery or well collateralized
- The speed with which the disease develops

- Whether the underlying process is primarily haemodynamic, thrombotic, atheroembolic or thromboembolic, or due to aneurysmal dilatation or dissection
- The presence of other co-morbidity and the general condition of the patient.

Anatomical site

The patient's symptoms and signs will depend upon the territory supplied by the affected artery:
- Coronary arteries: angina, myocardial infarction (MI)
- Cerebral circulation: stroke, transient ischaemic attack (TIA), amaurosis fugax, vertebrobasilar insufficiency (VBI)
- Renal arteries: hypertension, renal failure
- Mesenteric arteries: mesenteric angina, acute intestinal ischaemia
- Limbs: intermittent claudication (IC), chronic critical limb ischaemia (CLI), acute limb ischaemia.

Collateral supply

The clinical picture also depends upon whether the affected artery is the only supply to the distal tissues (e.g. coronary artery and the myocardium), or is one of several arteries supplying the part (e.g. internal carotid artery and the brain). This may vary between patients; for example, in a patient with a complete Circle of Willis, occlusion of one internal carotid artery may be asymptomatic whereas with an incomplete Circle, occlusion is more likely to cause a stroke.

Speed of onset

Where atheroma develops slowly over months or years, a collateral supply to the distal part may have the chance to develop, such that when the main artery finally occludes, there may be little change in the patient's clinical status. The most common example is where the profunda (deep) femoral artery (PFA) collateralizes around a diseased superficial femoral artery (SFA) in patients with IC (see below). By contrast, the sudden occlusion of a previously normal artery is likely to cause severe distal ischaemia (as there has been no time for collateral vessels to develop).

Mechanism of injury

The mechanism of injury has a major influence on the clinical presentation, prognosis and treatment of arterial disease (Fig. 21.2).

Haemodynamic mechanism

An atheromatous plaque must reduce the cross-sectional area of an artery by about 70% to cause an appreciable drop in flow at rest, a so-called 'critical stenosis'. However, on exertion – for example, walking – a much lesser stenosis may become flow limiting. The reason for this is that the pressure drop across a stenosis is proportional to the square of the velocity of the blood entering that stenosis; on exercise, blood velocity increases markedly. The clinical consequence of this is that the lesion only becomes symptomatic on exertion. This type of mechanism tends to have a relatively benign course; IC due to SFA stenosis is a common example.

Thrombosis

By the time a 'critical' stenosis occludes, the collateral supply may be so well developed that the event is clinically silent. However, if a plaque that has been causing little or no haemodynamic impairment suddenly ruptures, then acute thrombosis of the vessel can have severe consequences. Such an event can cause MI (coronary arteries) or stroke (internal carotid artery) in a previously asymptomatic patient.

Atheroembolism

The effect that embolizing plaque contents (predominantly cholesterol) or adherent thrombus (predominantly platelets) have upon the distal circulation depends upon the factors outlined above, as well as the embolic load. Perhaps the best-known example is atheroembolism from internal carotid artery plaque, which can cause small, discrete and temporary areas of cerebral and retinal ischaemia that manifest clinically as TIA and amaurosis fugax. If the embolic load is high, however, these emboli may cause irreversible occlusion of major distal vessels, leading to stroke and retinal infarction (monocular blindness).

Thromboembolism

The most common source of thromboembolism is the left atrium in association with atrial fibrillation (AF). The clinical consequences are usually dramatic as the thrombus load is often large and tends to suddenly and completely occlude a large or medium-sized vessel that has previously been healthy, and around which there is therefore no collateral supply. This is an important cause of stroke and acute limb ischaemia.

CHRONIC LOWER LIMB ARTERIAL DISEASE

Anatomy

The lower limb arterial tree comprises the aortoiliac segment above the inguinal ligament ('inflow'), the femoropopliteal segment and the infrapopliteal segment ('outflow') (Fig. 21.3).

Clinical features

Symptoms

Chronic lower limb ischaemia presents as two distinct clinical entities, IC and critical limb ischaemia (CLI), which have different epidemiologies, natural histories, treatments and prognoses (see below).

Examination findings

On examination, the chronically ischaemic limb is usually characterized by:
- Skin that is thin and dry
- Pallor, particularly on elevation. Upon dependency, the foot becomes bright red; this is known as dependent rubor or 'sunset foot', and is due to reactive hyperaemia (Buerger's test)
- Superficial veins that fill sluggishly in the horizontal position and empty upon minimal elevation (venous guttering)
- Nails that are brittle and crumbly
- Muscle wasting
- Reduced temperature
- Pulses that are weak or absent and sometimes associated with thrills on palpation and bruits on auscultation.

Pulse status

All patients admitted to hospital must have their pulse status recorded. In IC and CLI, the popliteal and pedal pulses are usually absent. If there is aortoiliac disease, then one or both femoral pulses will be weak or absent.

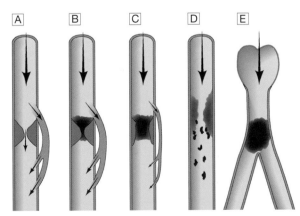

Fig. 21.2 Mechanisms of injury in atherosclerotic disease.
[A] Critical stenosis of main artery compensated for by collateral vessels; only symptomatic on exercise. [B] Acute thrombosis of a critical stenosis; little change in clinical status because of well-developed collaterals. [C] Acute thrombosis of a non-critical stenosis; severe symptoms because collateral supply is poorly developed. [D] Atheroembolism from ruptured, ulcerated plaque. [E] Thromboembolism from the heart; severe ischaemia because of lack of collateral supply.

21

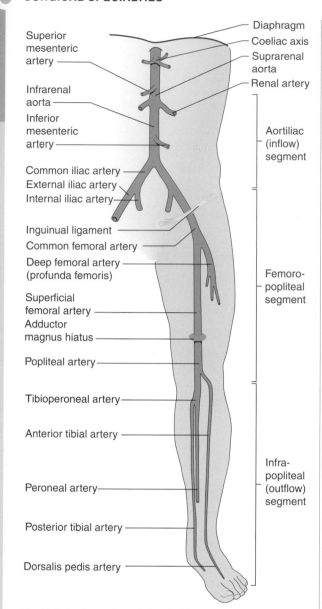

Fig. 21.3 Aortic and lower limb arterial anatomy.

Labels in figure:
Superior mesenteric artery
Infrarenal aorta
Inferior mesenteric artery
Common iliac artery
External iliac artery
Internal iliac artery
Inguinal ligament
Common femoral artery
Deep femoral artery (profunda femoris)
Superficial femoral artery
Adductor magnus hiatus
Popliteal artery
Tibioperoneal artery
Anterior tibial artery
Peroneal artery
Posterior tibial artery
Dorsalis pedis artery

Diaphragm
Coeliac axis
Suprarenal aorta
Renal artery
Aortiliac (inflow) segment
Femoro-popliteal segment
Infra-popliteal (outflow) segment

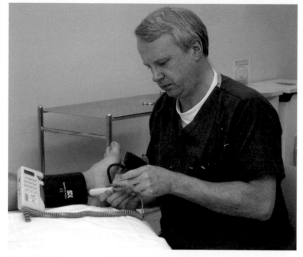

Fig. 21.4 Measurement of ankle:brachial pressure index (ABPI) using Doppler ultrasound.

Intermittent claudication

SUMMARY BOX 21.1

Intermittent claudication (IC)

- IC is the most common manifestation of peripheral arterial disease, affecting up to 1 in 20 people over 60 years of age
- Limb loss is uncommon (up to 1–2% per year), but myocardial infarction and stroke are three times more common than in a non-claudicant population (up to 5–10% per year)
- The mainstays of treatment are risk factor modification (most importantly, complete and permanent smoking cessation), statin and antiplatelet (aspirin, clopidogrel) therapy and (supervised) exercise. This so-called Best Medical Therapy (BMT) leads to a clinically significant improvement in walking distance in the majority of patients; it also improves health related quality of life and increases longevity
- Patients should not normally be considered for surgical or endovascular intervention until they have been compliant with BMT for at least 6 months; intervention in the face of continued smoking is very unlikely to produce meaningful or durable benefit and is cost-ineffective
- Intervention includes angioplasty, stenting and bypass surgery. Long-term results are generally much better in the aorto-iliac segment than below the inguinal ligament.

The presence of a thrill and/or bruit denotes turbulent flow. However, in the presence of effective collateralization, especially in younger patients, pulses may sometimes be present at rest despite significant proximal arterial disease.

Ankle to brachial pressure index (ABPI)

The severity of ischaemia in the leg can be simply estimated by determining the ratio between the ankle and brachial blood pressures. The latter is recorded in the normal way, the former using an ankle cuff and a hand-held Doppler device (Fig. 21.4).

In health, the ankle to brachial pressure index (ABPI) should be at least 1; that is, the pressure at the ankle should be at least as high as that in the arm. Patients with IC usually have an ABPI of 0.5–0.9, in CLI usually the ABPI is less than 0.5.

Clinical features

As lower limb arterial disease most frequently affects the SFA (Fig. 21.5), IC is usually characterized by pain on walking in the muscles of one or both calves. If the iliac arteries are affected then that pain may be felt in the thigh and even the buttock (internal iliac disease). The pain comes on after a reasonably constant 'claudication distance', and

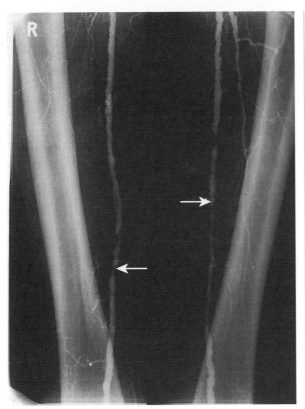

Fig. 21.5 Angiogram showing diffuse disease in both right and left superficial femoral arteries (arrows).

usually subsides rapidly and completely on cessation of walking. Resumption of walking causes the pain to return. These and other features distinguish it from neurogenic and venous claudication (Table 21.1).

Typically, the superficial femoral artery (SFA) first becomes narrowed at the adductor canal (Fig. 21.6A). Ankle pulses may be palpable but are diminished, and a bruit may be heard at or below the stenosis. The ABPI is often (near) normal at rest but reduced following exercise.

Over the next few months or years, collateral vessels arising from the PFA enlarge so that they carry a higher proportion of the blood flow to the lower leg. As a result, in the majority of patients, symptoms gradually improve or even disappear. But thrombotic occlusion of the SFA (Fig. 21.6B) may lead to a sudden deterioration in walking distance. Ankle and popliteal pulses will be absent at this stage.

Continued development of the collateral circulation may lead to an improvement in symptoms and walking distance. This phase of moderate claudication may remain apparently stable for several years. However, without 'best medical therapy' (BMT) (see below) and a change in the patient's lifestyle, the atherosclerosis will progress to involve other segments, such as the PFA, iliac and tibial vessels (Fig. 21.6C). The IC will progress to become severe, often forcing the patient to stop every 50–100 metres or so, and the scope for spontaneous improvement steadily diminishes. As the disease progresses further in severity and extent, symptoms are likely to worsen to a point where CLI develops due to multilevel disease (Fig. 21.6D). Such patients will often go on to develop night/rest pain and are at risk of tissue loss (see below).

An understanding of this cyclical pattern of exacerbation and resolution in IC is important as spontaneous improvement may mislead the patient into thinking all is well and that there is no longer a need to comply with medical advice (see below); and, in particular, that they can continue to smoke with impunity.

Epidemiology

IC affects up to 5% of people aged over 60 years. Provided patients comply with BMT only a small proportion (1–2%) of those affected by IC will deteriorate to a point where amputation and/or revascularization to prevent amputation is

Table 21.1 Differential diagnosis of claudication

	Arterial	Neurogenic	Venous
Pathology	Stenosis or occlusion of major lower limb arteries	Lumbar nerve roots or cauda equina compression (spinal stenosis)	Obstruction to the venous outflow of the leg due to iliofemoral venous occlusion secondary to deep venous thrombosis
Site of pain	Muscles: usually the calf but may affect thigh and buttock	Ill-defined; whole leg. Shooting in nature; may be associated with tingling and numbness	Whole leg. Bursting in nature
Laterality	Usually unilateral if femoro-popliteal, bilateral if aortoiliac disease	Often bilateral	Nearly always unilateral
Onset	Gradual onset after walking the 'claudication distance'	Often immediate upon walking or even on standing up	Gradual onset but may be present from the moment walking commences
Relieving features	On cessation of walking, the pain disappears completely in 1–2 minutes	On cessation of walking, the pain may gradually subside over 5–10 minutes. Often the patient has to sit down or lean against something to obtain relief	The subject usually needs to elevate the leg to obtain relief
Colour	Normal or pale	Normal	Cyanosed. Often visible varicose veins and venous skin changes
Temperature	Normal or cool	Normal	Normal or increased
Swelling	Absent	Absent	Always present
Pulses	Reduced or absent	Normal	Present, but may be difficult to feel because of swelling
Straight leg raising	Normal	Limited	Normal

Symptoms

Mild claudication

Moderate claudication

Severe claudication

Restpain
Ulcer
Gangrene

Pathology

A

B

C

D

Inguinal
ligament

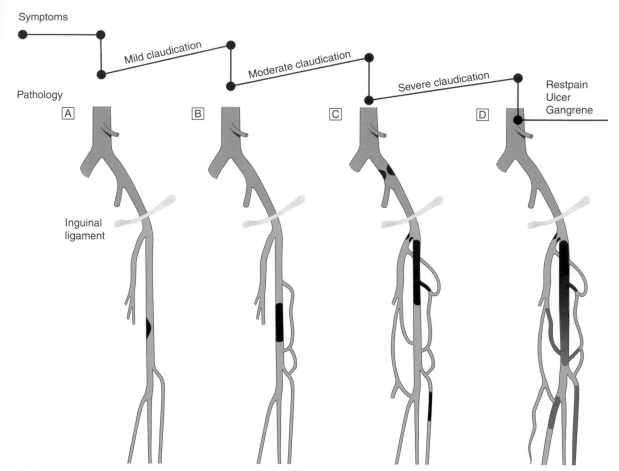

Fig. 21.6 Symptoms and pathology in intermittent claudication. A Superficial femoral artery (SFA) stenosis at adductor canal B Occlusion of the SFA and development of a collateral circulation between the deep femoral (profunda femoris) artery (PFA) and the popliteal artery C Iliac artery and PFA stenosis leading to worsening symptoms of IC and further collateralisation D Eventually CLI characterised by ischaemic rest pain and tissue loss develops due to multilevel disease affecting tibial arteries and collateral supply

required. However, the annual mortality rate is 5–10% per year, which is 2–3 times higher than an age- and sex-matched non-claudicant population. This is because IC is a powerful marker of widespread atherosclerosis, and most of these patients succumb to MI, stroke and limb loss. The emphasis is, therefore, on the preservation of life; in most patients, measures to reduce cardiovascular mortality and morbidity (MI, stroke) will also improve the functional status of the limb.

Critical limb ischaemia

Whereas IC is usually due to single-level disease, CLI (sometimes also termed severe limb ischaemia, SLI) is caused by multiple lesions affecting different arterial segments down the leg (Fig. 21.6D). These patients usually have tissue loss (ulceration or gangrene) and/or rest (night) pain; their ankle blood pressure is often 50–70 mmHg or less. Without revascularization, such patients will often lose their limb, and sometimes their life, in a matter of months.

Night and rest pain

Ischaemic 'night pain' typically develops in the forefoot a few hours after going to bed. The pain is due to the accumulation of metabolites (acidosis) as a result of reduced perfusion consequent upon the loss of the beneficial effects of gravity and the reduction in blood pressure and cardiac output that usually occurs during sleep. The pain is

severe and wakes the patient from sleep. At first the pain may be relieved by hanging the limb out of bed but, as the disease progresses, the patient has to get up and walk about to obtain relief. The patient then often takes to sleeping in a chair, which leads to dependent oedema. This increases interstitial tissue pressure and so further reduces arterial perfusion. The patient is then in a vicious cycle of increasing pain and sleep loss. At this point, even a trivial injury to the foot will fail to heal, and the entry of bacteria leads to infection and an increase in the metabolic demands of the foot. The result is the rapid formation of ulcers, gangrene and, without treatment, limb loss and death.

Diabetic vascular disease

Approximately 40% of patients with CLI have diabetes and such patients pose a number of unique problems for vascular specialists:

- Arteries are often calcified, which makes surgery and angioplasty technically difficult
- Calcification also leads to vessel incompressibility which results in spuriously high ankle pressures and ABPI measurements
- Reduced ability to fight infection
- Severe multisystem arterial disease (coronary, cerebral and peripheral), which increases the risks of intervention
- In the lower limbs, diabetic vascular disease has a predilection for the infrapopliteal vessels. Although vessels in the foot are often spared, the technical

challenge of performing a satisfactory bypass or angioplasty to these small vessels is considerable

- Frequent coexisting neuropathy may lead to foot ulceration in its own right but may also complicate peripheral ischaemia (see below).

The diabetic foot

This refers to the combination of ischaemia, neuropathy and immunocompromise that renders the feet of diabetic patients particularly susceptible to sepsis, ulceration and gangrene. Diabetic neuropathy affects the motor, sensory and autonomic nerves.

Sensory neuropathy

This renders the patient incapable of feeling pain. Minor trauma – for example, from a stone in the shoe – remains unnoticed. Even severe ischaemia and/or tissue loss that would lead a sensate patient to seek urgent medical advice may be completely painless. For this reason, diabetic patients often present late, with extensive destruction of the foot. Sensory neuropathy also affects proprioception such that, when walking, pressure is applied at unusual sites. This leads to ulcer formation and even joint destruction (Charcot's joint).

Motor neuropathy

The normal structure and function of the foot depends not only upon ligaments, but also upon the long and short flexors and extensors of the calf and foot. The former are affected more than the latter by motor neuropathy, leading to weakness and atrophy. The result is that the long extensors of the toes are unopposed and the toes become increasingly dorsiflexed. This exposes the metatarsal heads to abnormal pressure, and they are a frequent site of callus formation and ulceration (Fig. 21.7).

Autonomic neuropathy

This leads to a dry foot deficient in the sweat that normally lubricates the skin and contains antibacterial substances. The result is scaling and fissuring of the skin, and the creation of a portal of entry for bacteria. Abnormal blood flow in the bones of the ankle and foot due to loss of autonomic control may also contribute to osteopenia and bony collapse (Charcot's foot).

Management

If the blood supply to the foot is adequate, dead tissue can be excised in the expectation that healing will occur, provided infection is controlled and the foot is protected from

pressure (so-called off-loading). If there is ischaemia as well, the priority is to revascularize the foot, if possible. Sadly, many diabetic patients present late, with extensive tissue loss and 'unreconstructable' disease, which accounts for the very high amputation rate.

Management of lower limb ischaemia

Medical management

All patients with atherosclerotic vascular disease should be strongly urged to comply with BMT, which comprises:

- Immediate, absolute and permanent cessation from smoking. This is by far the most important intervention and prognostic factor. In the face of continued smoking, other treatments are rendered largely ineffective and disease progression, limb loss and death (usually from cardiovascular causes) within a few years are the likely outcome.
- Control of hypertension according to current guidelines (for example, see the British Hypertension Society, www.bhsoc.org).
- Control of hypercholesterolaemia according to current guidelines (for example, see the British Heart Foundation, http://www.bhf.org.uk). All vascular patients should be prescribed lipid lowering drugs, usually a statin, so that their baseline total cholesterol is reduced by a third (ideally to below 4 mmol/l). Statins also stabilize atheromatous plaques and prevent the development and progression of aneurysmal disease through as yet incompletely understood anti-inflammatory mechanisms.
- Prescription of an antiplatelet agent (for guidance see National Institute of Clinical and Health Excellence, http://www.nice.org.uk/guidance/index.jsp?action=folder&o=51201). This is normally aspirin (75 mg daily) but clopidogrel (75 mg daily) is a more effective and safer alternative (but is also more expensive). Anticoagulation with warfarin should normally be reserved for patients with AF.
- Regular exercise as possible; it is widely accepted that supervised exercise in a health care environment is more effective than (unsupervised) simple advice to exercise.
- Control of obesity. This will help to bring down blood pressure, cholesterol and the 'strain' of walking; diabetes will also be easier to control. Surgical and endovascular intervention is much more difficult and morbid in obese patients.
- The identification and active treatment of patients with diabetes. This includes foot care (for further information see, for example, Diabetes UK, http://www.diabetes.co.uk).

Compliance with BMT increases not only walking distance but also affords very significant protection against cardiovascular events, improves the patient's quality of life and life expectancy. Unfortunately, many patients fail to comply and, in particular, continue to smoke. Endovascular or open surgery for IC should not normally be considered until the patient is fully compliant with BMT and that therapy has been given adequate chance to effect symptomatic improvement. Intervention in the face of continued smoking is usually clinically and cost-ineffective and represents poor use of limited health care resources. Revascularization is in addition to, not instead of, BMT, a point that often has to be emphasized to patients anxious to return to their previous lifestyle.

By the time a patient develops CLI it is often (but not always) the case that, without surgical or endovascular revascularization, the limb will be lost. However, this does not in any way undermine the value of instituting BMT in

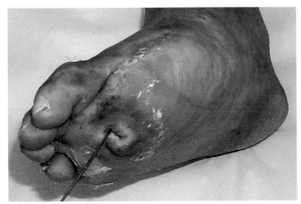

Fig. 21.7 Neuropathic ulceration of the first metatarsal head with sinus entering joint space.

such patients. On occasion, BMT may improve the condition of the leg such that intervention is not required or a lesser procedure becomes an option. In those undergoing intervention, BMT undoubtedly reduces the overall risks and increases the success of the procedure.

Endovascular management

Balloon angioplasty (BAP), with or without stenting, has been used successfully in the iliac, femoral, popliteal and crural arteries and is usually performed under local anaesthesia (Fig. 21.8). The arterial lesion to be treated (stenosis or occlusion) is identified and crossed with a wire. A balloon catheter is introduced over the wire and the balloon inflated. This enlarges the lumen by disrupting the atheromatous plaque. In occlusions and complex disease, metal stents may be deployed across the lesion to improve patency and reduce distal embolic complications. Sometimes these balloons and stents are coated with drugs that reduce the arterial scarring (neo-intimal hyperplasia) that follows such intervention and can lead to restenosis and reocclusion (so-called drug eluting balloons and stents). Endoluminal repair of the aortoiliac segment is the treatment of choice in most vascular units because of its high patency rates, and low morbidity compared to open surgery. Infrainguinal BAP and, less commonly, stenting is also widely used in the management of IC and CLI.

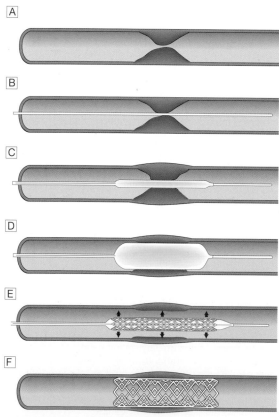

Fig. 21.8 Balloon angioplasty and stenting. [A] Critical arterial stenosis. [B] A guidewire is used to cross the lesion. [C] The guidewire is used to direct a balloon angioplasty catheter across the lesion. [D] The balloon is inflated. [E] A metal stent may be mounted on a catheter. The stent may be self-expanding or require expansion with a balloon. In many cases, the first manoeuvre is to cross the lesion with a stent and in this circumstance steps C and D may be omitted. [F] Metal stent holding open the stenosis.

Intermittent claudication

Endoluminal treatment (BAP, stent) should be used selectively in patients with IC because it may be associated with a 1–2% morbidity rate, rarely mortality, and many patients have a pattern of disease that is unsuitable for current endovascular technologies. There is controversy with regard to its role in the femoropopliteal and infrapopliteal segments because of a perceived lack of durability of benefit. In the future, this may be improved by the use of stents. By contrast, most vascular specialists believe that endoluminal therapy should be considered in patients with IC due to aortoiliac disease (absent or reduced femoral pulses) because they:

- tend to be younger, so that their symptoms have a greater impact on their quality of life and livelihood
- often have short-segment disease that is amenable to BAP, with or without a stent
- often have (relatively) normal infrainguinal arteries, so that restoring flow in the aortoiliac segment effects a dramatic improvement in the perfusion to their leg(s)
- tend to be more symptomatic, with shorter walking distances and bilateral symptoms
- may not achieve a satisfactory increase in walking distance with BMT alone, because the ability of the body to collateralize around aortoiliac disease is not as good as it is around femoropopliteal disease.

Furthermore, the long-term patency of BAP and stenting is optimal in high-flow, large-calibre vessels, leading to a durable clinical benefit in many patients.

Critical limb ischaemia

The role of BAP and stenting in CLI remains controversial and, with present technology, many such patients remain unsuitable for endovascular therapy. The only published randomized controlled trial to compare BAP and bypass surgery (BSX) (http://basiltrial.com) indicates that although BAP is safer and less expensive than BSX in the short term (12–18 months), BSX (with vein) offers a more durable and complete revascularization in the longer term (3–5 years) (EBM 21.1). At the present time, CLI patients expected to only live 1–2 years and who do not have a suitable vein for the construction of a bypass are probably best treated by BAP where technically possible; all other CLI patients are probably best served by BSX. The role for endovascular therapy may increase in the future as technology improves.

EBM **21.1 Bypass surgery (BSX) or balloon angioplasty (BAP) for severe limb ischaemia)**

'For patients who survived for at least 2 years after randomization, a BSX-first revascularization strategy was associated with a significant increase in subsequent overall survival and a trend towards reduced amputation free survival. BAP was associated with a significantly higher early failure rate than BSX. Many BAP patients ultimately required surgery. BSX outcomes after failed BAP are significantly worse than for BSX performed as a first revascularization attempt. BSX with vein offers the best long term outcome but BAP appears superior to prosthetic BSX.'

Basil Trial Investigators and Participants. Final results of the BASIL trial (Bypass Versus Angioplasty in Severe Ischaemia of the Leg) Journal of Vascular Surgery 2010; 51(5): 5S–17S.

Indications for arterial reconstruction

Intermittent claudication

Many surgeons are reluctant to perform infrainguinal bypass surgery for IC because:

- The risk of limb loss is very low with BMT
- Those patients who fail to comply with BMT (fail to stop smoking) are those most likely to press for surgery because of on-going symptoms. However, they are also those at greatest operative risk and those least likely to gain durable benefit from their bypass
- Surgery is associated with a significant risk of mortality and major morbidity, the size of that risk depending on the procedure and the patient but probably approaching 3–5% for infrainguinal bypass and 5–10% for aorto-bifemoral bypass
- As most patients have bilateral disease, even if they have unilateral symptoms, successful infrainguinal surgery on one side often reveals limiting IC symptoms on the other, requiring a second operation (the same for endoluminal treatment)
- Grafts have a finite patency, especially in those who fail to comply with BMT and, in particular, continue to smoke (the same for endoluminal treatment)
- As soon as a bypass graft is inserted, collaterals circumventing the original lesion shrink down. For this reason, when the graft occludes, usually suddenly, the patient is normally returned to a worse level of IC than before the operation. A patient who was previously a claudicant may now have acute limb-threatening ischaemia, which then forces the surgeon or radiologist to re-intervene. Secondary interventions are technically more difficult, are associated with higher risk and enjoy a lower patency rate.

As with BAP and stenting, the balance of risks and benefits for open surgery is different in patients with aorto-iliac disease. Although the risk of surgery is higher, the long-term patency rates of such grafts are excellent, and one operation deals with both legs. Whatever the treatment being considered, patients and their families must be made fully aware of the risks and benefits so that they can give fully informed consent. These discussions must always be faithfully recorded in the notes; it is good practice to send copies of this to the patient as well as the GP. Sadly, medicolegal activity continues to grow in the UK and clear and accurate verbal and written communication between the clinician, the patient and their family affords significant protection for all parties concerned.

Principles of arterial reconstruction

Endarterectomy

This involves the direct removal of atherosclerotic plaque and thrombus and is a relatively uncommon operation in modern vascular surgical practice except at the carotid and femoral bifurcations (Fig. 21.9).

Bypass grafting

For a surgical bypass operation (Fig. 21.10) to be successful in the long term, three conditions must be fulfilled:

- There must be high-flow, high-pressure blood entering the graft (inflow)
- The conduit must be suitable
- The blood must have somewhere to go when it leaves the graft (outflow or run-off).

Two main types of conduit are available:

- autogenous material, most commonly the ipsilateral great saphenous vein (GSV)
- prosthetic material, most commonly expanded polytetrafluoroethylene (ePTFE) or Dacron.

The main advantage of vein is that it is lined by endothelium that is actively antithrombotic and profibrinolytic, and therefore much less liable to induce coagulation than even the most inert of man-made materials. This translates into much better long-term graft patency. Vein is also much more resistant to infection (see below) and less expensive. It is generally agreed that, wherever possible, vein from the leg or arm should be used for infrainguinal reconstruction.

Extra-anatomic bypass

In most bypass operations, the new conduit more or less follows the course of the original artery – so-called anatomic bypass (Fig. 21.11). Where this is not possible and/or desirable, a so-called extra-anatomic bypass can be inserted (Fig. 21.12).

For example, if only one iliac artery is blocked, and the patient is unfit for abdominal surgery and unsuitable for endoluminal treatment, a femorofemoral crossover graft can be performed. If both iliac arteries are occluded, then an axillobifemoral graft can be inserted. In general, these extra-anatomic grafts do not have as good long-term patency as anatomic aortoiliac reconstructions. However, they are lesser procedures and so the preferred option in high-risk patients or those that have a limited life expectancy.

21

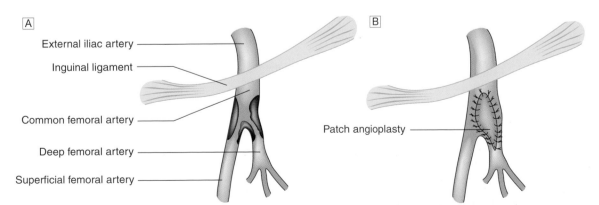

A
External iliac artery
Inguinal ligament
Common femoral artery
Deep femoral artery
Superficial femoral artery

B
Patch angioplasty

Fig. 21.9 Profundaplasty. A Focal atherosclerotic disease of the left common femoral artery is causing severe ischaemia because it is obstructing flow down the superficial and deep femoral (profunda femoris) arteries. B Local endarterectomy and closure of the profunda femoris using a vein or prosthetic patch (profundaplasty) restores normal flow to both vessels.

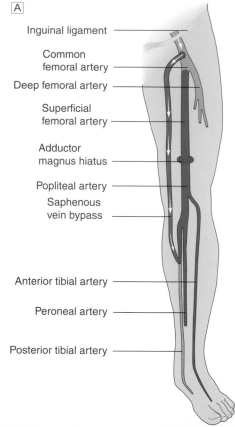

A
- Inguinal ligament
- Common femoral artery
- Deep femoral artery
- Superficial femoral artery
- Adductor magnus hiatus
- Popliteal artery
- Saphenous vein bypass
- Anterior tibial artery
- Peroneal artery
- Posterior tibial artery

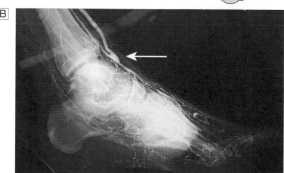

B

Fig. 21.10 Femorodistal bypass graft. A Diagram showing femoral to posterior tibial bypass graft. B On-table angiogram showing distal end of vein graft (arrow) anastomosed to the dorsalis pedis artery in the foot.

Complications of arterial reconstruction

The morbidity and mortality associated with vascular surgery is often high because vascular patients are usually elderly and unfit with widespread vascular disease, and the operations are often lengthy with significant blood loss. Meticulous perioperative care is essential for optimal results, and close liaison between the surgeon, the anaesthetist and the intensivist is essential. Longer term major complications include infection and graft occlusion for which outcome is better when identified early.

Although there is no strong evidence of benefit, many surgeons perform ultrasound scans of their grafts at regular intervals in the postoperative period, typically at 1, 3, 6, 12, 18 and 24 months. This so-called 'graft surveillance' is designed to pick up technical problems with the graft that are likely to increase the risk of failure. It is generally believed that it is better to correct a 'failing' graft before it has blocked than to try to resurrect one that has already failed.

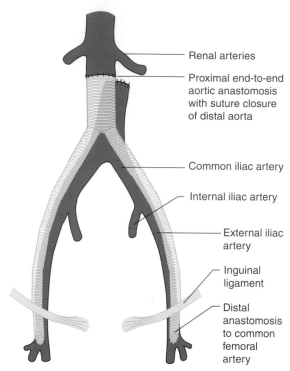

- Renal arteries
- Proximal end-to-end aortic anastomosis with suture closure of distal aorta
- Common iliac artery
- Internal iliac artery
- External iliac artery
- Inguinal ligament
- Distal anastomosis to common femoral artery

Fig. 21.11 Anatomic aortic bypass. Reconstruction of an occluded aortoilliac segment by means of aorto-bi-femoral bypass grafting.

Infection of prosthetic grafts is a serious and growing problem, largely due to the increasing prevalence of antibiotic-resistant organisms, including methicillin-resistant *Staphylococcus aureus* (MRSA). Once a prosthetic graft is infected, it must usually be removed to rid the patient of sepsis and/or to prevent life-threatening (anastomotic) haemorrhage. Graft removal of course renders the distal part ischaemic and, where possible, a new graft is inserted through fresh uninfected tissue. This can be extremely challenging, and on occasion is impossible. Measures to avoid graft infection include:

- Using vein wherever possible
- Peri-operative antibiotic prophylaxis
- Strict aseptic technique in the operating theatre and ward
- Always using gloves and washing hands between examining patients.

AMPUTATION

Indications

Amputation should only be considered where arterial reconstruction is considered by a vascular surgeon to be inappropriate or impossible. In some cases, patients are admitted profoundly unwell and septic from spreading gangrene and immediate amputation may be the only means of saving the patient's life.

Level of amputation

This is determined by local blood supply, the status of the joints, the patient's general health and his or her age. The broad principle is to amputate at the lowest level consistent with healing (Fig. 21.13). It is important to conserve the knee joint if at all possible, as the energy required to walk on a

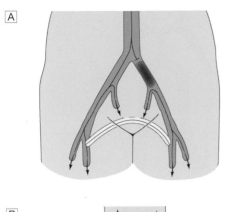

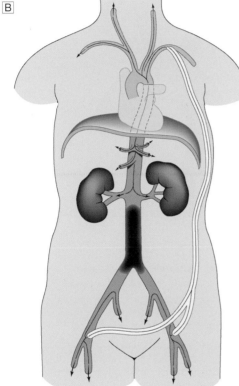

Fig. 21.12 **Extra-anatomic bypass.** A Unilateral iliac disease may be treated by femoro-femoral crossover graft. B Bilateral aorto-iliac disease may be treated with axillo-bifemoral bypass graft.

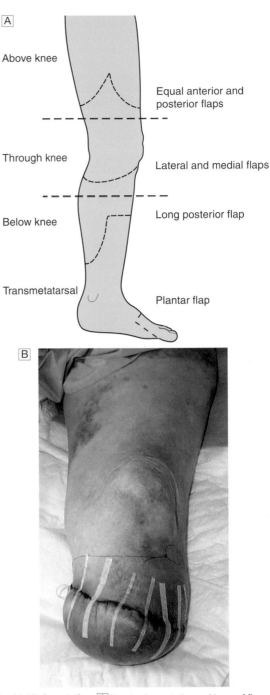

Fig. 21.13 **Amputation.** A Levels of amputation and types of flap used to close the residual defect. B Below-knee amputation.

below-knee prosthesis is much less that required to walk on an above knee prosthesis. However, if the patient has other co-morbidity or disability that would make walking with a prosthesis impossible, there is no point in attempting to conserve the knee joint at the expense of healing. A common situation is where a patient presents with a fixed flexion contracture of the knee. A below-knee amputation in such a patient is usually ill-advised because the contracture will prevent the patient from ever walking and will also result in the stump wound resting on the bed or chair, leading to poor healing and wound breakdown.

Surgical principles

A number of important principles must be observed if primary healing and satisfactory rehabilitation are to be achieved. The in-hospital mortality for major limb amputation approaches 20% and can exceed 30% in the elderly undergoing above-knee amputation. The decision to amputate, the level of amputation and the procedure itself require direct input from an experienced vascular surgeon. In some elderly patients, end of life care is more appropriate than amputation.

Rehabilitation and limb fitting

The speed of rehabilitation is variable but, typically, at about 1 week the patient should begin to bear weight on the other limb between parallel bars, and at 10 days begin to walk with a pneumatic walking aid. If healing is progressing well, a temporary prosthesis can be fitted at about 3 weeks. Final fitting of the artificial limb must await shaping and firming of the stump. Approximately 70% of below-knee amputees and 30% of above-knee amputees eventually walk although many of these do not persist with their prosthesis. It is important to appreciate that, because of the prolonged hospital admission, rehabilitation, home modifications and, in some cases, long-term care, amputation can be a much more expensive option than revascularization leading to limb salvage.

Phantom pain

Phantom limb pain can be a serious problem, especially if pain has not been well controlled before and after the amputation. With appropriate drug therapy, reassurance and time, it usually settles but can take a long time to do so. There is some evidence that if the patient goes to theatre pain-free, the risk of phantom pain can be reduced. For this reason, some surgeons request epidural anaesthesia prior to surgery. Input from a pain specialist can be invaluable.

ARTERIAL DISEASE OF THE UPPER LIMB

Overview

Occlusive arterial disease is about 10 times commoner in the leg than in the arm. Nevertheless, when the arm is affected, treatment can be difficult, and the loss of an arm (especially the dominant one) is even more devastating for the patient than loss of a leg.

The left subclavian artery just proximal to the origin of the vertebral artery is the most common site of disease. This may lead to:

- Arm claudication. This is relatively unusual, even when the subclavian artery is completely occluded, because of collateral supply, mainly from the vertebral artery
- Atheroembolism to the hand. Small emboli lodge in the vessels of the fingers and the hand and lead to symptoms that are often mistaken for Raynaud's phenomenon, except that in this case the symptoms are unilateral (see below)
- Subclavian steal. In this circumstance, when the arm is used, blood is 'stolen' from the brain, with retrograde flow via the vertebral artery. This leads to vertebrobasilar ischaemia (VBI), characterized by dizziness, cortical blindness and/or collapse when the arm is used (Fig. 21.14).

Management

Most subclavian artery disease can be treated by means of BAP and stenting, as the results are good and surgical access to the area is difficult. If surgery is required, then the usual operation is carotid–subclavian bypass.

CEREBROVASCULAR DISEASE

Definitions

Stroke

Stroke may be defined as an episode of focal neurological dysfunction lasting more than 24 hours, of presumed vascular aetiology.

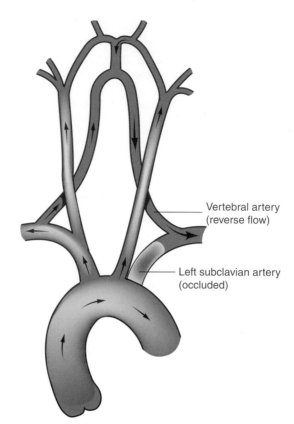

Fig. 21.14 Occlusion of the left subclavian artery, causing 'subclavian steal'.

Vertebral artery (reverse flow)

Left subclavian artery (occluded)

Transient ischaemic attack

When such symptoms last for less than 24 hours, the episode is described as a transient ischaemic attack (TIA).

Amaurosis fugax

This describes transient, usually incomplete, loss of vision in one eye owing to occlusion of a branch of the retinal artery by cholesterol emboli. The patient typically describes it as a veil or curtain coming across the eye, which remains for a few minutes and then disappears. Amaurosis fugax is never synchronously bilateral, as it is almost infinitely improbable that an embolus would enter both retinal arteries at exactly the same time. Bilateral visual loss is usually due to occipital ischaemia secondary to VBI (see below). Non-synchronous amaurosis fugax is, of course, possible in patients with bilateral carotid disease.

Carotid artery disease

Pathophysiology

Approximately 80% of strokes are ischaemic and about half of these are thought to be due to atheroembolism from the carotid bifurcation. The origin of the internal carotid artery is particularly prone to atheroma. The tighter the degree of stenosis, the more likely it is to cause symptoms. Athero-emboli entering the ophthalmic artery leads to amaurosis fugax or permanent monocular blindness on the same side (ipsilateral). If they enter the middle cerebral artery, they may cause hemiparesis and hemisensory loss on the opposite side (contralateral). If the dominant hemisphere is affected, there may also be dysphasia.

SUMMARY BOX 21.2

Carotid artery disease

- Up to 50% of all ischaemic strokes may be caused by atheroembolism from the carotid bifurcation
- Patients with carotid territory transient ischaemic attacks (TIA) and amaurosis fugax should be assessed by a vascular surgeon with a view to carotid endarterectomy (CEA)
- When compared to BMT alone, CEA in addition to BMT significantly reduces the risk of further ipsilateral ischaemic stroke in patients with high grade symptomatic internal carotid artery stenosis
- CEA for asymptomatic internal carotid artery stenosis is controversial; such patients should be discussed with a vascular surgeon
- Several large trials have shown that with current technology, carotid artery stenting (CAS) can be an effective treatment for carotid stenoses, and should be considered as an option, particularly in patients at high risk for surgery.

Assessment

The presence of a 'carotid' bruit bears no reliable relationship to the severity of underlying internal carotid artery disease and thus the risk of stroke. Such a bruit may arise from the external carotid artery or be transmitted from the heart. Furthermore, in the presence of a very tight internal carotid artery stenosis, flow may be so slow that no audible turbulence is present. It is important to exclude other causes of cerebral ischaemia and haemorrhage.

Colour flow Doppler (duplex) ultrasound (CDU) is the initial investigation of choice for imaging the carotid arteries (Fig. 21.15).

Magnetic resonance (MRA) or computed tomographic (CTA) angiography provide excellent images and are increasingly used to plan treatment (Fig. 21.16).

Intra-arterial digital subtraction angiography (IA-DSA) is associated with a small risk of TIA/stroke and nowadays is used rarely for diagnostic purposes.

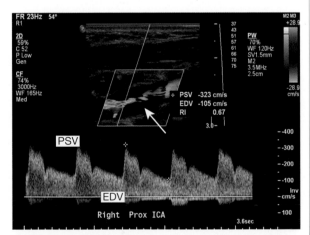

Fig. 21.15 Carotid ultrasound scan. The upper image shows the narrowing (arrow). By using Doppler ultrasound to measure the peak systolic velocity (PSV) (about 300 cm/s in this case) and end-diastolic velocity (EDV) (about 120 cm/s in this case) of the blood travelling through the stenosis it is possible to quantify the degree of narrowing. In this case the stenosis is estimated at greater than 70% and so further investigation with a view to surgery is warranted.

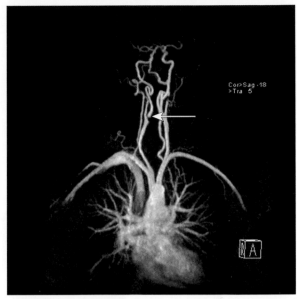

Fig. 21.16 Carotid magnetic resonance angiogram (MRA). The arterial blood to the brain from the origins of the great vessels from the aortic arch to the circle of Willis and cerebral arteries within the skull. The image confirms that there is a tight stenosis at the origin of the right internal carotid artery (arrow).

Management

Medical therapy

All patients should receive BMT.

Carotid endarterectomy (CEA)

Patients with completed major stroke and little in the way of recovery are not candidates for carotid intervention; nor are those with an occluded internal carotid artery. However CEA combined with BMT is associated with a significant reduction in recurrent stroke, compared with BMT alone in patients with amaurosis, TIA and stroke with good recovery, provided that:

- There is a high degree of internal carotid artery stenosis (usually taken as a greater than 60–70% diameter reduction)
- The patient is expected to survive at least 2 years
- The intervention can be undertaken with a stroke and/or death rate of less than 3–5%
- The intervention can be performed soon after the index event. The exact timing remains controversial and is matter of judgment for each patient but, in general, the sooner the better.

Patients who do not fulfill these criteria should, in most cases, be treated medically. The operation can be equally well performed under general or local anaesthetic.

> ### EBM 21.2 Carotid endarterectomy: general or local anaesthesia?
>
> 'A definite difference in outcomes between general and local anaesthesia for carotid surgery has not been shown. The anaesthetist and surgeon, in consultation with the patient, should decide which anaesthetic technique to use on an individual basis.'
>
> GALA Trial Collaborative Group. General anaesthesia versus local anaesthesia for carotid surgery (GALA): a multicentre, randomised controlled trial. The Lancet 2008; 372: 2132–42.

21

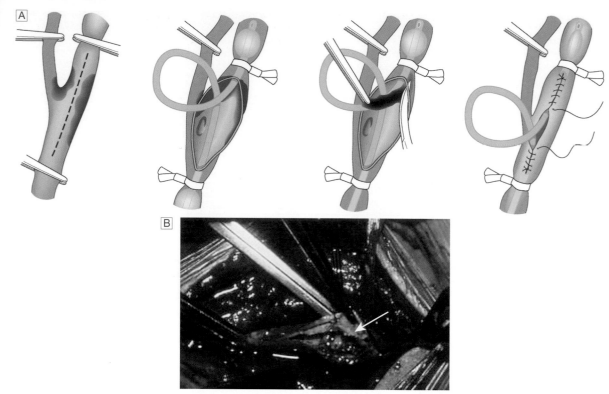

Fig. 21.17 Carotid endarterectomy. [A] Diagram showing carotid endarterectomy using a shunt in the internal carotid artery to maintain cerebral blood flow while the occluding plaque is removed and the artery repaired either by direct primary closure as shown here or, more usually, with a patch of vein or prosthetic material. [B] Operative photograph of plaque (arrow) being removed at carotid endarterectomy (no shunt being used in this case).

The carotid bifurcation is dissected, heparin is given and the arteries are clamped. If this may lead to cerebral ischaemia, a shunt is inserted. The plaque is shelled out (the endarterectomy) and the artery repaired with direct suture or a patch graft (patch angioplasty) (Fig. 21.17).

Carotid stenting

The role of carotid artery stenting (CAS) remains uncertain and controversial. While CAS avoids a neck wound and the risks of cranial nerve injury, and possibly reduces the risk of perioperative myocardial infarction, there is a growing body of evidence to show that the short-term risks of clinical and subclinical brain injury are greater than with CEA. For these reasons, most UK vascular specialists believe that CAS should be reserved for patients where CEA is either not possible or desirable because of anatomic and clinical factors (for example, recurrent stenosis after previous

surgery or radiation arteritis) optimal in the common carotid and inominate arteries.

Asymptomatic carotid disease

The evidence that undertaking CEA (or CAS) in addition to BMT confers clinical benefit in patients with asymptomatic ICA disease is weak. The risks of such people developing TIA/stroke are low (probably less than 10% at 5 years). So, even if one could halve that risk with intervention (*relative* risk reduction of 50%) the *absolute* risk reduction would be only 1% per year. This means the number of interventions needed to prevent one TIA or stroke is potentially quite large (perhaps 20–30 or more). By contrast, the *number needed to treat* for symptomatic disease is less than 10. CEA for asymptomatic carotid artery disease is, therefore, a highly cost-ineffective means of stroke reduction and a poor use of finite health care resources. Nevertheless, in many fee-for-service health care environments such as in the US, large number of CEA and CAS are still performed for asymptomatic carotid disease.

Vertebrobasilar disease

The vertebrobasilar system feeds the occipital cortex, cerebellum and brain stem. Patients with vertebrobasilar insufficiency (VBI) may complain of (bilateral) cortical blindness, vertigo and loss of balance. Few patients have focal, discrete disease amenable to vascular or endovascular intervention, and the great majority receive BMT only.

EBM **21.3 Carotid stenting**

'Completion of long-term follow-up is needed to establish the efficacy of carotid artery stenting compared with endarterectomy. In the meantime, carotid endarterectomy should remain the treatment of choice for patients suitable for surgery.'

International Carotid Stenting Study Investigators. Carotid artery stenting compared with endarterectomy in patients with symptomatic carotid stenosis: an interim analysis of a randomised controlled trial. The Lancet 2010; 375: 985–997.

RENAL ARTERY DISEASE

Pathophysiology

Atherosclerosis is by far the commonest cause of renal artery stenosis and usually affects the origin of the artery as part of aortic wall disease. Underperfusion of the juxtaglomerular apparatus leads to an increase in renin and angiotensin and the development of hypertension. The disease may also lead to ischaemic necrosis of the renal parenchyma and progressive renal failure. Fibromuscular hyperplasia is an uncommon condition that mostly affects young and middle-aged women. It may cause hypertension, but rarely renal failure.

Management

The indications for intervention remain controversial and, especially since the ASTRAL trial results were published (EBM 21.4), most patients with renovascular disease are treated medically in the UK. Although the evidence for benefit is weak, primary stenting for atherosclerotic renal artery disease may be considered in selected patients to:

- control hypertension that is refractory to medical therapy
- preserve renal function.

EBM 21.4 Intervention for renal artery disease

'Substantial risks but no evidence of a worthwhile clinical benefit from revascularization in patients with atherosclerotic renovascular disease was found.'

The ASTRAL Investigators. Revascularization versus Medical Therapy for renal-artery stenosis. New England Journal of Medicine 2009; 361: 1953–62.

Major complications (1–2%) include acute arterial occlusion, embolization and rupture. Surgical reconstruction is a major undertaking with significant associated morbidity and mortality that nowadays is rarely, if ever, performed. BAP alone is effective for fibromuscular hyperplasia.

MESENTERIC ARTERY DISEASE

Owing to rich collaterals between them, it is usually necessary for two of the three visceral vessels (coeliac axis, superior and inferior mesenteric arteries) to be occluded or critically stenosed before patients develop symptoms and signs. Typically, the patient develops severe central abdominal pain (mesenteric angina), sometimes with diarrhoea, 15–30 minutes after eating. Food avoidance and intolerance always leads to significant weight loss. The condition can mimic many much more common intra-abdominal pathologies. Surgery is associated with significant morbidity and mortality (5–10%), but the long-term symptom relief is usually excellent. BAP and stenting are increasingly used, particularly in patients with high operative risk and in those who have limited life expectancy.

Acute mesenteric ischaemia is usually caused by occlusion of the superior mesenteric artery (SMA) by embolus (usually from the heart in patients with AF) or acute thrombosis on top of pre-existing atherosclerosis. There is usually sudden onset of excruciating abdominal pain, collapse, bloody diarrhoea and peritonitis. Treatment comprises emergency SMA embolectomy (embolus) or SMA bypass (thrombosis) and resection of non-viable bowel. Unfortunately, extensive bowel necrosis is often already present at the time of surgery and mortality exceeds 50%. Endovascular techniques have little to offer, as the exclusion of bowel infarction requires a laparotomy.

SUMMARY BOX 21.3

Acute limb ischaemia

- Acute limb ischaemia is the most common vascular emergency
- The most common causes are embolus from the left atrium in association with atrial fibrillation and acute thrombosis at a site of long-standing atherosclerotic narrowing
- It is often but not always possible to distinguish these two conditions on clinical grounds alone
- The treatment of embolism is urgent embolectomy, usually without prior angiography
- Patients with thrombosis in situ should undergo angiography if possible; treatment comprises a combination of medical therapy, thrombolysis, angioplasty and bypass
- Paralysis, paraesthesia and muscle tenderness are the cardinal signs of complete acute ischaemia; when they are present, the limb must be revascularized within 4-6 hours if it is to be saved and full function restored. Fasciotomy should always be considered upon successful reperfusion to avoid compartment syndrome.

21

ACUTE LIMB ISCHAEMIA

Aetiology

Acute limb ischaemia is caused most frequently by acute thrombotic occlusion of a pre-existing stenotic arterial segment (60%), thromboembolism (30%) and trauma, which may be iatrogenic. Distinguishing between thrombosis and embolism is important because investigation, treatment and prognosis are different (Table 21.2).

Table 21.2 Embolus vs. thrombosis in situ

Clinical features	Embolus	Thrombosis
Severity	Complete ischaemia (no collaterals)	Incomplete ischaemia (collaterals)
Onset	Seconds or minutes	Hours or days
Limb	Leg 3:1 arm	Leg 10:1 arm
Multiple sites	Up to 15%	Rare
Embolic source	Present (usually AF)	Absent
Previous claudication	Absent	Present
Palpation of artery	Soft; tender	Hard/calcified
Bruits	Absent	Present
Contralateral leg pulses	Present	Absent
Diagnosis	Clinical	Angiography
Management	Embolectomy, warfarin	Medical, bypass, thrombolysis
Prognosis	Loss of life > loss of limb	Loss of limb > loss of life

More than 70% of peripheral emboli are due to AF. Thrombosis in situ may arise from acute plaque rupture, hypovolaemia, increased blood coagulability (for example in association with sepsis) or 'pump failure' (for example heart attack) (see below).

Classification

Limb ischaemia is classified on the basis of onset and severity (Table 21.3). Incomplete acute ischaemia (usually due to thrombosis in situ) can often be treated medically, at least in the first instance. Complete ischaemia (usually due to embolus) will normally result in extensive irreversible tissue injury within 6 hours unless the limb is revascularized. Irreversible ischaemia mandates early amputation or, if the patient is elderly and unfit, end-of-life care.

Clinical features

Apart from those that indicate 'loss of function', namely *paralysis* (inability to wiggle toes/fingers) and *paraesthesia* (loss of light touch over the dorsum of the foot/hand), the so-called Ps of acute ischaemia are non-specific and/or inconsistently related to its severity and should not be relied upon (Table 21.4).

Acute loss of limb function, of which vascular insufficiency is only one cause, must always be taken very seriously indeed; the patient should never be discharged

Table 21.3 Classification of limb ischaemia

Terminology	Definition/comment
Onset	
Acute	Ischaemia < 14 days
Acute-on-chronic	Worsening symptoms and signs (< 14 days)
Chronic	Ischaemia stable for > 14 days
Severity (acute, acute-on-chronic)	
Incomplete	Limb not threatened
Complete	Limb threatened
Irreversible	Limb non-viable
Severity (chronic)	
Non-critical	Intermittent claudication
Subcritical	Night/rest pain
Critical	Tissue loss (ulceration ± gangrene)

Table 21.4 Symptoms and signs of acute limb ischaemia

Symptoms/signs	Comment
Pain	May be absent in complete acute ischaemia; severe pain is also a feature of chronic ischaemia
Pallor	Also a feature of chronic ischaemia
Pulseless	Also a feature of chronic ischaemia
Perishing cold	Unreliable, as the ischaemic limb takes on the ambient temperature
Paraesthesia and paralysis	Loss of function is the most important feature of acute limb ischaemia and denotes a threatened limb that is likely to be lost unless it is revascularized within a few hours

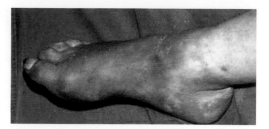

Fig. 21.18 Mottled right foot due to advanced acute limb ischaemia.

until a diagnosis has been made. In the presence of ischaemia, pain on squeezing the calf indicates muscle infarction and impending irreversible ischaemia.

At first, acute complete ischaemia is associated with intense distal arterial spasm and the limb is 'marble' white. As the spasm relaxes over the next few hours and the skin fills with deoxygenated blood, mottling appears. This is light blue or purple, has a fine reticular pattern and blanches on pressure: so-called 'non-fixed mottling'. At this stage, the limb is still salvageable. As ischaemia progresses, blood coagulates in the skin, leading to mottling that is darker in colour, coarser in pattern and does not blanch. Finally, large patches of fixed staining progress to blistering and liquefaction (Fig. 21.18). Attempts at revascularization at this late stage are futile and will lead to life-threatening reperfusion injury (see below).

Management

All suspected acutely ischaemic limbs must be discussed *immediately* with a vascular surgeon; a few hours can make the difference between amputation or death, and complete recovery of limb function. If there are no contraindications, such as trauma (especially head injury) or suspected aortic dissection, an intravenous bolus of heparin (typically 3000–5000U) is administered to limit propagation of thrombus and protect the collateral circulation. If ischaemia is complete, the patient proceeds directly to the operating theatre for attempted embolectomy (preferably under local anaesthesia). If ischaemia is incomplete, preoperative imaging is obtained wherever possible, as simple embolectomy or thrombectomy is unlikely to be successful; a 'road-map' for distal bypass is helpful; and it is often possible, at least initially, to manage the patient medically depending on the results of imaging.

Acute embolus

Embolic occlusion of the brachial artery is not usually limb-threatening and, in an elderly patient, non-operative treatment is reasonable. Younger patients should undergo embolectomy to prevent subsequent claudication, especially where the dominant arm is affected.

A leg affected by embolus is nearly always threatened and requires immediate surgical revascularization. Femoral embolus is usually associated with profound ischaemia to the level of the upper thigh because the deep femoral artery is also affected. Acute embolic occlusion of the aortic bifurcation (saddle embolus) leads to absent femoral pulses and a patient who is 'marble' white or mottled to the waist. Such patients may also present with paraplegia due to ischaemia of the cauda equina, which may be irreversible. Embolectomy can be performed under local/regional or general anaesthetic (Fig. 21.19).

Postoperatively, the patient should continue on heparin. Warfarin reduces the risk of recurrent embolism but is associated with an annual risk of significant bleeding of

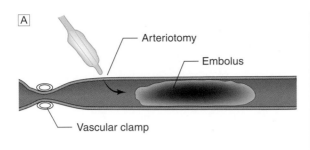

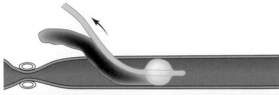

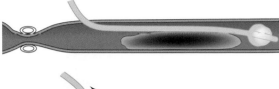

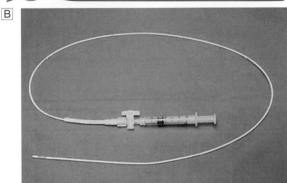

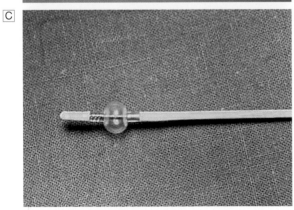

Fig. 21.19 Embolectomy. [A] Diagram showing removal of an embolus with a balloon catheter. The balloon is inflated once it is beyond the thrombus and then withdrawn. [B] Embolectomy catheter. [C] Tip of embolectomy catheter with balloon inflated.

1–2% in the long term. The in-hospital mortality from cardiac death and/or recurrent embolism, particularly stroke, is 10–20%.

Thrombosis in situ

There is usually a reason why the limb affected by stable chronic ischaemia suddenly deteriorates due to thrombosis in situ on top of atherosclerosis. These include 'silent'

or overt MI (drop in blood pressure); underlying, perhaps hitherto asymptomatic, malignancy (increase in thrombogenicity of the blood); septicaemia, particularly pneumococcal and meningococcal; and dehydration from any cause, which may be associated with widespread thrombosis. Many patients can be managed medically. If the limb remains threatened then it may be possible to clear the thrombus by open surgical or endoluminal means; to dissolve the clot by means of thrombolysis or bypass the affected segment. If urgent surgery is required the in-hospital limb loss rate may approach 30%; in hospital mortality is 10–20%

Popliteal aneurysm

Popliteal aneurysm can undergo thrombosis or act as a source of emboli. Bypass (or stent-grafting) should be performed to exclude the aneurysm (see below) and thrombolysis may be required to re-establish the distal run off. Acute thrombosis of popliteal aneurysm is associated with an in-hospital limb loss rate that can approach 50%.

Trauma

In the UK, acute traumatic limb ischaemia is frequently iatrogenic. The most common causes of non-iatrogenic injury are limb fractures and dislocations, blunt injuries occurring in the course of road traffic accidents, and stab wounds (gun shot wounds are mercifully rare in the UK but common in many other parts of the world). The presence of distal pulses emphatically does *not* exclude significant arterial injury, especially in otherwise young and fit trauma patients. Where there is any suspicion at all of major vascular injury, vascular imaging (e.g. MR or CT angiography) should be performed immediately; operating 'blind' is to be avoided if at all possible.

Intra-arterial drug administration

This leads to intense spasm and microvascular thrombosis. The leg is mottled and digital gangrene is common, but pedal pulses are often palpable. The mainstay of treatment is supportive care, hydration to minimize renal failure secondary to rhabdomyolysis, and full heparinization. Vascular reconstruction is almost never indicated, but fasciotomy may be required to prevent compartment syndrome (see below). Limb loss rates are high.

Thoracic outlet syndrome

Pressure on the subclavian artery from a cervical rib or abnormal soft tissue band may lead to a poststenotic dilatation lined with thrombosis, predisposing to occlusion or embolization. The distal circulation may be chronically obliterated and digital ischaemia advanced before the diagnosis is made. The diagnosis is confirmed on duplex scan and/or MRA. Treatment options include thrombolysis, thrombectomy/embolectomy, excision of the cervical rib and repair (replacement) of the aneurysmal segment.

Postischaemic syndromes

Reperfusion injury

Activated neutrophils, free radicals, enzymes, hydrogen ions, carbon dioxide, potassium and myoglobin released from reperfused tissue can lead to acute respiratory distress syndrome (ARDS), myocardial stunning, endotoxaemia and acute tubular necrosis, and in turn, to multiple organ failure and death.

21

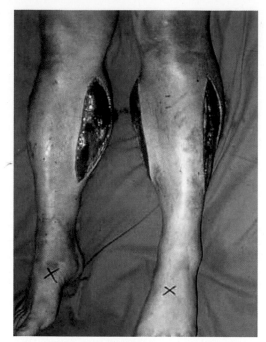

Fig. 21.20 Medial and lateral fasciotomy to decompress compartment syndrome in a patient who presented with bilateral acute limb ischaemia due to saddle embolus (the crosses marked on the skin indicate the position of palpable pulses) and underwent successful embolectomy.

Compartment syndrome

Endothelial cell injury during ischaemia leads to increased capillary permeability and oedema on reperfusion. In the calf, where muscles are confined within tight fascial boundaries, the increase in interstitial tissue pressure can lead to continuing muscle necrosis despite apparently adequate arterial inflow: the so-called compartment syndrome. There is swelling and pain on squeezing the calf muscle or moving the ankle or toes. It is very important to remember that palpable pedal pulses do not exclude compartment syndrome. The key to management is prevention through expeditious revascularization and a low threshold for fasciotomy to relieve the pressure (Fig. 21.20).

ANEURYSMAL DISEASE

Classification

An aneurysm may be defined as an abnormal focal dilatation of an endothelial-lined vascular structure (artery, vein, heart chamber). Arterial aneurysms are by far the most common. Aneurysms may be classified according to their site, underlying aetiology and morphology.

Site

Any artery can be affected. The most common site for aneurysmal disease requiring treatment is the infrarenal aorta; others include the popliteal, femoral and subclavian arteries.

Aetiology

Atherosclerotic

Most aneurysms are 'non-specific' in aetiology; in the past they were termed 'atherosclerotic'. However, it is now widely believed that aneurysmal disease is a distinct pathological process from occlusive arterial disease, although they share some of the same risk factors (smoking and hypertension) and may coexist in the same patient.

Mycotic

The term mycotic, meaning fungal, is a misnomer because fungi do not cause aneurysms. The term is used nowadays to include all aneurysms that are believed to be infectious in origin. The infection can be primary or secondary to other pathology. Arteries are generally resistant to infection, but two organisms, *Treponema pallidum* (syphilis) and salmonella, have a particular ability to produce primary mycotic aneurysms. Septic emboli from heart valves affected by subacute bacterial endocarditis may also lodge in the distal vasculature and produce secondary mycotic aneurysms. 'Non-specific' aneurysms and the layers of laminated thrombus within them may become infected in the course of a bacteraemia from another site. Lastly, infection of prosthetic grafts can lead to infected anastomotic aneurysms.

True aneurysms

All three layers of the arterial wall enclose a true aneurysm, which may be saccular or fusiform (Fig. 21.21).

False aneurysms

If the wall of an artery is damaged, the resulting surrounding haematoma can remain in continuity with the lumen leading to a pulsatile swelling whose wall comprises compacted thrombus and surrounding connective tissue. Small aneurysms (1–2 cm in diameter) often thrombose spontaneously but larger aneurysms tend to expand (especially if the patient is on aspirin, heparin or warfarin) and compress surrounding tissues. The most common site is the groin after common femoral artery instrumentation, and this may cause femoral vein compression and deep venous thrombosis (DVT). Surgery is increasingly being replaced by ultrasound-guided thrombin injection. Where such

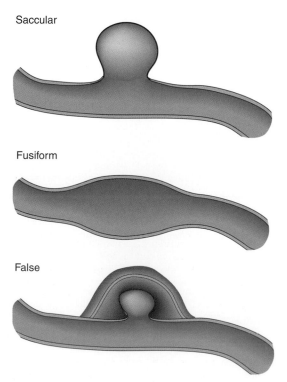

Saccular

Fusiform

False

Fig. 21.21 True and false aneurysms.

aneurysms develop in less accessible sites, such as the aorto-iliac segment, then the hole can be sealed using a covered stent introduced percutaneously or by blocking the artery (embolization) usually via the femoral artery.

Abdominal aortic aneurysm (AAA)

 SUMMARY BOX 21.4

Abdominal aortic aneurysm (AAA)

- AAAs are present in up to 5% of men aged over 70 years; more than half are asymptomatic and go undetected until they rupture
- Ruptured AAA is the 10th most common cause of death in men. Only a third of patients with ruptured AAA reach hospital alive and, of these, only about half survive surgery. The overall mortality for the condition therefore exceeds 80%. Population screening of men over the age of 65 years with ultrasound may reduce the number of ruptured AAAs by up to 50%
- Patients with asymptomatic AAA should be considered for repair if the maximum diameter reaches 5.5 cm and the surgeon believes the operation will be associated with a mortality of less than 5%
- An increasingly large number of AAAs are being treated by endovascular aneurysm repair (EVAR), which is associated with a significant reduction in peri-operative morbidity and mortality although questions still remain around long-term durability and protection from rupture.

Epidemiology

AAA is present in up to 5% of men aged over 70 years and is 2–3 times commoner in men than in women of the same age. In about 70% of cases, only the infrarenal aortic segment is involved. In the remainder, the rest of the abdominal aorta, the thoracic aorta or a combination of both is involved.

Clinical features

An AAA may present in the following ways:

- Asymptomatic (60%). The AAA may be detected incidentally on routine physical examination, plain X-ray or, most commonly, abdominal ultrasound scan conducted for another reason. Even a large AAA can be difficult to feel. Patients in whom an incidental finding of an AAA is made should be considered for treatment or surveillance.
- Symptomatic (10%). AAA may cause pain in the central abdomen, back, loin, iliac fossa or groin. Thrombus within the aneurysm sac may be a source of emboli to the lower limbs. Much less commonly, the aneurysm may undergo thrombotic occlusion. AAA may also become inflamed and then compress surrounding structures such as the duodenum, ureter and the inferior vena cava.
- Rupture (30%). AAA may rupture, usually into the retroperitoneum, but sometimes into the peritoneal cavity or rarely into surrounding structures, most commonly the inferior vena cava, leading to an aorto-caval fistula.

Studies have shown that screening for AAA by means of ultrasound results in a reduction in the number of deaths from rupture (EBM 21.5). The UK has begun introducing a national screening programme for AAA (http://aaa.screening.nhs.uk).

EBM 21.5 **Screening for AAA**

'The mortality benefit of screening for AAA in men aged 64–73 years was maintained in the longer term and screening was cost effective.'

Lindholt, J S. Long-term benefit and cost-effectiveness analysis of screening for abdominal aortic aneurysms from a randomized controlled trial British Journal of Surgery 2010; 97: 826–34.

Investigations

Ultrasound is the best way of establishing the diagnosis, of obtaining an approximate size, and of following up patients with asymptomatic AAAs that are not yet large enough to warrant surgical repair (Fig. 21.22). CT angiography (CTA) will provide much more accurate information about the size and extent of the aneurysm, involvement of visceral arteries and the surrounding structures, and whether there is any other intra-abdominal pathology. It is the standard prein-tervention investigation but is not suitable for surveillance because of the ionizing radiation and cost (Fig. 21.23).

Asymptomatic AAA

Trials have shown that the risks of open surgery generally outweigh the risks of rupture until an asymptomatic AAA has reached 5.5 cm in anteroposterior maximum diameter. It is, therefore, unusual in the UK for an AAA smaller than this to be operated upon in the absence of symptoms. Once a small AAA has been detected, the best way of following up the affected patient is by repeated ultrasound scans at regular intervals (depending on the size). Patients are encouraged strongly to comply with BMT, which affords the same benefits as it does in patients with occlusive disease (which often coexists). Ultrasound is only accurate to about 0.5 cm and tends to underestimate AAA size. Thus, many specialists will arrange for a CT when the AAA reaches 5.0 cm, along with other tests designed to assess fitness for surgery. Once the AAA reaches 5.5 cm and assuming the clinical assessment and investigations indicate that the patient is fit for surgery, the surgeon will normally begin discussions with the patient with a view to open repair (OR) or endovascular aneurysm repair (EVAR).

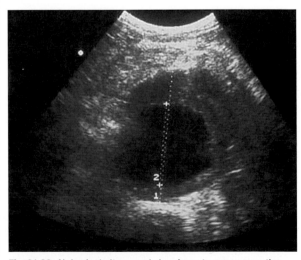

Fig. 21.22 Abdominal ultrasound showing a transverse section through a large abdominal aortic aneurysm. Measurement 1 shows the front to back (AP) diameter of the AAA from wall to wall while measurement 2 shows the diameter of the lumen through the thrombus lining the aneurysmal sac

21

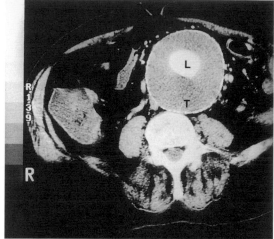

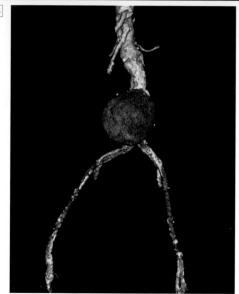

Fig. 21.23 Computed tomography (CT) in abdominal aortic aneurysm. **A** Transverse section (L = lumen, T = thrombus). **B** CT angiography (CTA): 3-D reconstruction.

Symptomatic AAA

All symptomatic AAAs should be considered for repair, not only to rid the patient of their symptoms, but also because pain often predates rupture. Distal embolization is a definite indication for repair, even if the AAA is small, as limb loss is common if the AAA is left untreated.

Ruptured AAA

This is the most common emergency presentation of AAA. Patients survive rupture for the following reasons:

- The rupture is usually into the retroperitoneum, which tamponades (restricts the extent of) the leak
- There is intense vasoconstriction of non-essential circulatory beds
- The patient develops an intensely prothrombotic state
- The patient's blood pressure drops, which helps to limit the blood loss.

Any medical intervention that upsets this delicate balance will convert a relatively stable, potentially salvageable patient into one unlikely to reach the operating theatre or to survive intervention. Specifically, large volumes of

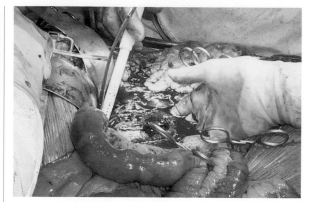

Fig. 21.24 Intraoperative photograph of repair of a ruptured abdominal aortic aneurysm.

intravenous fluid (saline or plasma expander) increase the patient's blood pressure, impair haemostasis and abolish vasoconstriction, and must therefore not be given. The only way of saving the patient is to either clamp and graft the aorta or insert a stent graft (EVAR) (if necessary having controlled the bleeding through angioplasty balloon occlusion of the thoracic aorta); there must be absolutely no delay in getting the patient to a hospital where this can be done (Fig. 21.24).

Open AAA repair (OR)

This entails replacing the aneurysmal segment with a prosthetic graft (Fig. 21.25). The 30-day major morbidity and mortality for this procedure is approximately 5–10% for elective asymptomatic AAA, 10–20% for emergency symptomatic AAA and up to 50% for ruptured AAA.

Endovascular aneurysm repair (EVAR)

EVAR involves placing a covered stent graft inside the aneurysm via a femoral arteriotomy, or percutaneously, under radiological guidance (Figs 21.26 and 21.27). The procedure can be performed under regional (epidural) or even local anaesthesia. Laparotomy and cross-clamping of the aorta are avoided. The patient is often fit to go home within 48 hours, as opposed to the 7–10 days that are typical following OR. Patients also usually make a rapid return (4–6 weeks) to their preoperative functional

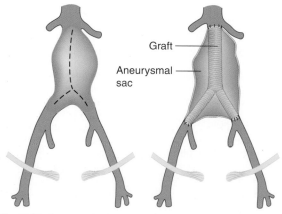

Graft

Aneurysmal sac

Fig. 21.25 Open repair of an abdominal aortic aneurysm. Diagram showing insertion of a 'trouser' bifurcation graft within the opened aneurysmal sac.

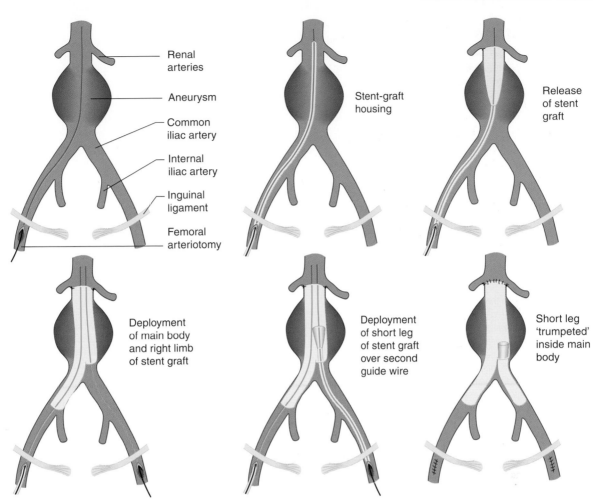

Fig. 21.26 Endovascular stent-graft repair of an abdominal aortic aneurysm. **A** A guidewire is passed through the aneurysm via an incision in the right common femoral artery. **B** A catheter containing the main body of the stent graft is passed over the guidewire and into position within the aneurysm. **C** The outer cover of the catheter is removed, allowing the upper part of the stent graft to spring open and become attached by hooks to the wall of the aorta just below the renal arteries. **D** The rest of the catheter is removed, allowing deployment of the main body of the graft and the right (long) limb within the common iliac artery. Note the short (left) limb of the graft. **E** Via an incision in the left common femoral artery a second guidewire is passed up through the short limb of the stent graft. A second catheter containing the rest of the stent graft is passed over the guidewire and into the main body of the stent graft. As before, retraction of the outer cover allows the top of the second limb of the stent graft to open within the short limb of the main body. **F** Deployment is complete and the aneurysm sac completely excluded from the circulation. The femoral arteries are closed.

status, whereas those who have undergone OR often take 4–6 months to feel as well as they did before their operation. Not surprisingly therefore, several trials have shown that EVAR is associated with a marked reduction in hospital mortality and morbidity, reduced hospital stay and improved early postoperative quality of life (EBM 21.6). There are, however, downsides; specifically, the devices are expensive (£5000 or more); a significant proportion of AAAs are unsuitable for the procedure with present technology; and there are still questions over durability in that the secondary intervention rate following EVAR is much higher than it is following OR, and EVAR appears to afford less protection from rupture than OR in the long term. In patients unfit for open surgery, the addition of EVAR to BMT is of no benefit when compared to BMT alone (EBM 21.6).

Over the coming years, the technology is likely to continue to improve, such that the morbidity and mortality associated with EVAR will fall even further; the second-ary intervention rates will also fall; and most patients can be treated by EVAR, which is likely to become the standard treatment. The technique also has applicability in patients with thoracic and thoraco-abdominal aneurysms and dissection. Several groups have published encouraging results of EVAR for ruptured aneurysms.

Peripheral aneurysms

Any peripheral artery, and very rarely vein, can be affected by aneurysmal dilatation. The aetiology, clinical features and treatment vary depending upon the site of disease.

Iliac aneurysms

In approximately 20% of patients, AAAs extend into one or both common iliac arteries and about a third of these extend into the internal iliac artery; the external iliac artery is rarely

Diagram labels (Fig. 21.26):
- Renal arteries
- Aneurysm
- Common iliac artery
- Internal iliac artery
- Inguinal ligament
- Femoral arteriotomy
- Stent-graft housing
- Release of stent graft
- Deployment of main body and right limb of stent graft
- Deployment of short leg of stent graft over second guide wire
- Short leg 'trumpeted' inside main body

EBM 21.6 Endovascular aneurysm repair (EVAR)

'Six years after randomization, endovascular and open repair of abdominal aortic aneurysm resulted in similar rates of survival. The rate of secondary interventions was significantly higher for endovascular repair.'

DREAM Study Group. Long-term outcome of open or endovascular repair of abdominal aortic aneurysm. New England Journal of Medicine 2010; 362(20): 1881–9

'In this large, randomized trial, endovascular repair of abdominal aortic aneurysm was associated with a significantly lower operative mortality than open surgical repair. However, no differences were seen in total mortality or aneurysm-related mortality in the long term. Endovascular repair was associated with increased rates of graft-related complications and re-interventions and was more costly.'

UK EVAR Trial Investigators. Endovascular versus open repair of abdominal aortic aneurysm. New England Journal of Medicine 2010; 362(20): 1863–71

'In this randomized trial involving patients who were physically ineligible for open repair, endovascular repair of abdominal aortic aneurysm was associated with a significantly lower rate of aneurysm-related mortality than no repair. However, endovascular repair was not associated with a reduction in the rate of death from any cause. The rates of graft-related complications and re-interventions were higher with endovascular repair, and it was more costly.'

UK EVAR Trial Investigators. Endovascular repair of aortic aneurysm in patients physically ineligible for open repair. New England Journal of Medicine 2010; 362(20): 1872–80

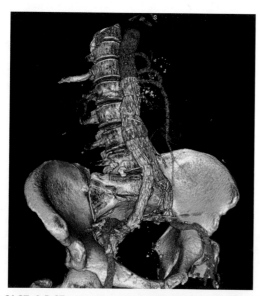

Fig. 21.27 3-D CT reconstruction of a stent graft deployed inside an abdominal aortic aneurysm. (Courtesy of Mr Donald Adam.)

affected. Isolated iliac aneurysms can also occur. The bifurcation of the aorta is at the level of the umbilicus, so that a pulsatile mass felt below that level is likely to be iliac in origin. Iliac aneurysms are most often treated in the course of AAA repair. Isolated iliac aneurysms should be considered for EVAR or surgical repair if they are causing symptoms or have reached twice the normal diameter of the native artery.

Femoral aneurysms

There are three main types of femoral aneurysm: iatrogenic false aneurysm (see above), non-specific aneurysm and anastomotic aneurysm. 'Non-specific' aneurysms of the common femoral artery are found in 10% of patients with AAA and also as an isolated occurrence. Patients presenting with a femoral aneurysm should have an AAA excluded by ultrasound scan. In 50% of cases they are bilateral. They are frequently asymptomatic but may cause pain and compression of surrounding structures (femoral vein and nerve); rupture is uncommon. If large (>3 cm) or symptomatic, they should be considered for surgical repair. Anastomotic false aneurysms are increasingly being seen in patients who have previously undergone bypass grafting for occlusive or aneurysmal disease. They may not present until many years after the original surgery, but once present, they usually grow inexorably and require repair. They are usually due to mechanical disruption of the anastomosis as a result of late suture failure or progressive disease of the femoral artery; less commonly, they are due to late graft infection.

Popliteal aneurysms

These are present in 20% of patients with AAA and their presence must be sought, if necessary with ultrasound, in all such patients. Around 50% are bilateral. If a patient presents with a popliteal aneurysm, there is a 50% chance that he or she also has an AAA, which again must be sought by ultrasound. The main complications of popliteal aneurysm are distal embolization and acute thrombosis; the latter is associated with limb loss in up to 50% of cases because the calf vessels are often chronically occluded, which makes surgical bypass difficult. The best treatment is by surgical bypass using the long saphenous vein. Sometimes, in severely ischaemic limbs, it is necessary to instill a thrombolytic agent at the same time as, or before, operative exclusion and bypass. Rupture of popliteal aneurysms is extremely rare. Occasionally, they can compress the popliteal vein and present as a DVT.

BUERGER'S DISEASE (THROMBOANGIITIS OBLITERANS)

This is an inflammatory obliterative arterial disease that is quite distinct from atherosclerosis. It is rare in Caucasians but more common in people from the Mediterranean, Asia and North Africa. It usually presents in young (20–30 years) male smokers and characteristically affects the peripheral arteries, giving rise to claudication in the feet or rest pain in the fingers or toes. Such pain in the feet on walking is often misdiagnosed as musculoskeletal in nature, whereas pain in the fingers or toes is often misdiagnosed as primary Raynaud's phenomenon. The condition also affects the veins, and superficial thrombophlebitis is common. Wrist and ankle pulses are usually absent, but brachial and popliteal pulses are palpable. Arteriography shows narrowing or occlusion of arteries below the diseased segment, but relatively healthy vessels above that level.

The condition often remits if the patient stops smoking; sympathectomy and prostaglandin infusions may be helpful. If amputation is required, it can often be limited to the digits at first. However, if the patient continues to smoke, then bilateral below-knee amputation is a frequent outcome. Although the disease is uncommon in the UK, it is very important to consider and exclude it in patients presenting with vascular symptoms in their legs and arms, especially if the symptoms are atypical and the patient is young (under 50 years of age). Failure to make the diagnosis often leads to avoidable limb loss and is a source of medicolegal activity.

RAYNAUD'S PHENOMENON

Raynaud's phenomenon describes digital pallor due to vasospasm of the digital arteries, followed by cyanosis owing to the presence of deoxygenated blood, then rubor due to reactive hyperaemia upon restoration of flow, in response to cold and emotional stimuli.

Primary Raynaud's phenomenon

Raynaud's disease affects 5–10% of young women in temperate climates, and usually appears between the ages of 15 and 30 years; a family history is common. It does not progress to ulceration or infarction. No investigation is necessary and the patient is given reassurance, advised to avoid exposure to cold, and treated in the first instance with nifedipine (a calcium channel blocker). The underlying cause is unclear.

Secondary Raynaud's phenomenon

This is also known as Raynaud's syndrome and tends to occur in older people in association with:

- connective tissue disease, most commonly systemic sclerosis
- vibration-induced injury, from the use of power tools (vibration white finger, hand-arm vibration syndrome)
- atherosclerosis, most commonly thoracic outlet obstruction from the cervical rib (see above).

Unlike primary disease that is due to reversible spasm, secondary disease is usually associated with fixed obstruction of the digital arteries. Fingertip ulceration and necrosis are often present. The fingers must be protected from cold and trauma, infection is treated with antibiotics, and surgery is avoided if possible. Vasoactive drugs have no clear benefit. Sympathectomy helps for a year or two. Prostacyclin infusions are sometimes beneficial. In the UK, hand arm vibration syndrome (HAVS) is a compensatable industrial occupational disease.

PATHOPHYSIOLOGY OF VENOUS DISEASE

Anatomy

The great (GSV) and lesser (LSV) (somewhat confusingly previously known respectively as the long and short) saphenous veins and their tributaries lie outside the deep fascia and in health carry about 10% of the venous return from the limb. The GSV begins at the medial end of the dorsal venous arch, crosses in front of the medial malleolus and ascends the medial side of the leg. It penetrates the deep (cribriform) fascia 2.5 cm below and lateral to the pubic tubercle to enter the common femoral vein at the saphenofemoral junction (SFJ). The LSV starts at the lateral end of the dorsal venous arch, passes posterior to the lateral

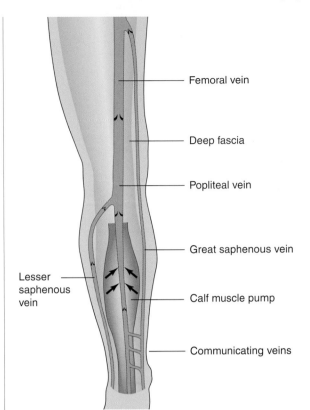

Fig. 21.28 Diagrammatic representation of the venous drainage of the lower limb.

malleolus, then ascends the median posterior line of the calf to join the popliteal vein at the saphenopopliteal junction (SPJ), usually just above the knee. Anatomical variations are very common.

The deep venous system comprises intramuscular veins and axial veins that accompany the main arteries; they are usually paired in the calf. Communicating veins perforate the deep fascia to connect the superficial and deep systems (Fig. 21.28).

Physiology

Weight-bearing compresses the veins in the sole of the foot, which propels blood into the calf ('foot pump'). Pushing off when walking is associated with calf muscle contraction and the compression of venous blood in the muscular sinuses and axial veins; this propels blood further up the leg ('calf pump'). When the leg is lifted off the floor and the muscles relax, blood is prevented from refluxing back down the leg by the closure of valves. During this relaxation phase, blood passes from the superficial to the deep veins via perforators, ready to be expelled during the next step. In motionless standing, the venous pressure at the ankle is approximately 100 mmHg: that is, the hydrostatic pressure exerted by the column of venous blood stretching from the ankle to the right atrium. However, upon walking, the mechanisms described above reduce the ankle pressure to less than 25 mmHg (ambulatory venous pressure, AVP). The symptoms and signs of lower limb venous disease are largely due to failure of these protective mechanisms and the presence of a high AVP.

Venous disease

- Varicose veins are present in over 50% of the adult population; approximately 10% have skin changes of chronic venous insufficiency; and the life time risk of chronic venous ulceration is about 1%
- Compression therapy is the mainstay of treatment for chronic venous insufficiency, but should never be implemented unless the arterial status of the leg is known to be satisfactory (palpable pedal pulses and/or an ABPI > 0.8)
- If patients with lower limb venous disease are being considered for surgical or endovenous treatment, they should undergo duplex ultrasonography to delineate the pattern of superficial and deep venous reflux and obstruction
- DVT in postoperative patients is often asymptomatic. Most postoperative patients developing (fatal) PE have normal legs on clinical examination. Duplex ultrasound or venography should be used to confirm the diagnosis of DVT; V/Q scan or CT pulmonary angiography can be used to diagnose PE
- All hospital patients, medical and surgical, should have their thromboembolic risk assessed and receive prophylaxis accordingly. PE remains the most common cause of potentially preventable death in hospital

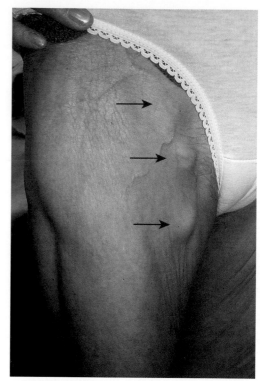

Fig. 21.29 Great saphenous varicose veins and saphena varix (arrow).

VARICOSE VEINS

Classification

Trunk varices

These involve the main stem and/or major tributaries of the GSV and LSV, are usually > 4 mm in diameter (and may be much larger); lie subcutaneously; are palpable; do not usually discolour the overlying skin; and are present in about a third of the adult population (Fig. 21.29).

Although 2–3 times more women than men present for treatment, the prevalence is roughly equal between the sexes. There appears to be a familial tendency; obesity, pregnancy, constipation and (occupational) prolonged standing may be aggravating factors.

Reticular varices

These lie deep in the dermis, are < 4 mm in diameter, are impalpable, and render the overlying skin dark blue. They are present in about 80% of the adult population, and may or may not be associated with trunk varices.

Telangiectasia

These are also called spider and thread veins. They lie superficially in the dermis, are usually 1 mm or less in diameter, are impalpable, and render the overlying skin purple or bright red. Again, they may be associated with trunk and reticular varices, and are present in 90% of adults. Like reticular veins, they appear to be more common in women, possibly because of poorly understood hormonal reasons.

Epidemiology

Varicose veins (VV) are so prevalent that they could almost be considered a variant of normal for a creature that spends its life on two as opposed to four legs. Their prevalence increases markedly with age and they are an almost universal finding in individuals over the age of 60.

Clinical features

The great majority of individuals with VV are asymptomatic, or at least they do not seek treatment. Those that attend the surgical clinic do so because they are unhappy about the appearance of their leg(s), and/or they associate lower limb symptoms with their VV, and/or they are concerned about developing complications.

Cosmetic issues

Many patients, especially young women, seek treatment because they consider their veins to be unsightly. Possibly because they are unwilling to admit that cosmesis is the main issue, they frequently complain of various lower limb symptoms as well.

Symptoms

A wide variety of lower limb symptoms have been attributed to VV. Lower limb symptoms are present in about half of the adult population, and there is an inconsistent relationship between these symptoms and the size and extent of VV on clinical examination and duplex ultrasound examination.

Complications

Only a proportion of patients with VV go on to develop the complications of chronic venous insufficiency (CVI): for example, leg ulcers, haemorrhage and thrombophlebitis. There is on-going controversy as to whether VV are a risk factor for DVT but in young, otherwise healthy individuals, they are probably not. However, in the elderly, in whom VV are more likely to be associated with skin changes of chronic venous insufficiency and in whom they may be a marker for coexistent deep venous disease, they probably are. At present, it is difficult to predict which patients will develop these complications and to know whether early VV surgery would prevent them, because the necessary longitudinal studies have never been done.

Indications for treatment

In correctly selected patients, it is clear that interventions for VV are associated with a marked improvement in health related quality of life (HRQL) and symptom relief. In patients with uncomplicated VV, surgeons must use their own judgment and experience to determine whether the patient truly does have symptoms, whether those symptoms are of venous aetiology, and, if so, whether they are likely to be relieved by intervention. Many VV interventions are performed in the private sector for purely cosmetic indications.

Aetiology

The true aetiology of VV remains unclear. The favoured hypothesis is that there is a structural defect in the vein wall, that may at least in part be inherited, which causes progressive dilatation in response to increased venous pressure consequent upon our bipedal posture and other factors. This leads to secondary incompetence of the valves (reflux), which in turn leads to more stress on the wall and more dilatation. These are sometimes termed primary VV. As in the deep venous system, thrombosis in the superficial veins (superficial thrombophlebitis) can destroy the valves leading to reflux. And lastly, deep venous obstruction, usually due to DVT, can lead to the appearance of superficial varices which act as collateral pathways around that obstruction. These are sometimes termed secondary VV. Such secondary VV should not be removed as that will result in a further reduction in the venous outflow of the leg leading to worsening post-thrombotic syndrome characterized by pain and swelling, especially on walking (venous claudication).

Examination and investigation

The patient should be examined standing in a warm room; the whole leg is visualized from toes to groin with the lower abdomen also exposed. The distribution of VV may indicate whether they are great or lesser saphenous or both. Various percussion and tourniquet based tests, such as the famous Trendelenburg test, are highly inaccurate and should not be performed these days. Some surgeons use hand-held Doppler probes to help delineate patterns of reflux but even in the best of hands the method lacks precision and accuracy. In reality, as duplex ultrasound machines become smaller, more portable, easier to use and cheaper, there is a move towards performing duplex examinations in the clinic on all patients being considered for intervention.

Severe VV, especially in children, of atypical distribution or associated with skin discoloration, soft-tissue hypertrophy or limb overgrowth, should raise the suspicion of congenital vascular malformations. Such patients should undergo MRI to assess the extent of the lesion and the arterial component.

Management

Conservative treatment

Many patients with uncomplicated VV can be managed conservatively in primary care. Elastic support hose, weight reduction, regular exercise and the avoidance of constricting garments and prolonged standing all help to relieve tiredness and reduce swelling. However, many patients, especially those seeking treatment for cosmetic indications, will refuse to wear unfashionable compression garments and seek surgical or endovenous treatment.

Surgery

VV surgery aims to remove varices and intercept incompetent connections between deep and superficial veins so that further varices do not form. In patients with GSV disease, the SFJ is ligated flush with the femoral vein (Fig. 21.30). Recurrence is very much less likely if the LSV is stripped out from knee to groin. Care must be taken not to damage the saphenous nerve, which joins and runs with the GSV below the knee. In patients with LSV disease, the SPJ is dealt with in a similar fashion. However, the LSV is not normally stripped for fear of injuring the sural nerve with which it runs. Remaining varices are avulsed through multiple tiny incisions.

Although such surgery has been the mainstay of VV treatment for many decades, even in the best of hands, the outcomes can be suboptimal with a significant incidence of minor but nevertheless undesirable complications and disappointing cosmetic results. It is salutary to note that VV surgery remains the commonest cause of litigation against vascular surgeons in the UK.

For these reasons, there has been a significant investment in time and money to try to find more satisfactory, non-surgical (endovenous) solutions.

Endovenous treatment

Surgery is being increasingly replaced by a range of minimally invasive endovenous treatments that can be performed under local anaesthesia as a day case or even as an outpatient procedure. The techniques include:

- Radiofrequency ablation (RFA)
- Endovenous LASER ablation (EVLA)
- Ultrasound guided foam sclerotherapy (UGFS) (Fig. 21.31).

Each of these techniques has pros and cons. However, performed correctly by appropriately trained clinicians, they appear to work at least as well as (often better than) surgery in many patients, and offer significant advantages in terms of less pain and a speedier return to normal activities. The catheter based techniques (RFA, EVLA) can deal with most truncal reflux but many patients require adjuvant treatment, such a stab avulsions or sclerotherapy, to deal with the varices themselves. UGFS has the advantage of being extremely versatile offering a complete treatment of truncal reflux and varices usually in one setting; foam is also much less expensive than RFA and EVLA and so more cost-effective.

21

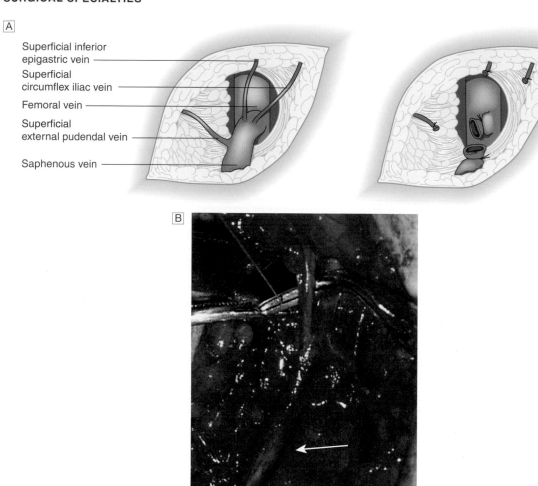

Superficial inferior epigastric vein

Superficial circumflex iliac vein

Femoral vein

Superficial external pudendal vein

Saphenous vein

Fig. 21.30 Saphenofemoral disconnection. **A** Diagram showing ligation of the tributaries of the great saphenous vein. **B** Operative photograph showing proximal great saphenous vein (arrow) and major tributaries.

Superficial thrombophlebitis

Inflammation and thrombosis of a previously normal superficial vein may result from trauma, from irritation due to an intravenous infusion or from the injection of noxious agents. Except when it arises from a septic puncture sites, superficial thrombophlebitis is usually non-bacterial. When it arises spontaneously, it almost invariably occurs in a VV. Redness and tenderness follow the line of the vein.

Thrombosis may spread through communicating channels into the deep veins and give rise to DVT and pulmonary embolism (PE).

Treatment comprises analgesia, anti-inflammatory drugs, support stockings and active exercise. Once the inflammation has settled down, it is usually wise to remove the underlying VV, as recurrence is common. Propagation towards the deep veins usually requires heparin therapy, and rarely thrombectomy or vein ligation. Recurrent migrating superficial phlebitis is occasionally seen in malignant disease.

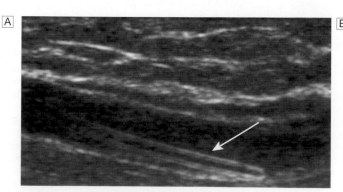

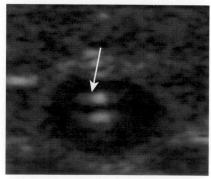

Fig. 21.31 Ultrasound guided foam sclerotherapy. **A** Cannula (arrow) inserted into great saphenous vein under duplex ultrasound control (longitudinal view). **B** Tip of cannula in varicose vein (longitudinal view).

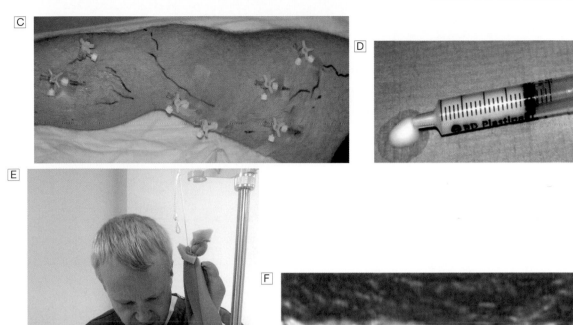

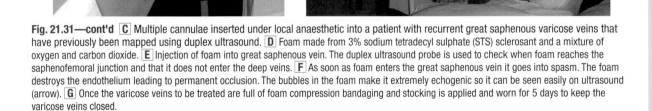

Fig. 21.31—cont'd C Multiple cannulae inserted under local anaesthetic into a patient with recurrent great saphenous varicose veins that have previously been mapped using duplex ultrasound. D Foam made from 3% sodium tetradecyl sulphate (STS) sclerosant and a mixture of oxygen and carbon dioxide. E Injection of foam into great saphenous vein. The duplex ultrasound probe is used to check when foam reaches the saphenofemoral junction and that it does not enter the deep veins. F As soon as foam enters the great saphenous vein it goes into spasm. The foam destroys the endothelium leading to permanent occlusion. The bubbles in the foam make it extremely echogenic so it can be seen easily on ultrasound (arrow). G Once the varicose veins to be treated are full of foam compression bandaging and stocking is applied and worn for 5 days to keep the varicose veins closed.

CHRONIC VENOUS INSUFFICIENCY

Pathophysiology

Chronic venous insufficiency (CVI) may be defined as the presence of (usually irreversible) skin damage (such as eczema, lipodermatosclerosis) in the lower leg as a result of sustained ambulatory venous hypertension. This hypertension is due to failure of the mechanisms (see above) that normally lower venous pressure upon ambulation, namely:

- Venous reflux due to valvular incompetence (90%). This may affect the superficial veins, the deep veins or both, and may be due to primary valvular insufficiency (as in VV) or to post-thrombotic damage.
- Venous obstruction (10–20%). This is usually post-thrombotic in nature and coexists with reflux.

CVI affects about 10% of the adult population and the lifetime risk of chronic venous ulceration (CVU) is around 1%.

Most patients with CVI and CVU (Fig. 21.32) are over 50 years of age and the incidence increases exponentially with advancing years. In 1992 it was estimated that the treatment of lower limb venous disease accounted for about 1–2% of health-care spending in the UK (£400–600 million per annum at the time). The female to male ratio is about 3:1. Approximately 70% of all leg ulcers are venous in aetiology and 20% are due to mixed arterial and venous disease. In many cases, the situation is aggravated by old age, poor social circumstances, obesity, trauma, immobility, osteoarthritis, rheumatoid arthritis, diabetes and neurological problems. It is usually possible to differentiate venous from arterial ulceration on clinical examination alone (Table 21.5).

The assessment and management of CVI and CVU should commence as follows: the patient first, then the leg, and then the ulcer.

371

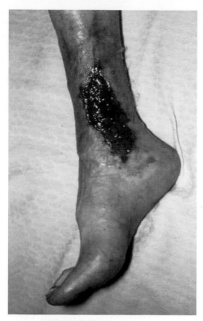

Fig. 21.32 Chronic venous ulcer.

Assessment

History

This should include the history of the present and previous episodes of ulceration; previous thrombotic episodes; previous venous and non-venous surgery to the leg, pelvis and abdomen; arterial symptoms; diabetes; autoimmune disease; other medical conditions; locomotor problems; current medications; and allergies.

Examination

This should include a description of the ulcer, concentrating on the features outlined in Table 21.5. Pulse status and ABPI should be recorded. Gait, particularly ankle mobility which is vital for the proper functioning of the calf muscle pump, should be assessed.

Investigations

All patients must undergo duplex ultrasound to define the nature and distribution of superficial and deep venous disease, as this has an important bearing on both treatment and prognosis. In patients with absent pulses and/or a low ABPI, ultrasound can also provide valuable information about the pattern of arterial disease. Patients may require a full blood count, standard biochemistry, thyroid function tests, blood glucose determination, lipid profile and rheumatoid serology to exclude underlying systemic conditions. If there is any suspicion that the ulcer might be malignant, multiple biopsies of the base and margins should be performed without delay.

Management

All patients with a break in the skin below the knee that has not healed within 2 weeks should be referred urgently (within a week) to a vascular surgeon for a full clinical, haemodynamic and duplex ultrasound assessment and consideration of surgical or endovenous treatment.

There is overwhelming evidence to indicate that the sooner an ulcer is diagnosed and appropriately treated, the more likely it is to heal and stay healed.

Medical therapy

Patients with leg ulcers often have multiple medical co-morbidities, the treatment of which must be optimal if the chances of ulcer healing are to be maximized. There are no drugs that have been proved to increase ulcer healing or reduce recurrence. Most ulcers are colonized with bacteria (often mixed faecal organisms or pseudomonas which explains the offensive smell) rather than infected, and antibiotics are usually contraindicated as they are ineffective and often select out resistant organisms. However, if the ulcer and surrounding skin are red and inflamed, or the ulcer is especially painful, then swabs should be taken.

Table 21.5 Differential diagnosis of leg ulceration

Clinical features	Arterial ulcer	Venous ulcer
Gender	Men > women	Women > men
Age	Usually presents > 60 years	Typically develops at 40–60 years but patient may not present for medical attention until much older; multiple recurrences are the norm
Risk factors	Smoking, diabetes, hyperlipidaemia and hypertension	Previous DVT, thrombophilia, varicose veins
Past medical history	Most have a clear history of peripheral, coronary and cerebrovascular disease	More than 20% have a clear history of DVT; many more have a history suggestive of occult DVT, i.e. leg swelling after childbirth, hip/knee replacement or long bone fracture
Symptoms	Severe pain is present unless there is (diabetic) neuropathy; pain may be relieved by dependency	About a third have pain, but it is not usually severe and may be relieved on elevation
Site	Normal and abnormal (diabetics) pressure areas (malleoli, heel, metatarsal heads, 5th metatarsal base)	Medial (70%), lateral (20%) or both malleoli and gaiter area
Edge	Regular, 'punched-out', indolent	Irregular, with neo-epithelium (whiter than mature skin)
Base	Deep, green (sloughy) or black (necrotic) with no granulation tissue; may involve tendon, bone and joint	Pink and granulating but may be covered in yellow-green slough
Surrounding skin	Features of severe limb ischaemia	Lipodermatosclerosis, varicose eczema, atrophe, blanche
Veins	Empty, 'guttering' on elevation	Full, usually varicose
Swelling	Usually absent	Often present

If β-haemolytic streptococcus or *Staphylococcus aureus* is cultured, oral antibiotics guided by sensitivities are indicated. Topical antibiotics and antiseptics are contraindicated. The best way to treat heavy, odorous colonization is to wash the leg regularly in warm tap water (no soap or disinfectant should be added) as 'the solution to pollution is dilution'.

Dressings

Of the available types of dressing, none has been proven to increase ulcer healing. Leg ulcer patients are notorious for developing contact sensitivity to all manner of substances present in ointments and dressings. Thus, the least expensive, simplest and blandest forms of non-adherent dressing are to be recommended.

Compression therapy

Although it is still unclear exactly how compression therapy works, it continues to be the mainstay of treatment and, correctly applied, is highly effective in healing the majority of venous ulcers and preventing recurrence (Fig. 21.33A).

To be maximally effective, compression should be:

- *elastic*, as this achieves the best and most durable pressure profile
- *multilayer*, as using many layers evens out the high- and low-pressure areas found under any bandage; the 'four-layer bandage' is a popular system
- *graduated*, with the pressure greatest at the ankle (*c*. 30–40 mmHg) and least at the knee (*c*. 15–20 mmHg).

It is vitally important to exclude arterial disease before compression is applied (Fig. 21.33B).

If pulses are not easily palpable, the ABPI should be measured (see above). Any patient with an ABPI of < 0.8 should be referred to a vascular surgeon. Such patients will have to be treated with modified compression or undergo revascularization to allow compression to be applied. Oedema is frequently present and significantly reduces the chances of healing. Even expertly applied graduated compression may fail to control severe oedema while the patient is still ambulant, and a period of bed rest for leg elevation may be required.

Elastic compression hosiery

Once the ulcer has been healed with compression bandaging, compression stockings will reduce the chance of recurrence and should be prescribed to all patients for life (assuming the arterial circulation is adequate).

Surgical and endovenous therapy

Eradication of superficial venous reflux by means of surgery or endovenous treatment in addition to compression therapy definitely reduces CVU recurrence and probably increases CVU healing rates when compared to compression alone (EBM 21.7).

EBM 21.7 **Surgery for chronic venous ulceration**

'*Eradication of superficial venous reflux in patients with chronic venous ulceration reduces recurrence at 2 years by over 50%.*'

Barwell JR, et al. Lancet 2004; 363(9424):1854–1859.

Although many of these patients are elderly, unfit for and/or do not want surgery, nowadays, most can be treated by endovenous methods. In particular, there is growing evidence that UGFS is not only as effective as surgery but also much less morbid. In patients with superficial

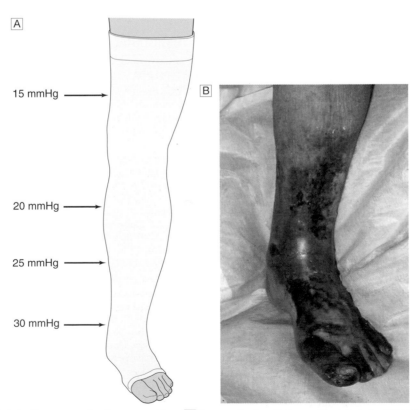

Fig. 21.33 Graduated elastic compression for venous ulcer. A Compression from the base of the toes to the tibial tuberosity usually suffices. B Extensive necrosis in a patient treated with compression for a venous ulcer in the presence of significant arterial disease. Above-knee amputation was required.

and deep venous reflux, especially where the latter is post-thrombotic in aetiology, the evidence that intervention for superficial reflux is beneficial is weaker. There is continuing controversy as to the benefit of ligating medial calf perforating veins either at open operation or endoscopically: so-called subfascial endoscopic perforator surgery (SEPS). The available data suggest that it adds little, if anything, to standard VV surgery in patients with isolated superficial venous reflux, and that it is as ineffective as VV surgery in patients with post-thrombotic deep venous disease. Some surgeons believe that performing split-skin or 'pinch' grafting speeds up ulcer healing. This is only likely to be the case if the underlying venous abnormality has been corrected successfully. Patients with arterial disease may require angioplasty or bypass surgery to relieve pain and allow compression therapy to be applied.

VENOUS THROMBOEMBOLISM (VTE)

Epidemiology

DVT is a common condition in medical and surgical patients and pulmonary embolism (PE) is consistently cited as the most common cause of potentially preventable death in the surgical patient. DVT also renders the leg prone to CVI and ulceration (the so-called postphlebitic limb or syndrome).

Pathophysiology

DVT probably begins in the calf in most cases. Clot may extend into the popliteal, femoral or iliac veins, and even the inferior vena cava. In some cases, DVT originates in the pelvic veins.

At first, the clot is free-floating within a column of flowing blood. The risk of PE is highest at this point. Later, when thrombus has completely occluded the vein and incited an inflammatory reaction in the vein wall, the clot becomes densely adherent and is unlikely to embolize. The classic 'text-book' features of DVT are due to this occlusion (leg swelling, dilated superficial veins) and thrombophlebitis (redness, pain and tenderness, heat). The important point is that most surgical patients developing a clinically significant postoperative PE do so on about the 7th to 10th day and nearly always have *clinically normal legs*. By the time a clinically apparent DVT has developed, the danger period for PE has largely passed; for this reason DVT prophylaxis must be considered in all thrombo-embolic prophylaxis must be considered in all patients undergoing open vascular or endovascular surgery

Aetiology

Three factors are traditionally associated with thrombogenesis (Virchow's triad): namely, venous stasis, intimal damage and hypercoagulability of the blood. Many of the recognized clinical risk factors for DVT relate to venous stasis: for example, immobility, obesity, pregnancy, paralysis, operation and trauma. In most instances of DVT no evidence of direct intimal damage can be detected. However, external trauma to a vein, for example, during a hip replacement operation, can provide a starting point for thrombogenesis. There is increasing interest in hypercoagulable states, also known as thrombophilias, which can be congenital (primary) or acquired (secondary). These include antithrombin, protein C and protein S deficiency, as well as factor V Leiden (activated protein C resistance, APCR). These should be sus-

pected if thrombosis occurs in a young patient (< 45 years), if there is a family history, or if thrombosis is recurrent or at an unusual site. Secondary hypercoagulable states include pregnancy, the puerperium, and malignancy. In some individuals the left common iliac vein may be compressed between the right common iliac artery in front and the spine behind. This is known as the May–Thurner syndrome and may be a cause of ileo-femoral DVT.

Diagnosis

Clinical examination alone is unreliable at confirming or excluding the presence of DVT. This means that the diagnosis of DVT cannot be made on clinical grounds alone, and that some form of investigation is required.

Colour flow duplex ultrasound

Colour duplex ultrasound imaging has largely replaced conventional venography in the diagnosis of DVT. It is non-invasive, avoids ionizing radiation and contrast, and is as accurate as venography in most cases. At times of doubt, MR (Fig. 21.34) or CT venography may be useful.

Venous gangrene

In certain circumstances, notably where there is underlying malignancy or severe sepsis, DVT may propagate to involve not only the main venous trunks, but also the venous collaterals and/or microcirculation (arterioles and venules). The former leads to an intensely swollen, cyanosed limb (phlegmasia caerula dolens), whereas the latter can lead to obstruction of the arterial inflow and the development of a swollen white leg (phlegmasia alba dolens). The patient may then go on to develop venous gangrene.

Prevention

Rationale

Because of our inability to diagnose DVT easily in its early asymptomatic but dangerous phase, prevention is very important. In this respect, it is helpful to determine which patients are at the highest risk and thus have the most to gain from prophylactic measures. The most important risk factors are a history of previous DVT or embolism, advanced age, malignant disease, obesity, and congenital or acquired thrombophilia. However, even patients at apparently low risk do develop DVT and PE, and prophylactic measures/ anticoagulation must be considered for all surgical patients (for further guidance see the National Institute of Clinical and Health Excellence, NICE, http://www.nice.org.uk/CG46).

General measures

Aspects of modern surgical care that help to reduce the likelihood of postoperative DVT include regional anaesthesia, accurate fluid replacement to avoid dehydration, effective pain control to facilitate early ambulation and, perhaps above all, the use of outpatient- or day-case-based minimally invasive (endovascular and endovenous) alternatives to traditional open surgery.

Physical methods

Graduated compression (thromboembolic deterrent, TED) stockings, which exert a pressure of about 20 mmHg at the ankle, augment flow in the deep veins and reduce the risk of thrombosis.

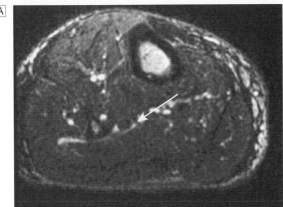

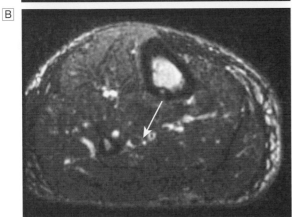

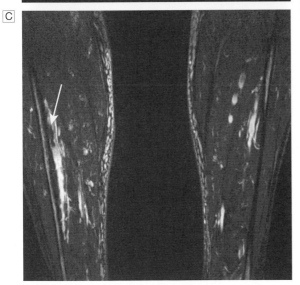

Fig. 21.34 Magnetic resonance venogram (MRV) showing deep vein thrombosis (arrows). The clot appears as a black "filling defect" within the white blood inside the deep veins of the right calf.

Pharmacological methods

Low-dose subcutaneous low molecular weight heparin (LMWH) protects against DVT and PE. The first dose may be given with the premedication (if an epidural is not being planned), and treatment is continued until the patient is fully ambulant. In high-risk patients, it can be continued following discharge and there is increasing evidence that this is of benefit in reducing venous thromboembolism and, probably therefore, the post-thrombotic syndrome.

Management

Overview

Before treatment is instituted, the diagnosis of DVT should normally have been established by means of ultrasound or MR (CT) venography. However, where the clinical suspicion of DVT and/or PE is high and there is no contraindication to heparin, the potential benefits of 'blind' treatment until the diagnosis is confirmed often outweigh the risks of withholding anticoagulation. The aims of treatment are to relieve the acute symptoms, protect against PE, and minimize the risk of recurrent thrombosis and post-thrombotic sequelae to the limb.

Uncomplicated DVT

If thrombus is confined to the calf, the patient is fully mobile and other risk factors are reversible, then an elastic stocking and physical exercise may be all that is required. However, the 'surgical' patient does not usually fulfill these criteria postoperatively and there is a real risk of thrombus extension into the femoropopliteal segment. In these cases, specific treatment is indicated.

For most uncomplicated DVT, it is now clear that:

- Bed rest is unnecessary and the patient can be mobilized immediately, wearing an appropriately fitted compression stocking.
- LMWH given by intermittent subcutaneous injection is more effective than unfractionated heparin given by infusion.

Thus, uncomplicated DVT is increasingly treated on an outpatient basis by protocol driven, specialist nurse run clinics

Complicated DVT

In a proportion of patients, however, treatment is more complicated because of one or more of the following:

- The DVT is more extensive (iliofemoral, vena cava, phlegmasia)
- The DVT is recurrent
- The patient has had a PE
- The patient has one or more major irreversible congenital and/or acquired thrombophilia
- Heparinization is contraindicated (heparin-induced thrombocytopenia, trauma – especially intracranial, recent haemorrhage).

In these circumstances, treatment must be tailored to the individual patient, and in selected cases it may be appropriate to use thrombolysis, insert a caval filter or consider thrombectomy. It is important to remember that a high proportion of patients with extensive DVT have an underlying malignancy, and reasonable steps should be taken to ensure that this is diagnosed and appropriately treated in order, hopefully, to reduce the thrombotic risk.

Thrombolysis

Catheter-directed intraclot thrombolysis (CDT) using recombinant tissue plasminogen activator (rTPA) has been advocated as a means of rapidly clearing the iliofemoral segment in patients with extensive proximal DVT. It is hoped that CDT will reduce the incidence of PE and postphlebitic syndrome (by reducing venous pressure and preserving valves). Although the rate and extent of clot clearance is certainly greater than with CDT than with heparin alone in the short term, it is not clear whether this results in improved patency and clinical outcome in the long term. CDT is also associated with a small risk of bleeding which can be serious or even life

21

threatening. The other potential role for CDT is in phlegmasia with venous gangrene. In this situation, not only is the rTPA given into the clot, it is also administered into the arterial circulation to try to clear the microcirculation. Again, although clot can be lysed in the short term, it is unclear whether this confers long-term benefit. Many of these patients have underlying malignancy and, unless the hypercoagulable state can be corrected, rethrombosis seems likely.

Surgical thrombectomy

In the UK, surgical thrombectomy to clear iliofemoral thrombus is very rarely performed nowadays.

Pharmacomechanical thrombectomy

There are now several catheter-based devices on the market that allow the thrombus to be isolated from the general venous circulation while being laced with thrombolytic (so reducing systemic effects) and at the same time disrupted mechanically. Trials are on-going to determine whether such pharmacomechanical thrombectomy (PMT) results in long-term benefits and if the cost is justified.

Venous stenting

If iliofemoral thrombus clearance reveals the May–Thurner syndrome as the likely cause of DVT, then a stent may be placed to help keep the left iliac vein open in the long term.

Caval filters

The rationale behind inserting an inferior vena cava filter (IVC) is that it will trap embolus that would otherwise have been destined for the lungs causing a PE. The use of IVC filters varies enormously around the world. In the UK, the accepted indications are in patients where:

- anticoagulation is contraindicated or has had to be discontinued owing to a complication of therapy
- PE are still occurring despite adequate anticoagulation
- compromised cardiovascular reserve means that even a small PE might have very serious clinical consequences.

Other forms of venous thrombosis

Superior vena cava thrombosis

Mediastinal tumours or enlarged lymph nodes (e.g. from breast or bronchial carcinoma) may obstruct the superior vena cava (SVC) and induce thrombosis. Central venous catheters for parenteral nutrition, pressure monitoring or haemodialysis may cause thrombosis of the SVC, or of the subclavian or axillary veins. The patient experiences an unpleasant bursting feeling in the head, neck and upper limbs. There is oedema, cyanosis and venous distension.

The obstruction is defined by CT or MR venography. In occlusion secondary to malignancy, percutaneous stenting, radiotherapy or chemotherapy may relieve malignant obstruction, and whilst the outlook remains poor, symptoms may be significantly relieved.

Subclavian and axillary vein thrombosis

Spontaneous axillary vein thrombosis is relatively common and usually occurs in otherwise healthy young adults following exercise, when it is termed 'effort thrombosis'. There may be a previous history of intermittent venous obstruction in the limb due to a mechanical cause at the thoracic outlet. A cervical rib, abnormal muscle or ligamentous band at the inner border of the first rib, or a narrow interval between the clavicle and the first rib (the costoclavicular scissors), may constrict the vein and lead to thrombosis.

The patient complains of an uncomfortable, heavy, cyanosed arm with venous engorgement. Venous collaterals develop over the shoulder and anterior chest wall. Upper limb venous duplex scanning and/or venography define the occlusion. The arm should be elevated, e.g. in a towel suspended from a drip stand. Heparin therapy followed by oral anticoagulants is standard treatment. CDT and PMT can be very effective in early cases. Many surgeons believe that after the axillary thrombosis has been cleared, the thoracic outlet should be explored and the first rib or other obstructing element removed. Once the rib is out, stenting of any underlying venous stenosis may be of value.

LYMPHOEDEMA

Pathophysiology

The lymphatic system removes excess water and protein from the interstitial space. Flow is directed centrally by intrinsic lymphatic contractions and endothelial valves, and is increased by muscle contraction. Lymph passes through lymph nodes before it re-enters the venous system, mainly through the thoracic duct. The total daily lymph flow is only 2–4 litres. Failure of this mechanism leads to the accumulation of protein-rich oedema fluid in the tissues (lymphoedema) (Fig. 21.35). Lymphoedema may be primary or secondary, and must be differentiated from other causes of leg swelling (Fig. 21.36, Table 21.6).

Primary lymphoedema

This often familial condition is estimated to affect 2% of the adult population and is caused by a developmental failure in which the lymphatics may be absent, hypoplastic, or varicose and dilated. It is usually categorized by the age of onset:

- Lymphoedema congenita. Swelling is present at birth or develops within the first year of life
- Lymphoedema praecox. Swelling develops between 1 and 35 years, usually during adolescence. It affects predominantly females, and may be unilateral or bilateral.
- Lymphoedema tarda. In patients developing lymphoedema after the age of 35, an underlying pelvic tumour (benign or malignant) compressing the proximal lymphatic (and venous) systems must be excluded.

Secondary lymphoedema

This develops when the lymphatic system is obstructed by tumour, recurrent infection or infestation (filariasis), or obliterated by surgery or radiotherapy.

Clinical features

Symptoms

The patient usually complains of gradual painless swelling of one or both legs. At first, lymphoedema is like other forms of oedema, in that it is present only upon dependency; that is, worse at the end of the day and absent in the morning. However, as the oedema fluid becomes more protein-rich, it is less and less affected by position. Lymphoedema nearly always commences distally on the foot and extends proximally, usually only to the knee.

Thus, there may be a complex interplay between nature and nurture; that is, many patients with apparently primary

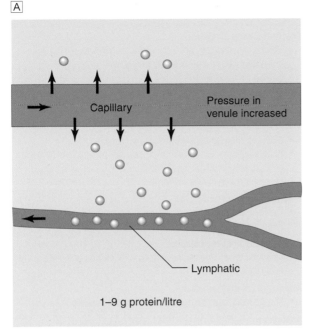

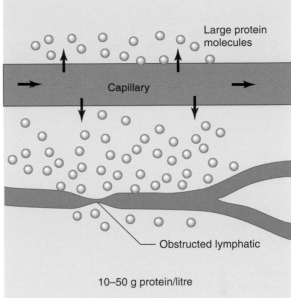

Fig. 21.35 Types of oedema. **A** Low-protein oedema due to abnormally high net fluid filtration. **B** High-protein oedema due to failure of lymphatics to remove interstitial protein.

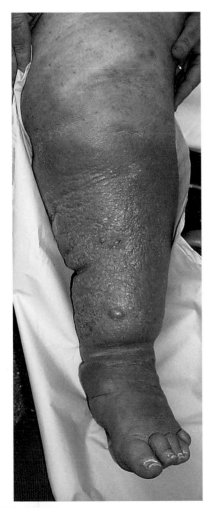

Fig. 21.36 Lymphoedema.

lymphoedema also have a secondary component. Some patients first present to medical attention because of acute cellulitis. Such patients are prone to recurrent episodes, each one of which damages the lymphatic system still further, leading to cycle of deterioration.

Signs

Unlike other types of oedema, lymphoedema characteristically involves the foot, as opposed to the lower calf and ankle. This is characterized by:

- infilling of the submalleolar depressions
- a 'hump' on the dorsum of the foot
- 'square' toes due to confinement by footwear; also, the skin on the dorsum of the toes cannot be pinched owing to subcutaneous fibrosis (Stemmer's sign).

Lymphoedema usually spreads proximally to knee level, and less commonly affects the whole leg. Lymphoedema will pit easily at first, but with time fibrosis and dermal thickening prevent pitting, except following prolonged pressure. Chronic eczema, fungal infection of the skin (dermatophytosis) and nails (onychomycosis), fissuring, verrucae and papillae are frequently seen in advanced conditions. Frank ulceration is unusual.

Investigations

Lymphoedema is essentially a clinical diagnosis and most patients require no further investigation.

Management

Physical methods

The patient should elevate the foot above the level of the hip when sitting, elevate the foot of the bed when sleeping, and avoid prolonged standing. Various forms of massage are

Table 21.6 Differential diagnosis of the swollen limb

Non-Vascular or Lymphatic	Post-thrombotic syndrome
General disease states • Cardiac, renal and liver failure • Hyperthyroidism (myxoedema) • Allergic disorders • Immobility and lower limb dependency	• Venous skin changes, secondary varicose veins on the leg and collateral veins on the lower abdominal wall • Venous claudication may be present
Local disease processes • Ruptured Baker's cyst • Myositis ossificans • Bony or soft tissue tumours • Arthritis • Haemarthrosis • Calf muscle haematoma • Achilles tendon rupture • Other trauma • Reflex sympathetic dystrophy	**Varicose veins** • Do not usually cause significant swelling
	Venous malformations • Most common is Klippel–Trenaunay syndrome • Abnormal lateral venous complex, capillary naevus, hypo(a)plasia of deep veins and limb lengthening • Lymphatic abnormalities often co-exist
Gigantism • Rare; all tissues are uniformly enlarged	**External venous compression** • Pelvic or abdominal tumour including the gravid uterus • Retroperitoneal fibrosis
Drugs • Steroids	**Arterial ischaemia-reperfusion** • Following lower limb revascularization for chronic and particularly acute ischaemia
Obesity • Lipodystrophy, lipoidosis	**Arteriovenous malformation** • May be associated with local or generalized swelling
Venous	**Aneurysm** • Popliteal • Femoral • False aneurysm following (iatrogenic) trauma
Deep venous thrombosis • The classic signs of pain and redness may be absent	

effective at reducing oedema. Intermittent pneumatic compression devices are also useful. The mainstay of therapy is graduated compression hosiery. Pressures exceeding 50 mmHg at the ankle may be required. Below-knee stockings are usually sufficient.

Drugs

Diuretics are of no value and are associated with side-effects, including electrolyte disturbance. No other drugs are of proven benefit.

Antibiotics

These should be prescribed promptly for cellulitis. Patients who suffer recurrent spontaneous episodes of cellulitis should be considered for long-term prophylactic antibiotic therapy. Fungal infection must also be treated aggressively. The feet must be dried after washing and the skin kept clean and supple with water-based emollients to prevent entry of bacteria.

Surgery

Only a small minority of patients will benefit from surgery. Operations fall into two categories: bypass procedures and reduction procedures. They are only rarely performed. The details of these procedures are beyond the scope of this book.

R.R. Jeffrey

Cardiothoracic surgery

22

BASIC CONSIDERATIONS

Pathophysiological assessment

Careful history and appropriate examination suggest the presence of possible cardiac pathology. The initial clinical assessment is then refined and specific investigations used to confirm and quantify any disease identified (Table 22.1).

Assessment of risk

As the risks of perioperative mortality and stroke are significantly higher with cardiac than with many other forms of surgery, a frank informed discussion of these risks, recognizing potential benefits of a successful operation, are essential elements of the preoperative consultation between the patient and surgeon.

Mortality

Risk stratification is important in cardiac surgery and Euroscore is a valuable tool for quantifying operative risk across all types of non-congenital cardiac surgery. Patient, condition, and procedure related factors contribute to a score which predicts 30-day mortality. Predicted operative mortality ranges from < 1% for routine elective procedures to more than 50% for complex emergency operations.

Stroke

Stroke risk varies from 1% to over 10%, and is associated with intracardiac thrombus and severe atheromatous disease of the proximal aorta and carotids. Patients with evidence of peripheral vascular disease have a higher risk of stroke and those with high-grade symptomatic carotid disease may benefit from carotid endarterectomy prior to cardiac surgery (Ch. 21).

Specific aspects of surgical technique

Cardiopulmonary bypass (CPB)

Modern cardiac and great vessel surgery became feasible with the development of cardiopulmonary bypass. Venous blood is drained via cannulae inserted into the right atrium or venae cavae and passes to a reservoir. It is then pumped through an oxygenator, which adds O_2 and removes CO_2, through a heat exchanger coil so that its temperature can be varied and finally, the blood is returned to the arterial circulation via a cannula in the ascending aorta or other suitable artery (femoral, axillary) (Figs 22.1, 22.2 and 22.3). Full anticoagulation with intravenous heparin is required to prevent blood clotting in the tubing, oxygenator and pump mechanisms. Roller or centrifugal pumps are used, as these minimize red cell trauma. Semipermeable membranes, or more commonly hollow fibres, form the blood–gas interface within the oxygenator. A trained perfusion technician controls the bypass machine.

CPB stimulates a systemic inflammatory response mediated by cytokine release, complement activation and white cell activation. These changes do not generally cause clinical problems but may be implicated in post-bypass pulmonary, renal and cerebral dysfunction. Cerebral damage occurs in about 1% of cases due to intracerebral bleeding, embolization of microbubbles or arterial debris, or inadequate cerebral perfusion. Subtle deterioration in cerebral function, as detected by psychological testing, is more frequent. Coagulopathy and haemolysis are associated with prolonged bypass.

Myocardial preservation

Cardioplegia

Cardioplegic arrest achieves a still bloodless heart. A cross-clamp is applied across the ascending aorta proximal to insertion of the arterial inflow cannula. This prevents blood flow into the coronary arteries. The heart is arrested by perfusing the coronary circulation with a cardioplegic solution, delivered either antegradely via the aortic root or coronary artery ostia utilizing the native coronary arteries, or retrogradely via a catheter placed in the coronary sinus.

The essential component of a cardioplegic solution is a high potassium concentration (circa 18 mmol/l), which causes the heart to arrest in diastole. Cardioplegia is typically delivered at a temperature of 4–6°C as either a crystalloid solution or using the patient's own blood as a vehicle. Blood-based solutions are believed to have buffering characteristics that are helpful in reducing the deleterious effects of ischaemic metabolites generated by the arrested myocardium. Cardioplegia solutions minimize myocardial energy requirements by abolishing energy expenditure on contraction and

Table 22.1 Specific assessments of cardiac pathophysiological status

Investigation	Yield
ECG	
Resting	Rhythm; conduction abnormalities; atrial and ventricular hypertrophy; established ischaemic changes; evidence of previous myocardial infarction
Exercise	Exercise-induced ischaemic changes or arrhythmias
Chest X-ray	Cardiac enlargement; valvular calcification; evidence of pulmonary oedema (Kerley B lines, pleural effusion, interstitial marking, hilar flare); absent or enlarged cardiac or great vessel structures
Thallium isotope scan	Areas of low radio-uptake indicative of impaired myocardial perfusion
Echocardiography	
Precordial	Ventricular contractility; valvular stenoses, regurgitation or leaflet abnormalities; intracardiac morphology, including septal defects and intracardiac masses; pericardial effusion
Transoesophageal	Enhanced views of posterior cardiac structures (aortic and mitral valves, ascending aorta, great veins and posterior septae); posterior pericardial fluid collections
Cardiac catheterization	
Chamber pressures	Assess left and right ventricular function via determination of left ventricular end-diastolic pressure; atrial pressures in valve disease; transvalvular gradients (Fig. 22.1)
Angiography	Coronary arterial anatomy; intracardiac anatomy; trans-septal flow
O_2 saturations	Intracardiac shunts
Cardiac output	Cardiac function and determination of secondary derived parameters, including peripheral and pulmonary vascular resistance

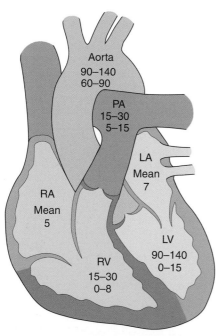

Fig. 22.1 Normal cardiac chambers. (LA = left atrium; LV = left ventricle; RA = right atrium; RV = right ventricle; PA = pulmonary artery).

by reducing basal cellular metabolism by local tissue cooling. Reducing core temperature on bypass to 26–34°C may enhance cardiac cooling. Cardioplegia combined with mild systemic hypothermia (32°C) provides the surgeon with a safe period of cardiac arrest of up to 120 minutes permitting surgery while minimizing the risk of myocardial damage.

Coronary bypass surgery (CABG) can be performed using a technique in which an aortic clamp is intermittently applied to cut coronary flow while the heart is electrically fibrillated so as to reduce movement. The resulting brief ischaemic episodes are tolerated. This cross-clamp fibrillation technique activates mechanisms within the myocardial cells that reduce damage caused by subsequent ischaemia (*preconditioning*).

In some circumstances, the surgeon may elect to leave the coronary arteries perfused while on bypass and to operate on a beating heart. Recently, there has been considerable interest in performing CABG on suitable patients without the use of CPB. Proponents of 'off-pump' surgery claim that the risks of artificial perfusion (particularly transient cognitive impairment) are avoided and that recovery may be quicker. Many surgeons, however, feel that the bloodless, still operative field resulting from cardioplegic arrest provides the optimum conditions for high quality accurate anastomoses.

Postoperative care

Intensive care

Postoperatively, patients are usually ventilated for a few hours until they are fully rewarmed, and have satisfactory stable haemodynamics, pulmonary gas exchange and acid–base status. Urine output is copious and potassium levels are, therefore, checked frequently so that potassium is administered intravenously to correct urinary losses. Invasive measurement of arterial and central venous pressure is standard. Pulmonary artery catheters may be used to measure pulmonary artery pressure, pulmonary artery capillary wedge pressure and cardiac output.

Complications

Other than death or stroke, established complications include:

- bleeding – multifactorial causes including hypothermia, platelet dysfunction, CPB and pharmacological (aspirin, clopidogrel)
- low cardiac output – poor myocardial protection, previous poor left ventricular (LV) function
- arrhythmias – atrial fibrillation occurs in up to 40%
- infection – wound, respiratory
- short-term memory impairment.

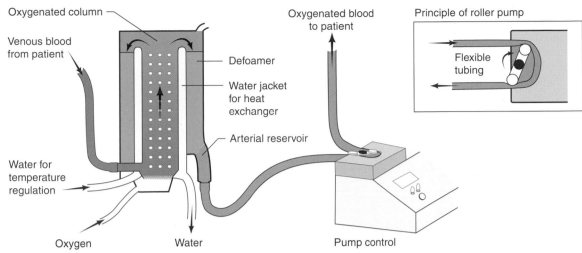

Fig. 22.2 Schematic of a bypass circuit.

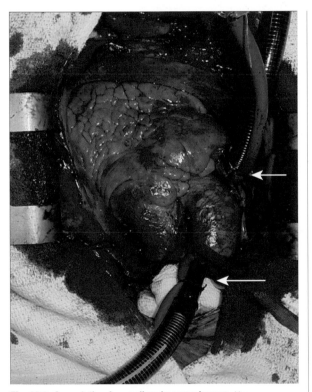

Fig. 22.3 Cannulation for cardiopulmonary bypass. Upper arrow from right atrium to pump. Lower arrow from pump to aorta.

Recovery time

Patients undergoing routine elective coronary or valve surgery will usually leave acute hospital care within one week. Those requiring more extensive surgery or emergency procedures may take longer to recover. Most patients will have undergone a median sternotomy (Fig. 22.4). This wound heals quickly and, as the sternal edges are approximated securely by wire or heavy sutures, chest discomfort eases rapidly. Leg vein donor sites may take longer to heal, particularly around the knee. By 2 weeks the patient should be able to walk a few hundred metres, and by 3 months should have returned to full activity, including work.

ACQUIRED CARDIAC DISEASE

Surgical intervention may be required in the management of:
- ischaemic heart disease
- cardiac valvular disease
- aortic aneurysm
- pericardial pathology
- cardiac trauma.

Ischaemic heart disease

Ischaemic heart disease encompasses coronary artery disease and its complications, principally acute mitral regurgitation, ventricular septal defect and left ventricular aneurysm.

Coronary artery disease (CAD)

Coronary artery atheroma (Ch. 21) results in narrowing of the vessels and most patients will present for surgery because of angina or previous myocardial infarction (MI).

Assessment

Exercise electrocardiography (ECG) is often used as an initial screening test for patients with suspected stable angina. Those with confirmed ischaemia then undergo coronary angiography and assessment of left ventricular function by means of angiography or echocardiography. Contrast medium is injected into the coronary circulation (Fig. 22.5) via a catheter that is usually inserted through the femoral or radial artery (Fig. 22.6). Images are obtained in several different planes so as to minimize the risk of missing eccentric lesions. Intervention is usually only advised for stenoses that exceed a 70% reduction in vessel diameter.

Indications

Elective surgery is indicated primarily for the control of angina that is refractory to medical treatment and is unsuitable for percutaneous intervention (PCI) usually with stent insertion. Historically, patients with three-vessel disease or left main stem disease have exhibited a high (c. 8% per year) risk of death from MI with medical therapy alone. Surgery improves long-term survival for such patients, particularly

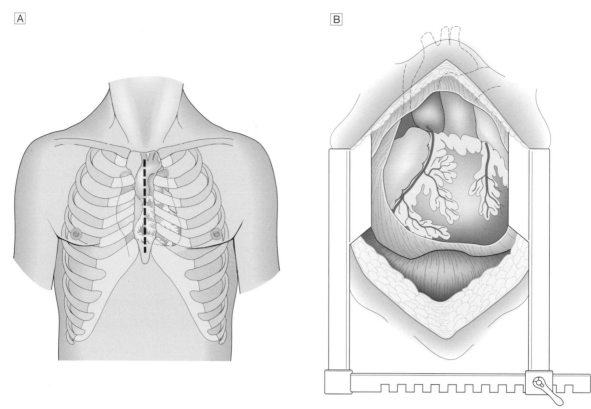

Fig. 22.4 Surgical approach to the heart. [A] Median sternotomy incision. [B] Right atrium and ascending aorta exposed.

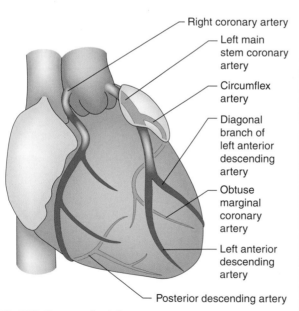

Right coronary artery

Left main stem coronary artery

Circumflex artery

Diagonal branch of left anterior descending artery

Obtuse marginal coronary artery

Left anterior descending artery

Posterior descending artery

Fig. 22.5 Coronary circulation.

when LV function is also impaired. PCI has an important role in the management of patients with acute coronary syndrome ranging from ST elevation myocardial infarction to unstable angina.

Some patients requiring other cardiac procedures may be shown to have significant coronary disease during cardiological assessment. In these cases, coronary surgery may be added to the primary procedure to improve perioperative survival and prevent future ischaemic problems. Emergency

coronary surgery is rare and patients with incipient or established MI fare better with PCI and supportive medical therapy, as the mortality of surgery in this setting is much increased.

Coronary bypass

A coronary artery bypass graft (CABG) delivers blood to the distal coronary artery beyond a stenosis. If the distal artery is obliterated by atheroma, an endarterectomy procedure may be performed to restore the lumen. Originally, nearly all grafts comprised reversed segments of the long saphenous vein anastomosed proximally to the ascending aorta and distally to the coronary artery. Such grafts have patency rates of around 70% at 5 years and 40% at 10 years. Venous graft failure occurs as a result of intimal hyperplasia, which is thought to be, in part at least, a response to arterial pressure. The relatively high rate of vein graft failure stimulated interest in arterial grafts and led to the almost universal use of the internal thoracic artery (ITA). This is usually employed as a pedicled graft when it is left attached to the subclavian artery proximally, but can also be used as a free graft in the same manner as vein. ITA graft patency exceeds 90% at 5 years and 70% at 10 years. A common combination is to use the left ITA for the left anterior descending artery and vein grafts for the other vessels (Fig. 22.7).

The radial artery is a possible option as a free graft for use in people with poor-quality saphenous vein and critical proximal occlusion of more than 70% in the target vessel, and may be used together with ITA grafts to achieve 'total arterial revascularization'. Occasionally, when there is a shortage of good conduit (e.g. in a 'redo' operation), the surgeon may consider using the right gastroepiploic artery, the short saphenous vein and the cephalic vein. Prosthetic grafts occlude early and are not used.

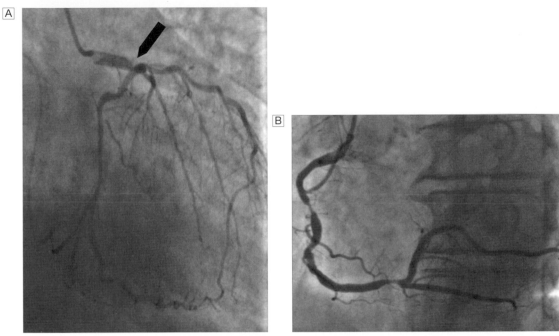

Fig. 22.6 Coronary angiography. [A] Left coronary angiogram demonstrating severe left main stem stenosis. [B] Right coronary angiogram demonstrating multiple stenoses.

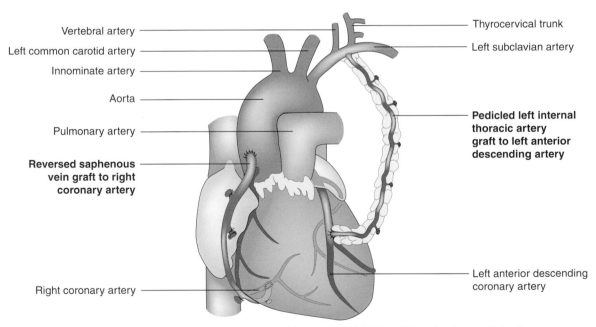

Vertebral artery

Left common carotid artery

Innominate artery

Aorta

Pulmonary artery

Reversed saphenous vein graft to right coronary artery

Right coronary artery

Thyrocervical trunk

Left subclavian artery

Pedicled left internal thoracic artery graft to left anterior descending artery

Left anterior descending coronary artery

Fig. 22.7 Completed coronary bypass procedure with venous and left internal thoracic artery grafts in situ.

Results

Uncomplicated coronary surgery should carry a 2–3% risk of mortality and a 1–2% risk of stroke. Angina is relieved completely in about 70% of cases, is significantly improved in the remainder, and recurs with a frequency of about 10% per year. Successful revascularization may also improve breathlessness if it is related to myocardial ischaemia, and survival is probably enhanced in patients with left main stem and triple vessel disease. The use of arterial conduits is associated with better graft patency and improved survival. Although there is a trend in that direction for patients with multiple arterial grafts followed up beyond 10 years, the added benefit over one ITA graft placed to the left anterior descending coronary is small. This may reflect the progression of native coronary disease. Secondary prevention is mandatory in all patients with CAD and includes antiplatelet medication (aspirin) and cholesterol reduction (statin) (EBM 22.1).

SUMMARY BOX 22.1

Coronary anatomy

- There are two coronary arteries (left and right), which have origin in the coronary sinuses: left or posterior sinus, right or anterior sinus
- The left main coronary artery passes behind the pulmonary trunk and divides into two large branches: the left anterior interventricular artery or left anterior descending (LAD), which supplies the anterior left ventricle and anterior two-thirds of the interventricular septum, and the circumflex coronary, which supplies the posterior and lateral walls of the left ventricle
- The right coronary artery passes down anteriorly in the right atrioventricular groove supplying the anterior right ventricle and acute marginal branches
- Either the right or circumflex may terminate as the posterior descending artery which supplies the inferior surface of both ventricles and the lower septum. This artery is then considered to be dominant
- The right, LAD and circumflex are each considered to be a 'vessel system'. Disease within any one of these three vessels or its branches is termed single-vessel disease. Similarly, two- and three-vessel disease indicates involvement of two and three systems, respectively.

EBM 22.1 Coronary bypass surgery

'Revascularization to improve long term prognosis.

Patients with significant left main stem disease should undergo coronary artery bypass grafting.

Patients with triple vessel disease should be considered for coronary artery bypass grafting to improve prognosis, but where unsuitable be offered percutaneous coronary intervention.

Drug interventions to prevent new vascular events.

All patients with stable angina due to atherosclerotic disease should receive long term standard aspirin and statin therapy.'

SIGN. Management of Stable Angina; Scottish Intercollegiate Guideline 96 (2007).

Surgery for the complications of coronary artery disease

Mitral valve regurgitation (MR)

Chronic

Chronic ischaemia may cause regurgitation, owing to papillary muscle fibrosis. Surgery may be indicated to repair or replace the valve as an elective procedure, usually concurrently with CABG. The operative mortality is around 8–11%.

Acute

Acute myocardial infarction involving a papillary muscle may cause this to rupture, causing gross regurgitation. The patient is usually very unwell with pulmonary oedema due to MR and low cardiac output due to infarction, and often requires emergency ventilation. Emergency mitral valve replacement and CABG is associated with a mortality of 15–40%, mainly due to poor ventricular function and secondary multiorgan failure (EBM 22.2).

EBM 22.2 Valve replacement

- Aortic valve replacement (AVR) is indicated for **symptomatic** patients with severe aortic stenosis (AS).
- AVR is indicated for patients with severe AS undergoing coronary artery bypass surgery (CABG) or surgery on the aorta or other heart valves.
- AVR is indicated for **symptomatic** patients with severe aortic regurgitation (AR) irrespective of left ventricular (LV) systolic function.
- AVR is indicated for asymptomatic patients with chronic severe AR and LV systolic dysfunction or while undergoing CABG or surgery on the aorta or other heart valves.
- Mitral valve (MV) surgery (repair if possible) is indicated in patients with symptomatic moderate or severe mitral stenosis.
- MV surgery is recommended for the symptomatic patient with acute severe mitral regurgitation (MR).
- MV surgery is beneficial for patients with chronic severe MR

Class I recommendations from ACC/AHA 2006 Guidelines for the Management of Patients with Valvular Heart Disease.

Postmyocardial infarction ventricular septal defect

Necrosis of the intraventricular septum due to MI may lead to a ventricular septal defect. Blood flows from the high-pressure left to the low-pressure right ventricle (left-to-right 'shunt'). This increases right ventricular work and pulmonary blood flow and decreases cardiac output. Typically, the patient complains of sudden, severe breathlessness 3–8 days after an MI and is noted to have developed a pansystolic murmur. The diagnosis is confirmed by echocardiography and coronary angiography is performed. Emergency repair is technically difficult due to the poor quality of the recently infarcted muscle to which the patch is attached. In addition, these patients have impaired cardiac function in the aftermath of an acute MI. Typically, such patients will require mechanical support of their ventricle with an intra-aortic balloon pump. Surgical mortality ranges from 20–50%. Patients with minor shunts are managed medically and may be considered for surgery some weeks later to allow cardiac function to stabilize. The margins of the defect will have healed by fibrosis, making patch repair relatively straightforward with more acceptable operative mortality (< 10%).

Left ventricular aneurysm

LV aneurysm complicates about 8% of MIs and occurs when a large left ventricular free-wall MI scar becomes aneurysmal as a result of intraventricular pressure. A large aneurysm impairs cardiac contraction and increases myocardial work. Complications include clot formation within the aneurysm, which may embolize, and arrhythmias generated within the zone of ischaemic myocardium around the periphery of the aneurysm.

At operation, the aneurysm is excised, the clot removed and the resulting defect usually closed by direct suture, reinforced by buttressing strips of Teflon felt or vascular graft. Occasionally, a small patch repair is performed to preserve the shape of the left ventricle. Surgery performed electively has a mortality of 6–10% and an increased risk of stroke.

Cardiac valvular disease

Valve disease may obstruct forward flow (stenosis) or permit reverse flow (incompetence/regurgitation), or both. The aortic and/or mitral valves are primarily affected; primary tricuspid pathology is rare and pulmonary valve disease is virtually unknown. Formerly, rheumatic fever following streptococcal infection was the most common aetiological factor. This remains the case in many developing countries, but in the UK it is rare.

Assessment

Transthoracic echocardiography provides useful data on forward gradients using Doppler techniques and can detect regurgitation. Transoesophageal echocardiography allows more detailed investigation of the valves and intracardiac anatomy. Coronary angiography is indicated in patients of middle age or older. Left ventricular angiography and aortic root angiography may allow the quantification of mitral and aortic regurgitation. A full catheterization study should include measurement of cardiac output and chamber and pulmonary artery pressures. Pressure gradients and orifice areas may be deduced from echocardiography parameters.

Surgical management

Options include valve replacement or repair. Replacement utilizes either a mechanical or a biological prosthesis. Mechanical valves have developed from the original ball-in-cage design through single disc designs to the current range of carbon bi-leaflet devices (Fig. 22.8). These should last indefinitely, but patients require lifelong warfarin to prevent thrombotic occlusion or embolism. Embolism risk is about 1–6% per year and is influenced by how accurately the INR is controlled. Mechanical valves produce audible clicks.

Biological valves are derived from:

- glutaraldehyde-preserved porcine aortic valves mounted on a frame (stent) (Fig. 22.9A)
- glutaraldehyde-preserved bovine pericardium formed into a three-leaflet valve and mounted on a stent
- glutaraldehyde-preserved porcine aortic unstented valves (Fig. 22.9B)
- human aortic root homografts removed from cadaveric hearts and preserved in antibiotic solution.

Unstented valves and homografts offer the advantage of a larger effective orifice area minimizing the residual pressure gradient. Warfarin is not required with biological valves provided the patient remains in sinus rhythm. However, such valves deteriorate over time and after 15 to 20 years may need replacement with an increased

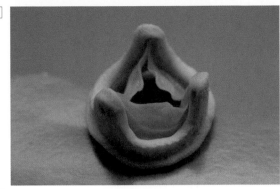

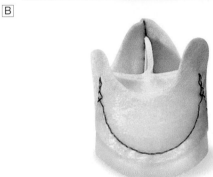

Fig. 22.9 Biological valve prostheses. A Stented. B Unstented.

operative risk. Unless there is a contraindication to anti-coagulation, mechanical valves are commonly used in a younger age group. In young women intending to have children it is usual to advise a biological valve, with the intention of replacing it with a mechanical device when the valve fails. This avoids problems with warfarin during pregnancy (placental separation and abortion, and teratogenicity).

Repair is the preferred surgical option in regurgitation and is largely restricted to the mitral and tricuspid valves. It is superior to valve replacement, as the problems associated with prosthesis are avoided. The techniques utilized for mitral incompetence include excision of portions of redundant leaflet, repositioning of the chordae and reduction in the size of the annulus (annuloplasty). Generally, only annuloplasty is applicable to the tricuspid valve. Rarely, isolated mitral stenosis without calcification may be found, in which case division of the fused leaflets under direct vision on bypass (commisurotomy) is performed.

Endocarditis

Abnormal native heart valves and artificial valves are prone to subacute bacterial endocarditis and prosthetic valve endocarditis, respectively. Controversial guidelines on antibiotic prophylaxis exist but it is reasonable to prescribe antibiotics in patients with prostheses who undergo any surgical or dental procedure.

Patients with endocarditis require prolonged parenteral antibiotic therapy which may be effective. However, surgery may be required if the infection does not respond or if the valve develops a significant paravalvular leak or annular abscess. Surgery is a high-risk venture as the patient is systemically septic, the perivalvular tissues are of poor quality

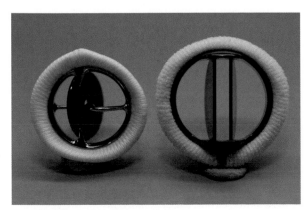

Fig. 22.8 Mechanical valve prostheses.

and the newly implanted prosthesis may itself become infected. Postoperative recovery is usually slow, with renal and ventilatory failure being common complications.

Aortic valve disease

Stenosis

Aortic stenosis is the commonest indication for valve surgery in the UK. Although rheumatic disease remains a common problem in underdeveloped countries, the most frequent aetiology in the Western world is calcific aortic stenosis which develops in the older population usually over 70 years. The normal aortic valve has three cusps but a congenital bicuspid valve usually calcifies from the sixth decade onwards (Fig. 22.10). Aortic stenosis causes left ventricular hypertrophy, effort angina, episodes of arrhythmia with syncope or even sudden death, and left ventricular failure.

Clinically, the patient has a slow rising pulse, a forceful apex beat and an ejection systolic murmur in the right upper parasternal area that may radiate to the root of the neck. Echocardiography will confirm a valvular gradient, which is considered severe aortic stenosis when this exceeds 60 mmHg. However, measurement of orifice area is independent of cardiac output and may be a more reliable measure. The onset of symptoms should initiate referral for surgery. Patients with cardiac failure have a low cardiac output and consequently a low gradient. In these cases, the decision to operate may be a difficult judgement, based on the absence of any other likely cause of poor left ventricular function and echocardiographic evidence of severe aortic valve disease.

In high risk patients e.g. the very elderly, those with patent ITA grafts or significant other co-morbidities, percutaneous replacement of the aortic valve may be considered (TAVI – transcatheter aortic valve insertion) where a biological valve on a holder is introduced percutaneously via the femoral artery or left ventricular apex.

Regurgitation

Native aortic regurgitation may be due to primary valve pathology (rheumatic fever, endocarditic valve destruction or, rarely, a bicuspid valve) or secondary to aortic root pathology with annular dilatation (see below). Prosthetic valve regurgitation can occur as a result of deterioration of a biological prosthesis, partial obstruction of a mechanical device, or paraprosthetic leakage. Chronic aortic regurgitation causes progressive left ventricular dilatation and hypertrophy.

Clinically, there is a wide pulse pressure – collapsing pulse, lateral displacement of the apex beat and a diastolic murmur in the left parasternal area. Chronic aortic regurgitation is well tolerated and often asymptomatic. In severe cases, the patient may complain of dyspnoea and angina, and may exhibit features of congestive cardiac failure. Surgery is advised to forestall the onset of cardiac failure due to irreversible myocardial damage. The timing of surgery is determined by serial echocardiography measurements demonstrating left ventricular dilatation.

Acute aortic regurgitation produces severe dyspnoea, with rapid onset of left ventricular failure and pulmonary oedema. The patient may require emergency ventilation and urgent surgery.

Surgical outcomes

Elective aortic valve replacement is a relatively straightforward procedure, with a mortality of about 3% and stroke rate of 1%. The risk is increased several-fold in cases that have progressed to cardiac failure, and in emergency cases with acute severe regurgitation.

Mitral valve disease

Stenosis

Although the incidence of rheumatic valvular heart disease is declining, the commonest pathological presentation is mitral stenosis which restricts the flow of blood into the left ventricle, which is consequently small and thin-walled. Cardiac output is also reduced. The left atrium is dilated and left atrial and pulmonary artery pressures are raised. Chronic pulmonary hypertension causes right ventricular hypertrophy and dilatation, and in advanced cases tricuspid incompetence may develop (see below).

Clinically, patients complain of shortness of breath on exertion and may experience palpitations. Chronic atrial fibrillation usually intervenes and the patient may be taking warfarin along with a diuretic therapy for pulmonary congestion. Examination reveals atrial fibrillation, a left parasternal heave due to right ventricular enlargement, and a diastolic murmur best heard at the lower left sternal edge, accompanied by a loud second heart sound. Chest X-ray shows right ventricular and atrial enlargement and the pulmonary artery is prominent. A progressive increase in heart size is often evident on serial annual films and renal function is frequently impaired.

The timing of surgery is a matter of judgement but an echocardiographic calculated mitral valve area below 1 cm^2 demonstrates severe stenosis and is an indication for surgery. Very occasionally, the patient may have echocardiographic evidence of leaflet fusion only, in which case percutaneous balloon valvuloplasty may be effective. Conservative surgery with separation of the fused leaflets (commissurotomy) and reconstruction of the valve is possible in some younger patients. Usually, however, there is extensive leaflet calcification, with involvement of the subvalvular apparatus. There is shortening and thickening of the papillary muscles and chordae tendinae, tethering the leaflets to the tips of the papillary muscles (Fig. 22.11). Valve replacement is therefore the only practical option.

Rarely, patients with a mechanical mitral prosthesis may develop thrombotic occlusion of their valve secondary to inadequate control of anticoagulation or to fibrous tissue (pannus) ingrowth from the sewing ring. This acute emergency causes catastrophic pulmonary oedema and a severe reduction in cardiac output. Emergency salvage valve replacement or debridement is required.

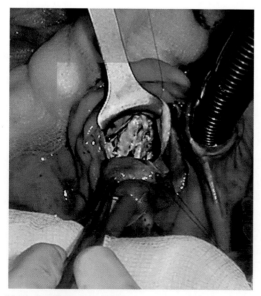

Fig. 22.10 Calcified aortic valve.

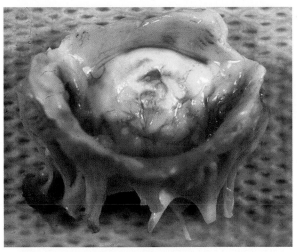

Fig. 22.11 Excised mitral valve showing the shortening and fusion of the papillary muscles and chordae tendinae in advanced mitral stenosis.

Regurgitation

Chronic mitral regurgitation occurs with rheumatic disease, ischaemic papillary muscle dysfunction, myxomatous degeneration of the mitral valve, a variety of systemic connective tissue disorders and chronic paraprosthetic valvular leakage. Acute regurgitation is much less common and follows acute MI involving a papillary muscle, as noted above, but can also result from spontaneous rupture of a chorda tendina, sudden failure of a bioprosthetic valve leaflet or perforation of an infected native valve. Chronic mitral regurgitation presents a volume load to the left ventricle, which ejects blood preferentially backwards through the incompetent mitral valve to the pulmonary circulation. This situation is often well tolerated for years, with patients typically complaining of shortness of breath on exertion and of occasional episodes of palpitation.

Clinical examination is often relatively unremarkable, apart from a pansystolic murmur radiating from the lower left sternal edge to the axilla and leftward displacement of the apex beat. Surgery is indicated where there is chest X-ray and echocardiographic evidence of left ventricular dilatation, as this process correlates with declining left ventricular function consequent upon the continued volume overload. Acute regurgitation causes pulmonary oedema and emergency surgery is necessary. Regurgitant mitral valves are frequently repaired but often prosthetic replacement is required.

Surgical outcomes

Elective mitral valve surgery for regurgitation is generally a low-risk procedure, with a mortality rate of 4–6% and a stroke rate of about 2%. The risk is much greater (10–15%) for patients with ischaemic regurgitation, owing to the concomitant coronary disease and previous myocardial damage. Valve replacement for mitral stenosis carries a significant mortality (8–12%) due to established pulmonary hypertension, right ventricular failure and poor renal function. The stroke rate is increased to 3–4%.

Emergency valve replacement for acute obstruction or regurgitation carries mortality of the order of 20%.

Tricuspid valve disease

Stenosis is very rare. Tricuspid endocarditis is occasionally encountered in intravenous drug abusers. Tricuspid incompetence secondary to enlargement of the tricuspid annulus is the most common pathology and occurs when the right ventricle is dilated, as in advanced mitral valve disease. Typically, the patient will have the features of the underlying mitral valve disease, an elevated jugular venous pressure with 'v' waves, an enlarged pulsatile liver, peripheral oedema and, occasionally, ascites. Liver function tests are frequently deranged and clotting is impaired. The preferred surgical option is to restore the normal dimensions of the valve through annuloplasty. It is uncommon to replace the tricuspid valve, except in rare cases of organic stenosis. If replacement is performed, a biological prosthesis is preferable, as the risk of mechanical valve thrombosis is increased in this position.

Multiple and repeat valve procedures

Multiple valve procedures are typically aortic and mitral valve replacement, or mitral replacement with tricuspid annuloplasty. Such operations attract a higher operative mortality (10% and 35%), as patients are often in poor general condition and may require prolonged periods of intensive care following surgery. Similarly, revisional valve surgery to replace a valve for a second time is technically more difficult and will involve a prolonged procedure against a background of impaired cardiac function or sepsis related to the defective prosthesis. Mortality is increased by two to three times the primary procedure risk, and ICU stay is prolonged.

Aortic aneurysm

Tubulosaccular aneurysms

These are 'true' aneurysms that form either a fusiform (tubular) or a focal (saccular) type of swelling (Fig. 22.12). They are lined by layered thrombus and most are due to medial degeneration secondary to smoking and hypertension (Ch. 21).

False 'aneurysms'

These result when bleeding from an aortic injury is contained within the mediastinum, so that the aneurysm wall is formed only by fibrous tissue and organized thrombus. There is usually a history of a road traffic accident or fall, which may have occurred many years previously.

Both true and false aneurysms may rupture and present as an acute emergency, with chest pain and catastrophic intrathoracic bleeding. However, they are often noted as incidental chest X-ray findings. Occasionally, an aneurysm may present with symptoms due to secondary pressure effects, such as dysphagia (oesophagus), stridor (left

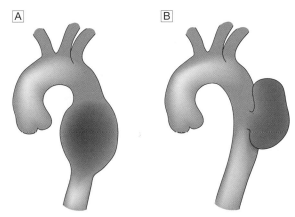

Fig. 22.12 Thoracic aortic aneurysm. **A** Tubular. **B** Saccular.

bronchus), chest wall pain (erosion of ribs), back pain (erosion of the vertebrae) or hoarseness (stretching of the left recurrent laryngeal nerve).

Aortic dissection

This is caused when blood enters into the wall of the aorta through a tear in the intima, creating a false lumen that spirals along the vessel within the medial layer but contained by the adventitia. The entry point is usually either just above the aortic valve or immediately beyond the left subclavian artery. However, the dissection process may extend along the entire length of the aorta into the iliac vessels. The false lumen may rupture through the adventitia into the mediastinum or pleural cavity, causing massive and frequently fatal haemorrhage, or into the pericardium, causing fatal tamponade. The origins of aortic side branches, which are encountered by the false lumen, tend to be encircled and occluded. This process can lead to widespread ischaemic damage to the heart (coronaries), brain (branches of the aortic arch), spinal cord (spinal arteries), kidneys (renal arteries), abdominal viscera (coeliac and mesenteric arteries) and the limbs. A dissection that involves the aortic root tends to lift the aortic valve leaflets away from the wall, leading to regurgitation. Finally, a dissected aorta may dilate over months to years, causing a progressive aneurysmal process. Acute dissection is often fatal prior to arrival at hospital. There may be severe interscapular pain, collapse, shock, aortic incompetence, unequal peripheral pulses, features of a left haemothorax, stroke, paraplegia, abdominal discomfort and lower limb ischaemia.

Dissections that originate distal to the left subclavian (Fig. 22.13 Type B), do not spread retrogradely to involve the aortic arch or ascending aorta, and are clinically stable, are usually managed conservatively by control of blood pressure, as the results of medical and surgical treatment are not different. Endovascular stent placement via the femoral artery under radiological control has an emerging role in this difficult situation and the decision to intervene on such patients is based on the development of rupture and organ/limb ischaemia.

In contrast, most patients with dissections that involve the ascending aorta (Fig. 22.13 Type A) or arch are offered emergency surgery to prevent rupture, stroke, MI and aortic valve incompetence. Surgery involves excising and replacing the portion of the aorta containing the entry point. This prevents more blood entering the false lumen and reapposes the layers of the aortic wall. Additional surgery to repair the aortic valve or to replace the aortic arch or descending aorta will be determined by individual circumstances.

Aorto-annulo ectasia

This is characterized by a flask-shaped aneurysmal dilatation of the aortic root and ascending aorta. This expanding aneurysm may rupture, initiate a dissection and lead to severe aortic regurgitation, with all the potential sequelae of these conditions. Aorto-annulo ectasia is frequently associated with connective tissue disorders, most commonly Marfan's disease.

Assessment

A patient with an incidentally discovered aneurysm should be thoroughly investigated, including tests of respiratory function and coronary angiography with contrast CT or MRI angiogram to fully delineate the extent of the aneurysm. Aneurysms that extend from the chest into the abdomen (thoracoabdominal aneurysm) require further investigations to clarify the relationship of the aneurysm to the renal and visceral vessels. Larger aneurysms (6 cm or greater) are more likely to rupture, and serial investigation will confirm whether or not an aneurysm is enlarging. Based on these considerations, a decision can then be taken regarding the potential benefit of surgery. In patients presenting with acute rupture of an aneurysm the diagnosis may have been made by one of the modalities described above or by transthoracic or transoesophageal echocardiography (Fig. 22.14). Surgery

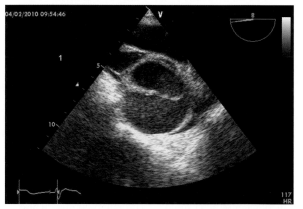

Fig 22.14 Transoesophageal echocardiography of aortic dissection.

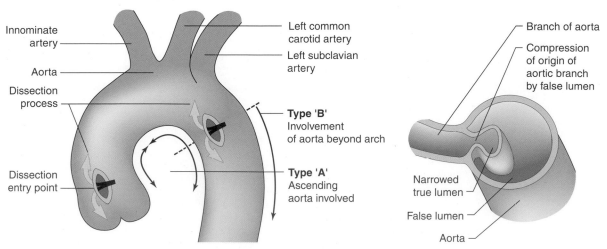

Fig. 22.13 Aortic dissection.

is recommended if they are potentially salvageable and considered likely to benefit from operative intervention.

Surgery for aortic pathology

Lesions of the aortic root and ascending aorta are repaired on bypass via a median sternotomy. A woven Dacron tube graft is used to replace an ascending aortic aneurysm, but in aortic annulo-ectasia a composite graft containing an aortic valve prosthesis is used to replace the whole aortic root. The coronary artery ostia are then attached as buttons onto side holes cut in the graft. Aneurysms involving the aortic arch require complex surgery. The patient is cooled to 16°C on bypass, the circulation arrested and the patient exsanguinated. Profound hypothermia protects against cerebral damage while the surgeon operates in a bloodless field. The brachiocephalic, left carotid and left subclavian arteries are anastomosed to the arch graft. Descending aortic aneurysms can often be repaired using a local shunt in order to deliver blood to the lower body. Clamps are applied to exclude the aneurysm, which is excised and replaced with a suitable length of graft. If a thoracoabdominal aneurysm is being repaired, the visceral arteries are also anastomosed to the graft.

Thoracic aortic aneurysm surgery is high-risk. Elective procedures carry a 5–15% mortality risk and a substantial risk of stroke. Procedures involving the descending aorta carry an additional 5–10% risk of paraplegia, owing to interference with spinal arterial supply. Emergency thoracic aneurysm surgery is in most cases a desperate measure. Mortality rates vary between 10% and over 60%, depending upon the extent of surgery required and, the degree of preexisting and acquired co-morbidities. It is not uncommon for the primary repair procedure to proceed satisfactorily, only for the patient to die later from multiorgan failure and/or stroke.

Pericardial pathology

Pericardial effusion

In chronic pericardial effusion, the pericardial sac will stretch and the clinical effects of the accumulated fluid may be modest. In contrast, a rapidly evolving effusion will prevent the heart from filling in diastole (tamponade) and lead to a low stroke volume. In order to maintain cardiac output and blood pressure, there is a tachycardia and intense peripheral vasoconstriction. The raised intrapericardial pressure leads to elevation of atrial pressure, and hence the central venous pressure rises in order to maintain a filling gradient. A pericardial effusion can often be drained percutaneously through a catheter placed under echocardiographic guidance. This may help clarify the diagnosis, but surgical drainage is likely to be required in infection, malignancy with reasonable life expectancy, and in chronic effusions. Chronic effusions are often drained into the left pleural cavity by creating a window in the left lateral pericardium either via an open left lateral thoracotomy or, more recently, as a minimal-access videothoracoscopic procedure. Acute and malignant effusions can be drained relatively simply into the peritoneal cavity via a short epigastric incision. Whichever approach is used, specimens of fluid and pericardium are sent for culture and histology.

Pericardial constriction

Chronic pericardial inflammation, often from tuberculosis, may heal by intense fibrosis and calcification (Fig. 22.15). This leads to chronic tamponade and investigations should include echocardiography, right heart catheterization with

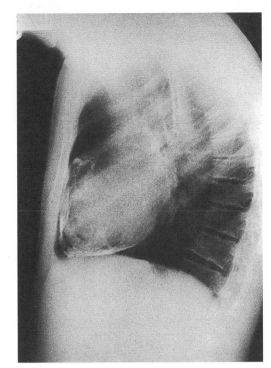

Fig. 22.15 Calcified constrictive pericardium.

record of chamber pressures and CT or preferably MRI. Surgery is undertaken via a median sternotomy to remove the parietal pericardium and any fibrotic visceral pericardium, and can be performed with or without CPB. Such surgery is difficult and can be accompanied by significant blood loss. The results are frequently disappointing because the patient may already have developed irreversible hepatic cirrhosis and myocardial function is poor.

Cardiac trauma

Cardiac tamponade with penetrating trauma

This is a surgical emergency and the clinical diagnosis is made from an elevated JVP, hypotension and the site of the wound which is commonly the result of an assault with a knife. Prompt anterior thoracotomy, relief of the bloody tamponade and digital control of the penetrating injury to the heart until suitable suture can be achieved may be life-saving. Major injuries to structures may require CPB.

CONGENITAL CARDIAC DISEASE

This may be classified as cyanotic or acyanotic, depending on the presence of central cyanosis. Those with cyanosis will have a right-to-left shunt, preventing complete oxygenation of systemic arterial blood. Some patients with high-flow left-to-right shunts develop severe pulmonary hypertension as a consequence of the massive pulmonary blood flow. This can result in pressures in the right heart chambers that are greater than those in the left heart and hence reversal of the shunt direction to right-to-left, causing cyanosis (Eisenmenger's syndrome). Primary repair is usually advised for congenital defects, but in some instances it may be helpful to delay definitive repair until the child is older, larger and fitter. In this situation, a temporizing palliative procedure is performed. This is usually designed to augment or restrict pulmonary artery blood flow.

22

Atrial septal defect

This is the most common abnormality, causing a left-to-right atrial shunt and hence an increase in right heart and pulmonary blood flow. Patients may be asymptomatic or may present with frequent chest infections. There is fixed splitting of the second heart sound and a pulmonary ejection systolic murmur. ECG demonstrates frequently right ventricular hypertrophy and echocardiography is diagnostic.

Small defects are of little haemodynamic significance, but if the pulmonary to systemic flow ratio exceeds 2:1, closure is recommended and may be undertaken percutaneously or by open operation depending on the size and morphology of the defect . Three anatomical types exist, named after the developmental area giving rise to the defect: *ostium secundum defects* are the most common, *sinus venosus defects* arise in the upper atrium adjacent to the superior vena cava and *partial atrioventricular canal defects* involve the anomalies of the mitral and tricuspid valves. Surgical repair in children carries a low mortality (< 1%), but adults presenting with pulmonary hypertension are at greater risk (10%).

Ventricular septal defect

Many ventricular septal defects are small and close within the first year of life. Larger lesions cause a left-to-right shunt and pulmonary congestion. Defects may again be subdivided according to their embryological origins, but most (85%) occur in the membranous septum. Infants with large defects may present with frequent respiratory infections but patients are often asymptomatic. A pansystolic murmur is audible, maximal at the left sternal edge. The second heart sound may be loud. Biventricular hypertrophy is present on ECG and pulmonary plethora may be noted on chest X-ray. Echocardiography is diagnostic. Asymptomatic defects are observed, but early operation is preferred for larger defects to prevent irreversible pulmonary hypertension. Repair is undertaken using a patch, with an operative mortality of 3–5%.

Patent ductus arteriosus

If the ductus arteriosus fails to close after birth, pulmonary blood flow is abnormally high, producing pulmonary congestion and hypertension. Infants have retarded growth and a continuous 'machinery' murmur is audible over the precordium and back. The chest X-ray shows pulmonary congestion, and echocardiography can exclude concurrent intracardiac defect(s). In premature children, the duct may close with an indomethacin infusion (prostaglandin E$_1$ inhibition), but clipping or division at left thoracotomy is definitive. Endovascular closure is an option in older children. The operative mortality is low in older children (< 1%) but high (25%) in preterm infants, who are generally very unwell.

Coarctation of the aorta

This condition is caused by a narrowing of the thoracic aorta, usually at the level of the ligamentum arteriosum. The lower body is perfused via extensive chest wall collaterals. Upper body hypertension develops and may lead to heart failure in infancy. Untreated adults develop hypertensive cerebrovascular and renal problems and accelerated coronary atheroma. Most children and young adults are asymptomatic and present with high blood pressure or an abnormal chest X-ray. The femoral pulses may be impalpable

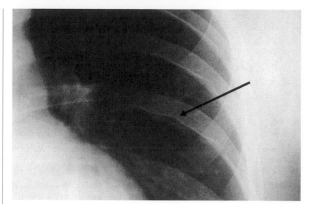

Fig. 22.16 Rib notching in coarctation.

or weak and delayed, and a systolic murmur may be audible over the back. LVH is seen on the ECG and the chest X-ray shows an enlarged heart, reduced aortic knuckle and characteristic rib 'notching', caused by enlarged and tortuous intercostal arteries eroding the ribs near the posterior angles (Fig. 22.16). Balloon angioplasty has been used to dilate some coarctations in infants, but surgical correction is usually required. At operation, the left subclavian artery may be used as an onlay patch. Older children and adults are usually managed with a Dacron bypass graft. Surgical correction tends to reduce upper body hypertension in children. It is less effective in adults but pharmacological control of hypertension becomes more reliable. The operative risk is about 5%.

Tetralogy of Fallot

This most common cause of cyanotic congenital heart disease comprises a high ventricular septal defect, an aorta that overlies the interventricular septum, pulmonary valvular and subvalvular stenosis, and right ventricular hypertrophy. Right ventricular outflow obstruction causes cyanosis as a result of right-to-left shunting across the ventricular septal defect. Clinical features depend upon the severity of the obstruction particularly the subvalvular component. The child may become blue and faint during feeding or crying.

Right ventricular hypertrophy is evident on ECG and the pulmonary artery shadow is small on chest X-ray. Echocardiography is diagnostic but is complemented by right ventricular angiography. Correction entails closing the ventricular septal defect with a patch, resecting muscle bands contributing to right ventricular outflow obstruction, and enlarging the right ventricular outflow tract with a patch placed across the pulmonary valve annulus and along the pulmonary artery if necessary. In those not fit for this procedure or in those with very small pulmonary vessels, a shunt is created in order to increase pulmonary blood flow and, hopefully, lead to further pulmonary arterial growth. Definitive correction may then be possible at a later stage. Operative mortality is about 10%.

THORACIC SURGERY

Assessment

This is concerned with confirming the diagnosis, determining in oncological cases whether resection is appropriate, and establishing that the patient is fit for the intended surgical procedure. The principal investigations are summarized

Table 22.2 Common thoracic surgical investigations

Investigation	Yield
ECG Resting	Rhythm; conduction abnormalities; atrial and ventricular hypertrophy; established ischaemic changes; evidence of previous myocardial infarction
Chest X-ray Posterior-anterior and lateral	Preliminary assessment of location of lesion; malignant involvement of phrenic nerve or ribs; presence of additional lesions or effusion; presence of pneumothorax or mediastinal air
Thoracic CT	Further refine radiological assessment of mass lesions as above; review mediastinum for enlarged nodes in bronchogenic carcinoma; inspect bronchi for dilatations in suspected bronchiectasis; determine areas of greatest disease in interstitial lung disease; locate intrathoracic collections; map out distribution of bullous/emphysematous lung disease
PET CT	Identify further disease elsewhere through metabolic uptake of ^{18}F-fluorodeoxyglucose not identified by conventional CT
Upper abdominal CT	Exclude or confirm liver abnormalities; identify adrenal metastases
Upper abdominal ultrasound	Determine probable nature of cystic hepatic lesions; provide guidance for biopsy of hepatic or adrenal lesions; review diaphragm motion in cases of suspected diaphragmatic rupture or phrenic nerve paralysis
MRI	Useful for assessing relationship of tumour to adjacent neural structures, e.g. detecting possible intraspinal extension of paravertebral neurogenic tumours or involvement of brachial plexus by superior sulcus (Pancoast) tumours
Isotope scans Bone Lung	Search for skeletal metastases; review chest wall for possible direct invasion by carcinoma Identify areas of low uptake indicative of impaired perfusion or ventilation
Pulmonary function tests FEV_1	Forced expiratory volume in 1 second; provides a measure of airway obstruction
FVC	Forced vital capacity; indicates presence of restriction of ventilation
CO transfer	Measures the diffusion capacity of the patient's lungs
Walking test	Measures distance walked by the patient in a set time period (4 mins) and the perceived exercise level achieved as assessed by the final heart rate; useful as an indicator of functional status in patients with poor FEV_1, as they may not comply well with the methodology of formal respiratory testing and hence underachieve
Arterial blood gas	Useful in demonstrating patients with CO_2 retention who should be excluded from surgical consideration

in Table 22.2. History can be instructive in suggesting advanced malignant disease and in providing evidence of the patient's functional status.

Bronchogenic carcinoma

Aetiology, pathology and presentation

This usually presents from the fifth decade onwards and is the leading cause of cancer death in the UK for both men and women. The principal risk factor is smoking; particularly cigarettes, but other rare causes include exposure to various chemicals. The combination of asbestos exposure and cigarette smoking produces a many-fold increase in risk.

With the exception of alveolar cell carcinomas, which arise from cells lining the alveoli, Primary lung cancers arise within the bronchial epithelium and are hence termed bronchogenic carcinoma. They are described as peripheral or central, according to their location within the lung (Figs. 22.17, 22.18 and 22.19). Peripheral lesions may grow to 8 cm or more before causing local symptoms such as chest wall pain. Many are detected as incidental findings on a chest film taken for unrelated reasons, or for non-specific symptoms such as weight loss. Central lesions tend to occlude the airways, causing varying degrees of pulmonary collapse and consolidation (Fig. 22.19). Nodal spread occurs to the intralobar, hilar and mediastinal nodes, and thence to the scalene nodes. Metastases occur in bone, brain, liver, adrenals and lung. Local direct spread may involve the chest wall, vertebrae, trachea, oesophagus and great vessels.

The approximate frequencies of the various cell types are: squamous 35%, adenocarcinoma 35%, undifferentiated 10%, small cell 15% and rare cancers 5%.

As small cell lung cancer is regarded as a systemic disease at presentation, patients are not usually referred for surgery and are therefore treated with chemotherapy. All other varieties are resected if possible (EBM 22.3). Therefore, for surgical treatment purposes, bronchogenic carcinoma is categorized into small cell and non-small-cell. However, cell type is important as recent advances in pathology have found genetic mutations that identify tumours that may be sensitive to new chemotherapeutic agents.

There may be no clinical features, but haemoptysis, pulmonary infection and weight loss are common presenting symptoms. Paraneoplastic syndromes are infrequent but well described, including ectopic hormone production (adrenocorticotrophic hormone (ACTH), parathyroid hormone (PTH), antidiuretic hormone (ADH)) and a painful periosteal reaction affecting the joints and long bones, termed hypertrophic pulmonary osteoarthropathy. Patients frequently have finger clubbing.

22

Assessment for pulmonary resection

Prior to referral to the surgeon, the diagnosis will often have been confirmed by sputum cytology, bronchoscopy or CT-guided needle biopsy, but approximately 30% of cases will be undiagnosed at this stage. Assessment addresses two questions:

• Is the patient fit for pulmonary resection?
• Is the disease potentially curable?

Fitness for resection

Fitness is determined by cardiorespiratory assessment. A history of angina or myocardial infarction does not preclude surgery, provided the symptoms are stable. However, patients with poor left ventricular function and/or unstable angina are not suitable for pulmonary resection. Respiratory investigations including the forced expiratory volume in one second (FEV_1) and carbon monoxide (CO) transfer data, will establish whether pulmonary reserve will be adequate following the intended resection. Patients with an $FEV_1 < 50\%$ predicted, prior to resection, are likely to be significantly breathless following surgery and may not be suitable candidates for surgical management. If the CO transfer value is low, implying poor alveolar gas exchange, the minimum FEV_1 figure would have to be revised upwards. However, resection of consolidated or collapsed lung does not affect residual respiratory capability.

Staging

Assessment of the potential for curative resection is determined by staging. Initial clinical assessment will normally filter out advanced disease and provide evidence of incurability because of local irresectability or disseminated disease (Table 22.3). Chest X-ray may reveal an elevated diaphragm, indicating phrenic nerve involvement, bone metastases or direct invasion of the rib cage. If an effusion is present, this should be aspirated; if malignant cells are noted on cytology, this would preclude resection.

Contrast-enhanced thoracic and upper abdominal CT will clarify the nature and position of the pulmonary mass and should exclude other pulmonary lesions that might represent

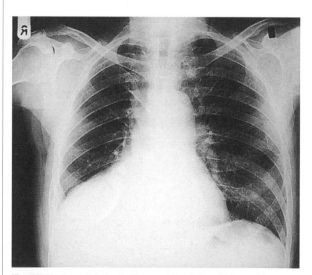

Fig. 22.19 Consolidation/collapse of the right middle and lower lobes associated with a central bronchogenic carcinoma.

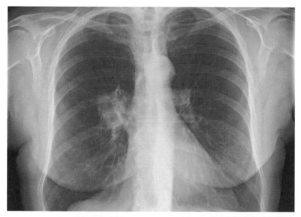

Fig. 22.17 Chest X-ray showing cancer in the right upper lobe.

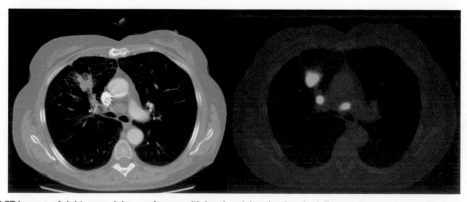

Fig. 22.18 PET CT images of right upper lobe carcinoma with local nodal and subcarinal disease. Same patient as Figure 22.17.

Table 22.3 Clinical indicators of locally irresectable or incurable lung cancer

Clinical finding	Pathological implication
Local inoperability	
Horner's syndrome	Involvement of upper sympathetic chain
Hoarseness	Involvement of left recurrent laryngeal nerve
Upper body venous congestion	Involvement of superior vena cava
Severe shoulder/inner arm pain	Involvement of brachial plexus (Pancoast tumour)
Disseminated disease	
Scalene node enlargement	Nodal spread out of operative field
Hepatomegaly	Hepatic metastases
Focal bone pain	Bone metastases
Skin deposits	Cutaneous metastases
Behavioural/balance disturbance	Cerebral/cerebellar metastases
Headache	

metastases or synchronous tumours. Mediastinal nodes < 1 cm in long axis are generally considered to be benign, but surgical sampling is necessary to confirm this. Where available, a combined thoracic CT/positron emission tomography (PET CT) scan is helpful in both locating and characterizing mediastinal lymph nodes (Fig. 22.18). A negative PET scan is highly accurate in predicting the absence of tumour involvement; a positive scan may indicate tumour but can also arise with inflammatory conditions, and, therefore, the positive glands must be sampled by mediastinoscopy. The liver and adrenals are common sites for metastases. Suspicious areas can be sampled by means of ultrasound-guided biopsy. Further investigations, such as bone or brain scans, will depend upon the clinical suspicion.

Surgical staging is concerned with further refining the intrathoracic assessment so as to ensure that thoracotomy will be associated with a reasonable chance of cure. In practical terms, this involves excluding those with involved mediastinal lymph nodes and, where possible, confirming the diagnosis and local operability. Techniques which are employed include:

- *Mediastinoscopy* is used to sample the paratracheal and subcarinal lymph nodes. A low anterior cervical incision is made just above the jugular notch and the mediastinoscope used to create a passage in the pretracheal region. The lymph nodes are dissected and biopsied. *EUS:* Under Endoscopic Ultrasound guidance, fine needle aspiration of mediastinal nodes may be performed either transbronchially or transoesophageally.
- *Mediastinotomy* is used mainly to assess lymph nodes within the concavity of the aortic arch or anterior to the aorta, as these areas cannot be reached at mediastinoscopy. Access is gained via a short left anterior second interspace incision.
- *Videothoracoscopy* is a technique that allows the surgeon to inspect the pleural cavity, biopsy the primary lesion and sample the lower mediastinal and aortic arch lymph nodes. The extent of resection likely to be required can also be assessed in relation to the patient's lung function. Videothoracoscopy may also reveal unforeseen causes of irresectability, such as pleural seedlings.

Resection

Lung tumours are normally removed en bloc with the surrounding parenchyma and local draining lymphatics. This involves either lobectomy or pneumonectomy. Occasionally, in unfit patients, small cancers are excised within a wedge or segment of lung but the risk of local recurrence is greater in these lung-sparing cases. An area of anterior chest wall directly invaded by tumour can be excised and replaced with synthetic patch, provided it is lateral to the posterior rib angles. Following assessment and surgical resection, the final pathological TNM stage (Table 22.4) is helpful in indicating prognosis and determining whether a patient might benefit from adjuvant therapy usually within the setting of a trial. Patients who are found to have positive mediastinal nodes following resection are routinely referred for adjuvant radiotherapy to the mediastinum in view of the high risk of recurrence in that area. Postoperative chemotherapy may improve 5-year survival across all resected stages by approximately 5%. Although still controversial, this form of adjuvant therapy is likely to become an increasingly common option for suitably fit patients. Operative mortality is about 2% for lobectomy and 6% for pneumonectomy.

Table 22.4 TNM classification of lung cancer

Tumour	
T1a	< 2cm
T1b	2–3 cm
T2a	3–5 cm
T2b	5–7 cm or within 2 cm of main bronchus or partial lung collapse
T3	> 7 cm, chest wall involvement, phrenic nerve involvement, whole lung collapse or > 1 tumour nodule in same lobe
T4	direct involvement of mediastinum or tumour nodules > 1 lobe
Nodes	
N0	No nodes
N1	Local node involvement
N2	Ipsilateral mediastinal nodes or sub carinal
N3	Contralateral mediastinal nodes or supraclavicular nodes
Metastases	
M0	No evidence of spread
M1a	Tumours in both lungs, malignant pericardial or pleural effusion
M1b	Distant metastases e.g. bone, adrenal, brain
Staging of lung cancer	
Stage 1A	T1a or T1b N0 M0
1B	T2a N0 M0
Stage 2A	Any T1 or T2 N1, T2b N0 M0
2B	T2b N1 M0 or T3 N0 M0
Stage 3A	Any T1 or T2 N2 M0, Any T3 N1 or N2, T4 N0 M0, T4 N1 M0
3B	Any T N3 M0 or T4 N2 M0 or T4 N3 M0
Stage 4	Any T or N with M1a or M1b

22

Survival

Reported 5-year survival data are approximately 60% for stage I, 35% for stage II and < 20% for stage IIIa disease. Relatively few patients (< 20%) with non-small-cell broncho-genic carcinoma are suitable for resection at presentation. One strategy to address this problem is the use of neoad-juvant preoperative induction chemotherapy to downstage tumours, although there are as yet no data to support the widespread use of this approach. The other obvious pos-sibility for improving resection rates would be to detect lung cancers at an earlier stage. Previous mass chest X-ray screening studies did not appear to show an improve-ment in long-term survival, but there is currently renewed interest in screening high-risk individuals (smoking history, > 50 years old) using CT as a more sensitive test.

Metastatic disease

Pulmonary metastases (Fig. 22.20) are the most common form of intrathoracic malignancy. A confirmatory diagnos-tic lung biopsy may be helpful for patients with no evident primary. A palliative pleurodesis in patients with associ-ated pleural effusion can be achieved by instilling an irritant such as aluminium silicate powder (kaolin) into the pleural cavity.

Rarely, a solitary metastasis (e.g. renal carcinoma) or lim-ited pulmonary metastases (e.g. in osteogenic sarcoma) may be found in patients without any other evidence of dissemi-nated disease. Increasingly patients with pulmonary metas-tases from colorectal cancer are considered for resection if there is evidence that intra-abdominal disease has been cleared and there is no increase in number or size of the metastases over a reasonable period.

Other lung tumours

These tend to present either as an incidental chest X-ray finding, in which case the concern is that they may in fact be malignant tumours, or as a cause of bronchial obstruc-tion and infection. True benign lung tumours are rare and can arise from all tissue elements within the lung architec-ture. If the lesion can be shown to be benign by transthoracic biopsy, no treatment is required. Where there is doubt, local

excision will be required. If a main bronchus is obstructed, lobectomy will be necessary to remove the tumour and the damaged portion of lung. Carcinoid tumours arise from argentaffin-containing cells within the bronchial epithe-lium. They are divided on histological grounds into 'typi-cal' tumours, which grow slowly locally, and 'atypical' tumours, which grow more quickly and can metastasize. Resection is by lobectomy. As local recurrence may occur up to 15 years following resection, good local clearance is essential. Unlike abdominal carcinoids, thoracic carcinoids do not secrete vasoactive substances.

An adenochondroma is a hamartoma, a tumour that develops from residual embryological tissue within the lung parenchyma. It presents as an incidental chest X-ray finding and is typically partly calcified and has a very smooth out-line. CT-guided needle biopsy should provide the diagno-sis, and surgery is only undertaken when the diagnosis is in doubt.

Mesothelioma

This causes progressive thickening of the parietal and vis-ceral pleura, with subsequent encasement of the lung and the formation of a large pleural effusion. In the later stages, the growth penetrates the chest wall, causing pain, and involves the mediastinal structures and abdominal cavity. Metastatic spread is rare until an advanced stage is reached. Mesothelioma is strongly related to a history of asbestos exposure, (e.g. boiler makers) but there is usually a latent period of 20–40 years before the onset of symptoms. The patient commonly presents with shortness of breath, owing to a large pleural effusion. In many cases, the diagnosis is made by a percutaneous pleural biopsy but, if this is not successful, thoracoscopy or open pleural biopsy is useful. The main differential diagnosis is disseminated adenocar-cinoma involving the pleural cavity. It can be difficult to distinguish these two pathologies on light microscopy, and diagnosis may be delayed while immunohistochemistry and electron microscopy studies are performed. Surgical resection by excision of the parietal pleura, lung, diaphragm and pericardium (pleuropneumonectomy) is not generally reported to offer a survival benefit, except possibly in very early lesions. Radiotherapy and chemotherapy have no curative value. Therapy is, therefore, usually directed towards controlling symptoms. If the lung re-expands after drainage of the effusion, kaolin may be instilled in order to promote pleurodesis and so prevent recurrence. Life expectancy varies from 1–4 years from initial presentation, depending on age, the rate of tumour growth and the stage at presentation.

Mediastinum

Mass lesions

Benign and malignant masses may arise in the mediasti-num. Some clue to the likely diagnosis is provided by the location of the lesion (Fig. 22.21) within the mediastinum. Where the diagnosis is in doubt, tissue may be obtained by CT-guided needle biopsy. If this is either not feasible or is unsuccessful, a surgical biopsy can be obtained using mediastinotomy, mediastinoscopy or videothoracoscopy. The clinical features vary considerably, with some quite large masses being asymptomatic and identified on routine chest films. Non-specific symptoms include vague chest pain, cough, weight loss, fever and general malaise. Other lesions may cause direct pressure effects, such as tracheal compression by a retrosternal thyroid goitre or oesophageal

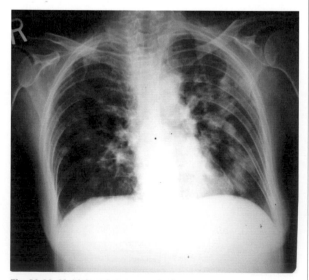

Fig. 22.20 Multiple pulmonary metastases.

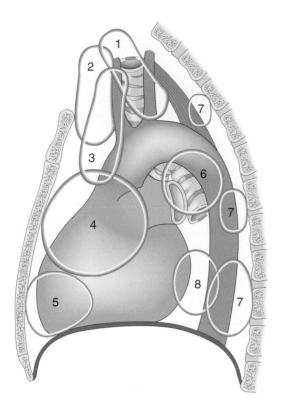

1 Goitre
2 Lymph node tumours, primary and metastases
3 Thymoma
4 Dermoid/teratoma
5 Pleuropericardial cyst
6 Bronchogenic cyst
7 Neurogenic tumour
8 Enterogenous cyst

Fig. 22.21 Topography of mediastinal lesions.

compression by malignant lymphadenopathy. Thymomas may be identified during the evaluation of patients with myasthenia gravis and resection of these may improve their neurological symptoms.

Wherever possible, primary mediastinal tumours are resected, although in many cases this is precluded because the growth involves the great vessels and mediastinal viscera. Benign cysts are usually resected or, less commonly, marsupialized in order to prevent pressure effects or the development of infection. Surgery is generally undertaken via a median sternotomy for anterior lesions or a thoracotomy for mid- and posterior lesions.

Infection

Mediastinal infection is an uncommon but serious condition that is associated with a rapid onset of septicaemia and septic shock. It is almost always a consequence of oesophageal or pharyngeal leakage, which may follow perforation or breakdown of an oesophageal anastomosis (see Ch. 13).

Pneumothorax

Pneumothorax occurs when air enters the potential space between the visceral and parietal pleura through either an external chest wound or an internal air leak. External air entry occurs with a traumatic chest wall defect, and the resulting open pneumothorax is often associated with a 'sucking wound', where air moves in and out of a chest wound with respiration. Internal air leakage may follow oesophageal perforation or anastomotic breakdown, as air can enter the pleural cavity via the mouth.

However, the most common cause of pneumothorax is leakage of air from the lung, due either to a traumatic puncture wound or to spontaneous leakage from a large (bulla) or small (< 1 cm, 'bleb') air sac on the lung surface. Occasionally, the pulmonary leak point may have a flap valve mechanism that allows air out of but not back into the lung, causing a rapid build-up of pressure within the pleural cavity (*tension pneumothorax* – Fig. 22.23). This can be fatal, as the high intrapleural pressure completely flattens the ipsilateral lung while deviating the mediastinum to the opposite side, impeding venous return.

Spontaneous pneumothorax is described as primary or secondary. Primary pneumothorax typically occurs in young (15–35 years) individuals with essentially normal lungs apart from a few apical bullae or blebs. Secondary pneumothorax develops in elderly patients (55–75 years) with a background of emphysema and chronic obstructive pulmonary disease. It is caused by rupture of a bulla.

Management

Initial management may involve aspiration or the insertion of a chest drain connected to an underwater seal into the pleural space (Fig. 22.24). This allows the lung to re-expand. In most cases of primary pneumothorax, air leakage stops within 48 hours or so, after which the drain can be removed. If the pneumothorax recurs or the air leakage does not stop, thoracoscopic surgery is indicated. The lung is inspected and any blebs or bullae are stapled. These are usually found at the apices of the upper or lower lobes (Fig. 22.22). Pleurodesis is then performed either by using an abrasion technique to scarify the parietal pleura, or a pleural strip (pleurectomy), or by insufflation of kaolin. Bullectomy and abrasion or pleurectomy carry about an 8% risk of further recurrent pneumothorax. This is reduced to 1–2% with kaolin insufflation, but as this technique involves leaving foreign material in the chest of a young person, it is usually kept in reserve for recurrent pneumothorax or for patients with no obvious culprit bulla or bleb.

22

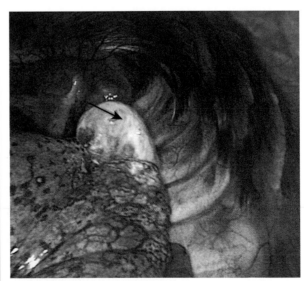

Fig. 22.22 Typical moderate sized apical bulla seen at thoracotomy.

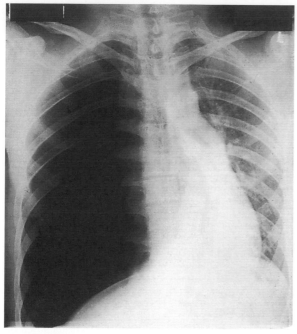

Fig. 22.23 Radiographic appearance of a right-sided tension pneumothorax (note the mediastinal shift to opposite side).

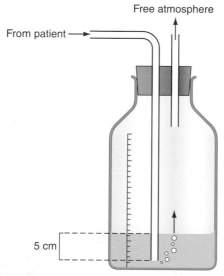

Fig. 22.24 Underwater seal drain. The water acts as a hydraulic valve. This allows air to escape from the pleural cavity with ease but the pressure required to cause reverse air flow is much greater, being increased by the ratio of the surface areas inside and outside the tube that enter the water.

Secondary pneumothorax may not settle rapidly, owing to the poor quality of the underlying lung tissue. It typically occurs in individuals who are poor candidates for general anaesthesia and major thoracic surgery. It is customary, therefore, to wait for 1–2 weeks to see if the air leak will stop spontaneously. If not, videothoracoscopy is undertaken in better-risk patients to inspect the lung for a leaking bulla, which can be closed by stapling. Alternatively, kaolin mixed with local anaesthetic can be inserted as slurry up the drain. This option avoids general anaesthesia but results in significant pain. Either treatment is associated with an appreciable mortality of 5–10%, owing to respiratory and cardiovascular complications.

Emphysema

Emphysema is characterized by progressive loss of interalveolar septae. Large air spaces form throughout the lungs, which become grossly enlarged with severely affected areas that are neither ventilated nor perfused. This causes progressive loss of respiratory function, culminating in respiratory failure and death. Recurrent infection and pneumothorax are common.

This is typically a smoking-related disease affecting patients from the fourth or fifth decade onwards, with a tendency towards an upper lobar distribution. In less than 10% of cases, however, it can also result from a deficiency of α_1-antitrypsin, affecting younger patients from the third decade and having a lower lobar distribution. Medical treatment with bronchodilators and steroids may improve symptoms but transplantation is the only definitive cure. This is only an option for younger patients, and even in these it should be postponed for as long as possible.

Lung volume reduction surgery aims to improve lung function by excising parts of the worst-affected areas, typically the upper lobes. This removes the space-occupying effect of these non-functional areas and allows the overall lung volume to return towards normal, thereby improving diaphragmatic and chest wall function. The improvement in respiratory function is modest in absolute terms, being in the order of 0.5 litres for FEV_1. However, patients eligible for this surgery typically have FEV_1 values of less than 1 litre, so that the relative improvement and hence the perceived benefit can be significant. The procedure may be performed either as a videothoracoscopic operation or through a median sternotomy. The clinical improvement only lasts for a few years, as lung function continues to fall, reflecting the progressive nature of emphysema. Case selection is important as the operative mortality is high (6–12%), reflecting the generally very poor condition of these patients.

Interstitial lung disease

This can arise from many causes and correct treatment depends on an accurate pathological diagnosis. Transbronchial biopsy can be effective in some instances, particularly sarcoidosis, but provides only a small tissue sample, which may not be diagnostic. It is usually preferable to use videothoracoscopic techniques to excise a wedge of affected lung. The patient is typically allowed home on the first postoperative day.

Pleuropulmonary infection

Empyema

This is a collection of pus within the pleural cavity. It commonly follows pneumonia due to secondary infection of a reactive parapneumonic effusion. In the initial phase, the infected fluid is thin and may be completely evacuated by a low intercostal drain. The empyema quickly becomes thick and loculated as a result of the deposition of fibrin, and at this stage formal surgical drainage is required. The collection is typically placed posteriorly towards the base of the pleural cavity and causes a D-shaped shadow on the chest film (Fig. 22.25). Drainage in this phase may be achieved by videothoracoscopic techniques or by excising a 2 cm segment of rib over the lowest part of the empyema and suctioning and curetting the cavity clean. As dense fibrosis surrounds an empyema, drainage creates a fixed cavity. In elderly or unfit patients, a simple open tube drain is left in

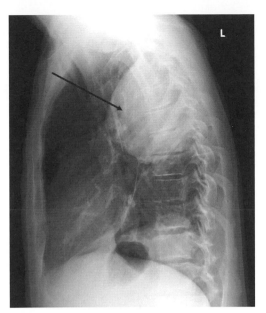

Fig. 22.25 Lateral X-ray of empyema. This film shows the D-shaped outline of a typical empyema with fluid level (arrow).

situ for many months, during which the cavity gradually shrinks and finally obliterates. In younger patients, open formal thoracotomy with decortication allows the fibrous cavity to be excised and any cortex over the lung removed. This returns more lung function to the patient and avoids prolonged open drainage, so that recovery is more rapid.

Other causes of empyema include postsurgical bronchial or oesophageal suture line leakage, oesophageal rupture or perforation, repeat aspiration of pleural effusion, secondary infection of a clotted haemothorax and, rarely, a subphrenic abscess.

Bronchiectasis

Dilatation of bronchi and bronchioles can follow childhood infections e.g. measles or pertussis. The stagnant pools of secretions that collect are subject to continued infection, resulting in episodes of acute pulmonary infection or pneumonia and, more rarely, in haemoptysis. Management is by antibiotic therapy, physiotherapy and daily postural drainage. Evaluation by CT usually demonstrates that the condition is fairly widespread throughout the lungs, but occasionally one lobe may be particularly badly affected. This is more likely when the bronchiectasis is secondary to chronic bronchial obstruction by an inhaled object or, more rarely, from external glandular compression. In this relatively uncommon situation, lobectomy may result in a gratifying decrease in chronic sputum production and in the frequency of recurrent infection. Resection can be technically difficult, as dense vascular adhesions surround the affected lobe.

Chest wall deformities

Sternal protuberance (pectus carinatum) or retraction (pectus excavatum) may be obvious and corrected in childhood. Pectus excavatum can be associated with connective tissue disorders such as Marfan's syndrome, and with unilateral breast hypoplasia. There is often a mild degree of scoliosis present and patients characteristically stand with a hunched posture. Often, however, patients with these deformities present in their early teenage years. At this time,

the deformity is exacerbated by accelerated growth and the individual becomes extremely sensitive about his or her appearance. Neither deformity is of physiological significance, and correction is only indicated when the patient's quality of life is clearly impaired because of appearance.

Correction involves major surgery. Open operation with resection of the costal cartilages from the third rib downwards bilaterally mobilizes the sternum so that it can be repositioned. In addition, a steel bar is implanted behind the elevated sternum for excavatum cases so as to maintain the new sternal position. Alternatively the bar may be introduced with a minimally invasive technique through bilateral small incisions avoiding division of the costal cartilages (Nuss procedure). The patient and family must be advised that, as with all major thoracic surgery, this procedure can be associated with serious postoperative complications, including death. Also, the sternum must be given time to fuse in the corrected position, and so contact or vigorous sports are not permitted for about 9 months after surgery. In general, if repair is to be undertaken, it is best delayed until the patient is at least 17 years old, as major growth has stopped by this time, thereby reducing the chance that further deformation could follow repair.

Postoperative care

The majority of major thoracic surgery is performed through a lateral thoracotomy incision, which is inherently much more painful than a median sternotomy. Patients are not electively ventilated, as this is not helpful to healing lung or to lung function. Patients undergoing major thoracic surgery are therefore usually cared for in a high-dependency unit (HDU) for the first 24–48 hours following surgery. The key objectives are to enable the patient to breathe effectively and to clear secretions properly.

Pain control

Pain management during the HDU phase is achieved normally by placement of an epidural catheter. It can have disadvantages related to increased fluid requirement, nursing care, and marked pain appreciation when the epidural infusion is stopped. Many units prefer not to place an epidural catheter and to rely instead on a combination of patient-controlled morphine infusion supplemented by parenteral non-steroidal analgesics and local intercostal nerve blocks. These can be conveniently given via a paravertebral catheter inserted at surgery.

Management of secretions

It is vital that patients cough and clear secretions. This requires humidification of oxygen to prevent the secretions becoming excessively viscous, effective pain control, and considerable input from physiotherapy since many patents have pre-existing impaired lung function. Excessive secretions may require to be removed by suction bronchoscopy under light general anaesthesia, and a mini-tracheostomy tube may be inserted via the cricothyroid membrane. In severe cases, ventilation and formal tracheostomy may be required.

Fluid management

Following major thoracic surgery, the pulmonary alveolar-capillary membrane becomes relatively leaky, so that fluid tends to accumulate within the pulmonary interstitial spaces. This decreases lung compliance and increases the work of breathing. A degree of postoperative fluid restriction for the first 48 hours ensures that the left atrial pressure is kept low, thereby decreasing pulmonary venous pressure and the transcapillary gradient.

22

Late management

All patients receive subcutaneous heparin as prophylaxis for deep venous thrombosis until fully mobile, because the risk of thrombosis is high in thoracic surgery and the consequences of pulmonary embolism are that much worse when lung has been resected. Drains are withdrawn when air leakage stops, and patients are mobilized as rapidly as possible. In an uneventful recovery, discharge home should occur about 6–9 days after major open resection, and after 1–5 days following a video-thoracoscopic minimal-access procedure. The patient's age, general health and social circumstances will influence these estimates.

Cardiac and pulmonary transplantation

Transplantation for end-stage cardiac and pulmonary disease is discussed in Chapter 25.

L.H. Stewart
S.M. Finney

23

Urological surgery

ASSESSMENT

General points

Patients may present with symptoms clearly related to the urinary tract but seemingly unrelated symptoms may be urological; backache from metastatic prostatic carcinoma, fever of unknown origin from renal carcinoma, lethargy and anaemia from obstructive renal failure.

Urinary tract symptoms

Pain

Afferent innervation of the urinary tract is rudimentary and as such pain originating from these organs, though characteristic, may not easily be localized. Renal pain occurs in the angle between the 12th rib and the sacrospinalis muscles. Ureteric pain (or colic) typically radiates forwards and downwards towards the groin, testes or labia, following the dermatomes relating to the nerve roots from which the sympathetic innervation of the ureter originates (i.e. T10–L2). Acute bladder obstruction usually causes central lower abdominal pain. By contrast, chronic bladder obstruction may be virtually asymptomatic. Disease of the bladder and prostate causes ill-defined perineal or penile pains. A prostate that is grossly enlarged can cause rectal symptoms, including tenesmus.

Disorders of micturition

The history aims to distinguish between obstruction (e.g. poor stream), storage problems (e.g. urgency), infection (e.g. frequency, dysuria) and malignancy (e.g. dark, discolored or brown urine). Frequency is recorded numerically: D/N 6/3 (by day, six times; by night, three). Hesitancy, poor stream and dribbling are characteristic of urinary outflow tract obstruction. Urgency, a sudden uncontrollable desire to void, may be associated with incontinence (urge incontinence). Stress incontinence relates to the involuntary loss of urine due to coughing, sneezing or straining. Dysuria describes painful micturition.

Examination

Examination should not be confined to the urinary system, as cardiological, neurological and gynaecological problems may be associated with urological symptoms and signs. Many urological patients are elderly and require an assessment of their fitness for further investigations and operative treatment. Furthermore, the patient's cardiovascular status may be relevant to subsequent treatment: for example, administration of oestrogens for carcinoma of the prostate.

With the patient relaxed, the kidney can be balloted; lifted with one hand placed behind the loin and compressed by the other hand pressing downwards (Fig. 23.1). The ureter cannot be palpated. An enlarged bladder rises centrally out of the pelvis, is dull to percussion and may even be visible. In men, the hernial orifices, cords, testes and epididymes are examined with the patient standing and lying. If the foreskin is uncircumcised, it must be confirmed that it retracts and that the glans and meatus are normal. In women, the vulva, urethra and vagina must also be examined. A speculum examination should be carried out if there is any suspicion of vaginal or cervical abnormality. A full pelvic bimanual examination, whether in males or females, is best carried out under general anaesthesia with a muscle relaxant. A rectal examination is mandatory, not only to examine the prostate but also to detect abnormalities of the anal margin (haemorrhoids, fissures) and lower rectum (carcinoma).

Investigations

Urine

In the absence of infection, urine is normally almost protein-free. Proteinuria of more than 150 mg/24 hrs mandates further investigation. Glycosuria suggests the presence of diabetes. Screening for urinary tract infection may also be done by Dipstix. Microscopic examination may detect casts or tubular epithelial cells associated with renal parenchymal

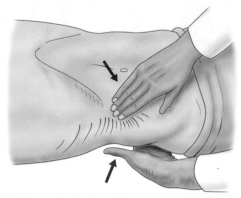

Fig. 23.1 Bimanual palpation of the right kidney.

disease, crystals in patients with renal calculi, or ova in schistosomiasis. Cytology and, more recently, urinary cellular markers are useful in the diagnosis and follow-up of bladder (and other urothelial) cancers. For microbiological examination, the patient is asked to pass some urine into the toilet. Then, without interrupting the flow, the next part is directed into a special container, and the remainder into the toilet; hence the term midstream specimen of urine (MSU). If it is necessary to store the specimen, it should be kept at 4°C. To exclude contamination, fine-needle suprapubic aspiration of a full bladder may be required.

Blood tests

Creatinine is a breakdown product of skeletal muscle and serum levels do not begin to rise until the glomerular filtration rate (GFR) is halved. Creatinine clearance can be used to estimate GFR. Patients with chronic renal disease often have disordered erythropoiesis leading to normocytic, normochromic anaemia in addition to disordered calcium metabolism. The erythrocyte sedimentation rate (ESR) can be markedly raised in idiopathic retroperitoneal fibrosis, a cause of ureteric obstruction. Human chorionic gonadotrophin (HCG), α-fetoprotein (AFP) and prostate-specific antigen (PSA) are useful tumour markers.

Intravenous urography (IVU)

A plain X-ray of the abdomen and pelvis is obtained to outline the areas of the kidneys, ureters and bladder (KUB film). The lumbar spine and pelvis, as well as stones in the region of the urinary tract, will be shown. An intravenous urogram (IVU) involves injecting iodine-containing contrast material intravenously and taking serial X-rays (Fig. 23.2) to demonstrate the renal pelvis and calyces, the rate of kidney emptying, the calibre of the ureters and the bladder outline. Once the bladder has filled, a 'post-micturition' film will demonstrate bladder emptying and the amount of residual urine.

Ultrasonography

This is another means of first-line imaging (Fig. 23.3), tending to give superior information about the renal parenchyma but less about the collecting system. It also allows visualization of other related organs, such as the liver, spleen and gynaecological organs.

CT Urogram

The IVU is largely becoming superceded by the 'plain' CT KUB, a non contrast enhanced CT, which has a higher specificity and sensitivity for the detection of renal and ureteric calculi. Furthermore, CT urography allows the

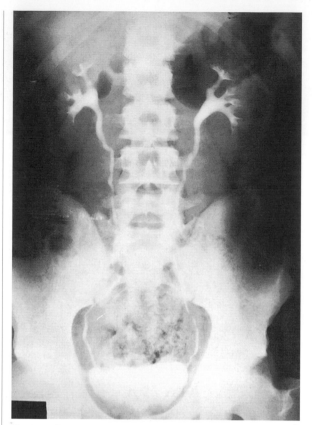

Fig. 23.2 Normal intravenous urogram (IVU).

ureters to be delineated by contrast, as in an IVU, but also allows other structures within the abdomen to be assessed.

Special radiological investigations

In certain circumstances a retrograde ureteropyelogram may be necessary. This involves retrograde injection of contrast material through a catheter placed in the lower ureter (Fig. 23.4). Abnormalities of the renal vessels can be demonstrated by renal angiography. Computed tomography (CT) is now the preferred method for imaging renal tumours. A micturating cystourethrogram (MCU) will outline the bladder, detect ureterovesical reflux and examine the bladder neck and urethra. The bladder is filled with contrast material (via a catheter) and emptying is then studied by X-ray screening. An *ascending* urethrogram, in which contrast medium is injected into the urethra, can be used to define strictures. When used in conjunction with a MCU, a *descending* urethrogram can also be obtained.

Nuclear imaging

Radio-labelled substances are used for two main purposes:

1. *Detecting bony metastases from carcinoma of the prostate (bone scan).* ^{99m}Tc-labelled methylene diphosphonate (MDP) is the most reliable method.
2. *Measurement of renal function (scintigraphic renography).* Occasionally 'how a kidney looks' does not correlate with 'how it behaves', e.g. hydronephrosis does not always mean the presence of obstruction. Renography allows assessment of obstruction to a kidney (e.g. from a pelviureteric obstruction), differential kidney function (i.e. how

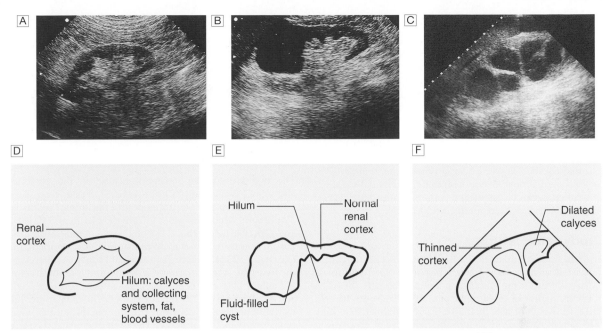

Fig. 23.3 Renal ultrasound. **A** Normal kidney. **B** A simple cyst occupies the upper pole of an otherwise normal kidney. **C** The renal pelvis and calyces are dilated by a chronic obstruction to urinary outflow. The thinness of the remaining renal cortex indicates chronicity. **D**, **E** and **F** The diagrams beneath show the anatomical features.

23

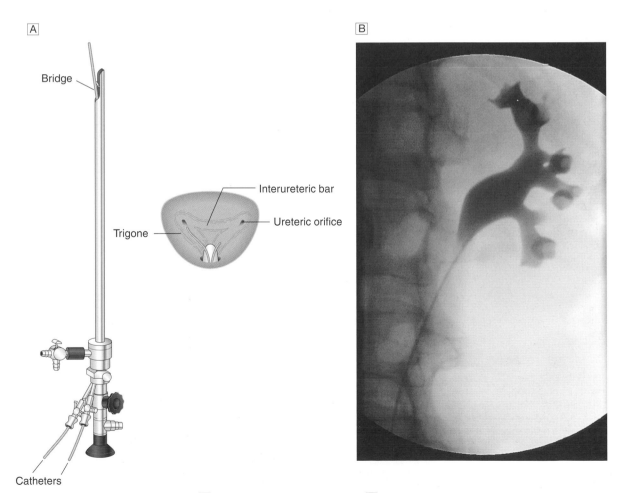

Fig. 23.4 Retrograde ureteropyelography. **A** Cystoscope and ureteric catheterization. **B** The best views of the normal collecting system are shown by pyelography. A catheter has been passed into the left renal pelvis at cystoscopy. The anemone-like calyces are sharp-edged and normal.

much each kidney is contributing to overall function), assess non-functioning areas of renal parenchyma (e.g. scarring) and allow accurate assessment of GFR. Radio-labelled mercaptuacetyltriglycine (MAG-3) has largely superseded technetium labeled diethylenetriamine pentaacetic acid (Tc-DTPA) for dynamic scanning. It is secreted from the renal tubules and is used in the identification of obstructed kidneys and to assess differential function. Dimercaptosuccinic acid (DMSA) is concentrated in the renal tubules and static imaging can be carried out some 2–3 hours after injection. Parenchymal defects such as scars, haematomas, lacerations or ischaemia may be demonstrated. Differential renal function can be quantified from measuring the DMSA concentration/density in each kidney.

Urodynamic studies

The maximum urinary flow rate during micturition can be measured using a flow meter when the voided volume is at least 150 ml or the values may be misleadingly low. The norm in males is 15–30 ml/s and in females 20–40 ml/s and a flow rate of less than 10 ml/s is abnormal. The flow rate pattern can help to determine the cause of obstruction (Fig. 23.5). Measurements of flow rate can be combined with cystometry to provide a measure of residual urine, bladder capacity, the capacity at which a desire to void occurs, and the detrusor pressures when the bladder is full and during maximum flow. Spontaneous detrusor contractions during bladder filling may indicate an unstable bladder, a cause of urgency and urge incontinence.

Semen analysis

Microscopic examination of the semen is a basic investigation in infertile males. The specimen is collected following a period of abstinence of at least 3 days and is examined within 2 hours. Normal semen has a volume of > 2 ml and a sperm concentration of $> 20 \times 10^6$/ml. More than 50% of the sperm should be motile at 2 hours. The morphology, biochemistry and viability of the sperm may also be studied. In selected cases, immunological tests may help to determine the cause of infertility.

Biochemical screening for stones

Recurrent urinary tract calculi should raise the suspicion of hyperparathyroidism, idiopathic hypercalciuria, hyperoxaluria or cystinuria. Serum calcium, phosphate, oxalate and uric acid should be measured. If more detailed investigation is required a 24-hour collection of urine for determination of calcium, phosphate, oxalate and uric acid excretion can be obtained. The composition of passed or removed stones should be analysed to determine their metabolic type.

UPPER URINARY TRACT (KIDNEY AND URETER)

Anatomy

The two kidneys lie retroperitoneally on the posterior abdominal wall. Each is approximately 12 cm long, 6 cm wide and 3 cm thick. The upper pole of the kidney lies on the diaphragm, which separates it from the pleura and the 11th and 12th ribs. Below this, it lies on the psoas, quadratus lumborum and transversus abdominis muscles from medial to lateral (Fig. 23.6). Anteriorly, the right kidney is covered by the liver, the second part of the duodenum and the ascending colon. The spleen, stomach, tail of pancreas, left colon and small bowel overlie the left kidney. The renal hilum lies medially and transmits from front to back the renal vein, renal artery and renal pelvis. The ureter begins at the renal pelvis and runs for 25 cm to the bladder. The abdominal ureter lies on the medial edge of the psoas muscle, which separates it from the tips of the transverse processes. It then crosses the bifurcation of the common iliac artery, which separates it from the sacroiliac joint, to enter the pelvis. The pelvic ureter runs on the lateral pelvic wall to just in front of the ischial spine, when it then turns medially and forward to enter the bladder. In the male, it is crossed by the vas deferens. In the female, it lies close to the lateral fornix of the vagina and is crossed by the uterine vessels, where it is vulnerable to damage during hysterectomy. The section of ureter that lies within the bladder wall functions as a flap valve to prevent reflux. Stones tend to impact at the three points where the ureter narrows: namely, the pelviureteric junction, the pelvic brim and the ureteric orifice.

Physiology

The healthy kidney can produce between 0.3 and 17 ml of urine per minute, depending on the state of hydration, but on average produces 1 ml of urine per minute. This is

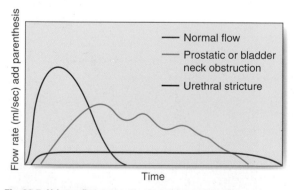

Fig. 23.5 Urinary flow rates. The normal flow rate shows a rapid rise to maximum high-peak flow. In a typical bladder outflow obstruction due to benign prostatic hyperplasia, there is a slow rise to poor maximum flow rate and prolonged variable flow. In a typical urethral stricture, there is prolonged flow with little variability, giving a plateau- or box-shaped curve.

Legend in figure:
- Normal flow
- Prostatic or bladder neck obstruction
- Urethral stricture

Y-axis: Flow rate (ml/sec) add parenthesis
X-axis: Time

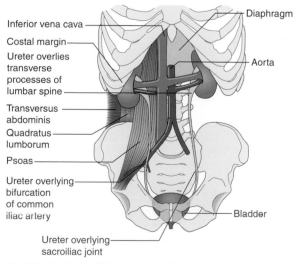

Fig. 23.6 Anatomy of kidneys and ureters.

Labels in figure:
- Diaphragm
- Inferior vena cava
- Costal margin
- Ureter overlies transverse processes of lumbar spine
- Aorta
- Transversus abdominis
- Quadratus lumborum
- Psoas
- Ureter overlying bifurcation of common iliac artery
- Bladder
- Ureter overlying sacroiliac joint

transported down the ureter by 4–5 peristaltic waves per minute to reach the bladder, where it is stored without refluxing up the ureters.

Renal cysts

Simple cysts

These are usually single, almost always asymptomatic, and often found incidentally on ultrasound where they can usually be differentiated from carcinoma. Complex cysts containing multiple septa raise the suspicion of malignant change

Polycystic kidney disease

An autosomal dominant congenital anomaly affecting both kidneys that often leads to chronic renal failure in middle life. Despite their very large size, the cystic kidneys cause few symptoms. Infection or bleeding may occur in a cyst causing pain or haematuria.

Benign tumours

Renal adenomas are small and are usually an incidental finding. Haemangiomas are a rare cause of dramatic haematuria.

Nephroblastomas

Epidemiology

This tumour usually occurs in children under 4 years of age, and is the most common childhood urological malignancy, with an incidence of 7 per million children per year. Growth is rapid and there is early local spread, including invasion of the renal vein. Invasion of the renal pelvis occurs late, and so haematuria is seen in only 15% of cases. Distant metastases most commonly appear in the lungs, liver and bones. Tumours presenting in the first year of life have a better prognosis.

Clinical features

The cardinal sign is a large abdominal mass. Some of the unusual clinical features associated with a renal carcinoma in adults, such as fever or hypertension, may be present.

Investigations

CT of the abdomen and chest is essential for diagnosis and staging. The main differential diagnosis to consider is adrenal neuroblastoma, but other causes of a large kidney, such as hydronephrosis and cystic disease, must also be considered. The tumour is bilateral in 5–10% of cases.

Management

The diagnosis is confirmed by biopsy. Chemotherapy is followed by transabdominal nephrectomy with wide excision of the mass. Further chemotherapy ± radiotherapy is performed dependent upon the histopathological features of the removed tumour; the 5-year survival rate is in the region of 70–90%.

Renal adenocarcinoma

Epidemiology

This tumour arises from the renal tubules and is the most common malignant tumour of the kidney. The incidence is 16 cases per 100 000, being twice as common in males.

It is uncommon before the age of 40 years and has a peak incidence between 65 and 75 years of age. There can be spread into the renal pelvis, causing haematuria. Invasion of the renal vein, often extending into the inferior vena cava, can also occur. Direct spread into perinephric tissues is common, so that the whole fascial envelope and kidney should be removed en bloc. Lymphatic spread occurs to para-aortic nodes, but blood-borne metastases (which may be solitary) may develop almost anywhere. In the lungs, these characteristically give the appearance of 'cannon ball' metastases.

Clinical features

The triad of pain, haematuria and a mass is an important, albeit late, feature occurring in only 15% of cases. Historically, 60% present with haematuria, 40% with loin pain and only 25% with a mass, but increasing access to ultrasonagraphy and CT has increased incidental diagnosis. Patients may present with pyrexia of unknown origin, raised ESR, polycythaemia, disorders of coagulation, and abnormalities of plasma proteins and liver function tests, or with neuromyopathy due to secretion of renin, erythropoietin, parathormone and gonadotrophins.

Investigations

The initial investigation is ultrasound, followed by a staging contrast CT of the abdomen and chest (Fig. 23.7).

Management

Organ confined renal adenocarcinoma should be treated with curative intent, either by laparoscopic or open nephrectomy. Metastatic renal adenocarcinoma is relatively radio and chemoresistant. Immunotherapy, in the form of interferon, gives a modest survival benefit (3–5 months) but angiogenesis inhibiting drugs, such as tyrosine kinase inhibitors, are showing more promising results. A further modest survival benefit may be seen in metastatic disease by reducing the tumour burden if nephrectomy is performed prior to starting immunotherapy.

23

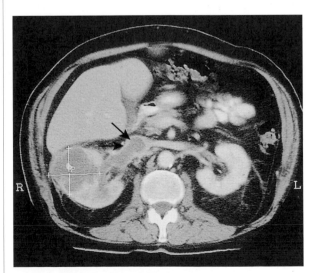

Fig. 23.7 Contrast-enhanced CT of renal cancer. The right kidney is expanded by a low-density cancer that fails to take up the contrast. Tumour is seen extending into the renal vein and inferior vena cava (arrow).

Renal carcinoma

- Renal adenocarcinoma is the most common malignant renal tumour and is twice as common in males
- The carcinoma arises in the renal tubules and spreads early to the renal pelvis, producing haematuria. Later spread involves the renal vein (with bloodstream dissemination), perinephric invasion and lymphatic spread
- The clinical presentation is very varied. The triad of pain, haematuria and a mass may be late features, and early systemic effects include fever, polycythaemia, disordered coagulation and pyrexia of unknown origin
- The key investigations are ultrasonography, chest X-ray and contrast CT
- Treatment consists of radical nephrectomy; the tumour is not radiosensitive. The natural history of renal carcinoma is very variable and excision of solitary metastases may be worthwhile.

Renal and ureteric calculi

Mechanism of stone formation

A *solute* dissolves in a *solvent* to form a *solution* but when the concentration of solute in solution reaches a certain level, termed the solubility product, the compound precipitates out to form crystals. This initial crystal formation (*nucleation*) may progress such that crystals clump together (*aggregation*) to form calculi. There are substances in urine that act to keep compounds in solution by inhibiting nucleation (*inhibitors*) but, above a certain concentration of solute, nucleation will occur despite their presence (*formation product*). Where the concentration of a compound lies between the solubility product and the formation product, being kept in solution solely by the action of inhibitors, it is described as being *metastable*. A solution with a concentration above

the formation product is described as being *supersaturated*. The ability of urine to keep compounds in solution, and prevent calculus formation is a balance between forces keeping the solute in solution and those that promote nucleation. Therefore, stones form when the amount of solute increases (e.g. hypercalcuria), the amount of solvent decreases (e.g. dehydration) or the concentration of inhibitors falls (e.g. decreased citrate excretion). Foreign bodies, anatomical abnormalities, and calculi can all act as a nidus for nucleation and promote further stone formation.

Types and causes of stone formation

The commonest stone types are; calcium oxalate (85%), uric acid (10%), mixed calcium phosphate/calcium oxalate (10%), magnesium ammonium phosphate (5–15%) and cystine (1%). Calcium oxalate stones are commonly caused by hypercalciuria, hypercalcaemia, hyperoxaluria or hypocitraturia. Uric acid stones are formed due to increases in uric acid formation either through gout or myeloproliferative disorders. Approximately 50% of patients with urate stones have gout but only 20% of patients with gout develop urate stones. Calcium phosphate stones are generally secondary to renal tubular acidosis. Magnesium ammonium phosphate (struvite) stones are usually due to urinary tract infection by pathogens that can break urea down into CO_2 and ammonia, thereby alkalinizing the urine.

Clinical features

Renal pain, renal colic and ureteric colic are characteristically unilateral. Renal pain is dull and aching, whereas ureteric colic is acute and severe, occurring in waves. A stone may cause bleeding or there may be symptoms of urinary tract infection. However, a stone in the kidney may remain silent, even one large enough to fill the pelvis and calyces ('staghorn' calculus).

Investigations

IVU or CT KUB provides all the necessary information on the position of the stone (Fig. 23.8). Routine hematological and biochemical tests are needed to assess renal function

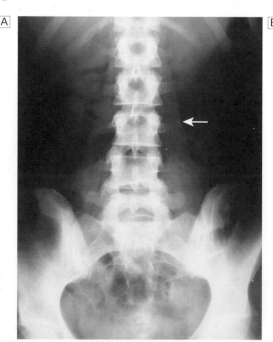
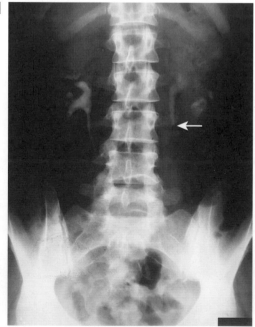

Fig. 23.8 IVU showing ureteric stone. **A** Eighty percent of stones are visible on a plain X-ray (arrow). **B** The contrast excreted by the kidney in an IVU clearly shows the obstruction caused by the stone in the ureter (arrow).

and to exclude metabolic causes. A urine sample is cultured to determine whether there is infection. If obstruction is acute, its relief is the prime clinical need; if it is chronic and has caused renal damage, the surgical approach depends on the function of the affected kidney. This is best determined by radioisotope methods (renography).

Management

Symptomatic treatment should be instituted as soon as the diagnosis is confirmed. Intramuscular diclofenac, a nonsteroidal anti-inflammatory, is the most effective analgesic; pethidine is an alternative. The likelihood of spontaneous passage depends on the size of the stone and on its smoothness. A stone less than 0.5 cm in diameter should pass. Immediate treatment should be considered in cases of ongoing pain, renal obstruction or, more importantly, where there are signs of sepsis (infected obstructed kidney). Extracorporeal shock-wave lithotripsy (ESWL), the technique of focusing external shock waves to break up stones, has revolutionized the treatment of renal and ureteric stones. If a stone can be visualized on X-ray or ultrasound, then it can be treated by ESWL. Other stones can be visualized directly by passing a fine telescope up the ureter (ureteroscope) and the stones may be either broken up or removed intact. Some stones in the kidney that are unlikely to pass even if broken up are best treated by direct puncture of the kidney, insertion of a sheath and removal under vision with a nephroscope (percutaneous nephrolithotomy, PCNL). It is now very rare to remove stones from the renal tract at open operation. In cases of acute obstruction leading to sepsis (infected obstructed kidney) or renal impairment, decompression of the kidney either via insertion of a ureteric stent or percutaneous nephrostomy is required. Stones and infection within a kidney can be the cause of renal destruction and if the kidney contributes less than 10% of total renal function, then a nephrectomy is recommended.

Upper tract obstruction

Obstruction may be due to extrinsic, intrinsic or intraluminal causes (Table 23.1). In the kidney, stones within the pelvicalyceal system and a congenital abnormality of the pelviureteric junction (see below) are the main causes of obstruction leading to hydronephrosis. More rarely, a sloughed renal papilla, blood clot or tumour may be the cause.

Pelviureteric junction obstruction (idiopathic hydronephrosis)

Narrowing of the junction between the renal pelvis and the ureter is a common cause of hydronephrosis. As the aetiology is obscure, the term 'idiopathic' hydronephrosis is appropriate. This condition is seen in very young children.

Table 23.1 Causes of urinary tract obstruction

Extrinsic
- Retroperitoneal fibrosis
- External pressure (e.g. carcinoma of the cervix, prostate)

Intrinsic
- Transitional cell tumours
- Tuberculosis / schistosomiasis
- Ureterocoele
- Ectopic ureter

Intraluminal
- Calculi

It is likely to be congenital and can be bilateral, but gross hydronephrosis may present at any age.

Clinical features

Idiopathic hydronephrosis may produce a large painless mass in the loin; in its grossest form, the volume of urine in the hydronephrotic sac may simulate free fluid in the peritoneal cavity. The more usual moderate hydronephrosis causes ill-defined renal pain or ache that may be exacerbated by drinking large volumes of liquid (Dietls' Crisis). The patient may regard these symptoms as 'indigestion'. Rarely, there may be no symptoms.

Investigations

IVU or a CT urogram (CTU) provides sufficient information in many cases. The calibre of the ureter is normal. There are a few patients in whom there is doubt as to whether the dilatation of the pelvis and calyces is truly obstructive in nature. In these cases a MAG-3 renogram is performed.

Management

Either laparoscopic or open pyeloplasty is performed to remove the obstructing tissue and refashion the pelviureteric junction (PUJ) so that the lower part of the renal pelvis drains freely into the ureter (Fig. 23.9). It is not possible to predict the degree of recovery of renal function after the relief of obstruction, but a kidney contributing less than 10% of total renal function should be removed.

Retroperitoneal fibrosis

Pathology

Fibrosis of the retroperitoneal connective tissues may encircle and compress the ureter(s), causing hydroureter and hydronephrosis. Fibrosis occurs in three groups of conditions:
- *Idiopathic.* The aetiology is unknown, although it may be associated with methysergide or analgesic abuse

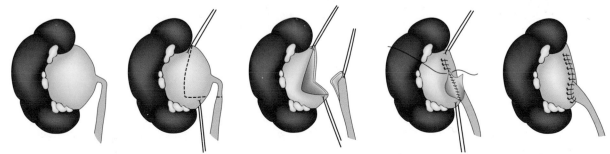

Fig. 23.9 Anderson–Hynes pyeloplasty.

Mediastinal fibrosis and Dupuytren's contracture may coexist
- *Malignant infiltration.* The fibrosis contains malignant cells that have metastasized from primary sites such as the breast, stomach, pancreas and colon
- *Reactive fibrosis.* Radiotherapy, resolving blood clot, or extravasation of sclerosants can lead to fibrotic change in the retroperitoneum.

As the gross appearance of fibrosis in all three groups may be similar, biopsy of the tissue is essential for diagnosis.

Clinical features

Ureteric obstruction may cause symptoms similar to idiopathic hydronephrosis: namely, ill-defined renal pain or ache, and low backache.

Investigations

IVU or CTU shows hydronephrosis and usually hydroureter down to the level of the obstruction. The ureter is often difficult to define, but it is usually pulled medially. A markedly raised ESR is found in more than 50% of cases with idiopathic fibrosis.

Management

Relief of obstruction may be difficult. Where ureteric stenting fails to give adequate drainage uretrolysis can be performed; the ureter is dissected out of the fibrous sheet of tissue (ureterolysis) and wrapped in omentum to prevent further involvement.

 SUMMARY BOX 23.2

Urinary tract obstruction

Common causes of obstruction of the lower outflow tract
- Benign prostatic hyperplasia
- Prostatic cancer
- Bladder cancer involving the bladder neck
- Bladder-neck obstruction (dyssynergia, infection, neurological disorders)
- Urethral obstruction (congenital posterior urethral valves, blocked urinary catheter, trauma, infection, stricture).

Common causes of obstruction of the upper urinary tract
- Renal and ureteric calculi (80% are calcium oxalate/phosphate stones)
- Pelviureteric junction obstruction (idiopathic hydronephrosis)
- Retroperitoneal fibrosis (idiopathic/malignant infiltration/radiotherapy)
- Transitional cell carcinoma (with or without bleeding and clot)
- Congenital abnormalities (e.g. ectopic ureter, ureterocoele)
- Infections (notably schistosomiasis and tuberculosis).

LOWER URINARY TRACT (BLADDER, PROSTATE AND URETHRA)

Anatomy

The bladder is a muscular reservoir that receives urine via the ureters and expels it via the urethra. In children up to 4 years of age, it lies predominantly in the abdomen; in the adult it is a pelvic organ, well protected in the bony pelvis. Superiorly, the bladder is covered with peritoneum, which separates it from coils of small bowel, the sigmoid colon and, in the female, the body of the uterus. Posteriorly lie

the rectum, the vas deferens and seminal vesicles in the male, and the vagina and supravaginal cervix in the female. Inferiorly, the neck of the bladder transmits the urethra and fuses with the prostate in the male and with the pelvic fascia in the female.

The bladder is composed of whorls of detrusor muscle, which in the male become circular at the bladder neck. They are richly supplied with sympathetic nerves that cause contraction during ejaculation, thereby preventing semen from entering the bladder (retrograde ejaculation). There is no such sphincter in the female. The bladder is lined with specialized waterproof epithelium, the urothelium. This is thrown into folds over most of the bladder, except the trigone where it is smooth.

The male urethra is 20cm long; the prostatic urethra descends for 3cm through the prostate gland, and the membranous urethra is 1–2cm long and intimately associated with the main urethral sphincter, the rhabdosphincter. The spongy urethra is 15cm long and is surrounded by the corpus spongiosus throughout its complete length, opening on the tip of the glans penis as the external meatus. The spongy urethra is further subdivided into the proximal bulbar urethra and the distal penile urethra. The female urethra is 3–4cm long, descending through the pelvic floor surrounded by the urethral sphincter and embedded in the anterior vaginal wall to open between the clitoris and the vagina.

In the male, the prostate is pyramidal, with its base uppermost. It resembles the size and shape of a chestnut and surrounds the prostatic urethra. Traditionally described as having a median and two lateral lobes, it is better considered as being composed of a small central and a larger peripheral zone (Fig. 23.10).

Physiology

Neurological control of micturition

Detrusor contraction is mediated through cholinergic parasympathetic nerves arising from the nerve roots S2–S4, and relaying through ganglia lying predominantly within the detrusor. Sympathetic nerves arise from T10 to L2 and relay via the pelvic ganglia. Their exact role in the control of micturition is unclear. It is known that α-adrenergic receptors and their nerve terminals are found mainly in the smooth muscle of the bladder neck and proximal urethra. The α-receptors respond to noradrenaline (norepinephrine) by stimulating contraction, thereby maintaining closure of the bladder neck.

The distal sphincter mechanism is innervated from the sacral segments S2–S4 by somatic motor fibres that reach the sphincter either by the pelvic plexus or via the pudendal nerves. Afferent nerves are carried in both the parasympathetic and pudendal pathways and transmit sensory impulses from the bladder, urethra and pelvic floor. These sensory impulses pass to the cerebral cortex and the micturition centre, where they produce reflex bladder relaxation and increased tone in the distal sphincter, so helping maintain continence. Cortical control is a basic part of the micturition cycle described below. The higher centres suppress detrusor contractions and their main function is to inhibit micturition until an appropriate time.

The micturition cycle

The micturition cycle has two phases.

Storage (or filling) phase

Due to the high compliance (elasticity) of the detrusor muscle, the bladder fills steadily without a rise in intravesical pressure. As urine volume increases, stretch

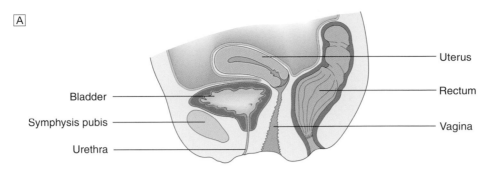

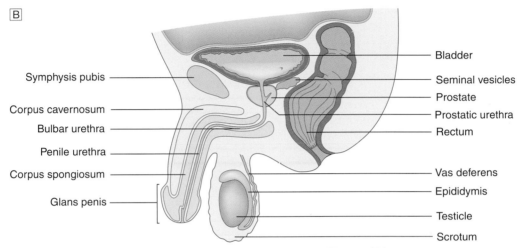

Fig. 23.10 Anatomy of the lower urinary tracts. [A] Female. [B] Male.

receptors in the bladder wall are stimulated, resulting in reflex bladder relaxation and reflex increased sphincter tone. At three-quarters of bladder capacity, sensation produces a desire to void. Voluntary control is now exerted over the desire to void, which temporarily disappears. Compliance of the detrusor allows further increase in capacity until the next desire to void. Just how often this desire needs to be inhibited depends on many factors, not the least of which is finding a suitable place in which to void.

Emptying (or micturition) phase

The act of micturition is initiated first by voluntary and then by reflex relaxation of the pelvic floor and distal sphincter mechanisms, followed by reflex detrusor contraction. These actions are coordinated by the pontine micturition centre. Intravesical pressure remains greater than urethral pressure until the bladder is empty.

The normal control of micturition requires coordinated reflex activity of autonomic and somatic nerves, as described above. These responses depend on normal anatomical structures and normal innervation. There are thus two main types of disorders of micturition: structural and neurogenic. Examples are extensive carcinoma of the prostate that has damaged the sphincter mechanism (structural), and spinal cord injury that has damaged the innervation (neurogenic).

Trauma

Bladder

Open injuries

The bladder may be damaged as a result of a penetrating injury to the lower abdomen, or through the course of pelvic surgery; during which damage to the urethra, rectum, vagina or uterus may also occur. Unrecognized damage during surgical procedures may lead to a wound fistula, a vesicovaginal fistula or a vesicocolic fistula.

Closed injuries

Intraperitoneal rupture typically occurs in a patient who has been drinking alcohol, has a full bladder and is assaulted and kicked in the abdomen. The dome of the bladder ruptures and urine extravasates into the peritoneum, causing intestinal ileus and abdominal distension. Extraperitoneal rupture is usually due to a major road traffic accident in which the pelvis has also been fractured when the bladder is not full, but may follow endoscopic resection of the prostate or a bladder tumour (Fig. 23.11).

Clinical features

The ileus and distension that occur with intraperitoneal rupture of the bladder are often detected late because of the circumstances surrounding the injury. However, the patient

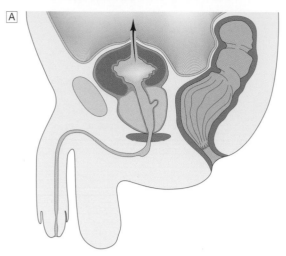 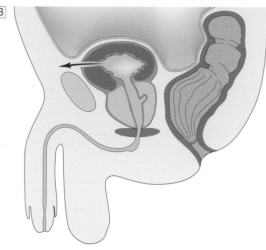

Fig. 23.11 Rupture of the bladder. A Intraperitoneal. B Extraperitoneal.

will be aware of the inability to pass urine and seek advice. Extraperitoneal extravasation of urine, if part of a major accident, adds to what already are severe pelvic injuries. When the leak occurs during an endoscopic procedure, the patient later complains of suprapubic pain with varying degrees of lower abdominal tenderness.

Investigations

Generally, the circumstances of the bladder injury establish the diagnosis. If confirmation of injury is required, water-soluble contrast is injected via a urethral catheter and the bladder examined on the X-ray screen (cystogram).

Management

Intraperitoneal rupture demands laparotomy and repair. Extraperitoneal rupture in the absence of other injuries tends to be managed conservatively through drainage of the bladder with a urethral catheter left in situ for 6–10 days. Occasionally, surgical exploration is required.

Urethra

Open injuries

Penetrating injuries resulting in damage to the anterior or posterior urethra are rare.

Closed injuries

Damage to the anterior urethra is typically due to falling astride a hard object, although a kick can cause a similar injury. The mechanism of injury to the posterior urethra is similar to that of extraperitoneal rupture of the bladder. In the majority of cases, posterior urethral injuries are associated with a fracture of the pubis or fracture-dislocation of the pelvis. Both the posterior urethra and bladder are damaged in 10% of cases.

Clinical features

Anterior urethral injuries are usually located at the bulb, so that the patient presents with a perineal haematoma. If this becomes infected, there may be sloughing of the skin, urethra and even the scrotal tissues. Because of the mechanism of injury, patients with posterior urethral tears are usually shocked and require resuscitation before a detailed assessment can be made. If the patient has passed clear urine, the bladder and urethra are probably intact. If there is blood at the external meatus, urethral injury must be suspected. A distended bladder can occur because of spasm of the urethral sphincter or because of a torn posterior urethra.

Investigations

If the physical signs suggest an anterior urethral injury, and the patient has passed clear urine, no further steps need be taken. If there is blood at the external meatus or the urine is blood-stained, a urethrogram using water-soluble contrast material may demonstrate the extravasation (Fig. 23.12). A catheter should never be passed in the emergency room. If urine is blood-stained, retrograde urethrography may be carried out but the radiological distinction between a rupture of the membranous urethra and an extraperitoneal bladder rupture may be difficult.

Management

All patients with an injury to the bulb of the urethra have a perineal haematoma. If the injury is only a contusion, this will resolve, but prophylactic antibiotics are indicated. A large haematoma may require drainage if the urethra has been lacerated. The extent of injury should be defined and

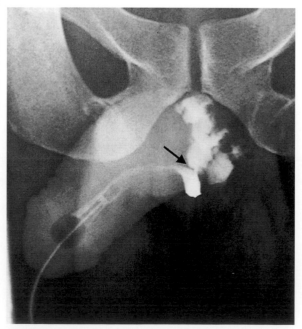

Fig. 23.12 Ascending ureterogram in urethral rupture. Contrast is seen extravasating at the site of the disrupted urethra (arrow).

the urethra repaired if possible. A urethral or suprapubic catheter drains the bladder. Treatment of a posterior urethral injury depends on the expertise available. It is quite acceptable to perform a suprapubic cystostomy and deal with the injury to the urethra at a later date. If laparotomy is necessary for other reasons, this may give an opportunity to pass a catheter. If the rupture is incomplete, the catheter will act as a splint. If the rupture is complete, the ends of the urethra can be approximated and splinted by the catheter. The late complications of these injuries are stricture and impotence.

Bladder tumours

Pathology

The vast majority of bladder tumours arise from the urothelium or transitional cell lining, which it shares in continuum with the renal pelvis and the proximal urethra. The urothelium is exposed to chemical carcinogens excreted in the urine, such as naphthylamines and benzidine, which were extensively used in the chemical and dye industries in the past. The bladder is more susceptible to urinary carcinogens, as urine is stored in the bladder for relatively long periods of time.

Almost all tumours are transitional cell carcinomas. Squamous carcinoma may occur in urothelium that has undergone metaplasia, usually due to chronic inflammation or irritation caused by a stone or schistosomiasis. An adenocarcinoma is a rarity but may occur in an urachal remnant in the dome of the bladder, or from local infiltration, e.g. bowel cancer. The prevalence of transitional cell carcinoma in the bladder is 45 cases per 100 000, and it is three times more common in men than women. The appearance of a transitional cell tumour ranges from a delicate papillary structure to a solid ulcerating mass. Papillary tumours are less aggressive superficial cancers, whereas those that ulcerate are much more aggressive.

Staging

Biopsy is essential to confirm the diagnosis (*cell type*), determine the degree of cell differentiation (*grade*), and assess the depth to which the tumour has penetrated the bladder wall

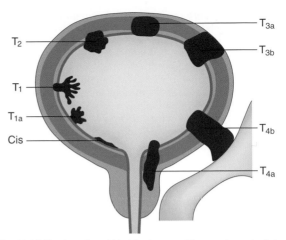

Fig. 23.13 T categories of bladder tumour. (Cis = carcinoma in situ)

(*stage*). The TNM system of tumour classification is applicable to bladder tumours. Assessment of the primary tumour (T) is of prime clinical importance and requires bimanual examination under anaesthesia to judge the degree of penetration through the bladder wall. This is especially important for T_2 and T_3 tumours (Fig. 23.13). Clinical examination, urography and CT are used to assess the involvement of regional and juxtaregional lymph nodes (N). Assessment of distant metastases (M) requires clinical examination and CT. Histopathological examination guides the choice of treatment. Biopsy gives accurate information on superficial tumours, but depth of invasion of invasive tumours cannot be assessed precisely as the biopsy does not examine the full thickness of the bladder wall.

Clinical features

More than 80% of patients have haematuria, which is usually painless (Fig. 23.14). It should be assumed that such bleeding is from a tumour until proved otherwise. In women, symptoms of cystitis are so common that occasional bleeding may be thought to be part of an infective

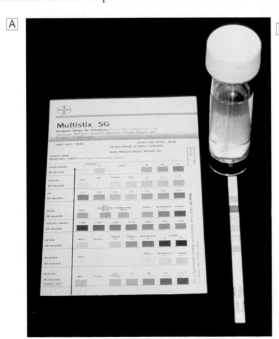
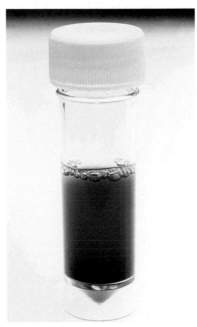

Fig. 23.14 Haematuria. A Microscopic. B Macroscopic.

problem. Therefore, in cases of haematuria, MSSU is mandatory with further investigation required if no growth is found. In men, symptoms of bladder outflow obstruction are common and may include bleeding. Bleeding at initiation of micturition suggests a prostatic, or urethral, origin. Haematuria throughout micturition suggests either a bladder or upper tract cause. A tumour at the lower end of a ureter or a bladder tumour involving the ureteric orifice *may* cause obstructive symptoms. However, frank haematuria may be the only presenting symptom. Examination is usually unhelpful. Rectal examination detects only advanced tumours.

Investigations

Because upper tract tumours are much less common, they may be overlooked in the presence of an obvious bladder tumour. Both may occur together, and the whole of the urothelium must be examined on the IVU or CTU (Fig. 23.15). If there is any suspicious filling defect in the ureter, a retrograde ureteropyelogram is necessary. In cases of frank haematuria, investigations consist of flexible cystoscopy, peformed under local anaesthesia, and either an ultrasound of the kidneys with an IVU or a CTU. Where a lesion is found within the bladder, cystourethroscopy and examination under anaesthesia are performed (Fig. 23.16). With the patient relaxed under general anaesthesia, the bladder and tumour are examined bimanually to determine the depth of spread. The physical features of the tumour(s) are noted, the normal bladder mucosa is inspected and the tumour is fully resected if possible. If not, biopsies are taken from the tumour and any other suspicious areas.

Management

Superficial bladder tumours (T_a, T_1)

Ideally these are treated by formal transurethral resection of the blabber tumour (TURBT) down to and including detrusor muscle; however, they can also be treated solely by endoscopic diathermy if required. Intravesical chemotherapy (mitomycin C) is useful to treat multiple low-grade bladder tumours and to reduce recurrence (EBM 23.1).

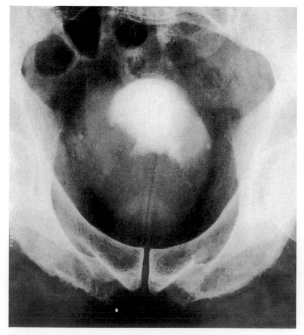

Fig. 23.15 Filling defect on IVU due to bladder tumour.

Regular check cystoscopies are required. Recurrences are mostly treated by repeat diathermy or resection but, if they become very frequent and excessive, cystectomy may be advisable. Carcinoma in situ (Cis) may be present in mucosa that appears normal or in association with a proliferative tumour. Cis can also exist as a separate entity, when there may be only a generalized redness (malignant cystitis). Cis should be considered in patients with ongoing irritative urinary symptoms associated with pain or symptoms suggestive of ongoing urinary tract infection, both in the absence of urinary tract infection upon MSSU culture. Untreated patients with Cis have a high risk of progression to invasive cancer. Cis responds well to intravesical bacille Calmette-Guérin (BCG) treatment. However, if there is any doubt about the response, and especially if there is any pathological evidence of progression, more aggressive treatment is warranted.

EBM	**23.1 Role of intravesical chemotherapy in superficial bladder cancer**
	'A single dose of intravesical mitomycin C following transurethral resection of a bladder tumour reduces the risk of subsequent recurrence.'
	Tolley DA, et al. J Urol 1996; 155(4):1233–1237.

Invasive bladder tumour (T_2–T_{3s})

Management is controversial. For patients under 70 years of age, radical cystectomy is recommended. In older patients, radiotherapy may be a better option. Unfortunately, this may not always cure the tumour and 'salvage' cystectomy may be needed. Cystectomy always necessitates urinary diversion. Where the urethra can be retained, it may be possible to construct a new bladder from colon or small bowel (orthotopic bladder replacement), so achieving continence. Alternatively, the urine is collected in an internal reservoir that is connected to the body surface via a continent conduit (ileum or appendix), through which the patient drains the urine at regular intervals with a catheter. In less favourable circumstances, an ileal conduit should be performed (Fig. 23.17). In some countries where an 'ostomy' is not acceptable, the ureters can be implanted into the sigmoid colon (ureterosigmoidostomy). However, renal infection and metabolic disturbances are potentially serious complications of this procedure. An invasive T_4 tumour, fixed to the pelvis or surrounding organs, is inoperable and only palliative treatment can be given.

Prognosis

Outlook depends on tumour stage and grade. Superficial disease carries a much better prognosis with a 5-year survival of 70–90%. Muscle invasive disease has a 5-year survival of 10–60%.

Carcinoma of the prostate

Epidemiology

In the UK, this is the fourth most common malignancy in males, with a prevalence of 50 cases per 100 000 population, and is increasing in frequency. It is the second most common cause of cancer death in men in the UK. The tumour is common in northern Europe and the USA (particularly in the black population), but rare in China and Japan. It rarely occurs before the age of 50 and is uncommon before the age of 60. The mean age at presentation is approximately 70 years. The aetiology is unknown, but genetic, hormonal and possibly viral factors are implicated.

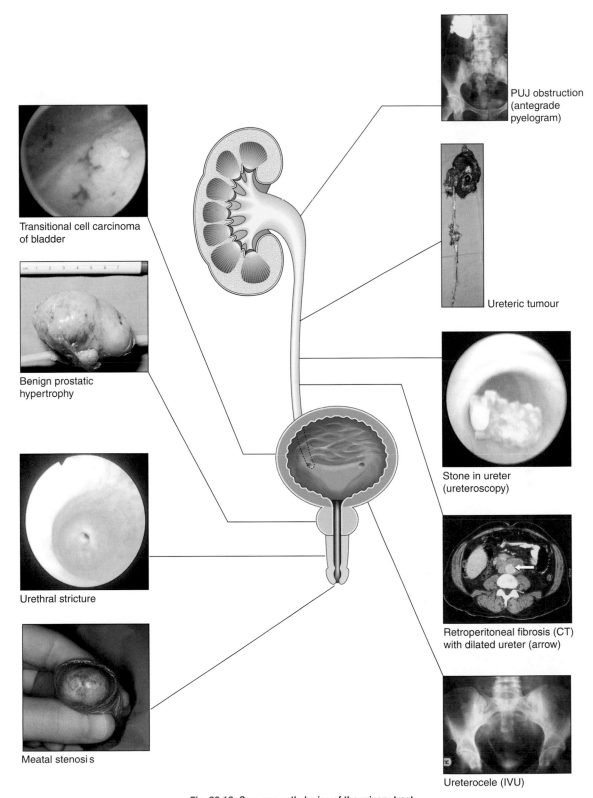

PUJ obstruction
(antegrade
pyelogram)

Ureteric tumour

Transitional cell carcinoma
of bladder

Benign prostatic
hypertrophy

Stone in ureter
(ureteroscopy)

Urethral stricture

Retroperitoneal fibrosis (CT)
with dilated ureter (arrow)

Meatal stenosi s

Ureterocele (IVU)

Fig. 23.16 Common pathologies of the urinary tract.

Pathology

Almost all malignant tumours of the prostate are carcinomas with the most common being adenocarcinoma (> 95%). If a prostate is examined by serial section, a small malignant focus is detected in almost all men over the age of 80. Thus, there is a very high prevalence of histological prostate cancer and many men will die with a cancer of the prostate – but not *from* that cancer. It is estimated that the prevalence of focal histological cancer in men aged 50–75 is approximately 40%, whereas the prevalence of clinical prostate cancer is approximately 8%, one-quarter of whom will die from that cancer. The TNM system is used in classification

23

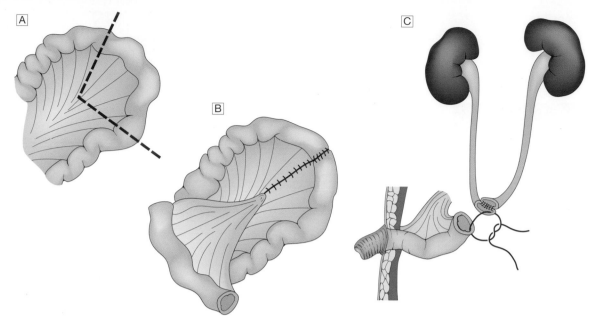

Fig. 23.17 Ileal conduit urinary diversion. A and B Isolation of segment of terminal ileum. C Fashioning of uretero-ileal anastomosis. The stoma is made to protrude from the skin to minimize skin contact with urine and so reduce irritation.

 SUMMARY BOX 23.3

Urothelial tumours

- The urothelium or transitional cell epithelial lining of the urinary tract extends from the renal papilla to the distal urethra
- The incidence of urothelial cancer is increasing, possibly because of increasing exposure to occupational carcinogens, smoking and analgesic abuse
- Almost all urothelial cancers are transitional cell tumours and the vast majority occur in the bladder. Squamous cancers are rarer and are associated with chronic irritation or inflammation (e.g. calculi and schistosomiasis). Adenocarcinomas are extremely rare
- Frank haematuria is present in 80% of cases
- Transitional cell cancers of the bladder are treated as follows:
  - Carcinoma in situ (Cis) may respond to intravesical BCG but is unpredictable and may require more aggressive treatment
  - Superficial tumours (Ta, T1) are usually treated by transurethral resection ± intravesical chemotherapy
  - Invasive tumours (T2, T3) may be best dealt with by radical cystectomy (or by radical radiotherapy)
  - Invasive T4 tumours with fixation to the pelvis or surrounding organs are dealt with by palliative radiotherapy.

(Table 23.2). Metastatic spread to pelvic lymph nodes occurs early. One-third of clinically localized tumours at the time of presentation will have spread to regional nodes. Metastases to bone, mainly the lumbar spine and pelvis, occur in some 10–15% of cases.

The Gleeson score is also used to grade prostate adenocarcinoma. Cells are graded 1–5 depending upon their level of differentiation (grade 1 = most differentiated, grade 5 = least or most anaplastic). The pathologist uses the two most common malignant cell types to determine a

'Gleeson score'; (most common type + second most common type = Gleeson score). Therefore, Gleeson scores range from 2–10 and are always expressed as an equation (e.g. $4 + 3 = 7$).

Table 23.2 TNM classification of prostate cancer*	
T (Tumour)	
• T_0	No evidence of primary tumour
• T_x	Primary tumour cannot be assessed
• T_1	Tumour clinically inapparent and not palpable
• T_{1a}	Incidental finding following TURP in < 5% prostate chips
• T_{1b}	Incidental finding following TURP in > 5% prostate chips
• T_{1c}	Prostate cancer detected by prostate biopsy
• T_{2a}	Palpable nodule involving half of one lobe
• T_{2b}	Palpable nodule involving one lobe
• T_{2c}	Palpable nodule involving both lobes
• T_{3a}	Extracapsular extension of prostate cancer
• T_{3b}	Prostate cancer involving the seminal vesicles
• T_{4a}	Prostate cancer involving the bladder neck and/or external sphincter and/or rectum
• T_{4b}	Prostate cancer involving the lateral pelvic wall
N (Nodes)	
• N_0	No regional lymph node metastasis
• N_x	Regional lymph nodes cannot be assessed
• N_1	Regional lymph node metastasis
M (Metastases)	
• M_0	No distant metastasis detected
• M_x	Distant metastasis cannot be assessed
• M_{1a}	Metastasis to non-regional lymph nodes
• M_{1b}	Skeletal metastasis present
• M_{1c}	Metastasis to other sites

*Sobin LH, Wittekind C, eds. TNM classification of malignant tumours, 6th edn. Chichester: John Wiley; 2002.
(TURP = transurethral resection of the prostate)

Clinical features

The presentation of patients with prostatic carcinoma is similar to benign prostatic hyperplasia (BPH); one-quarter present with acute retention (Fig. 23.18). Occasionally, the tumour extends posteriorly around the rectum and causes alteration in bowel habit. Presenting symptoms and signs due to metastases are much less common, but include back pain, weight loss, anaemia and renal failure secondary to ureteric obstruction. On rectal examination, the prostate feels nodular and stony hard but many irregular prostates, even those with nodules, are not malignant. Conversely, 50–60% of malignant prostates are not palpably abnormal on rectal examination.

Investigations

As most patients present with outflow tract obstruction, ultrasound and serum creatinine determinations are performed to assess the urinary tract. An X-ray of the pelvis or lumbar spine (to investigate backache) may show osteosclerotic metastases as the first evidence of prostatic malignancy. Whenever possible, the diagnosis is confirmed by needle biopsy, usually performed under transrectal ultrasound (TRUS) guidance, or by histological examination of tissue removed at endoscopic resection if this is needed to relieve outflow obstruction. The patient is assessed for distant metastases by a radioisotope scan. Prostate-specific antigen (PSA) is the main serum marker for the detection of prostate cancer. A PSA of < 4.5 is generally regarded as normal although there has been a move to regard < 3.5 as being normal if less than 65 years of age. Metastatic disease is exceptional when the PSA level is < 15, but levels > 100 ng/ml almost always indicate distant bone metastases. PSA is the main test for monitoring response to treatment and disease progression. A bone scan may be carried out at follow-up to localize and define the extent of metastases, whereas CT is useful to assess pelvic lymphadenopathy.

Management

Prostatic cancer is sensitive to endocrine influences (EBM 23.2) as testoterone is a trigger for moving prostate cells through the cell cycle thereby stimulating mitosis. Management is best considered in three clinical groups, as follows.

Organ confined / localized disease

With increasing use of PSA, a raised value may be the only abnormality that leads to the diagnosis of cancer confirmed by a needle biopsy. A patient with a small focus of well-differentiated carcinoma may be managed by an active surveillance policy, as usually these patients remain unaffected by their prostate cancer for between 10–15 years. In younger patients with a longer life expectancy (i.e. > 10 years), or in patients with a large tumour with a less well-differentiated cell pattern (Gleeson score 7 or more) there is an increased risk of progression. In these cases, treatment with curative intent by either surgery or radiotherapy is suggested. The prostate can be removed laparoscopically, robotically or by the traditional open route. Radiotherapy can be performed by external beam radiotherapy (EBRT) or by the insertion of radioactive seeds in the prostate (brachytherapy). There are no data to support one treatment over the other in terms of overall survival. However, each treatment modality has a different side effect and complication profile. Therefore, the choice of treatment tends to be based upon patient preference. In active surveillance, patients tend to have regular PSA measurements and only undergo treatment if the level rises.

Locally advanced disease; no evidence of bone metastases

This term refers to cases where the prostate cancer has invaded directly outside the prostate but has not metastasized. Surgery does not confer a cure in this situation. However, EBRT along with hormonal therapy has shown some survival benefit. In patients not able to tolerate EBRT, hormone therapy alone or palliative treatment can be considered.

Metastatic prostate cancer

Approximately half of the men diagnosed with prostate cancer will have metastatic disease. The basis of treatment in these cases is castration either physically by androgen depletion (orchiectomy) or chemically, by androgen suppression (gonadotrophin-releasing hormone analogues) and/or androgen receptor antagonists. A small number of patients fail to respond to endocrine treatment; a larger number respond for a year or two, but then suffer disease progression. PSA levels are a useful marker of response, ideally falling to < 0.01 in well controlled cases. Oestrogens are useful but are limited by their thromboembolic effects. Chemotherapy with taxanes has shown a marginal improvement in both symptoms and survival. Radiotherapy is an effective treatment for localized bone pain. For severe generalized bone pain, intravenous [89]Strontium may give effective palliation, but the basis of treatment remains pain control by analgesia.

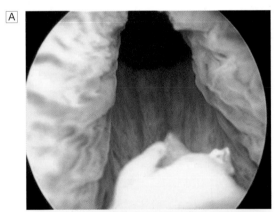

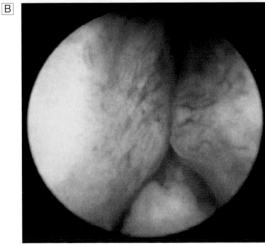

Fig. 23.18 Endoscopic view of prostate. **A** Normal. **B** Obstructed.

23

Prognosis

The life expectancy of a patient with an incidental finding of focal carcinoma of the prostate is that of the normal population. With tumours localized to the prostate, a 15-year survival rate of 56–87% can be expected; if metastases are present, this falls to < 10%. PSA is a very useful marker to determine response to treatment in addition to monitoring disease progression or recurrence.

SUMMARY BOX **23.4**

Prostatic cancer

- In the UK this is the second most common cancer in men, presents at a mean age of 70, and is increasing in incidence
- The carcinoma may be incidental (i.e. found on histological examination), clinically apparent (bladder outflow obstruction and a hard craggy prostate) or occult (metastatic disease)
- Metastatic spread may occur early; one-third of clinically confined cancers have spread to lymph nodes, and 10–15% of all new cases have bony spread (to lumbar spine and pelvis)
- Treatment of prostatic cancer varies:
  - *Incidental* or focal cancer. If well differentiated, then life expectancy can be normal with a watch-and-wait policy. If the cancer contains undifferentiated cells, then either radical surgery or radiotherapy is considered
  - Localized cancer with no evidence of bony metastases. Treated by either radical surgery or radiotherapy, keeping endocrine therapy in reserve
  - Metastatic cancer. Treated by androgen depletion (orchiectomy) or androgen suppression (gonadotrophin releasing hormone analogues)
  - Tumours localized to the prostate and amenable to radical curative treatment have a 10-year survival rate of 60–75%.

Benign prostatic hyperplasia

Pathology

From about the age of 40 years, the prostate undergoes enlargement as the result of hyperplasia of periurethral tissue, which forms adenomas in the transitional zone of the prostate. Normal prostatic tissue is compressed to form a surrounding shell or capsule. There is considerable variation in the growth rates of the adenomas and in the proportions of stromal and epithelial tissue. A prostate that has been infected previously or has a preponderance of stromal tissue is firm and fibrous on rectal examination. Adenomas with an epithelial preponderance can grow to form large discrete masses weighing more than 100 g, and have a characteristic

rubbery consistency, referred to as benign prostatic hyperplasia (BPH). Enlarging adenomas lengthen and obstruct the prostatic urethra, causing outflow obstruction and detrusor muscle hypertrophy. The muscle bands of the bladder form trabeculae, between which saccules form diverticula (Fig. 23.19). Occasionally, a diverticulum may become quite large, even larger than the bladder. Bladder diverticula empty poorly and are liable to the three main complications of urinary stasis: infection, stones and tumour. With progressive inability to empty the bladder completely (chronic retention), the risk of urinary infection and stone formation increases. Eventually, the residual urine volume may exceed one litre, resulting in progressive obstruction and dilatation of the ureters (hydroureter) and pelvicalyceal system (hydronephrosis). This ultimately leads to obstructive renal failure.

Clinical features

Frequency, nocturia, urgency, dysuria and poor stream are common. Straining may cause vessels at the bladder neck to bleed. Clinical features may be due to obstruction (slow stream and hesitancy) and those due to detrusor instability (urgency and urge incontinence). In isolation, the latter symptoms are not an indication for prostatectomy. Increasing frequency may deceive the patient into believing that an adequate amount of urine is passed, whereas the bladder has a small functional capacity and may be almost full all of the time (chronic retention). Frequency may progress to continual dribbling incontinence leading over time to signs and symptoms of obstructive uraemia, including drowsiness, anorexia and personality changes. Urinary

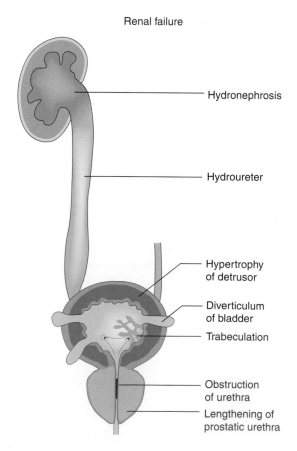

Fig. 23.19 Late sequelae of prostatic obstruction.

infection, cold weather, anticholinergic drugs or excessive alcohol intake can cause sufficient congestion of the bladder neck to provoke acute or acute-on-chronic retention. If the patient has a bladder stone, he may have obstructive symptoms during micturition, and there may also be bladder pain at the end of micturition. Examination reveals little except rubbery, symmetrical and smooth prostatic enlargement, with a median groove between the two lateral 'lobes'. Asymmetry or a hard consistency raises the suspicion of malignancy. In a patient with acute painful retention of urine, the size of the prostate is more difficult to determine. In patients with chronic retention, the painless, enlarged bladder rises out of the pelvis, almost to the umbilicus. The overlying area will be dull on percussion. In addition, the patient with chronic retention may be ill from obstructive uraemia.

Investigations

A good history and examination are paramount. Further mandatory assessment includes blood for renal function, haemoglobin and electrolytes, urine culture and PSA. Prostatic cancer can occur with normal PSA values (0–4 ng/ml) while BPH can cause elevated values, so careful interpretation is required (Table 23.3). If digital rectal examination raises suspicion, needle biopsy is indicated. Ultrasound can detect bladder diverticula, intravesical stones and measure residual urine volume. A urine flow rate will quantify a reduction in urinary stream. A symptom score sheet will quantify the degree of inconvenience and bother. In some patients, especially the elderly, neurological or pharmacological causes for the changes in micturition must be considered. A pressure-flow urodynamic assessment may be necessary.

Management

Patients can be divided into three clinical groups, each requiring a different approach to management.

Symptomatic only

The patient's assessment of the severity of symptoms is influenced by his age, the social inconvenience caused, and the frequency and progression of symptoms. A young man may be greatly inconvenienced by symptoms that are quite acceptable to one who is elderly. If the exact role of the prostate in causing symptoms is difficult to determine, urodynamic studies may be helpful, especially if the symptoms appear to be irritative rather than obstructive. Initial management should be medical once prostate carcinoma and renal failure are excluded and it is established that the

---

Table 23.3 Factors affecting the level of prostate-specific antigen (PSA)

Causes of increase in PSA
- Increase in age
- Acute retention of urine
- Urethral catheterization
- Transurethral resection of the prostate (TURP)
- Prostatitis
- Prostate cancer
- Large benign prostatic hyperplasia
- Prostatic biopsy

Cause of decrease in PSA
- Patient taking a 5-α reductase inhibitor (finasteride, dutasteride)

---

prostate is the principal problem. Alpha-blockers can relax the smooth muscle of the bladder neck and prostatic capsule, and are useful in small prostates; 5α-reductase inhibitors block the intraprostatic conversion of testosterone to dihydrotestosterone, resulting in shrinking of the prostate, and are useful in large glands. Prostatectomy (transurethral or open) is reserved for medical failures.

Acute retention

This condition usually requires emergency admission to hospital. If there is a history of bladder outflow obstruction, conservative measures aimed at encouraging micturition (sedation, a warm bath) only delay the inevitable requirement for catheterization. A self-retaining Foley catheter (size 16 Fr) is passed using strict asepsis and connected to a closed drainage system. If it is not possible to pass a urethral catheter, the bladder is entered directly by puncture with a trocar/cannula (suprapubic cystostomy). A specimen of urine is cultured and, if there is microbiological evidence of an infection, antibiotics are given. If the history of urinary symptoms is short, the catheter can be removed after 12 hours (*trial without catheter*), following which normal voiding may occur. This is more likely if the patient is given α-blockers (EBM 23.3). If retention recurs, then definitive treatment with TURP is performed.

EBM **23.3 Benign prostatic hyperplasia: α-blockers in patients with acute urinary retention**

'Alfuzosin 10 mg/day increases the likelihood of successful trial without catheter (TWOC) in men with a first episode of spontaneous urinary retention.'

McNeill SA, et al. Urology 2005; 65(1):83–90.

Chronic retention

It is essential to determine whether the patient has any complications of obstruction, especially renal damage. Although the upper urinary tracts may be dilated, renal function is not necessarily impaired. If the patient is well, with no haematological or biochemical disturbance, there is no indication for preliminary bladder drainage and prostatectomy may be planned in the usual way. If the patient is uraemic, his general fitness for operation must be assessed. Uraemia alone is not a contraindication to surgery, but hyperkalaemia, dehydration or other evidence of fluid and electrolyte disturbance must be corrected. The bladder is catheterized and prostatectomy is carried out as soon as the patient is fit. Relief of chronic obstruction is almost always followed by a diuresis, due partly to an osmotic (urea) diuresis and partly to renal tubular changes resulting from back pressure. Accurate intake/output fluid charts in addition to daily weights can detect these losses. The blood pressure, both lying and standing, should be monitored and intravenous fluid replacement may be necessary. Medical therapy is contraindicated in patients who present with renal failure secondary to BPH; these patients should be managed either by long-term catheter or TURP.

Open prostatectomy

Open procedures are now reserved for very large adenomas. Apart from the length of hospitalization (7–10 days) and the presence of an abdominal wound, enucleation of smaller adenomas may damage the external sphincter and cause incontinence. This is a particular problem with more fibrous glands and those that contain a focus of cancer.

23

Closed (endoscopic) prostatectomy

During transurethral resection of the prostate (TURP), the prostate is removed piecemeal by electroresection using a resectoscope. The advantages are patient acceptance, short hospitalization (2–3 days) and the precision of removal of the obstructing tissue. However, serious damage can be inflicted on the prostatic sphincter mechanism by inexpert use of the resectoscope. Prolonged resection can result in excessive absorption of irrigating fluid and electrolyte imbalance (TURP syndrome). Recent alternatives using minimally invasive techniques to TURP include transurethral radiofrequency needle ablation (TUNA), transurethral microwave thermotherapy (TUMT), and transrectal high intensity focused ultrasound (HIFU). The focused energy within the prostate causes coagulative necrosis and subsequent sloughing of prostatic tissue. However, improvement in symptoms is only modest and no long-term outcome data are available. More favourable results are seen with laser prostatectomy but again no long-term follow-up data is available. The different types of laser prostatectomy are: holmium only laser ablation of the prostate (HoLAP), holmium laser resection of the prostate (HoLRP), and holmium laser enucleation of the prostate (HoLEP).

Retrograde ejaculation is a common sequel to any operative procedure on the prostate and all patients should be advised preoperatively of this effect. Any associated bladder stone may be crushed with a lithotriptor or removed by suprapubic lithotomy. After prostatectomy, the bladder must be allowed to drain freely via a urethral catheter while the prostatic bed heals and bleeding stops. After TURP, the catheter is normally removed on the second postoperative day and after an open procedure, the fifth postoperative day. The main postoperative hazard is bleeding. In an open procedure, blood vessels at the bladder neck are sutured but bleeding within the capsule is less easy to control. With TURP, coagulation of the blood vessels is more precise but not always complete. If postoperative bleeding is excessive, clot may lead to obstruction (*clot retention*). This hazard can be minimized by continuous irrigation through a three-way urethral catheter. The results of all forms of prostatectomy continue to improve, but TURP has the lowest morbidity and mortality (< 1%) and requires a shorter hospital stay (50% less) than other procedures.

Bladder neck obstruction

Occasionally, the obstruction to the outflow tract appears to be at the bladder neck and the prostate is often quite small. The cause may be an infective condition such as prostatitis or schistosomiasis, or a neurological disorder such as diabetes or a prolapsed intervertebral disc. Endoscopic incision or excision of the bladder neck is preferable to long-term drug treatment, but surgery is relatively contraindicated if the risk of retrograde ejaculation and hence infertility is of concern to the patient.

Urethral obstruction

Pathology

Obstruction of the urethra may be congenital, or due to a stricture or malignancy (Fig. 23.20). Foreign bodies, including urinary stones, may also be responsible. The complications include infection with periurethral abscess, fistulation and stone formation. Congenital valves in the posterior urethra occur only in boys. They lie at the level of the verumontanum and may cause gross obstructive changes in the bladder and upper urinary tracts at birth. Increasingly, this diagnosis is being established during pregnancy by ultrasound examination. If the diagnosis is established after birth, it is confirmed by micturating cystourethrography. Treatment consists of endoscopic incision of the valves. Urethral diverticulum is a rare cause of obstruction. More commonly, it is secondary to obstruction and infection in women. Urethral trauma or infection may result in a stricture, the severity of which is related to both the site and the extent of the insult. A posterior urethral stricture following major trauma may be surrounded by dense fibrous tissue, whereas healthy tissues may surround a stricture of the bulb of the urethra. The former requires major reconstructive surgery but urethral dilatation or incision can readily manage the latter. Rough inexpert use of any instrument (including a catheter) in the urethra can cause stricture formation. The principal organism responsible for inflammatory scarring and stricture of the urethra is *Neisseria gonorrhoeae*. Long-term use of a self-retaining catheter, although not necessarily associated with infection, can also cause an inflammatory reaction in the urethra.

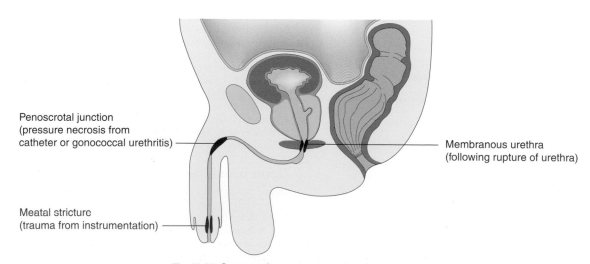

Penoscrotal junction
(pressure necrosis from
catheter or gonococcal urethritis)

Membranous urethra
(following rupture of urethra)

Meatal stricture
(trauma from instrumentation)

Fig. 23.20 Common sites and causes of urethral stricture.

Clinical features

The diagnosis should be considered if there is a history of urethral infection, instrumentation or trauma. The external meatus must always be examined and, if the foreskin is present, it should be retracted for full inspection. The urethra is palpated. It is still possible for a patient to pass urine, albeit with difficulty, in the presence of a urethral stone.

Investigations

Urinary flow rate will help differentiate urethral strictures from bladder neck and prostatic obstruction, the former giving a uniformly low and prolonged (box-like) pattern (see Fig. 23.5). Post-micturition ultrasound may exclude an increased residual volume. An ascending and descending urethrogram will adequately demonstrate the urethral anatomy. The final investigation to assess a urethral lesion is cystourethroscopy.

Management

Many simple strictures are easily treated by repeated dilatation with metal bougies, or may be incised under direct vision using an urethrotome. Most short strictures in the region of the bulb respond well, but recurrence is common (50%) and operative reconstruction (urethroplasty) may be required. Short strictures can be excised and the healthy urethra re-anastomosed. Longer strictures can be patched with full-thickness skin flaps or buccal mucosal grafts, to restore normal calibre.

DISORDERS OF MICTURITION – INCONTINENCE

Overview

Incontinence is defined as the involuntary leakage of urine. It may be due to problems in storage, resulting in urge and stress incontinence or continual incontinence with fistulae, or to problems in emptying, resulting in chronic retention with overflow incontinence. In stress incontinence, leakage occurs because passive bladder pressure exceeds normal urethral pressure. This may be because of poor pelvic floor support, because of a weak urethral sphincter or an element of both. In urge incontinence, leakage usually occurs because detrusor overactivity produces an increase in bladder pressure that overcomes the urethral sphincter. A hypersensitive bladder (sensory urgency) resulting from urinary tract infection (UTI) or bladder stone may also drive urgency in the absence of overactive bladder contractions. Incontinence in these circumstances is less common. Stress incontinence and urge incontinence may coexist (mixed incontinence). All of the above terms, with the exception of a fistula, are descriptive only and do not accurately diagnose the underlying pathophysiology, which can only be determined by urodynamic testing.

Structural disorders

Clinical assessment

Abnormalities of function of the lower urinary tract are notoriously difficult to assess because there is frequently dual underlying pathology. Incontinence in an elderly man may be due to cerebral cortical degeneration, but could also be due to chronic outflow tract obstruction resulting from prostatic hyperplasia. The history is important but may

be deceptive and the exact character of the urinary abnormality must be determined so that structural causes can be separated from neurological ones. Details of drug treatment are noted since diuretics and drugs with anticholinergic side-effects may tip the balance when there is already dysfunction. Urine is tested for glycosuria and infection. In addition to intravenous urography, there is now a range of more specific methods for assessing micturition, but not all are required for a diagnosis. They include radiology (cystourethrography), urodynamic studies (uroflowmetry, cystometrography and urethral pressure measurement) and direct inspection (cystourethroscopy and pelvic examination under anaesthesia). A full history and physical examination, with cystourethroscopy and bimanual examination, remain the basic initial investigation of structural disorders.

Structural causes of incontinence in males

Postprostatectomy

Disordered control of micturition occurs in 3–5% of patients after prostatectomy. In this operation, any inadvertent damage to the external sphincter can lead to difficulties with continence. Stress incontinence may occur, but as the damage to the sphincter is usually incomplete, it usually responds to physiotherapy. If not, insertion of an artificial urinary sphincter can be considered.

Chronic outflow obstruction

Changes within the bladder (detrusor hypertrophy) due to chronic obstruction commonly lead to secondary urgency and detrusor overactivity. Relief of obstruction alone is usually sufficient to correct the associated urgency and urge incontinence, but in about 10% of cases the instability is primary and antimuscarinics may be necessary. Chronic retention may also lead to overflow or dribbling incontinence. It must be emphasized that continence requires normal cortical control, and in an elderly patient this may be impaired. Possible abnormalities of both structure and innervation need to be considered in these patients.

Carcinoma of the prostate

Tumour may involve the external sphincter, preventing it from closing. Repeated transurethral resections for recurring obstruction may convert the posterior urethra into a rigid tube so that dribbling incontinence occurs. An indwelling catheter or condom incontinence appliance may be necessary.

Postmicturition dribble incontinence

This is very common, even in relatively young men, and is caused by a small amount of urine becoming trapped in the 'U-bend' of the bulbar urethra. This then leaks out passively when the patient moves. The condition is more pronounced if associated with a urethral diverticulum or urethral stricture.

Chronic illness and debility

Especially in the elderly, incontinence may arise from poor tone in the periurethral striated muscle of the pelvic floor and from difficulty in getting to the toilet. This may be worsened by loss of cortical inhibition of micturition.

Structural causes of incontinence in females

Incontinence is more prevalent than generally suspected; approximately 14% of all women have been incontinent at some time, half of them within the last 2 months. This figure rises rapidly in older patients, and reaches 50–70%

23

in geriatric units. Only a proportion of younger women seek advice, either because of embarrassment or because of stoical acceptance of some incontinence as being normal.

Childbirth and operations

Multiparous women commonly lose some of the tone in the pelvic floor muscles with each pregnancy. Symptoms may range from occasional stress incontinence to almost continual dribbling incontinence. Examination shows weakening of the pelvic floor muscles and anterior vaginal wall (cystocoele). It is important to distinguish stress incontinence from urge incontinence. The former responds well to pelvic floor exercises and to surgical procedures designed to support the bladder neck, but the latter should be treated by bladder retraining and drug therapy. Stress incontinence is characterized by an involuntary loss of urine during coughing, laughing, sneezing or any other activity that suddenly raises the intra-abdominal pressure. A cough, however, may stimulate involuntary detrusor contractions (cough-induced detrusor instability), which causes urge incontinence. This differential diagnosis can be made only by urodynamic assessment. In parts of the world where obstetric services are poor, prolonged labour may lead to a vesicovaginal fistula, which presents as continuous dribbling incontinence. The association with delivery is usually clear, but a small fistula may be missed. Investigation of dribbling incontinence must distinguish between urethral damage and a fistula. Treatment consists of closing the fistula through a vaginal or suprapubic approach.

Cystitis

Cystitis is common in women and, in addition to causing frequency, urgency and dysuria, sometimes causes sensory urge incontinence. Treatment of both the infection and the bladder spasm is required. Interstitial cystitis (painful bladder syndrome) is a chronic inflammatory condition that, in addition to causing frequency and dysuria, may also cause urgency and urge incontinence. Treatment is often unsatisfactory. Hydrostatic dilatation may be effective.

Ectopic ureter

Dribbling incontinence in a child should raise the suspicion of an ectopic ureter, in which the lower of the two ureters opens outside the control of the urethral mechanism. The abnormal ureter must be relocated in the bladder.

Cervical cancer

Carcinoma of the cervix or its treatment by radiotherapy may cause vesicovaginal fistula and incontinence.

Neurogenic disorders

Clinical assessment

A full history, including an interview with relatives, is required. Examination must include assessment of the plantar reflexes and the sensation and tone of the anal canal. Glycosuria and urinary infection should be excluded. Urodynamic, radiological and electromyographic studies may all be required.

Aetiology of abnormal micturition
Impaired cortical control

Diseases affecting the frontal lobe can alter the pattern of micturition by increasing or decreasing its frequency, or by affecting the social awareness of incontinence. There may also be failure to inhibit initiation of micturition. The paracentral lobule controls the activity of skeletal muscle, so that lesions in this area may cause sustained pelvic and perineal

muscular contraction. It must be remembered that a disorder of micturition may be accentuated by, or may even be due to, the physical inability to prepare for micturition such as poor mobility.

Emotional state

This may affect the postponement of micturition, giving rise to 'giggle' incontinence and possibly to enuresis in some patients. Incontinence with epilepsy is also due to a loss of inhibitory control. Excessive sensory stimuli, as with the pain of cystourethritis in women, may cause 'sensory urge incontinence'.

Drugs

Drugs, including alcohol, may alter cortical control of micturition. Sedatives can affect the postponement phase and precipitate incontinence, especially at night. The intoxicated patient may lack the mental alertness to maintain continence, or may continually suppress the desire to void, leading to prostatic congestion and retention.

Damage to the spinal cord

Two aspects of disease or injury to the spinal cord influence disordered micturition: namely, the level of the disease and the completeness of the damage.

Injury at or below the sacral outflow (S2, 3, 4) may be due to a fracture of the spine at the level of T12 and L1 which damages the conus medullaris, a central prolapsed intervertebral disc leading to cauda equina injury, or to spinal stenosis. The bladder distends without sensation, the external sphincter is weak and little detrusor contraction is seen upon urodynamic assessment. The patient develops retention with overflow, but emptying is possible with abdominal straining or hand pressure.

Injury between the sacral segment and the pontine micturition centres (upper motor neuron lesions) may be due to fractures of the spine; tumours that compress the cord; surgical removal of such a tumour; and diseases of the cord itself, such as multiple sclerosis, transverse myelitis and cervical cord stenosis. If these central connections are disrupted, the patient develops a reflex bladder with impaired or absent cortical control; that is, the bladder loses the coordination imposed by the pontine micturition centre. The detrusor becomes overactive and attempted voiding results in detrusor contraction occurring synchronously with that of the external sphincter (detrusor-sphincter dyssynergia). The net result is poor bladder emptying and the development of a thick, trabeculated bladder wall. The resultant high-pressure bladder will, over time, lead to renal impairment. Usually the central connections are not completely disrupted and there may be some sensation and some cortical inhibition.

Damage to pelvic nerves may occur in the course of surgery, especially when dissection involves the side walls of the pelvis, as in radical dissection of the rectum or the uterus. Similarly, aneurysm surgery may disrupt neural pathways in the pelvis. Diseases affecting the autonomic system, principally diabetes mellitus, also affect the control of micturition. With the loss of sensation and contraction, the bladder becomes atonic, prone to the complication of stasis infection. The external sphincter remains closed by uninhibited tonic contractions, but the internal sphincter is partly open as it, to some extent, depends on detrusor activity.

Primary failure of the detrusor has been described, but it is usually secondary to chronic overdistension. Atonic myogenic bladder is caused by prolonged outlet obstruction and is found in the late stages of bladder decompensation. The most common cause is silent prostatic obstruction, where progressive loss of the desire to void results in overflow incontinence. In women, conscious postponement can lead to a large atonic bladder.

Principles of management

More than one mechanism may account for disordered micturition and urodynamic assessment is mandatory in all patients with a suspected or proven neuropathic bladder.

Neurologically intact patients

Patients with congenital defects or fistulae should have these repaired surgically if possible. If the fistula is malignant or the surrounding tissues are poor because of radiation, urinary diversion is preferable. Stress incontinence in both males and females should be treated initially with pelvic floor exercises. If it persists in males, it is best treated by the insertion of an artificial urinary sphincter. In females, the urethra and bladder neck should be returned to their natural positions and supported by means of colposuspension or a pubovaginal sling. The injection of bulking agents at the bladder neck can improve continence, but remains under evaluation. Urge incontinence should be treated initially by bladder retraining, supplemented by anticholinergic drugs. If this fails, good results can be obtained by intravesical injection of botulinum toxin type A via flexible cystoscopy. Alternatives are insertion of a sacral nerve stimulator device, a detrusor myectomy which typically involves stripping off a substantial proportion of the detrusor muscle (myectomy) or splitting the bladder in half and suturing a strip of small bowel to augment the bladder (clam ileocystoplasty). Patients with atonic bladders are best managed by regular intermittent self-catheterization (ISC).

Neuropathic patients

These patients are prone to urinary infection and renal impairment, and preservation of renal function takes priority. The patient's overall condition is important and those that are poorly motivated or immobile with poor cognition and hand function are best managed by suprapubic catheterization or urinary diversion. Highly motivated intelligent patients should be treated in much the same way as the neurologically intact, although the results are often less good.

SUMMARY BOX 23.5

Micturition

- Micturition requires parasympathetic innervation (S2–S4) of the detrusor, sympathetic innervation (T10–L2) of the bladder neck and proximal urethra, and somatic innervation (S2–S4) of the bladder, pelvic floor and urethra
- Structural causes of disordered micturition in the male include prostatic enlargement, prostatectomy (dribble, stress and urge incontinence) and chronic illness/debility
- Structural causes of disordered micturition in the female include childbirth, surgery, radiotherapy and cystitis (infection, chronic interstitial cystitis and urethral syndrome)
- Neurogenic causes of disordered micturition are:
  - impaired cortical control
  - alcohol abuse and drugs
  - spinal cord damage (at/below T12–L1 – flaccid bladder with overflow; above T12–L1 – overactive bladder with incoordination of urinary sphincter, which results in poor bladder emptying)
  - pelvic nerve damage (surgery, diabetic autonomic neuropathy)
  - atonic myogenic bladder (prolonged outlet obstruction).

EXTERNAL GENITALIA

Anatomy

In the male, these comprise the penis, testicles and scrotum; in the female, the mons pubis, labia majora, labia minora and the clitoris (Fig. 23.21).

The penis consists of three cylinders of erectile tissue. The ventral corpus spongiosum is expanded proximally as the bulb and distally as the glans penis, and transmits the urethra. Two dorsolateral corpora cavernosa attach to each side of the inferior pubic arch as the crura. They form the body of the penis and become embedded in the glans.

The penile skin is hairless, free of fat, and extends over the glans as the prepuce or foreskin. Blood is supplied from the internal pudendal arteries. The scrotum is a thin rugose pouch of skin containing the two testicles. Each testicle is contained within a tough capsule (tunica albuginea) and has the epididymis attached to it posteriorly. This highly coiled tubular structure arises from the rete testis, where some 20 small tubules enter it. This head of epididymis is considerably larger than the lower tail, from which the vas deferens arises to traverse the spermatic cord and finally to open into the prostatic urethra as the ejaculatory duct. The testicle and epididymis are invaginated into the tunica vaginalis, which lies anteriorly, so providing a potential space where a hydrocoele may form. The testicular arteries supply the testes. Venous blood drains along the spermatic cord

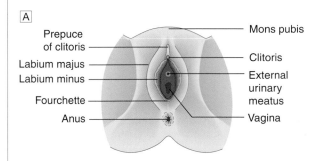

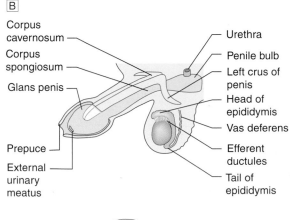

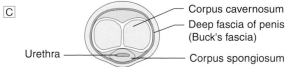

Fig. 23.21 Anatomy of the external genitalia. A Female. B Male. C Cross-section through the penis.

23

as the pampiniform plexus. The scrotum drains lymph to the inguinal lymph nodes, and the contents of the scrotum drain along the spermatic cord to nodes in the pelvis and abdomen.

In the female, the mons pubis is the fatty elevation over the pubis from which the labia run backwards, enclosing between them the vestibule into which open the vagina and urethra. The clitoris lies above the urethral opening and is a smaller replica of the penis, with the same erectile tissues.

Physiology

Parasympathetic stimulation leads to erection through the release of nitric oxide, with resultant vasodilatation of the arterioles, increased penile blood flow and passive closure of the venules. After sufficient stimulation, sperm from the epididymis and seminal fluid from the seminal vesicles are emptied into the prostatic urethra. Sympathetic stimulation is responsible for this emission, and also closes the bladder neck to prevent leakage of semen into the bladder. Ejaculation proper is due to rhythmic contraction of the bulbospongiosus muscles expelling the semen out through the urethra.

Circumcision

The foreskin is normally non-retractile for the first few months of life. By the end of the first year, half will retract, but it may be 3–4 years before all do so. Provided the parents are reassured, there is no reason, apart from religious grounds, to remove the foreskin within the first few years of life. In some children, the foreskin remains non-retractile and has to be treated by division of preputial adhesions or by circumcision. Otherwise, secretions collect under the foreskin, leading to infection (balanitis) and narrowing of the orifice (phimosis).

Severe phimosis may obstruct urinary flow and if a poorly retracting foreskin remains retracted, it can act as a tight band and cause engorgement and oedema of the glans (paraphimosis). This demands urgent treatment. It may be possible to compress the glans and draw the foreskin forwards, but if this fails, the tight band must be incised under general anaesthesia. Later, elective circumcision is advocated.

Congenital abnormalities of the penis

Hypospadias

Failure of the embryonic folds to fuse results in abnormal placing of the external urinary meatus on the ventral surface of the penis. The opening may be coronal, penile, scrotal or even perineal. The corpus spongiosum may be scarred and fibrosed, leading to a ventral curvature or chordee of the penis. The aim of treatment is to correct the chordee by excising the fibrosis, and then to construct a new urethral opening in the normal position on the glans. This procedure should be ideally completed before the boy goes to school.

Epispadias

In this condition the external urinary meatus opens on the dorsal surface of the penis. The extent of the malformation varies from an isolated penile abnormality to gross malformation of the bladder and urethra. The mucosa of the bladder and the ureteric orifices may be exposed and form the infraumbilical part of the abdominal wall (exstrophy). The urethra then lies opened out like a gutter. Other associated abnormalities include separation of the symphysis pubis and rectal prolapse. Reconstruction of these deformities is not always successful, and urinary incontinence may remain a major problem and require urinary diversion.

Disorders of erection (impotence)

Impotence may be psychogenic, organic or drug-induced. Psychogenic problems, the most common cause, can usually be established from a careful history that includes details of sexual habits. Organic impotence is associated with diabetes mellitus, neurogenic disorders, major pelvic injury or operations, vascular disease of the pelvic vessels (Leriche's syndrome), priapism and Peyronie's disease. Most of these conditions constitute irreversible impotence. Drug-induced impotence occurs with hormonal manipulation for prostatic cancer; some antihypertensive drugs may cause loss of erection or inability to ejaculate, and barbiturates, benzodiazepines, corticosteroids, phenothiazines and spironolactone may affect libido. Medical treatment is by oral sildenafil (Viagra), intracavernosal (self)-injection of papaverine, or prostaglandin E. Vacuum suction devices or a prosthesis implanted into the corpora cavernosa are effective alternatives.

Priapism

This is a painful maintained erection unassociated with sexual desire. It is associated with intracavernosal self-injection for impotence (the most common cause), leukaemia, disorders of coagulation, renal dialysis and sickle-cell trait, and is believed to be due to venous sludging in the corpora cavernosa. (The corpus spongiosum and glans are unaffected.) Aspiration and intracavernosal injections of vasoconstrictors (phenylephrine) may be effective, especially in self-injection cases. If these fail, the creation of a venous shunt within 6–12 hours gives satisfactory results, and the patient can achieve normal erections subsequently. If treatment is delayed or incomplete, the erectile tissue is damaged and the patient will be impotent.

Peyronie's disease

This is the occurrence of a hard fibrous plaque (or plaques) in the wall of a corpus cavernosum, causing curvature of the penis. The cause is obscure but is possibly related to trauma, leading to the formation of hard scar tissue. In addition to the deformity, the patient complains of pain during intercourse. Various treatments, including cortisone injections, vitamins and radiotherapy, have met with little success. Excision of the plaque and replacement by a dermal patch graft, or excision of a wedge of tissue on the convex (opposite) border of the penis, may be effective.

Carcinoma of the penis

This uncommon tumour has a prevalence of 1.5 cases per 100 000 and is generally attributed to poor hygiene associated with a non-retractile foreskin (Fig. 23.22). It is very rare in circumcised men and almost always occurs in the elderly. The cancer may be a papillary or an ulcerating squamous cell carcinoma. Local spread occurs early and the tumour may ulcerate and fungate. Lymphatic spread to inguinal lymph nodes is common; associated infection may also lead to lymphadenopathy. The patient may present with a

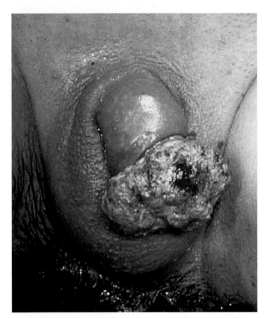

Fig. 23.22 Penile carcinoma.

purulent or blood-stained discharge. Unfortunately, many patients do not seek help until the lesion is advanced – some only when much of the penis is already destroyed and the inguinal lymph nodes are involved. The diagnosis must be confirmed by biopsy. Circumcision may cure early tumours confined to the prepuce. Early tumours confined to the glans may be treated by excision of the glans and skin grafting. Advanced tumours will require partial or total penile amputation, and often bilateral block dissection of the inguinal lymph nodes. Inoperable tumours are treated by radiotherapy.

Inflammation of the penis

Inflammation of the glans penis (balanitis) usually also involves the prepuce (posthitis) and is common in children with poorly retractile foreskins. Circumcision usually cures recurrent non-specific balanitis. Balanitis xerotica obliterans (BXO) is the local manifestation of lichen sclerosus et atrophicus of the glans and prepuce. It causes typical white scarring of the prepuce and glans, and may involve the urethral meatus and distal urethra. Meatal stenosis occurs as a result of recurrent infection, trauma or BXO. It may respond to removal of the inflammation (by circumcision) and meatal dilatation; alternatively, it may require meatotomy or meatoplasty.

Undescended testes (cryptorchidism)

Retractile testis

Normally, both testes are in the scrotum by 6 months of age. However, they may be excessively mobile and readily retract towards the external inguinal ring, even into the inguinal canal, especially when the patient is examined in a cold room. Such retractile testes may easily be misdiagnosed as being incompletely descended. Care must be taken to examine the baby in a warm room or after a bath. True undescended testes are of two types:

1. *Incomplete.* Such a testis is arrested in its normal pathway to the scrotum. Usually this is within the inguinal canal, more rarely within the abdomen.

2. *Ectopic.* An ectopic testis has developed normally, but after passing through the external inguinal ring its further descent is impeded. It either remains in the superficial inguinal pouch (common) or is transposed to perineal, femoral or prepubic sites (rare).

Torsion of the testis

Torsion of the cord can occur where the visceral layer of the tunica vaginalis completely covers the testis so that it lies suspended within the parietal layer. The patient, usually a teenager, presents with sudden onset of testicular pain and swelling. There may be a history of minor trauma, or previous episodes of pain due to partial torsion. On examination there is a red, swollen hemiscrotum that is usually too tender to palpate. Misdiagnosis of the swelling as epididymo-orchitis, which is rare in teenagers, is a serious error. Torsion of the testis is a surgical emergency; if the blood supply is not restored within 12 hours, the testis infarcts and must then be excised. If at operation the testis is found to be viable, it is sutured to the parietal tunica to prevent recurrence. As the underlying abnormality of the tunica is bilateral, the other testis must be fixed at the same time.

Testicular tumours

Pathology

Tumours of the testes are uncommon, with a prevalence of 5 cases per 100 000. They most commonly affect men between 20 and 40 years of age. Seminoma and teratoma account for 85%; malignant lymphoma, yolk-sac tumours, interstitial cell tumours and Sertoli cell/mesenchyme tumours make up the remainder. Seminomas arise from seminiferous tubules and are of relatively low-grade malignancy. Metastases occur mainly via the lymphatics and may involve the lungs. Teratoma (non-seminomatous tumour) arises from primitive germinal cells. It may contain cartilage, bone, muscle, fat and a variety of other tissues, and is classified according to the degree of differentiation. Well-differentiated tumours are the least aggressive; at the other extreme, trophoblastic teratoma is highly malignant. Occasionally, teratoma and seminoma occur in the same testis. A history of undescended testis increases the risk of malignancy in the ipsilateral testis. Orchidopexy does not reduce this risk but it does allow the testis to be moved into a position where it allows regular self examination.

Clinical features

The most common presentation is the incidental discovery of a painless testicular lump. The history is often vague, however, and symptoms may be attributed to an injury, or there may be pain and swelling suggesting inflammation. The patient may have wrongly received treatment for 'acute epididymitis'. Very rarely, patients with teratoma may complain of gynaecomastia. Irrespective of the history, any new painless testicular lump in a young man must be regarded with suspicion. A hydrocoele in a young man also demands investigation, as testicular tumours may be accompanied by blood-stained effusion in the tunica vaginalis.

Investigations

All suspicious scrotal lumps should be imaged by ultrasound, which provides a high degree of accuracy. As soon as a tumour is suspected, and before orchiectomy, serum levels of AFP, β-HCG and LDH should be determined. The levels of these 'tumour markers' are increased in extensive

Table 23.4	Royal Marsden classification for testicular cancer
• Stage 1	Tumour confined to testis
• Stage 2	Tumour spread only to lymph nodes below diaphragm
• Stage 3	Tumour spread only to lymph nodes above and below diaphragm
• Stage 4	Tumour spread to inguinal lymph nodes or distant metastases

disease. Accurate staging is based on CT of the lungs, liver and retroperitoneal area, and an assessment of renal and pulmonary function (Table 23.4).

Management

Through an inguinal incision the spermatic cord is divided at the internal ring; only then is the testis removed. Radiotherapy is the treatment of choice for early-stage seminoma, as this tumour is very radiosensitive. The management of a teratoma depends on the stage of the disease. Early disease confined to the testes may be managed without further treatment, provided that there is close surveillance for at least 2 years; tumour progression is treated by chemotherapy. More advanced cancers are managed initially by chemotherapy, usually with a combination of bleomycin, etoposide and cisplatin. Retroperitoneal lymph node dissection is now only performed for residual or recurrent nodal masses. AFP, β-HCG and LDH each offer a valuable means of monitoring response to treatment and detecting recurrent disease. These markers should be monitored in all patients with testicular tumours for at least 2 years after they are considered to be tumour-free. CT is used to follow the response of enlarged lymph nodes to treatment.

Prognosis

The 5-year survival rate for patients with seminoma is 90–95%. The more variable prognosis of teratomas depends on tumour type, stage and volume. With more favourable tumours the 5-year survival rate may be as high as 95%, but in more advanced cases 60–70% is more usual.

SUMMARY BOX 23.6

Testicular tumours

- In the UK, there are about 1000 new cases of testicular tumour per year and the 20–40-year age group is predominantly affected
- Seminomas and teratomas account for 85% of all testicular tumours
- Seminomas arise from the seminiferous tubules, are of relatively low-grade malignancy, spread mainly via the lymphatic system and are very sensitive to radiotherapy
- Teratomas arise from germinal cells, their differentiation reflects their aggressiveness (well-differentiated tumours being the least aggressive) and they are not radiosensitive
- Treatment consists of radical orchiectomy (with division of the spermatic cord at the level of the deep inguinal ring). Radiotherapy is used if the tumour proves to be a seminoma, whereas chemotherapy (bleomycin, etoposide and cisplatin) is used for teratomas that are advanced or recurrent
- Seminomas have a 5-year survival rate of 90–95%, whereas teratomas have a more varied prognosis (60–95% 5-year survival rate).

Epididymo-orchitis

Acute epididymo-orchitis is usually the appropriate term, as both testis and epididymides are involved in the acute inflammatory reaction. The spermatic cord is also often thickened (funiculitis). After infection has subsided, the epididymis alone may remain thickened and irregular, so that chronic epididymitis may be diagnosed. Thus a late effect of tuberculosis is an irregularly hard (craggy) epididymis. Apparent involvement of the testis alone may be a feature of viral infections such as mumps orchitis. The usual cause of epididymo-orchitis is bacterial spread, either from infected urine or from gonococcal urethritis. The affected side of the scrotum is swollen, inflamed and very tender. In all cases, the urine or urethral discharge must be cultured. Sometimes there is no evidence of a bacterial cause and a viral aetiology is then likely. Treatment consists of antibiotics, analgesia, bed rest and a scrotal support. The choice of antibiotic depends on the results of culture and sensitivity determination of the organism responsible. If there is any doubt about the diagnosis, the testis should be explored. Abscess formation is now rare, but if signs of localization or fluctuation develops, the pus should be drained. Infertility is an important late complication of epididymo-orchitis.

Hydrocoele

This is a common condition, especially in older men, in which fluid collects in the tunica vaginalis, resulting in an enlarged but painless scrotum. The inconvenience of its size usually leads the patient to seek advice. The cause of most hydrocoeles is unknown (idiopathic). The fluid is straw-coloured and protein-rich. In some patients, a hydrocoele develops as a reaction to epididymo-orchitis. Rarely, it may develop with a malignant testis (secondary hydrocoele) and the fluid may then be blood-stained. On examination of the scrotum, a normal spermatic cord can be palpated above a smooth oval swelling. Typically, an idiopathic hydrocoele transilluminates (Fig. 23.23), but where it is long-standing this may be difficult to elicit, owing to fibrosis and thickening of its wall. It is important always to seek this physical sign and also to examine the neck of the scrotum carefully to exclude an inguinal hernia as the cause of the swelling. It may be possible to palpate the testis and confirm that it is normal, but this is unusual as it lies behind and is enveloped

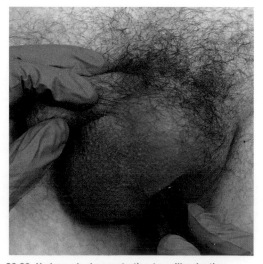

Fig. 23.23 Hydrocoele demonstrating transillumination.

by the hydrocoele. If there is any doubt about the diagnosis, then an ultrasound should be performed. Injury to the scrotum may result in a swelling that resembles a hydrocoele but does not transilluminate because the tunica has filled with blood (haematocoele). Aspiration alone does not cure an idiopathic hydrocoele and the tunica soon refills. It is possible to obliterate the sac by injecting a sclerosant after aspiration, but surgical excision and eversion is associated with a much lower recurrence rate. If the hydrocoele fluid becomes infected, incision and drainage of the pus is necessary. Similarly, a haematocoele may require treatment by incision and drainage.

Hydrocoele is a common abnormality in children. It is due to failure of closure of the processus vaginalis after descent of the testis. This patent processus vaginalis (PPV) allows fluid to drain into the scrotum around the testis. Most congenital hydrocoeles of this sort resolve before the first birthday. Those that persist require surgical treatment comprising ligation of the PPV through a small groin incision.

Cyst of the epididymis

Cysts in the epididymis arise from diverticula of the vasa efferentia. The distinction between a cyst of the epididymis and a hydrocoele is easy. Epididymal cysts are almost always multiple and, therefore, nodular on palpation; they are located above and behind the testis, which is palpably separate from the cysts, and always transilluminate brightly. A solitary epididymal cyst may even resemble a testis, so giving rise to fables of three testes and the term 'pawnbroker's sign'. Sometimes the fluid within an epididymal cyst is opalescent and contains sperm (spermatocoele). Usually the fluid is clear. It is best to leave these cysts alone unless increasing size warrants excision. Careful dissection is needed to remove the cyst completely. Often several other little cysts are present which, if not removed, will eventually increase in size and produce a so-called recurrence. If all the cysts are removed, the pathway for sperm will almost certainly be damaged. Bilateral operations can result in sterility.

Varicocoele

The veins of the pampiniform plexus are dilated and tortuous, producing a swelling in the line of the spermatic cord that resembles a 'bag of worms'. It is more common on the

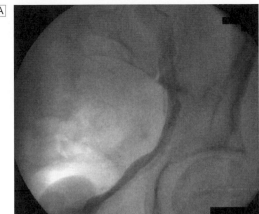

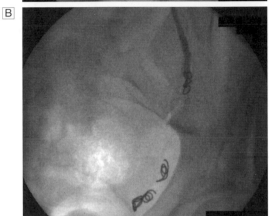

Fig. 23.24 Varicocoele. A Before treatment. B After radiological coil embolization.

left side, possibly because the right-angled drainage of the left testicular vein into the renal vein renders it more liable to stasis. In some men, varicocoele is associated with infertility. A dragging sensation in the scrotum may cause concern. Treatment is by ligation of the spermatic vein, which may be done surgically (laparoscopically) at the internal inguinal ring. Alternatively, the feeding veins can be obliterated radiologically by means of coil embolization (Fig. 23.24).

I.R. Whittle
L. Myles

Neurosurgery

CHAPTER CONTENTS

INTRODUCTION

Over the last 50 years, neurosurgery has witnessed major advances in imaging, anaesthesia, instrumentation, pharmacology, microsurgery and, most recently, computer-assisted surgery. In particular, the application of computed neuroimaging with frameless image-guided surgery has facilitated many operations. These advances have considerably reduced mortality and morbidity for many conditions.

SURGICAL ANATOMY AND PHYSIOLOGY

The skull

The skull is made up of the skull base and the calvarial skeleton, which comprises the frontal bone, the paired parietal and temporal bones and the occipital bone. The frontal and parietal bones are joined by the coronal suture, the parietal bones by the sagittal (midline) suture, and the parietal and occipital bones by the squamosal sutures. These sutures close at about 18 months, and thereafter the brain is enclosed in a rigid container. The skull base comprises the orbital roof, cribriform plates and sphenoid bones (anterior cranial fossa); sphenoid wings and petrous temporal bone (middle cranial fossa); and the squamous occipital bones, the clivus and petrous temporal regions (posterior cranial fossa). The cranial cavity is subdivided by thick folds of dura. The falx separates the two cerebral hemispheres and the tentorium separates the middle from the posterior cranial fossa. At the base of the posterior cranial fossa is the foramen magnum, through which the medulla projects inferiorly towards the spinal cord.

The spine

The bony axial spinal skeleton comprises 7 cervical, 12 thoracic and 5 lumbar vertebrae, as well as the sacrum and coccyx. Although vertebral structure varies between regions, the vertebrae are basically comprised of a body, pedicles, lamina and a posterior spine. The bony spinal canal is formed by the body (anteriorly), the pedicles (laterally) and the lamina (posteriorly). The canal contains the spinal dura, the spinal cord and, inferiorly, the cauda equina. The vertebral bodies are joined by fibroelastic discs and articulate via facet joints.

The brain

The brain is a gelatinous structure that, in adults, weighs about 1.4 kg. It comprises the paired cerebral hemispheres, the brain stem and the cerebellum. Primary fissures divide the brain into lobes (frontal, parietal, occipital, temporal and limbic). The temporal lobe is separated from the frontal and parietal lobes by the sylvian fissure, and the rolandic (central) sulcus separates the frontal from the parietal lobes. Commissural fibres, the largest of which is the corpus callosum, connect the cerebral hemispheres. Cortical grey matter lies on the surface of the brain and comprises laminae of neurons that project into the white matter (tracts). Important deep cortical nuclear regions include the basal ganglia, thalamus and hypothalamus. The brain stem comprises the midbrain, pons and medulla. The cerebellum attaches to the back of the pons and is responsible for movement, coordination, balance and posture.

The meninges and cerebrospinal fluid

The brain and spinal cord are encased by the meninges. The outer layer is like leather and is called the dura. The two inner layers are much finer: a spider's web-like tissue, the arachnoid, and a very thin layer over the surface of the brain called the pia, which bound the cerebrospinal fluid (CSF) space. The CSF is secreted from the choroid plexus and extracellular fluid from the brain that passes across the ependyma. The paired lateral ventricles, which are lined by ependyma, are the large CSF-containing spaces within the hemispheres. They communicate via the foramen of Munro with the third ventricle, which in turn communicates via the aqueduct with the fourth ventricle in the pons and medulla. Outflow foramina (Luschka and Magendie) connect with the basal and spinal subarachnoid spaces. There are several large CSF cisterns around the base of the brain (e.g. cisterna magna, cerebellopontine cistern). CSF flows over the hemisphere to be reabsorbed in the arachnoid granulations.

The cranial nerves

The 12 paired cranial nuclei arise from the base of the brain. The olfactory nerve (cranial nerve – CN I) transmits the sense of smell via the olfactory bulbs and tracts to the rhinencephalon ('old smell brain') in the temporal lobes. Vision is conveyed from the retina by the optic nerves (CN II) that connect through the optic tracts to the lateral geniculate body of the thalamus. The oculomotor (CN III) and trochlear (CN IV) nerves project from the midbrain and control ocular motility. The trigeminal nerve (CN V) provides sensation to the face, as well as innervating the muscles of mastication. The abducens nerve (CN VI) controls abduction of the eye. The facial nerve (CN VII) arises from the pontomedullary junction and controls the facial musculature, conveys taste from the anterior two-thirds of the tongue, and is secretomotor to the lacrimal and submandibular glands. The vestibulo-cochlear nerve (CN VIII) conveys hearing from the cochlea and balance from the labyrinth. Nerves IX (glossopharyngeal), X (vagus), XI (accessory) and XII (hypoglossal) project from the medulla to innervate the tongue, pharynx, larynx, bronchus and intestines.

The spinal cord

The spinal cord consists of central grey (neurons) and white (tracts) matter, and gives off 8 cervical, 12 thoracic, 5 lumbar and 4 sacral paired spinal roots. Each root comprises a ventral and a dorsal rootlet. The spinal cord is enlarged in the lower cervical region and at the thoracolumbar (conus), and terminates at about L1–L2 level. It continues as the cauda equina in the lower spinal canal to innervate the lower limbs, bladder and genitalia.

BLOOD SUPPLY

The brain requires a large blood flow (800 ml/min, 16% of cardiac output) to satisfy its oxygen and glucose requirements. The cortex receives about 50 ml/100 g/min, and white matter about 20 ml/100 g/min. Cerebral blood flow (CBF) is largely pressure-autoregulated (i.e. for mean arterial pressures between 60–140 mmHg, CBF remains constant), but is directly related to P_aCO_2. Other compounds, such as nitric oxide and endothelin, also

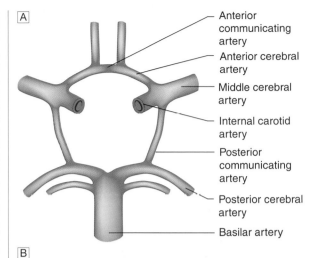

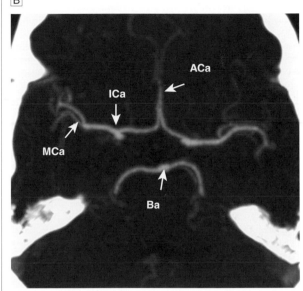

Fig. 24.1 Circle of Willis. Ⓐ Diagram outlining the major arteries. Ⓑ View on a CT angiogram. The basilar artery (Ba) bifurcation, carotid bifurcation (ICa), anterior cerebral arteries (ACa) and middle cerebral arteries (MCa) can all be clearly seen.

regulate local CBF. The anterior and posterior circulations of the brain communicate with each other and across the midline through the circle of Willis (Fig. 24.1). In some circumstances, occlusion of a major artery can be compensated for by collateral flow.

Anterior circulation

The major vessels supplying the anterior circulation of the brain are the paired internal carotid arteries. These arise from the common carotid artery, pass through the skull base and cavernous sinus, and divide into the anterior and middle cerebral arteries. Smaller but important branches include the posterior communicating artery, which interconnects the anterior and posterior circulations, the anterior choroidal arteries, and fine perforating vessels to the inferior part of the brain. The anterior cerebral arteries supply large parts of the frontal and medial parts of the parietal lobes. The middle cerebral artery supplies the posterior frontal region and most of the temporal and parietal regions.

24

Posterior circulation

The posterior cerebral circulation arises from paired vertebral arteries that pass through the cervical foramina, enter the skull and join to form a single midline basilar artery. This divides terminally into the paired posterior cerebral arteries. The posterior cerebral arteries communicate with the anterior circulation through the posterior communicating arteries. The posterior circulation supplies the brain stem, cerebellum, occipital lobes and inferior parts of the temporal lobes. Because many of these are 'end-arteries', occlusion often leads to a well-defined stroke syndrome.

INTRACRANIAL PRESSURE

The brain is enclosed within a rigid bony container. Intracranial pressure (ICP) therefore depends on the relative volumes of intracranial blood, CSF and brain parenchyma. ICP also fluctuates in response to changes in intrathoracic pressure (e.g. increased by coughing, defaecation) and cardiac pulsation. These transient increases do no harm. In a normal supine adult, ICP is the same as the CSF pressure obtained at lumbar puncture (5–15 cm H_2O, 4–10 mmHg). In patients with intracranial mass lesions (tumour, haemorrhage), oedema or CSF obstruction, the extra volume is at first compensated for by a reduction in cerebral blood volume and CSF volume. However, a critical point is soon reached where no further compensation is possible, and any additional volume insult will lead to exponential rises in ICP (Fig. 24.2).

Generalized or localized increases in ICP may lead to marked displacement of intracranial structures (brain herniation syndromes) and can compromise brain perfusion. The cerebral perfusion pressure (CPP) equals mean arterial pressure (MAP) less the ICP (CPP = MAP – ICP). Progressive rises in ICP lead to increases in MAP and reflex bradycardia. However, if there is a severe and sustained elevation of ICP, autoregulation will be ineffective and cerebral perfusion may be focally or generally compromised, leading to cerebral ischaemia and infarction. A CPP of > 60 mmHg is generally required to sustain adequate cerebral perfusion. Although children and young adults can tolerate lower levels, the consequences of a profound, prolonged lowering of CPP are

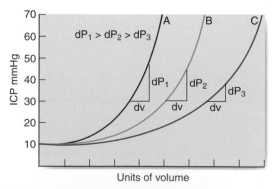

Fig. 24.2 Diagrammatic representation of the effects of a mass lesion on intracranial pressure (ICP). Generally, ICP increases exponentially with the mass lesion. However, the shape of the pressure-volume curves varies depending on the brain. Thus curve A would represent a mass lesion in a young healthy brain (limited compensation), curve B the brain of a middle-aged patient, and curve C a patient with brain atrophy who is thus able to compensate for a large intracranial mass lesion before ICP rises.

often devastating (e.g. following severe head injury with raised ICP, or after cardiac arrest). The rate of increase in the volume of intracranial mass is crucial to the shape of the ICP pressure–volume curve (Fig. 24.2). With more chronic, slow-growing lesions such as brain tumours, abscesses or congenital abnormalities, extraordinary degrees of compensation can occur. In some situations, even massive lesions can lead to minimal symptoms and signs, despite brain herniation.

Brain herniation syndromes

Subfalcine (cingulate gyral) herniation

With a parasagittal mass, the ipsilateral cingulate gyrus may herniate beneath the free edge of the falx (Fig. 24.3A). The anterior cerebral artery may be compressed sufficiently to cause medial hemispheric infarction, but otherwise there are no obvious clinical signs except deteriorating conscious level.

Transtentorial (uncal) herniation

With large ipsilateral brain lesions, the medial part of the temporal lobe is pushed down through the tentorial notch to become wedged between the tentorial edge and the midbrain (Fig. 24.3B). The opposite cerebral peduncle is pushed against the sharp tentorial edge, and the midbrain and uncus become wedged at the tentorium. The aqueduct is compressed, obstructing CSF flow, and venous obstruction leads to midbrain haemorrhage. The clinical features of an uncal herniation, most often due to a traumatic intracranial haematoma, are:

- The Glasgow Coma Score (GCS) falls (Table 24.1)
- The motor component of the GCS becomes asymmetrical
- The ipsilateral pupil dilates and becomes non-reactive to light
- The blood pressure rises
- The pulse slows
- The respiratory rate falls and the patient become apnoeic.

Foraminal (tonsillar) herniation

With mass lesions of the posterior cranial fossa, the cerebellar tonsils and medulla are displaced downwards through the foramen magnum (Fig. 24.3A and C). Cerebellar impaction leads to medullary compression. Following traumatic or spontaneous haematomas, this can lead to a dramatic decrease in the GCS, acute hypertension, bilateral extensor responses and bilateral fixed dilated pupils, followed by sudden respiratory arrest. A similar syndrome may occur following the removal of CSF at lumbar puncture in patients with raised ICP due to a posterior fossa tumour, and is also known as 'coning'. There is a rapid deterioration in conscious level, with decerebration. Lumbar puncture must not be performed in patients suspected of having raised ICP due to a mass lesion.

INVESTIGATIONS

Plain X-ray

Plain X-rays of the skull and spine may reveal evidence of metastatic tumour spread, narrowing of the intervertebral discs, congenital abnormalities, bony erosion due to tumour (e.g. of the pituitary fossa) or abnormal vascular markings. Calcification of the pineal gland or choroid plexus may allow displacement to be detected, and abnormal calcification can develop in certain cysts and tumours. This investigation has, however, largely been superseded by computed tomography and magnetic resonance imaging.

Computed tomography (CT)

Although CT does not image brain tissue as well as magnetic resonance imaging, it is particularly good for visualizing bony tissue and has the advantage that images can be acquired more simply and rapidly. It is the investigation of choice following trauma and for imaging spontaneous intracerebral haematomas. Modern spiral CT scanners allow the craniofacial skeleton and blood vessels (CT-angiography, or CT-A) to be reconstructed in remarkable detail.

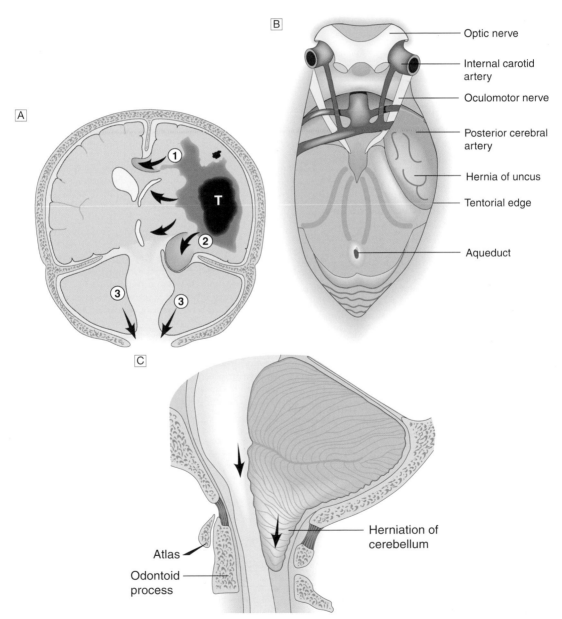

Fig. 24.3 Herniation syndromes. **A** Coronal diagram of the dynamics of an intracranial mass lesion. Tumour (T) causes mass effect that compresses the midline and the ventricles (unnumbered arrows), provoking subfalcine or cingulated herniation (arrow 1), and transtentorial herniation (arrow 2). If the mass effect is uncontrolled, tonsillar herniation may also occur (arrows 3). **B** Transtentorial herniation in the axial plane (plane of dotted line in Fig. 24.3A). **C** Foraminal herniation.

Table 24.1 Glasgow Coma Scale

Eyes open	
• Spontaneously	4
• To verbal command	3
• To pain	2
• No response	1
Best motor response	
To verbal command	
• Obeys verbal command	6
To painful stimulus	
• Localizes pain	5
• Flexion withdrawal	4
• Abnormal flexion (decorticate rigidity)	3
• Extension (decerebrate rigidity)	2
• No responses	1
Best verbal response	
• Orientated and converses	5
• Disorientated and converses	4
• Inappropriate words	3
• Incomprehensible sounds	2
• No response	1
Total number of points (minimum 3, maximum 15)	

Magnetic resonance imaging (MRI)

Magnetic resonance images can be reconstructed in axial, coronal or sagittal planes. As the water in bony tissue is tightly bound, the cranium is not as well visualized as it is with CT. However, as the cortical grey matter comprises approximately 78% water and white matter approximately 68% water, these two areas, as well as subnuclei within the brain, can be clearly distinguished. CSF is also well imaged. By using different magnetic pulse sequencing techniques, the anatomy of the normal and abnormal brain can be imaged in millimetre detail. With both CT and MRI, an intravenous enhancing agent can be administered (iodine-based compounds with CT and gadolinium-based for MRI). Both of these compounds are normally excluded from the brain parenchyma by the blood–brain barrier (BBB). However, with either neoplastic, inflammatory or ischaemic breakdown of BBB integrity or the development of tumour neovascularity, enhancement will be seen in areas involved with the pathological process. MRI is limited by certain conditions (cardiac pacemakers, early pregnancy, some metallic aneurysm clips).

CT and MR angiography

By employing certain contrast agents and rapid sequence imaging, both MRI and CT can be used to perform angiography (MRA, CT-A). In some circumstances, these non-invasive techniques are replacing conventional intra-arterial digital subtraction angiography (IA-DSA). More complex imaging sequences can be used to show white matter disorders, subtle changes in brain water (diffusion tensor imaging) and chemical signals from the brain (magnetic resonance spectroscopy). The function of brain tissues can also be evaluated, since active areas of the brain will have increased blood flow (functional MRI).

CEREBROVASCULAR DISEASE

Stroke is a common major clinical disorder in clinical neuroscience practice. Occlusive disease often affects the extracranial vessels and is a common cause of stroke and transient ischaemic attack, usually managed by vascular surgeons (Ch. 25). Most forms of embolic and ischaemic stroke are dealt with by medical neurologists, whereas many large primary intracerebral haemorrhages and, more importantly, subarachnoid haemorrhage (SAH) are dealt with by the neurosurgeon. Brain tissue metabolism is vitally dependent on a consistent delivery of oxygen and glucose substrates for energy. If there is cessation of substrate delivery, the brain tissue will either die (if CBF is below a threshold of 12–15 ml/100 g/min) or stop functioning (if CBF is between 15 and 25 ml/100 g/min). These ischaemic thresholds are very important in terms of the extent of stroke (i.e. the amount of tissue that will die) and the penumbra (i.e. tissue that is damaged but still able to recover from these acute events). Urgent thrombolysis in ischaemic stroke is possible if the patient reaches hospital within 4 hours of onset of symptoms and can improve prognosis. Decompressive craniectomy can also save life in selected cases if raised intracranial pressure due to ischaemic brain swelling is a problem.

Subarachnoid haemorrhage

Spontaneous SAH affects 100 persons per million per year and most frequently (70%) results from the rupture of an intracranial 'berry' aneurysm. Other causes include arteriovenous malformation (AVM), cavernoma, tumour, infection and trauma. Typically, the patient complains of a sudden onset of severe headache that peaks in intensity within 1 minute. Patients often describe it as like being 'hit on the head with a hammer' or as 'the worst headache they have ever had'. There is usually associated neck stiffness and photophobia. A positive Kernig's sign denotes meningism. In some cases, a small 'herald' bleed may go unnoticed, or is only remembered when a major bleed occurs. Nausea and vomiting are common. The patient's conscious level is variably affected, ranging from mild disorientation to coma to rapid death.

Grading of SAH depends on the coma score of the patient at time of presentation. The most widely used system, and also the easiest to use, is the World Federation of Neurosurgical Societies' (WFNS) grading, which goes from grade 1 to grade 5 (Table 24.2). When the SAH has produced a syndrome of grade 2–5, it is quite apparent that some neurological catastrophe has occurred. However, when the syndrome is of a grade 1 haemorrhage, differential diagnosis is quite extensive and not infrequently the primary event is overlooked. SAH can mimic atypical migraines, thunderclap headache, coital cephalgia, pituitary apoplexy and meningitic-like syndromes. Sudden death is not uncommon

Table 24.2 World Federation of Neurosurgical Societies (WFNS) grading system for subarachnoid haemorrhage

WFNS grade	Glasgow Coma Score	Focal neurological deficits
1	15	No
2	13–14	No
3	13–14	Yes
4	9–12	–
5	3–8	–

when an aneurysm ruptures into the brain substance rather than the subarachnoid space. The focal signs depend upon the vessel affected. When symptoms and signs are mild, the differential diagnosis is quite extensive and diagnosis depends on having a high index of suspicion.

Saccular intracranial aneurysms

Risk factors include smoking, hypertension, polycystic disease of the kidney and female gender. The median age of affected patients is 47 years, although familial aneurysms may rupture earlier. Most aneurysms (85%) affect the anterior circulation and 15% of patients have more than one. The majority have no symptoms until rupture occurs, although a few may suffer compressive symptoms, and ectatic aneurysms may not rupture at all but cause symptoms by embolic phenomena. The most common compressive clinical signs are features of oculomotor nerve (CN III) palsy due to an aneurysm of the posterior communicating artery. Many intracranial aneurysms are now discovered as incidental findings when the brain is imaged.

Investigations

The standard investigation is CT, which characteristically shows blood in the CSF basal cisterns in the acute phase (Fig. 24.4). As CSF blood is broken down, the CT detection rate falls after the first 72 hours. If the diagnosis is in doubt, then a lumbar puncture should be performed, but only in patients whose clinical condition is good and in whom CT has excluded an intracranial mass lesion or midline shift. If this is performed early, the CSF will be uniformly blood-stained; later it will contain haem pigments that will be apparent on naked-eye inspection (xanthochromia) or can be detected by spectrophotometry.

Next, a search must be made for the site of the bleeding. About 80% of aneurysms involve the anterior circulation. Conventionally, carotid or vertebral angiography has been performed (Fig. 24.5). However, CT and MR angiography are equally good at revealing aneurysms greater than 5 mm, and are non-invasive and so associated with less morbidity. As the consequences of missing a diagnosis of SAH are serious, there is a tendency to perform angiography in

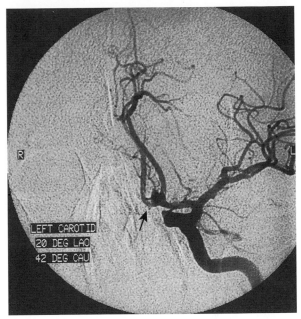

Fig. 24.5 Intra-arterial digital subtraction angiogram outlining the cerebral vasculature and showing an aneurysm of the anterior communicating artery (arrow).

patients in whom the diagnosis is equivocal. For that reason, a source of bleeding will be identified in only 70% of angiograms. This is usually an aneurysm, less commonly an AVM or a cavernoma. In 30% of cases, no source is found. In the majority, this is a 'true' negative, and many of these patients will have a condition called perimesencephalic SAH, which is of unknown aetiology.

Management of aneurysmal SAH

The medical management of SAH includes intravenous fluids; the calcium antagonist, nimodipine (EBM 24.1); analgesia; and antiemetics. Patients in coma will usually be intubated and managed in a neurointensive care unit. Having initially been quite well, many patients begin to exhibit signs of focal or global cerebral ischaemia 4–10 days following an SAH. This has been attributed primarily to vasospasm and can be ameliorated by the prophylactic use of nimodipine; however, clinical deterioration may occur due to hydrocephalus, seizures, metabolic abnormalities and systemic infections.

> **EBM** **24.1 Nimodipine and subarachnoid haemorrhage (SAH)**
>
> 'Nimodipine, a calcium channel antagonist, significantly reduces both death and stroke following SAH.'
>
> Pickard JD, et al. BMJ 1989; 298:636–642.

Rebleeding is a major cause of morbidity and mortality following aneurysm rupture. Until recently, standard management was occlusion of the aneurysm from the cerebral circulation by surgically clipping its neck (Fig. 24.6 and EBM 24.2). However, it is now possible to place detachable coils within the aneurysm via a catheter passed from the femoral artery into the cerebral circulation (Fig. 24.7). The coils unwind in the aneurysm and induce thrombosis. Coiling is a much less invasive procedure than open surgery and a recent prospective randomized controlled trial showed that, when an aneurysm can be treated by surgery or coiling, the latter is safer (EBM 24.3). Previously, only a proportion of aneurysms were suitable for coiling.

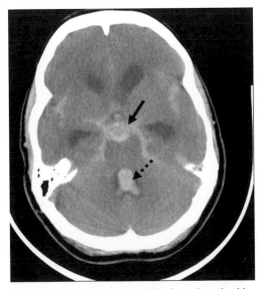

Fig. 24.4 Axial CT scan of a patient following subarachnoid haemorrhage. Blood is seen in the basal cisterns as a white lesion (solid arrow), and also in the fourth ventricle (broken arrow). There is early enlargement of all ventricles. Courtesy of Dr R Gibson.

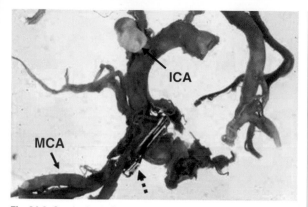

Fig. 24.6 Cerebral arteries at postmortem showing a surgical clip (broken arrow) on a ruptured middle cerebral artery aneurysm (MCA). There is also a non-ruptured carotid bifurcation aneurysm (arrow). (ICA = internal carotid artery)

EBM	24.2 Aneurysm clipping after subarachnoid haemorrhage (SAH)

'The timing of aneurysm clipping after SAH made little difference to outcome.'

Kassell NF, et al. J Neurosurg 1990; 73:37–47.

EBM	24.3 Coiling for ruptured intracranial aneurysms

'Coiling ruptured intracranial aneurysms is superior to clipping (the ISAT trial).'

Molyneux AJ, et al. Lancet 2005; 366:809–817.

However, improvements in coil, stent and basket technology mean most aneurysms can now be coiled.

Even when an aneurysm has been successfully excluded by means of coiling or surgery, the patient can still suffer stroke. Although nimodipine has significantly decreased the risk of stroke (to 23%) and death (to 22%), there is still no effective treatment for delayed cerebral ischaemia following SAH. Clinical practice has included induced hypertension and plasma volume loading (to keep up CPP), as well as haemodilution (to reduce blood viscosity in the hope of increasing flow), but this triple therapy has its own problems, such as heart failure. The outcome following aneurysmal SAH is heavily dependent upon the condition of the patient on admission and the CSF blood load (the more blood, the worse the outcome). Patients admitted in good condition (grade 1) enjoy a complete recovery in about 90% of cases. By contrast, about 50% of those admitted in coma (grade 5) die or are severely disabled. The outcome of intermediate patients is unpredictable and not necessarily dependent on the clinical excellence of either the attending surgeon or interventional neuroradiologists. Hypotension and fever are also associated with poorer outcome.

Primary intracerebral haemorrhage (ICH)

Primary ICH is becoming an increasing problem as the population of many developed countries ages. It is four times more common than SAH and, in about 30% of cases, is associated with amyloid angiopathy. Most cases are caused by hypertensive rupture of small arterioles in the basal ganglia or cerebellum which have been damaged by chronic hypertension. Many haemorrhages are small and deep; others may be very large and cause death by raising ICP and provoking uncal or tonsillar herniation syndromes. Other causes of primary ICH include the rupture of a saccular aneurysm or AVM. The onset is usually abrupt, with many patients developing a flaccid hemiparesis or brain stem-cerebellar syndrome. One-third of patients die within a few weeks and many of those who survive are permanently disabled. Emergency removal of the haematoma was not uncommon neurosurgical practice in an effort to save life. However, the results of a recent prospective multicentre international randomized controlled trial of surgery for ICH (STICH) have shown that there are no significant differences in outcome with either medical or surgical management of spontaneous, non-aneurysmal, supratentorial ICH (EBM 24.4).

EBM	24.4 Surgical evacuation of intracerebral haemorrhage

'Surgical evacuation of intracerebral haemorrhage is not superior to medical management (the STICH trial).'

Mendelow AD, et al. Lancet 2005; 365:387–397.

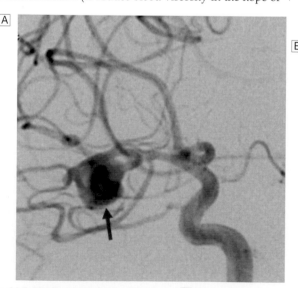

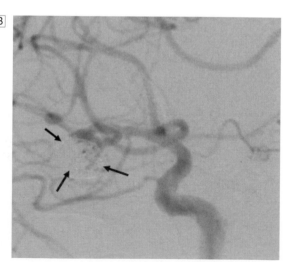

Fig. 24.7 Middle cerebral artery aneurysm. A Digital subtraction angiogram showing the aneurysm (arrow). B Its occlusion from the cerebral circulation after coiling (arrows).

Arteriovenous malformations

Cerebral AVMs are congenital abnormalities of the capillary system that lead to a direct arteriovenous communication (fistula). This leads to gross dilatation of the draining cerebral veins, as well as ectasia and occasionally aneurysmal dilatation of the feeding artery. AVMs can lead to cerebral ischaemia (because blood preferentially enters the venous system, bypassing the tissues), focal seizures and haemorrhage. Rupture of an AVM typically causes a spontaneous intracerebral haemorrhage rather than an SAH. As the haematoma is under less pressure, the overall prognosis is better than for aneurysmal SAH. The diagnosis is confirmed on CT or MRI and angiography (Fig. 24.8). If the AVM can be excised, then the risk of further haemorrhage is removed, and the incidence and frequency of seizures is considerably reduced. Sometimes, however, the AVM is large and in an important or inaccessible location. In these cases, endovascular 'glueing' or stereotactic radiosurgical treatment is appropriate. The latter is a focused form of X-ray therapy that leads to fibrosis over a 2-year period. AVMs may also affect the spine and lead to cord ischaemia. Symptoms are often progressive and include pain, weakness and, ultimately, paraplegia. Nowadays, the treatment is usually occlusion by interventional neuroradiology.

SUMMARY BOX 24.2

Vascular disorders and the central nervous system

- Symptoms due to occlusive vascular disease most often originate from blockage of extracranial vessels by atherosclerosis. Intracranial occlusion can be thrombotic or embolic
- Transient ischaemic attacks are associated with a high risk of major stroke within 5 years unless treatment is instituted (e.g. by carotid endarterectomy or aspirin therapy)
- Intracranial haemorrhage may be extradural, subdural, subarachnoid or intracerebral. Extradural and subdural haemorrhage are usually the result of trauma; subarachnoid bleeding is due to rupture of an aneurysm in around 70% of cases; and intracerebral bleeding is frequently associated with hypertension and amyloid angiopathy
- Patients with subarachnoid haemorrhage from an aneurysm should be considered for either clipping or coiling of the aneurysm to avoid recurrent bleeding.

Cavernomas

These are well-circumscribed collections of small vascular channels (usually capillaries). Patients typically present with headaches, focal neurological deficits or epilepsy, owing to small, recurrent focal haemorrhages. The haemorrhages are usually small in volume and cause a clinical syndrome less dramatic than that associated with SAH or AVM rupture. CT and angiography often miss these lesions, but the lesions have a characteristic appearance on MRI and may be much more common than was previously appreciated. Those causing epilepsy or haemorrhage are usually excised, unless they are in a vital and/or inaccessible place (e.g. brain stem). The risk of rebleeding from cavernomas and AVMs is poorly documented, and prospective natural history studies are under way so that the risks and benefits of intervention can be better defined.

NEUROTRAUMA

Head injury comprises a large proportion of emergency neurosurgical practice. Severity can range from a minor concussive injury through to severe craniocerebral trauma associated with high-velocity motor vehicle accidents. The head injury may be associated with direct injury to scalp or face, and may be penetrating (open) or non-penetrating (closed). From the neurosurgical perspective, the important objective in the management of head injury is to minimize the events that can occur secondary to the primary head injury. Primary brain injury occurs as a direct result of trauma. It may be diffuse or focal and of varying severity, and is essentially irreversible. Secondary brain injury occurs after the primary trauma as a result of hypotension, ischaemia, hypoxia, pyrexia, infection and raised ICP. Secondary brain damage can have a devastating effect on what may initially have been a relatively minor injury and amenable to prevention and treatment.

Assessment

Glasgow Coma Score

The GCS is a measure of conscious level that has greatly facilitated the classification and objective management of head-injured patients. It is used internationally and records

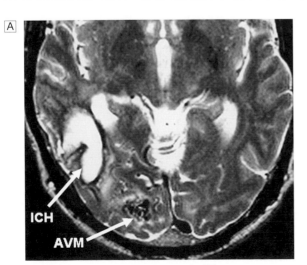
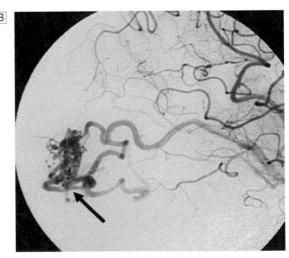

Fig. 24.8 Arteriovenous malformation (AVM). [A] MRI scan showing an AVM that has bled, causing an intracerebral haematoma (ICM). [B] Angiogram of the same AVM (arrow).

24

the best verbal response, best motor response and eye open- ing. The maximum score is 15 and the minimum is 3. Change in GCS over time is much more informative than an absolute reading at any one point in time. The Glasgow Coma Scale can be used in children of all ages, although the 'best verbal' component of the scale needs to be modified to take into account the age of the child, particularly in children under the age of 4 years. The best postresuscitation GCS is used to classify severity of head injury. Mild injury is GCS from 15 to 13; moderate is from 12 to 9; and less than 8 is classified as severe. Coma is also defined as a GCS of 8 or less.

Neurological examination

This should include routinely an assessment of pupil size and reaction; a search for CSF leaks from nose, mouth and ears; a survey of the scalp for penetrating injuries; signs of a basal skull fracture (Battle's sign, raccoon eyes); and an assessment of the maxillofacial skeleton. Peripheral neurological examination will give a guide to focal brain injury, spinal injury or peripheral nerve injury.

Other systems

Patients with head injury often have extracranial injury. It is important to remember that head injury alone never causes hypovolaemic shock. The management of systemic complications such as severe chest injury, intra-abdom- inal haemorrhage or major volume loss is a priority in treatment, since these phenomena will lead to secondary cerebral ischaemia and hypoxia and thus secondary brain damage.

Management

As with all injured patients, management commences with airway, breathing and circulation. The neck should be immobilized until a cervical spine injury has been excluded. The GCS should be documented on arrival and following resuscitation, and the findings of a neurological survey recorded. Many patients with head injury are under the effects of alcohol and other drugs that affect conscious level. If in doubt, assume that depressed consciousness is due to brain injury. Continued monitoring of conscious level over time by means of GCS is a key aspect of management, and sedatives must be avoided.

In general, patients with a GCS of 8 or less are intubated and ventilated; to prevent hypoxia and aspiration pneu- monitis, and to allow hyperventilation, which reduces the P_aCO_2 and so lowers ICP through cerebral vasoconstriction. Following resuscitation, stabilization and prioritization of injuries, a head CT is performed to visualize intracranial haematoma, brain contusions (bruises), depressed bone fragments, intracranial air and associated maxillofacial frac- tures. Mass lesions such as extradural haematoma, subdural haematoma and haemorrhagic contusions may cause brain swelling and shift, and are often surgically evacuated. In many cases, an ICP monitor is inserted for postoperative or elective ICP monitoring. Indications for clot evacuation are > 5 mm midline shift, significant impairment of GCS, or pro- tracted headache or vomiting. Compound cranial wounds need to be surgically explored, dead tissue and foreign bod- ies removed, depressed bone fragments elevated, haemo- stasis secured and the dura closed in a watertight fashion. Depending of the age of the wound, bone fragments may be either cleaned and replaced or discarded.

Brain injury evolves over several days and the principal aim of management is to limit secondary damage due to ischaemia and brain herniation caused by raised ICP,

hypoxia and hypotension. ICP is often severely elevated following neurotrauma because of oedema, haematoma, contusions, engorgement of the brain vasculature, hydro- cephalus or even infection. A sustained ICP that exceeds 25 mmHg is associated with a poorer outcome. Severely brain-injured patients are therefore kept sedated and ven- tilated and their ICP is monitored. Hyperventilation, man- nitol and barbiturates are used to reduce ICP, and the systemic blood pressure may be raised using fluids and inotropes (EBM 24.5). CBF is often directly related to MAP after head injury due to loss of autoregulation, and a CPP of > 60 mmHg is generally required to sustain adequate cerebral perfusion. Although children and young adults can tolerate lower levels, the functional consequences of profound and prolonged lowering of CPP are often devastating. Prolonged rehabilitation is required for many neurotrauma patients.

EBM 24.5 **Dexamethasone after head injury**

'Dexamethasone after head injury is harmful (the CRASH trial).'

Edwards P, et al. Lancet. 2005; 365:1957–1959.

Skull fracture

The presence of a skull fracture is an important pointer to the likelihood of significant primary and/or secondary brain injury, especially if accompanied by a depressed GCS. However, the absence of a fracture does not exclude life- threatening brain injury, particularly in young children. A patient without a fracture who has a GCS of 15 has a risk of intracranial haematoma of 1:6000. If a fracture is present, this figure rises to 1:30; if the GCS is 14 or less, the figure is 1:4. Plain X-ray will miss many fractures, particularly of the skull base. CT is the investigation of choice after head injury, and certainly should be performed if there is a skull fracture.

Extradural haematoma

This is usually the result of a skull fracture with tearing of a meningeal artery (Fig. 24.9A). It is most common in the mid- dle fossa after a temporal fracture and middle meningeal artery tear. The primary brain injury is often minimal, with a typical 'lucid' interval followed by rapid deterioration as the haematoma enlarges. The prognosis after treatment is usually good.

Subdural haematoma

This is more common than extradural haematoma and is due to laceration of vessels (especially small cerebral veins) on the brain surface, or 'bursting' of the brain. CT shows a haematoma that is concave on its inner surface (Fig. 24.9B). Craniotomy is performed to remove the hae- matoma and arrest the bleeding. Morbidity and mortality are often high because of the severity of the primary brain injury. An increasingly common problem with the ageing population is chronic subdural haematoma (CSDH). This is a collection that varies in viscosity from breaking-down clot to bloodstained CSF-like fluid, and which can collect after relatively minor head trauma. Patients with cerebral atro- phy who are on aspirin or anticoagulants are predisposed to CSDH. Because the collection can occur slowly, there may be significant midline shift and sometimes very few signs and symptoms. CSDH can mimic most neurological

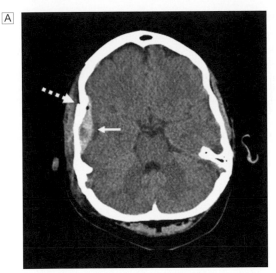 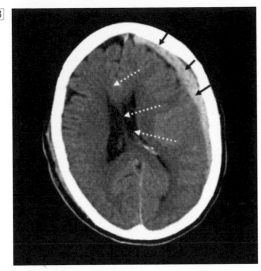

Fig. 24.9 Extradural and subdural haematoma. [A] Axial CT scan showing an acute extradural haematoma. The extradural clot is lens-shaped (solid arrow), and is associated with a skull fracture and a small amount of intracranial air (broken arrow). [B] Axial CT scan showing a subdural haematoma. The subdural clot (black arrows) is compressing the brain and causing significant midline shift and subfalcine herniation (white arrows).

syndromes in their presentation. Treatment involves drainage of the collection through burr holes or mini-craniotomy, with or without drainage of the subdural space.

Intracerebral haematoma and contusions

Trauma can cause focal intracerebral haematoma or, more commonly, foci of contusions or small areas of brain bruising. Such lesions can cause cognitive and focal deficits in the longer term, but acutely can be associated with severe pericontusional brain oedema.

Diffuse axonal injury

This type of injury is caused by rotational head movements. It is common after high-speed motor vehicle accidents. The GCS is usually low. Paradoxically, the CT may appear normal, or there may be only small punctate brain contusions. The ICP is often normal. However, because of the diffuse nature of the brain injury, severe neurological deficits are common.

 SUMMARY BOX 24.3

Head injury

- Grading (Glasgow Coma Score, GCS): minor, GCS 13–15; moderate, GCS 8–12; severe, GCS < 8
- May cause extradural haematoma, subdural haematoma, intracerebral haematoma, cerebral contusions, diffuse axonal injury
- Avoidance of hypotension, hypoxia, hypercapnia, pyrexia and ICP > 25 mmHg minimizes secondary brain damage.

Traumatic spinal injury

Injury to the spinal cord may arise as a result of sports injury, following accidents with or without severe craniocerebral neurotrauma, or following relatively minor falls in the elderly. The important factors are whether there is spinal axis instability, and whether there has been spinal cord or nerve root injury. The latter is invariably a consequence of the former; however, many cases of spinal axis injury are not associated with neural injury. This is particularly the case for odontoid fractures and pedicular fractures of C2, and many burst fractures of L1. Prompt recognition of cases with an unstable bony injury is required to avoid a devastating spinal cord injury.

Cervical spinal injury

This is commonly caused by trauma that produces subluxation of the cervical vertebra, often C5 on C6, a crush fracture of a cervical vertebral body, or hyperextension or hyperflexion injury in a patient with a narrow cervical spinal canal. The resulting neural injury may cause quadriparesis or a complete cord transection syndrome. A common pattern of injury in the elderly is a central cord syndrome, in which the segmental grey matter is contused but the fibre tracts are relatively spared. This produces weakness in the upper limbs, but relative sparing of the lower limbs.

Management consists of prompt recognition of the injury. Patients will have variable neurological deficits. With cord transection, there may be hypotension and bradycardia (due to loss of peripheral sympathetic tone), areflexia, hypotonicity and paresis. Sensory examination provides a clue to the level of spinal injury. Initially, investigations usually consist of cervical spinal X-rays and then MRI. The spine is then immobilized and, if necessary, spinal realignment is obtained with traction. High-dose steroids can also be given. Surgical stabilization of the spine is then usually performed. Neurorehabilitation is important.

INTRACRANIAL INFECTIONS

Infection of the central nervous system and its meninges acquires surgical importance if it produces a mass (abscess or oedema), hydrocephalus or osteomyelitis, or if it occurs as a result of a breach in, or absence of, the coverings of the brain. In developed countries, intracranial infections are relatively uncommon in immunocompetent patients. However, immunocompromised patients, particularly those affected with HIV, frequently suffer from a range of

24

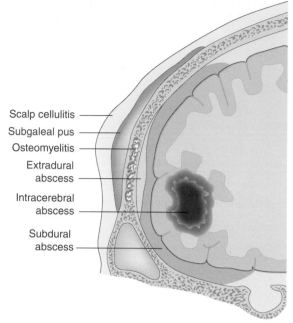

Scalp cellulitis
Subgaleal pus
Osteomyelitis
Extradural abscess
Intracerebral abscess
Subdural abscess

Fig. 24.10 Types of bacterial cranial infection.

opportunistic organisms: for example, toxoplasmosis and tuberculosis. Infection may affect the scalp, cranium and meninges, as well as the brain itself (Fig. 24.10).

Bacterial infections

The brain is relatively resistant to infection but abscesses or subdural empyema (SDE) may form. Initially, there is cerebritis (encephalitis), following which the brain necroses to form pus surrounded by a tough glial capsule. There may be an obvious source of concurrent or contiguous infection (e.g. SDE complicating frontal sinusitis, temporal lobe abscess complicating mastoiditis, brain abscess via haematogenous spread in patients with bronchiectasis), but in many patients the infection appears to arise de novo. Brain abscess and SDE usually present in a subacute or acute manner with headache, seizures and focal neurological deficit. Meningism and pyrexia are common with SDE but are not infrequently absent with brain abscess.

Treatment is a medicosurgical emergency. As well as loculations of pus, the major problems are severe peri-ilesional brain oedema and the propensity to venous sinus thrombophlebitis. CT permits the rapid diagnosis and localization of pus and greatly facilitates surgical drainage. The latter is usually done by image-directed surgery using a frame (stereotactically) or frameless system for an abscess, or craniotomy or burr holes for an SDE. Epidural infections and osteomyelitis of the skull are now very rarely seen in Europe. If the abscesses are multiple, they can mimic metastatic neoplasia radiologically.

High-dose intravenous antibiotics are necessary and pus is sent for Gram staining, culture and sensitivity. Anaerobic streptococci are the most common agents, although infections due to middle ear disease are often mixed. Dexamethasone can be used to reduce the brain oedema. Although the mortality from brain abscess and subdural empyema has fallen considerably owing to earlier diagnosis, patients frequently have significant neurological sequelae and there is a high incidence (50–60%) of post-infective seizures. Anticonvulsants are prescribed routinely and are often required indefinitely.

Postsurgical infection

Postcraniotomy wound infections occur in less than 1% of procedures and are generally due to staphylococcus. Once the flap is colonized and a nidus of osteomyelitis has developed, the infection will not usually be eradicated by antibiotic therapy. Quite frequently, a sinus will develop along the line of the craniotomy scar and intermittently discharge pus. In most cases, the flap needs to be removed and some form of cranioplastic procedure is performed 9–12 months later. Fortunately, infection of the brain itself following surgery is extremely rare, even following the implantation of prosthetic material.

Meningitis

Although most forms of meningitis are treated by physicians, some involve neurosurgeons. For example, a dural tear following a skull-base fracture leads to the egress of CSF into the paranasal sinuses (cranionasal fistula) or mastoid air cells. From there, the CSF can pass through the Eustachian tube into the nasopharynx (cranioaural fistula). Under these circumstances, pneumococcal infection can occur, either early or extremely late following injury. Early treatment of post-CSF fistula meningitis is important, as this generally leads to a very satisfactory outcome. Conversely, failure to recognize the disorder can result in death. With post-traumatic CSF fistula, there is no evidence that prophylactic antibiotics reduce the incidence of meningitis. If the CSF leak continues, then the site of leakage needs to be surgically repaired.

INTRACRANIAL TUMOURS

Tumours of the skull

This is an uncommon group of tumours. The differential diagnosis of skull lumps includes osteomas, meningiomas with hyperostosis, metastatic malignancy, fibrous dysplasia, histiocytosis and Paget's disease. Most are painless and diagnosis involves a combination of skull imaging with CT and MRI and systemic investigations.

Gliomas

This group comprises the most common (60%) primary intracranial tumour. Gliomas arise from the brain-supporting cells. Glioma is a generic non-specific term applied to such diverse tumours as glioblastoma, astrocytoma, oligodendroglioma and ependymoma. These are infiltrating tumours and are graded using the WHO four-point scale:

- *Grade I tumours* (e.g. pilocytic astrocytoma, dysembryoplastic neuroepithelial, ganglioglioma) are on the borderline between hamartomas and extremely low-grade tumours. They are often cured by surgery.
- *Grade II tumours* (astrocytoma, oligodendroglioma and ependymoma) have variable intrinsic malignancy and survival periods are usually long (median 8.5 years after surgery, radiotherapy and chemotherapy).
- *Grade III tumours* are prefixed anaplastic (e.g. anaplastic astrocytoma, anaplastic oligodendroglioma) and frequently have median survival periods of around 3 years after multimodality treatment (Fig. 24.11). As with grade II tumours, oligodendrogliomas tend to be more responsive to therapies than astrocytomas.
- *Grade IV tumours* are highly malignant and comprise glioblastoma and gliosarcomas.

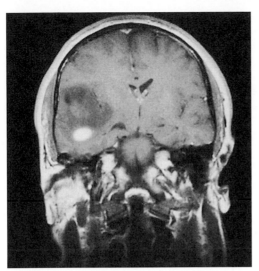

Fig. 24.11 Coronal MRI scan showing a right temporal mass lesion of low signal intensity, with an oval-shaped region of gadolinium enhancement. The latter suggests malignancy. This tumour was an anaplastic astrocytoma.

- Grade III and grade IV tumours have features suggestive of malignant transformation (e.g. vascular endothelial proliferation, nuclear pleomorphism, high mitotic rate). Despite multimodality treatment, median survival with glioblastoma is around 9–12 months, depending on age (younger patients do better), performance status (patients in good condition do better) and history of seizures.

Meningiomas

These arise from the dura (Fig. 24.12) and account for 20% of all primary intracranial tumours. They commonly arise from the skull convexity, skull base or sagittal sinus region. They may compress the adjacent brain and cause seizures. They are generally slow-growing (90% are WHO grade I

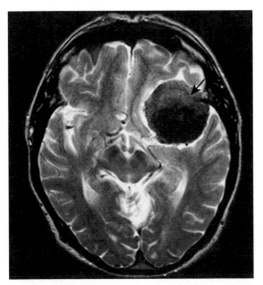

Fig. 24.12 Axial MRI showing a large sphenoid wing meningioma (arrow). There is no associated brain oedema. This tumour caused troublesome seizures.

tumours) but may spread widely over the dura ('en plaque' tumours), and may invade the skull to form a palpable mass. The treatment is excision and prognosis is usually good. However, recurrences are not infrequent with WHO grade II (atypical) or WHO grade III (anaplastic) meningiomas, or following subtotal excision of a grade I tumour.

Schwannomas

Cranial nerve tumours account for 10% of intracranial tumours and virtually all of them affect the vestibulocochlear nerves (acoustic neuroma or vestibular schwannoma) (Fig. 24.13). The tumour grows within, expands and erodes the internal auditory meatus. The VIIth and VIIIth nerves become stretched over its surface as it grows into the cerebellopontine angle. Early VIIIth nerve symptoms include progressive nerve deafness, tinnitus and vertigo. Larger tumours may involve the trigeminal nerve, leading to diminished facial sensation, as well as the pons and cerebellum, leading to ataxia and nystagmus. Displacement of the fourth ventricle and aqueduct may lead to hydrocephalus. Patients are often misdiagnosed as having Ménière's disease and the tumour may reach a large size before it is discovered. Treatment options include microsurgical excision, stereotactic radiosurgery or observation.

Pituitary tumours

These account for 10% of all intracranial tumours. Histologically, most are benign. They produce symptoms through local pressure on the visual apparatus (e.g. distortion of the optic chiasma leads to bitemporal hemianopia) and endocrine effects (by secretion of hormones). They may be treated medically, by trans-sphenoidal hypophysectomy and by radiotherapy.

Brain metastasis

Metastatic tumours are present at postmortem in 20% of patients dying of cancer, and in 50% they are multiple (Fig. 24.14). They most commonly arise from the lung, breast, kidney, melanoma and colon. Such metastases may be the presenting feature or appear only late in the course of a previously diagnosed primary cancer. Prostate cancer classically spreads to the cranium and never involves the brain parenchyma. Conversely, gliomas very rarely spread beyond the central nervous system.

24

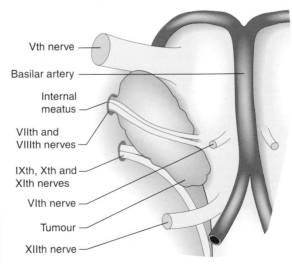

Vth nerve

Basilar artery

Internal meatus

VIIth and VIIIth nerves

IXth, Xth and XIth nerves

VIth nerve

Tumour

XIIth nerve

Fig. 24.13 Right acoustic neuroma.

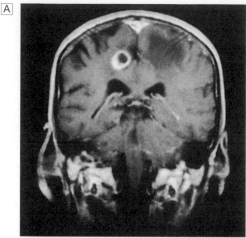

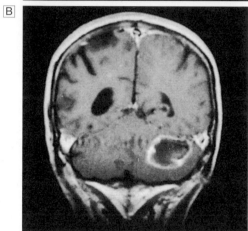

Fig. 24.14 Coronal MRI scans showing two gadolinium-enhancing lesions in the brain. **A** The smaller lesion is in the cingulate region of the cerebral hemisphere. **B** The larger lesion is in the cerebellum. Both have low signal intensity centres, suggesting necrosis. The multiplicity of the lesions is highly suggestive of metastatic neoplasia. This MRI appearance can also be seen with multiple brain abscesses.

Clinical features of intracranial tumours

Symptoms of raised ICP

Intracranial tumours commonly present as an intracranial mass lesion, either from tumour volume itself or from surrounding peritumoral oedema. This classically leads to morning headache that is aggravated by bending or straining. If the lesion is large, there may be psychomotor slowing; that is, the patient does everything normally but does it slowly and apathetically. This is a generalized sign of brain hypofunction.

Focal neurological deficit

This refers to any sign or symptom that indicates focal neuronal hypofunction. The most common is hemiparesis due to dysfunction of the motor cortex. Dysphasia occurs in about 50% of dominant hemispheric brain tumours and may be receptive, expressive or mixed. Visual field defects, dyslexia, dysgraphia and dyspraxia are also common.

Seizures

These represent local neuronal hyperfunction. The disorder may be generalized, partial or focal, and the precise nature of the seizures will reflect the anatomical position of the lesion. Seizures are more common with lower-grade tumours and meningiomas, and may respond well to anticonvulsant therapy and excision of the tumour.

Personality disintegration

There may behavioural disturbances, cognitive decline and problems with insight, judgement, memory and planning abilities. The patient usually has no insight into this progressive decline and may be referred initially to a psychiatrist.

Endocrinopathy

Secondary amenorrhoea, galactorrhoea or (in men) loss of libido caused by a prolactin-secreting pituitary adenoma is the most common example. Acromegaly, Cushing's syndrome, diabetes insipidus and precocious puberty may also occur.

Diagnosis

MRI of the brain parenchyma, before and after the administration of contrast agents, usually clarifies the locality and neuropathology of neoplastic cranial lesions. In most malignant tumours, there is a neovascular capillary bed so that with anaplastic change, tumours will enhance (see Fig. 24.11). However, some low-grade tumours (e.g. pilocytic astrocytomas) also enhance, even though these are, in fact, grade I tumours. Meningiomas, which have a mesodermal origin, do not have a BBB and therefore enhance. With the better resolution of MRI, apparently solitary lesions on CT are not infrequently found to be multifocal. A feature of the anaplastic and malignant tumours is peritumoral brain oedema. This fluid occurs in the interstitial white matter due to the neoplastic endothelium not having the integrity of the normal BBB.

Management

The management principles of surgical neuro-oncology generally rely on:

- obtaining tissue diagnosis
- undertaking appropriate surgery to relieve patients' signs and symptoms
- using appropriate radiotherapy and chemotherapy
- providing support services for the patient and family.

The groups of operations that can be performed for brain tumours generally include biopsy, craniotomy and tumour resection. A range of surgical adjuncts, such as awake craniotomy and intraoperative localization techniques, are now employed. The surgical procedure to be undertaken is influenced by the neuroradiological findings (i.e. the likely tumour pathology) and the patient's age, symptomatology and functional status, as well as the accessibility and multiplicity of the lesional pathology.

If peritumoral brain oedema is a feature, the administration of dexamethasone can lead to a dramatic reduction in symptoms and signs over a 12–24-hour period. How steroids work in brain tumours is not well understood, but their preoperative use has led to a major reduction in surgical morbidity and mortality. If the clinical and radiological parameters suggest only diagnosis is required, then stereotactic or image-guided frameless biopsy is the procedure of choice. This relatively simple procedure involves obtaining special CT or MRI images, entering this detailed information into a computer and then performing the biopsy. Surgery requires a 2.5 cm incision in the head, drilling a burr hole and either affixing a stereotactic frame to the cranium or using a computer image-directed biopsy system. The settings are adjusted so that the biopsy needle is directed at the chosen tumour target. Such systems are accurate to within 1 mm and the tumour diagnostic rate is around 98%. Because this is a minimally invasive procedure, the associated morbidity is generally very low (around 5%) and the 30-day mortality is usually less than 2%. Much of the latter is, however, related to the primary disease process rather than direct complications of the surgery.

Excision of the lesion is warranted to reduce mass effect, control seizures and restore lost brain function. If the pre-operative neuroradiology suggests a malignant glioma, then extensive resection may provide optimal symptomatic control, a smoother course during radiotherapy and a reduction in steroid requirement. A recent phase III study has shown survival benefit for patients with malignant gliomas who have had nitrosurea-impregnated biodegradable wafers (Gliadel) placed in the resection cavity (EBM 24.6). If the lesion is a meningioma, then a total excision is generally planned, as this is a benign lesion. Similarly, if a posterior fossa lesion looks like a vestibular schwannoma, complete excision may be the treatment of choice. During excisional surgery, a whole variety of adjunctive techniques can be used, ranging from surgical ultrasonic aspirators to intraoperative localization techniques, as well as cortical stimulation of the brain of the awake patient with neurophysiological assessment. The latter technique is extremely useful in operating in areas of eloquent brain, such as the language cortex and motor region.

EBM **24.6 Use of biodegradable chemotherapeutic wafers for malignant glioma**

'Biodegradable chemotherapeutic wafers placed after resection of malignant glioma significantly improve survival.'

Westphal M, et al. Neuro-oncol 2003; 5:79–88.

Outcome after surgical resection is influenced by many factors but, for malignant gliomas, the 30-day mortality is around 5% and neurological morbidity around 10%. Common complications include iatrogenic neurological deficits, cavity and extradural haematomas, and superficial wound infections. Outcome for primary intracranial tumours depends largely on tumour type (see above). Outcome following surgical excision of brain metastases depends on the state of the primary disease, as well as the locality and multiplicity of intracranial disease. Excision plus radiotherapy of a solitary metastasis is typically associated with a median survival of 7 months.

 SUMMARY BOX 24.4

Tumours affecting the skull and its contents

- Common tumours involving the skull are osteomas and metastatic deposits
- Intracranial tumours have a bimodal age distribution (peaks at 6–7 years and the fifth decade). Almost 50% of intracranial tumours are metastatic (the most common primary sources being lung and breast)
- Primary cerebral tumours arise from the supporting cells of the brain (gliomas), from the walls of ventricles (ependymomas) and from the roof of the fourth ventricle (medulloblastomas). They constitute about 60% of intracranial tumours
- Meningiomas account for 20% of intracranial tumours (90% of meningiomas are supratentorial), grow slowly, can cause focal seizures, and are treated by excision
- Pituitary and parapituitary types account for 10% of all intracranial tumours. Pituitary tumours may be functional, both types can cause pressure effects and both types are best removed surgically
- Neurinomas of the cranial nerves account for 10% of all intracranial tumours. Acoustic neurinomas develop in the internal auditory meatus and involve the VIIth and VIIIth cranial nerves, to cause deafness, tinnitus, vertigo and facial weakness. Involvement of the Vth nerve may cause loss of facial sensation.

Paediatric neuro-oncology

Tumours of the central nervous system are the second most common tumours of childhood after leukaemia. The incidence of paediatric central nervous system tumours in the UK is 15 per million of the paediatric population. In children under the age of 2 years, the most common tumours are teratomas, astrocytomas or primitive neuroectodermal tumours (PNET), and these can occur anywhere in the neuraxis. Between the ages of 2 and 15 years, the most common site for tumours is the posterior fossa, and most tumours are PNETs (also known as medulloblastomas (Fig. 24.15) when found in the posterior fossa), astrocytomas and ependymomas.

There may be an insidious onset of symptoms, such as lethargy, nausea and vomiting, with progressive ataxia in posterior fossa tumours. The symptoms of raised ICP (headache, drowsiness, nausea and vomiting) due to hydrocephalus or to the mass effect of the tumour itself may be the factors precipitating admission. Not infrequently, children with posterior fossa tumours present with a torticollis, which is persistent and not related to trauma. General surgeons may be asked to see a child because of persistent vomiting and weight loss, with no other symptoms or signs. Suprasellar tumours, such as craniopharyngioma, may present with visual failure, hydrocephalus or endocrine dysfunction. Brain-stem gliomas may present with cranial nerve deficits.

One should take seriously the information that a previously well child has lost ground or fallen behind his or her peers. A clumsy child may have ataxia. Endocrine dysfunction may show as short stature, obesity or cachexia. Optic atrophy or papilloedema should always be looked for, as visual problems are difficult to diagnose in small children and visual failure may be profound at the time of presentation. Hemiparesis is occasionally the presenting feature of a hemispheric neoplasm. Spinal cord tumours, although rare in children, may present with back pain, scoliosis, limb weakness or bladder dysfunction. Occasionally, children will present in coma because of a catastrophic bleed into

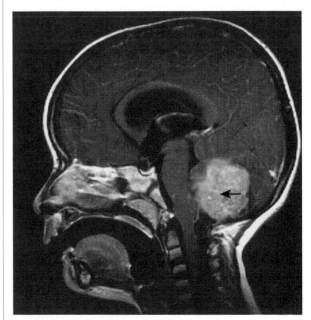

Fig. 24.15 Sagittal MRI of a medulloblastoma. The tumour (arrow) can be seen filling the fourth ventricle between the pons anteriorly and the cerebellum posteriorly. There is associated obstructive hydrocephalus due to blockage of CSF flow through the fourth ventricle.

24

a tumour or the rapid onset of obstructive hydrocephalus. The investigation of choice is MRI, but a CT with contrast will often make the diagnosis. MRI should image the spine in order to exclude spinal metastases.

Treatment consists of a combination of surgery, chemotherapy and radiotherapy. Surgical excision remains the mainstay of treatment in most cases, but is usually not curative by itself in malignant tumours, e.g. PNET, ependymoma, malignant astrocytoma. Surgery alone may be curative in the benign tumours (e.g. pilocytic astrocytoma, pineocytoma). Radiotherapy cannot be used in children under the age of 3 because of the risk of damaging the developing brain. Between 3 and 8 years of age, radiotherapy may cause loss of IQ and other neurodevelopmental delays, but to a lesser extent. Many tumours (e.g. PNET and ependymoma) are radiosensitive and radiotherapy is used as treatment after surgery in older children. Some tumours are chemosensitive (e.g. germinomas). Most childhood brain tumours have a disappointing response to chemotherapy, but it may be used as adjunctive treatment and for recurrent disease. Chemotherapy after radiotherapy in PNET has been shown to improve the prognosis and is now standard practice. The prognosis for PNET is improving. In those children who are older than 3 years at the time of presentation, with no CSF seeding or metastatic disease and with a gross total excision of tumour at the time of surgery, the prognosis is reasonably good, with 5-year survival as high as 70%. Pilocytic astrocytomas of cerebellum usually do well with complete surgical excision alone, and 90% 10-year survival is the norm.

SPINAL DYSRAPHISM

This is a congenital abnormality of the spinal axis, with or without abnormalities of the spinal cord, meninges and nerves, owing to failure of the neural tube to close (Fig. 24.16). Closure usually begins in the mid-dorsal region and extends cranially and caudally. Thus, thoracic defects are rare and cervical defects uncommon, and most affect the lumbar/lumbosacral region. Fortunately, maternal folate supplementation and prenatal screening for raised serum α-fetoprotein at 16 weeks' gestation have reduced the incidence of myelomeningocoele. There are two categories of dysraphism: open and closed.

Open spinal dysraphism

This is known as classic spina bifida aperta or myelomeningocoele. The child has an obvious open spinal defect and lower motor neuron signs below the level of the lesion, with numbness, weakness and a neuropathic bladder. These children often develop hydrocephalus following surgical closure of the spinal lesion and require ventriculo-peritoneal shunting. Around 90% of these children have an associated abnormality of the hindbrain known as a Chiari II malformation, which may cause respiratory or feeding difficulties. They may develop scoliosis as they grow. These children require lifelong follow-up in a multidisciplinary clinic, where the renal tract, neurological status and orthopaedic deformities can be regularly reviewed.

Closed spinal dysraphism

This is also known as spina bifida occulta and encompasses lesions such as lipomyelomeningocoele, meningocoele, tight filum terminale syndrome, sinus tracts and intradural dermoids, split cord malformations and caudal agenesis. The condition may be apparent at birth owing to the characteristic

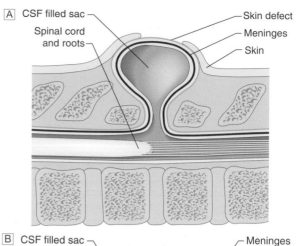

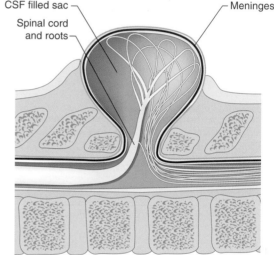

Fig. 24.16 Spinal dysraphism. **A** Simple meningocoele. **B** Myelomeningocoele.

overlying skin lesions, which include midline lumbar lipomas, hairy patches, dimples and sinuses. However, the diagnosis may not be noted until later in childhood, when the child develops neurological symptoms (often following minor trauma or a growth spurt), pain in the legs and/or recurrent urinary tract infections. Late neurological deterioration and/or bladder dysfunction are due to tethering of the developing spinal cord at the level of the lesion. The treatment is surgical untethering. Other causes include splitting of the cord by a bony projection from the posterior surface of the vertebral body (diastematomyelia), which can be removed, and the presence of intracord lipomas, which are often diffuse and multiple and whose removal is difficult and hazardous. In severe cases, one foot may be smaller than the other. Dural sinus tracts may lead to meningitis. In general, affected individuals do not develop hydrocephalus and there is no association with the Chiari malformation. Low-lying sacral dimples, within the natal cleft, are much more benign and rarely signify serious intradural pathology.

HYDROCEPHALUS

Aetiology and clinical features

Hydrocephalus is the accumulation of CSF within the ventricles or over the surface of the brain. This may rarely be due to overproduction of CSF (because of a choroid

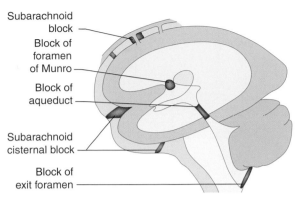

Fig. 24.17 Hydrocephalus: sites of cerebrospinal fluid (CSF) blockage.

plexus papilloma), but the vast majority are due to reduced drainage secondary to obstruction of normal CSF flow (Fig. 24.17). Obstruction may be congenital, such as in aqueduct stenosis (Fig. 24.18), or acquired, as a result of tumour or arachnoidal adhesions and fibrosis secondary to intraventricular or subarachnoid haemorrhage. Hydrocephalus due to obstruction of flow within the ventricular system, leading to dilatation of the ventricles, is termed 'internal', 'non-communicating' or 'obstructive'. In 'external' or 'communicating' hydrocephalus, the ventricular system is patent but there is reduced flow through the basal cisterns or absorption of CSF by the arachnoid granulations. This is commonly due to fibrosis following meningitis or subarachnoid haemorrhage, or to sagittal sinus thrombosis. In this type, the ventricles and the CSF spaces around the surface of the brain will be enlarged. In adults, chronic hydrocephalus may cause the 'normal pressure hydrocephalus' syndrome of gait ataxia, incontinence and cognitive decline. Diagnosis is often difficult in the elderly because brain atrophy causes ex-vacuo dilatation of the ventricles due to loss of brain substance, mimicking hydrocephalus. Cognitive decline can be asso-

ciated with Alzheimer-like pathology or cerebrovascular disease, and urinary disturbances may be related to prostate problems.

Congenital hydrocephalus usually presents at birth or in early infancy. The cranial sutures may start to open and the fontanelle will be tense and bulging. The veins of the scalp and the bridge of the nose will be dilated. As the hydrocephalus worsens, the eyes may become downcast (sunsetting). The child may be floppy and develop apnoeic spells and episodes of bradycardia. In older children and children with closed fontanelles, the symptoms are those of raised ICP (headache, vomiting and drowsiness). The eyes may develop a squint owing to VIth cranial nerve palsy. Papilloedema may be present and, if severe or chronic, may lead to blindness.

Management and prognosis

Treatment consists of relieving the pressure by bypassing the block to CSF drainage. In some cases of aqueduct stenosis, this can be done in a minimally invasive way by endoscopic third ventriculostomy. In this procedure, using an endoscope a small hole is formed in the floor of the third ventricle, allowing CSF to flow into the basal cisterns. In most cases, however, a ventriculo-peritoneal (VP) shunt will have to be inserted (Fig. 24.19). This consists of a catheter in the lateral ventricle, which drains CSF through a valve (that sits on the skull under the scalp) into the peritoneal cavity. The risk

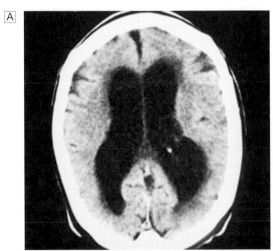

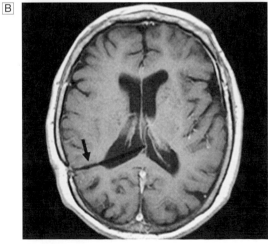

Fig. 24.19 Hydrocephalus. A CT showing adult hydrocephalus. B MRI after operation (ventriculo-peritoneal shunt, arrow). There has been dramatic resolution of the hydrocephalus.

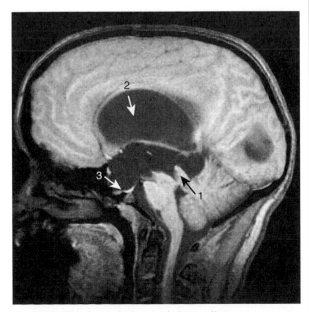

Fig. 24.18 MRI of aqueduct stenosis (arrow 1). This is an example of an obstructive hydrocephalus. There is gross ventricular enlargement (arrow 2) and herniation of the floor of the third ventricle into the interpeduncular cistern (arrow 3).

24

24

of bleeding into the ventricular system or brain during the insertion or removal of a VP shunt is of the order of 1–2%. There is also a risk of early infection, usually with skin commensal organisms such as *Staphylococcus epidermidis*. Shunts can become blocked or malfunction, causing a rapid return of symptoms, and this can be a medical emergency. Shunts can also become infected many months or years after insertion, in which case the shunt has to be removed and reinserted once the infection has cleared. Occasionally, a shunt will over-drain the ventricles, leading to premature closure of the cranial sutures and microcephaly. Over-drainage may be symptomatic, with headache and vomiting. It also predisposes to blockage of the ventricular catheter.

The long-term prognosis depends very much on the underlying cause of the hydrocephalus. In cases of simple aqueduct stenosis treated early, the prognosis for normal IQ and normal neurological function is good. Repeated episodes of raised ICP or ventriculitis can lead to loss of IQ and neurological deficit.

MALFORMATIONS OF THE SKULL

Abnormalities of the scalp and skull are often a source of worry for parents. The common problems are moulding at the time of birth, which is self-limiting, and scalp haematomas caused by ventouse extractions. These usually resolve spontaneously. Subgaleal haematomas in infants, often related to underlying skull fractures, can be extensive and can cause the haemoglobin to drop significantly. Growing skull fractures are peculiar to infancy and are caused when a fracture is associated with an underlying dural tear. The CSF pulsations cause the edges of the bone at the fracture site to absorb, and the child may present some months later with a palpable skull defect in the line of the fracture. The treatment is to repair the dura. The defect can be repaired with bone, but this is not always required.

Craniosynostosis

This refers to the premature closure or absence of a cranial suture. Several intramembranous ossification centres occur in the skull vault and form plates of bone. Sutures form where these plates of bone meet each other. This is where further bone growth occurs. Overall bone growth is driven by the expanding brain. The brain has reached 85% of its adult size by the age of 2 years but continues to grow slowly after this time. The midline frontal metopic suture fuses at the age of 2 years. Premature fusion of a suture will lead to asymmetrical skull growth. Fusion of a single suture is associated with certain typical head shapes, depending on the particular suture affected (Fig. 24.20). The common ones are scaphocephaly and plagiocephaly (premature fusion of the sagittal and coronal sutures respectively). Plagiocephaly may also be caused by fusion of a lambdoid suture but this is much rarer. Many cases of plagiocephaly are due to head moulding, when the baby lies on its back to sleep. This usually resolves when the child starts to sit and walk.

Sometimes, more than one suture can be affected. This can be syndromal (e.g. Crouzon's or Apert's syndrome). These syndromes are associated with characteristic craniofacial deformities. Craniosynostosis may also lead to a reduction in cranial volume, causing raised ICP. Surgery can be undertaken to remodel the skull into a more acceptable shape or to increase the cranial volume.

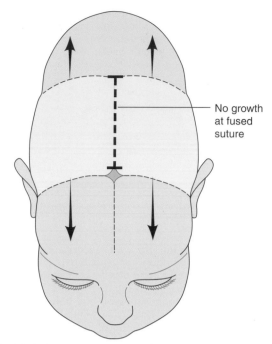

Fig. 24.20 Sagittal suture craniosynostosis. The sagittal suture is prematurely fused (broken line). Growth normally occurs perpendicular to the suture line. In this case, the skull cannot widen, as there is no growth at the fused suture, which may be palpable as a ridge in the midline. There is compensatory growth at the coronal and lambdoid sutures, leading to an elongated head shape (scaphocephaly), with bulging of the forehead (frontal bossing) in severe cases.

No growth at fused suture

Cranial dermal sinuses and angular dermoids

Dermal sinuses are midline tracts lined with squamous epithelium that may communicate with the intracranial cavity and may predispose to meningitis. They are also found in the spine. In the head, most are found in the occipital region; 70–80% are associated with inclusion dermoids and 80% extend subdurally. In the face, because of the complex embryology, dermoids can be found at the tip of the nose and the lateral aspect of the eye.

FUNCTIONAL NEUROSURGERY

A relatively small but highly specialized branch of neurosurgical practice involves the treatment of movement disorders, intractable epilepsy and even certain cases of psychiatric disorder. The aim of surgery in such cases is to modify brain function.

Movement disorders

Stereotactic surgery for movement disorders such as tremor (Parkinson's disease, essential tremor), dystonia, chorea and tics involves selecting a target within the central nervous system for either ablation or stimulation. The latter is thought safer and is thus preferred. Neural transplantation is still being evaluated and involves the implantation of neural tissues into the target brain areas in the hope that

Epilepsy

The types of seizure disorder that can be helped by neurosurgical intervention are those that, firstly, are intractable to medical therapies; secondly, have a focal onset of seizure disorder; and thirdly, have a structural disorder of the brain associated with the seizure disorder that relates to the seizure focus. The most common indications for neurosurgery are in patients with refractory complex partial seizures usually known as temporal lobe epilepsy. Many of these patients will have either a hamartoma, a low-grade neoplasm or a condition termed hippocampal sclerosis, which leads to chronic seizures. Resection of the involved temporal tissues and hippocampus leads to resolution of the seizure disorder in about 70% of cases. The success rates for surgery in non-temporal epilepsy are lower. However, successful treatment of chronic refractory childhood epilepsy associated with hemispheric dysgenesis is often found following hemispherectomy in young children. Rather surprisingly, resection of the anatomically and physiologically abnormal hemispheric tissues leads to resolution of the seizure disorder and often dramatic improvements in both motor and developmental milestones. Vagal nerve stimulators can also be useful for refractory epilepsy.

VERTEBRAL COLUMN

Spinal degenerative disease

Aetiology and clinical features

Degenerative changes in the intervertebral discs and reactive changes in the vertebral bones are common in the lumbar and cervical regions. Disc degeneration is associated with loss of 'disc space' height. This throws abnormal strain on the intervertebral (apophyseal) joints, leading to osteophyte formation and narrowing of the intervertebral foramina. This condition is known as spondylosis and is associated with chronic disc herniation; it may lead to nerve root (lateral recess stenosis), cord (spondylitic myelopathy) or cauda equina (lumbar canal stenosis) compression. These may result in a radiculopathic (i.e. a specific nerve root syndrome), myelopathic or lumbar claudication-type syndrome, with or without low back or neck pain.

In response to acute trauma, the nucleus pulposus may protrude (herniate) through a tear in annulus (Fig. 24.21). Posterolateral protrusion usually compresses the adjacent nerve root or radicle, causing a sciatica (lumbar) or brachialgic (cervical) syndrome, with or without neurological deficit. Leg pain may be exacerbated by coughing and sneezing, and arm pain by neck movement. There is usually loss of normal lumbar lordosis, and a scoliosis often develops that is concave to the affected side. Straight leg raising is diminished. The neck may have paravertebral spasm. Tendon jerks and muscle power are diminished according to the site of the lesion Thus a L5/S1 prolapse affects the S1 nerve root and produces pain down the back of the thigh, the lateral side of the calf and the lateral border of the foot. There is sensory loss in the latter region. The ankle

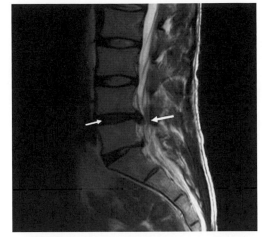

Fig. 24.21 Sagittal MRI scan of the lumbar spine showing bulging and herniation of the L4/5 disc (arrows).

jerk may be diminished or absent and, as plantar flexion of the ankle is weak, the patient may have difficulty standing on tiptoe. With an L4/L5 disc prolapse, the L5 root is compressed. Pain radiates down the back of the thigh, the lateral aspect of the calf and the dorsum of the foot into the great toe. There may be accompanying sensory loss; the ankle jerk is normal but ankle dorsiflexion is weak.

A surgical emergency occurs if the disc prolapses or herniates directly into the spinal canal (Fig. 24.22). In the cervical region, this will cause a progressive myelopathy, with numb, clumsy hands and spasticity. In the lumbar region, it is usually associated with severe pain in both lower limbs, loss of foot function, urinary retention and numbness up the back of the legs and around the genitalia, anus and buttocks (saddle anaesthesia). A rectal examination should be performed to assess anal tone. These features, known as a cauda equina syndrome, may be unilateral if the disc prolapse is asymmetrical.

SUMMARY BOX 24.5

Acute lumbar disc prolapse

- The condition is most common in the fourth and fifth decades, and men are most often affected
- The annulus fibrosus ruptures, allowing protrusion of the central nucleus pulposus. The prolapse most commonly occurs posterolaterally, and compresses and angulates the spinal nerve(s) as it leaves the spinal canal. Less commonly, the disc ruptures posteriorly, with compression of the cauda equina
- The most common levels for disc prolapse are L4–5 and L5-S1
- Pain is the predominant symptom and is exacerbated by coughing and sneezing. Tendon jerks and muscle power are diminished, straight leg raising is restricted (e.g. from 80–90° to 30°) and lumbar lordosis is flattened, with scoliosis concave to the side of the lesion
- Most cases settle on conservative therapy, but those with major protrusions or persistence of symptoms beyond 6 weeks should be considered for removal of the prolapsed material
- The cauda equina syndrome (severe back pain, urinary retention and weakness bilaterally below the knees) requires urgent surgical relief.

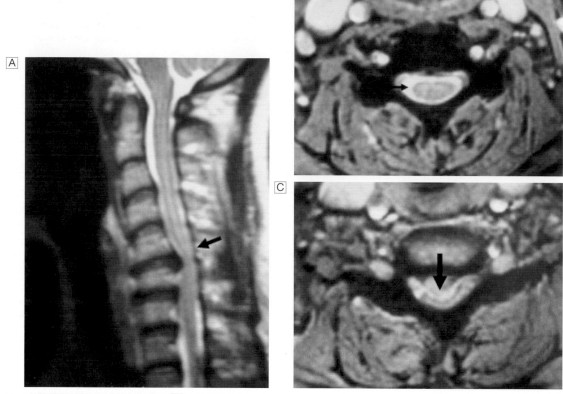

Fig. 24.22 MRI of the cervical spine. A The sagittal image shows severe spinal cord compression by a central disc prolapse (arrow). B Axial image showing the spinal canal, cord and CSF (arrow) at a normal level. C Axial image at the level of compression. The posterior disc herniation (arrow) is easily seen.

Management

Degenerative lumbar and cervical spine problems are extremely common, but the majority of problems respond to analgesia, physiotherapy and acupuncture. About 90% of cases of acute sciatic pain will settle with conservative treatment within three months. Persistent pain associated with signs of neural compression may require surgical decompression. The investigation of choice is spinal MRI. Flexion and extension X-rays may occasionally be useful if there is a spondylolisthesis and any question of spinal instability contributing to the clinical syndrome but X-rays are not indicated in uncomplicated cases of back pain or sciatica. In some cases, unusual pathology, such as metastatic tumours, neurofibromas and spinal ependymomas or meningiomas are the cause of pain or neurological disability.

The type of surgery is determined by the clinical syndrome and radiological investigations. A microdiscectomy may be performed for a simple posterolateral disc prolapse causing a sciatica-radicular syndrome. A posterior foramenotomy or anterior cervical discectomy, with or without fusion and plating, may be performed for a cervical disc prolapse. For multiple-level spinal canal stenosis, a laminectomy may be required in either the cervical or lumbar region. For lumbar spondylolisthesis associated with canal stenosis or radicular signs, decompression and fusion with pedicle screws for stabilization may be necessary. Results depend on many parameters.

PERIPHERAL NERVE LESIONS

Lesions of the peripheral nerves can be classified as: traumatic, compressive, metabolic, inflammatory, autoimmune, neoplastic and genetic. The neurosurgeon will see many compressive lesions, a small amount of trauma and the occasional nerve tumour. The common compressive neuropathies are carpal tunnel syndrome, ulnar nerve compression at the elbow and meralgia paraesthetica.

Carpal tunnel syndrome

The syndrome consists of symptoms of pain and numbness in the distribution of the median nerve in the hand. It is more common in patients with diabetes, hypothyroidism, acromegaly and pregnancy. Symptoms may be intermittent, are usually worst at night, and may be relieved by shaking the hand while holding it in a dependent position. The symptoms are often provoked by wrist flexion. On examination, there are usually no signs. Occasionally, there may be wasting of the thenar eminence, weakness of the abductor pollicis brevis, and diminished or altered sensation in the median nerve distribution. Tapping over the nerve in the carpal tunnel may elicit paraesthesia in the median nerve distribution (Tinel's sign). Phalen's test involves acutely flexing the wrist and holding it in this position. This may precipitate paraesthesia or numbness, and this is abnormal if it occurs within 1 minute. The diagnosis can be confirmed using electrophysiology to measure nerve conduction velocity and distal motor latency. Treatment depends on severity of symptoms. Splinting the wrist or injections of steroid into the carpal tunnel provide relief in a third of cases. If this fails, the transverse carpal ligament can be divided surgically, and in many cases this can be performed as a day case under local anaesthetic.

Ulnar nerve compression at the elbow

This is usually due to acute and chronic trauma, osteoarthritis or rheumatoid arthritis. The nerve may suffer repeated dislocation over the medial epicondyle on flexion of the elbow. Sometimes, the nerve may be compressed by the aponeurosis between the two heads of flexor carpi ulnaris. There is pain in the forearm and wasting of the small muscles of the hand, leading in the worst cases to an ulnar 'claw' hand. There may be reduced sensation in the ulnar distribution of the hand. The diagnosis may be made clinically, but electrophysiology is recommended to confirm the diagnosis. Treatment consists of surgically releasing and decompressing the nerve.

Meralgia paraesthetica

This is numbness and painful paraesthesia in the lateral thigh caused by compression or injury of the L2/3 sensory lateral cutaneous nerve. The nerve emerges from the lateral border of the psoas muscle just above the iliac crest and crosses the iliacus to pass beneath or through the inguinal ligament, 1 cm medial to the anterior superior iliac spine, to pass into the thigh. Seat belts, pregnancy, trauma and postsurgical scar tissue, to name but a few, can cause mechanical compression. Diabetes is present in up to 10% of cases. The clinical diagnosis can be confirmed by injecting local anaesthetic into the inguinal region 1 cm medial to the anterior superior iliac spine. Treatment includes weight loss, the removal of constricting clothes and belts, nonsteroidal anti-inflammatory drugs, ice packs and injections of corticosteroid. Most cases will settle within 2 years. Surgical decompression is reserved for those that do not.

EVIDENCE-BASED NEUROSURGERY

Much of neurosurgery lacks an evidence base but is performed because the results are considered generally satisfactory. There are, however, many areas of controversy and there is an increasing demand for evidence-based practice. Where randomized controlled trials (RCTs) have been performed, the results have usually led to significant improvements in practice and a softening of entrenched opinion (see the EBM boxes throughout this chapter). There are many other areas, such as the management of low-grade and malignant gliomas, where evidence from RCTs is urgently required in order to optimize patient treatments.

24

25

L.P. Marson
J.L.R. Forsythe

Transplantation surgery

CHAPTER CONTENTS

INTRODUCTION

For many patients, the optimal treatment of their end-stage renal failure (ESRF) is kidney transplantation because it not only improves quality of life but may also confer survival benefits (EBM 25.1). Liver, heart and lung transplantation can be truly life-saving, as often no alternative treatments are available. The two main obstacles to transplantation are overcoming the recipient's immune response and a shortage of donor organs.

EBM 25.1 **Transplantation versus dialysis in renal failure**

'Recent studies have demonstrated a significant survival benefit for renal transplantation compared with dialysis for virtually all ages. In addition, long-term dialysis is a major risk factor for graft loss, with best outcomes occurring in those patients transplanted early in the course of end-stage renal failure.'

Wolfe RA, et al. N Engl J Med 1999; 341 (23):1725–1730. Oniscu GC, Brown H, Forsythe JL. J Am Soc Nephrol 2005; 16(6):1859–1865. Meier-Kriesche HU, Kaplan B. Transplantation 2002; 74(10):1377–1381.

TRANSPLANT IMMUNOLOGY

The basis of transplant immunology is the host's recognition of foreign tissue and its subsequent response to that. Our understanding of the molecular basis of this response has developed significantly over the last 50 years, which has allowed clinical transplantation to expand enormously. The process of transplant rejection, caused by infiltrating leucocytes, exhibits both specificity and memory and is prevented by lymphocyte depletion.

The major histocompatibility complex (MHC) encodes the predominant transplant antigens responsible for acute rejection, and these are identical to serologically defined human leucocyte antigens (HLA).

The recipient's immune response to the donor organ

Early events

Inflammation lies at the heart of the rejection process and is activated through early events around the time of transplantation. Brain-stem death and retrieval of organs, as well as cold ischaemic time (while the organ is stored on ice) and a period of warm ischaemia (while the vascular anastomoses are completed) stimulate an early inflammatory response to the transplanted organ. Reperfusion is associated with endothelial activation and the infiltration of inflammatory cells, particularly macrophages. The importance of this early ischaemia reperfusion injury (IRI) in shaping the patient's subsequent course is illustrated by the superior outcome observed following living donor transplantation, despite more significant major histocompatibility (MHC) mismatching, and the adverse impact of a more prolonged cold ischaemic time on graft outcome. Indeed, the severity of this inflammatory injury modulates the subsequent alloimmune response, generating a 'danger signal' which primes the immune response to the transplanted organ. Thus, IRI impacts upon long-term outcome: it leads to a delay in primary graft function, increases acute rejection rates and reduces long-term graft survival (EBM 25.2). The crucial role of IRI in mediating transplant-associated injury has become more apparent as acute rejection rates fall with the introduction of new and highly effective immunosuppressive agents, and has led to an increasing interest in how IRI may be reduced through preconditioning strategies.

EBM 25.2 Impact of delayed graft function on long term outcome

'Delayed graft function, defined as the requirement for dialysis during the first week following transplantation is associated with:

41% increased risk of graft loss at 3 years

Higher serum creatinine at 3.5 years

38% relative increased risk of acute rejection,

Compared with patients that have primary function'

Yarlagadda SG, Coca SG, Formica RN Jr, Poggio ED, Parikh CR. Association between delayed graft function and allograft and patient survival: a systematic review and meta-analysis. Nephrol Dial Transplant. 2009 Mar;24(3):1039-47. Epub 2008 Dec 22.

The afferent arm of the immune response

The immune response to the transplanted organ can be divided into afferent and efferent arms: the afferent arm includes presentation of donor antigen to recipient T cells, T cell receptor (TCR) binding and costimulation, which leads to T cell activation. The efferent arm describes the sequence of events that occurs as a result of T cell activation.

Antigen presentation

Donor MHC antigens are recognized as foreign (allo-recognition) by recipient T cells following presentation upon donor (direct) or recipient (indirect) antigen-presenting cells (APCs) (Fig. 25.1).

T-cell receptor binding and costimulation

MHC antigen-binding to the T-cell receptor (TCR) in the presence of certain co-stimulatory molecules leads the T cells to undergo clonal expansion. Engagement of the TCR can result in a number of possible outcomes, depending on the costimulatory stimulus, and leads to T-cell proliferation,

apoptosis or anergy. Costimulatory blockade is an interesting therapeutic strategy which has recently been introduced into clinical practice, with some benefit.

T-cell activation

Antigen binding and costimulation leads to the activation and clonal expansion of T cells. T cells differentiate into helper (CD4-positive) and effector (CD8-positive) cells that are able to secrete cytokines and kill target cells. Engagement of the CD4-positive T (helper) cells play a central role in initiating and amplifying the rejection response.

The efferent arm of the immune response

Donor organ damage can be mediated via cellular or antibody-mediated (humoral) mechanisms. The latter depends on B-lymphocyte maturation and the production of antibodies that activate complement. The former, also known as delayed-type hypersensitivity (DTH), involves cytotoxic T cells, natural killer (NK) cells, macrophages and neutrophils.

Patterns of allograft rejection

Hyperacute rejection

This is usually apparent following removal of the vascular clamps as the donor organ becomes swollen and discolored, leading to graft destruction within 24 hours. It results from the presence of preformed cytotoxic antibodies directed against donor HLA antigens, but has largely been overcome by screening for such antibodies and crossmatching.

Acute rejection

This occurs in up to 50% of grafts, usually in the first 6 months. Acute rejection is diagnosed on renal transplant biopsy and is classified according to Banff 07 diagnostic criteria (Table 25.1).

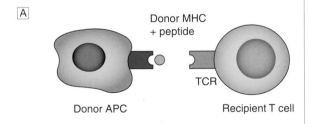

A

Donor MHC + peptide

TCR

Donor APC   Recipient T cell

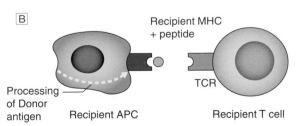

B

Recipient MHC + peptide

TCR

Processing of Donor antigen   Recipient APC   Recipient T cell

Fig. 25.1 Antigen presentation. [A] Direct. [B] Indirect. (APC = antigen-presenting cell; MHC = major histocompatibility complex; TCR = T-cell receptor)

Table 25.1. Banff 07 diagnostic criteria for renal allograft biopsies

1. Normal
2. Antibody mediated rejection (AMR)
   a. Acute AMR
      i. ATN-like-C4d+, minimal inflammation
      ii. Capillary margination and/or thromboses, C4d+
      iii. Arterial-v3, C4d+
   b. Chronic active AMR. Glomerular double contours and/or peritubular capillary basement membrane multilayering and/or interstitial fibrosis/tubular atrophy and/or fibrous intimal thickening in arteries, C4d+
3. Borderline changes: suspicious for T-cell mediated rejection, no intimal arteritis, foci of tubulitis
4. T-cell mediated rejection
   a. Acute T-cell mediated rejection
   b. Chronic active T-cell mediated rejection
   c. Chronic allograft arteriopathy
5. Interstitial fibrosis/tubular atrophy (IF/TA), no evidence of specific aetiology Grade:
      I. Mild IF/TA (< 25% cortical area)
      II. Moderate IF/TA (26-50%)
      III. Severe (> 50%)
6. Other: changes not considered to be due to rejection

25

Chronic allograft damage

This usually occurs after 6 months and often leads to a progressive decline in, and eventually loss of, organ function. The aetiology of chronic allograft damage is multifactorial: immune-mediated injury, ischaemia–reperfusion injury, toxicity from immunosuppressive agents and viral infections. Histologically it is characterized by cellular atrophy and fibrosis, and there are currently no therapeutic strategies to combat it.

Testing for histocompatibility

The immune system has evolved specifically to recognize and destroy harmful agents such as bacteria and viruses, but it is this in turn which has acted as an obstacle to successful allotransplantation. There are two main genetic systems involved: ABO blood groups and the human leucocyte antigen (HLA) system. There are two classes of HLA genes involved in the immune response to transplantation, class I and II. Potential donors and recipients are tested for class I (HLA-A, B and Cw) and class II (HLA-DR, DQ and DP) to facilitate organ allocation, such that the national allocation system for kidney transplantation places high priority on HLA matching, as the better match the kidney is to the recipient, the better the outcome.

In addition to this tissue typing process, a cross-match is undertaken immediately prior to renal transplantation to ensure that there is no reactivity between donor and recipient cells. There are two types of cross-match techniques: the complement-dependent cytotoxicity cross-match (CDC-XM), which, when positive in the presence of IgG antibodies, is likely to result in rapid rejection of the transplanted kidney. The flow cytometry cross-match (FC-XM) is a more sensitive test, which, if positive, may represent an increased risk of rejection. A decision should then be made as to whether or not to proceed with transplant following discussion between surgical and histocompatibility experts. The FC-XM is clinically relevant only in renal transplantation.

Immunosuppression

The challenge is to minimize the risk of graft rejection with as few side effects as possible. Various strategies are adopted: induction therapy, maintenance immunosuppression and treatment of rejection. The mechanisms of action of the common immunosuppressive drugs are outlined on Figure 25.2.

Immunosuppressive drugs

Steroids

Corticosteroids play an important role in induction and maintenance and are the first-line treatment for acute rejection. The side effects of steroids are numerous and are responsible for many of the long-term complications of immunosuppressive therapy (Table 25.2). This has led to attempts to withdraw steroid therapy some time after transplant, or to minimize their use.

Antiproliferative agents

Azathioprine

Azathioprine (AZA), along with corticosteroids, was the earliest immunosuppression medication used for prevention of acute cellular rejection in renal transplant recipients. AZA is a prodrug of 6-mercaptopurine, which exerts its

Table 25.2 Side effects of corticosteroids
• Hypertension
• Diabetes mellitus
• Osteoporosis
• Peptic ulceration
• Cushingoid features
• Pancreatitis
• Poor wound healing
• Psychiatric disorders

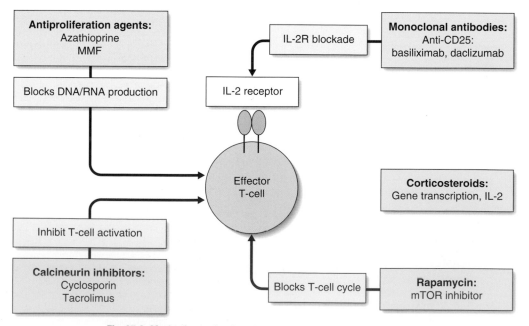

Fig. 25.2 Mechanisms of action of common immunosuppressive agents.

action by directly inhibiting purine synthesis. AZA is given as a single daily dose of 1–3 mg/kg/day. Side effects of azathioprine include severe myelosuppression resulting in neutropenia and gastrointestinal symptoms.

Mycophenolate mofetil

Mycophenolate mofetil (MMF) was developed in the 1990s, and is a prodrug for mycophenolic acid (MPA). MPA prevents lymphocyte activation through inhibiting DNA formation. MMF has replaced AZA in many renal transplant patients, following the publication of several randomized trials which demonstrated decreased treatment failure at 6 months post-kidney transplant compared with AZA. The most common side effects are gastrointestinal disturbances, leucopenia, thrombocytopenia and anaemia.

Calcineurin inhibitors (CNIs)

Cyclosporin

Cyclosporin (CYA) was introduced in the early 1980s, and this led to dramatic improvements in short- and long-term outcomes in transplantation. Its role in maintenance therapy was not challenged for a little over 10 years. CYA inhibits the production of key cytokines for early T-cell activation, such as interleukin-2. The main side effects are nephrotoxicity, hypertension, hyperlipidaemia and hyperglycaemia.

Tacrolimus

Tacrolimus, the second CNI to be introduced into clinical practice, resulted in significantly improved one-year outcome in liver transplant patients (EBM 25.3), and this has been borne out in studies in renal transplantation. Tacrolimus now forms the mainstay of many immunosuppressive regimens. It too carries the risk of nephrotoxicity, and serum levels must be monitored closely. Other side effects include neurotoxicity, diabetes and alopecia.

EBM | **25.3 Tacrolimus versus cyclosporin in renal and liver transplant patients**

'Treatment with the calcineurin inhibitor, tacrolimus, reduces acute and steroid-resistant rejection rates when compared with cyclosporin following renal transplantation, and results in better long-term function. In liver transplant patients, tacrolimus is the agent of choice, with improved outcomes in patient and graft survival.'

Margreiter R, European Tacrolimus vs Ciclosporin Microemulsion Renal Transplantation Study Group. Lancet 2002; 359(9308):741–746.
O'Grady JG, et al. Lancet 2002; 360(9340):1119–1125.

Sirolimus

Sirolimus inhibits T cell activation and proliferation and early evidence supported its use for the prevention of acute cellular rejection. However, increasing concern about synergistic nephrotoxicity with the CNIs and other side effects such as impaired wound healing and increased incidence of lymphoceles, has limited its use.

Antibody therapies

Antibody therapies may be used as induction therapy or for treatment of acute rejection. Induction therapy, given at the time of transplantation, provides immediate immunosuppression after transplantation. Antibody therapy for acute rejection is usually selected in steroid resistant rejection.

Antibody therapies may be depleting, in which the target cells are removed from the peripheral blood, or non-depleting, in which the function of the target cells is affected.

Depleting antibodies include rabbit antithymocyte globulin (ATG) and alemtuzumab, and they may be used as induction therapy, or to treat steroid-resistant rejection. Non-depleting antibodies, such as the interleukin-2 receptor antibody, basiliximab, are used as induction therapy, and reduce acute rejection rates, with few side effects.

General risks of immunosuppresssion:

Infection

The risk of infection is related to the dose of immunosuppression and patients are therefore at greatest risk early after transplantation. Bacterial infections are most common during the first month. Viral infections are most common between 1 and 6 months and, of these, cytomegalovirus (CMV) is the most clinically relevant; it can be prevented by using prophylactic antiviral agents such as valganciclovir. Opportunistic infections with protozoa and fungi are also important and most patients receive up to 6 months' co-trimoxazole prophylaxis against *Pneumocystis jirovecii* (formerly *carinii*).

Malignancy

The risk of developing skin cancer is particularly high following transplantation, with squamous cell carcinoma being 20 times more common in transplant patients than in the normal population. Post-transplant lymphoproliferative disorders (PTLDs) are usually related to infection with Epstein–Barr virus and are associated with a high risk of developing B-cell lymphoma. Treatment of PTLD involves reduction in immunosuppression and, in some cases, chemotherapy.

The future of immunosuppression

Tolerance is defined as the coexistence of a transplanted organ or tissue within a recipient without the need for continuous, long-term immunosuppression, whilst maintaining an otherwise intact immune system, and is one of the major goals of transplant research.

Other, perhaps more realistic goals of treatment, are to reduce the use of corticosteroids, and of CNIs. Several groups have explored steroid withdrawal, undertaken some time after transplantation, steroid avoidance, in which steroids are stopped a few day postoperatively and steroid-free regimens. Whilst the benefits of reduced steroid use have been observed in these studies, steroid-free and steroid-withdrawal were associated with increased incidence of biopsy-proven acute rejection at 12 months post-transplant.

Complete CNI elimination has been associated with higher rejection rates, without improvements in renal or metabolic side effects. The ELITE symphony study compared low dose CYA, low dose tacrolimus, low dose sirolimus and standard dose tacrolimus, and demonstrated superiority in the low dose tacrolimus group, in terms of acute rejection, renal function and allograft survival at one year.

 SUMMARY BOX **25.1**

The immune response

- The immune response to a transplanted organ is largely mediated by T cells, and these are the target for immunosuppressive therapy
- Acute rejection is seen in up to 50% of grafts and episodes are treated with high-dose steroids
- Chronic rejection has a multifactorial aetiology and results in significant graft loss over the months and years following transplantation.

25

ORGAN DONATION

The shortage of organs for transplantation remains a major challenge to the transplant community, with demand consistently outstripping supply over many years (Fig. 25.3). Such a shortage has led to significant changes in practice over the last decade, with an increasing number of patients undergoing transplants from living donors, and from marginal or extended criteria deceased donors. These will be discussed in this section.

Deceased donation

The identification and selection of potential donors and the subsequent approach to the family has been the focus of much attention within the United Kingdom. A UK Organ Donor Taskforce has made a series of recommendations which are aimed at increasing donor numbers. The donor transplant co-ordinators, now known as Specialist Nurses in Organ Donation, play a pivotal role in organ donation; they are now embedded within critical care areas, involved in the education of critical care staff on organ donation and transplantation, in addition to their key roles in donor management and discussion with donor families.

Current UK legislation is based on an 'opt in' policy, so that lack of objection must be obtained from the family in order to proceed. Other countries adopt an 'opt out' policy of presumed consent. There is a real need to raise public awareness of organ donation and to encourage individuals to carry organ donor cards.

Few absolute contraindications for organ donation exist; those that do are directed against the avoidance of disease transmission from donor to recipient (Table 25.3).

Donor management

Specific criteria must be met in order to make the diagnosis of brain-stem death (Table 25.4). Events leading up to brain death may impact upon the quality of the retrieved organs. Initially,

---

Table 25.3 Donor contraindications to organ donation

General contraindications
- Age > 90 years
- HIV disease (not HIV infection; no AIDS defining illness)
- disseminated cancer (above and below the diaphragm)
- melanoma (except local melanoma treated > 5 years before donation)
- treated cancer within 3 years of donation (except non-melanoma skin cancer and in-situ cervical cancer)
- nvCJD and other neurodegenerative diseases associated with infectious agents

Organ-specific donor contraindications
Liver
- acute hepatitis (AST > 1000 IU/L)
- cirrhosis
- portal vein thrombosis

Kidney
- chronic kidney disease (CKD stage 3B and below, eGFR < 45)
- long-term dialysis, (that is, not relating to acute illness)
- any history of renal malignancy
- previous kidney transplant, > 6 months previously

Pancreas
- insulin dependent diabetes (excluding ICU associated insulin requirement)
- any history of pancreatic malignancy

---

at the point of brainstem death, compression associated with coning results in hypertension and bradycardia, known as the Cushing reflex. An autonomic storm ensues, characterized by the massive release of catecholamines, with resultant hypertension and hypoperfusion. The effect on cardiac function is the deterioration of ventricular systolic function, the liver and kidneys are affected by hypoperfusion, and it is likely that these changes contribute to non-specific endothelial cell damage, which increases the immunogenicity of the organs.

Thus the clinical management of the donor focuses on providing cardiovascular stability and maintaining organ function. The first principle is to ensure optimal fluid management, maintaining blood pressure with minimal

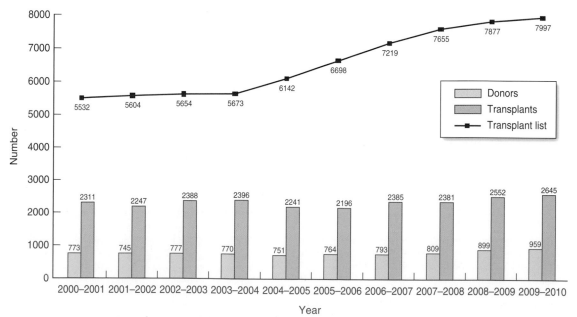

Fig. 25.3 Number of cadaveric donors and transplants in the UK, 1 April 1995 to 31 March 2009, and patients on the waiting lists at 31 March each year (ODT statistics).

Table 25.4 Criteria for diagnosis of brain-stem death

Preconditions
- Ventilated and in a coma
- Known diagnosis for coma
- Sufficient length of time on ventilator to determine severity of brain injury
- Optimization of condition, to reverse injury
- Interval of 6–24 hours from latest intervention and testing

Exclusions
- Drug or alcohol intoxication require a delay appropriate to half-life of drug
- Time for clearance of neuromuscular blocking agents
- Primary hypothermia, metabolic and endocrine disturbances
- Coma of unknown aetiology

Investigation
Absent brain-stem reflexes
- No papillary response to light
- Absent corneal reflexes
- Absent vestibulocochlear reflexes: caloric tests
- No motor response in cranial nerve distribution
- No gag reflex

Apnoea testing
- No attempt to breathe despite arterial $PCO_2 > 6.65$ kPa following pre-oxygenation with 100% oxygen

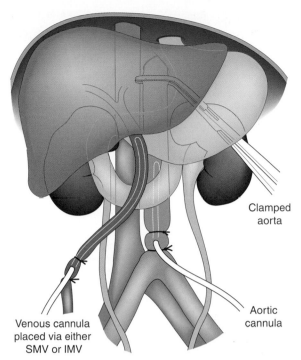

Fig. 25.4 Multiorgan retrieval, showing placement of intra-abdominal cannulae. (IMV — inferior mesenteric vein; SMV = superior mesenteric vein)

25

inotropic support. The use of thyroxine replacement is controversial, and insulin may be required.

Multiorgan retrieval

Donors following brain death (DBD) are indistinguishable from other critical care patients so it is essential that the lead surgeon identifies the patient in the operating theatre prior to commencement of surgery. The preoperative check must also ensure complete documentation of brain-stem death tests, consent and donor blood group.

Organ retrieval begins with opening the abdomen (midline incision) and the chest (sternotomy). Once other pathology has been excluded and the liver mobilized, exposure of the inferior mesenteric vein and the aorta allows insertion of the perfusion cannulae (Fig. 25.4). Cold perfusion is commenced and the vena cava is divided in the mediastinum. Crushed ice is placed throughout the peritoneal cavity, with particular emphasis on the organs to be retrieved. The heart and lungs are excised. The pancreas is usually retrieved in conjunction with the liver. The kidneys are excised with ureters and the renal arteries on aortic patches. A portion of spleen and mesenteric lymph nodes are excised for the purpose of tissue typing and cross-matching, and the iliac vessels are excised and preserved for formation of conduits if necessary. The operation is completed by careful wound closure, application of dressings and patient cleaning. The procedure must be carefully documented in the patient's notes.

Organ preservation

Organ preservation is an important factor in ensuring viability of the organ and in optimizing outcomes. Following cessation of the blood supply, cell damage will occur due to the depletion of adenosine triphosphate (ATP) and a failure of the sodium potassium pump. This leads to cell swelling and anaerobic metabolism. Cold storage is the most commonly adopted method of organ preservation, and comprises intravascular flush with chilled preservation fluid to promote organ cooling, washout of blood components and

rapid equilibration of the fluid with the tissues. Preservation fluids include Marshall's, University of Wisconsin (UW) and Eurocollins solution. UW solution is the preservation solution of choice in liver and pancreas donors, whilst Marshall's solution is used for kidney-only donors.

An alternative to cold storage is hypothermic machine perfusion, which may be associated with a reduction in delayed graft function, but no impact on graft survival has been observed. Although recent improvement in cold preservation fluids allows extended preservation times (e.g. kidneys up to 24 hours and livers up to 20 hours) prolonged cold ischaemia remains a significant cause of primary non-function or delayed graft function.

Until recently the vast majority of deceased donors were those who have been diagnosed as brain-stem dead following an intracerebral event. Due to the shortage of organs for transplantation, there has been an increase in the number of donations following circulatory death (DCD).

Donation after circulatory death

Recent years have seen the development of DCD programmes (previously known as non-heart beating donors) and this has resulted in the cincrease in numbers of deceased donors. Donors after circulatory death are categorized according to the Maastricht criteria (Table 25.5). The majority of such donors in the UK are category III donors, with successful outcomes for renal, liver, pancreas and lung transplant patients.

The techniques for procurement for DCD vary: the essential principles are to flush and cool the organs as rapidly as possible. The open technique involves a rapid access laparotomy and cannulation of the aorta at its bifurcation. The inferior vena cava is vented and the aorta clamped just below or above the diaphragm. The alternative technique relies on the use of an intra-aortic balloon catheter which is placed via the femoral artery through a groin incision. Venous exsanguination is performed via the femoral vein.

25

Table 25.5 Maastricht criteria for donation after circulatory death

Category 1: Dead on arrival at hospital. The moment of sudden death must be witnessed and the time documented.

Category 2: Unsuccessful resuscitation. Usually in the Accident and Emergency department.

Category 3: Awaiting cardiac arrest. Patients in whom cardiac arrest is inevitable, but they do not fulfil criteria for brain-stem death testing.

Category 4: Cardiac arrest in a brain-stem dead individual.

Category 5: Unexpected death in a patient in ITU or critical care unit.

EBM **25.4 Non-heart-beating versus heart-beating kidney donors**

'Initial concerns about poorer long-term outcome from non-heart-beating donor kidneys have not been borne out, with recent studies demonstrating no significant differences in 5- and 10-year graft survival. However, one study has demonstrated a significantly higher serum creatinine at 5 and 10 years in the non-heart-beating donor group compared with kidneys from donors with a heart beat, suggesting some irreversible damage has been sustained.'

Metcalfe MS, et al. Transplantation 2001; 71(11):1556–1559.
Weber M, et al. N Engl J Med; 2002; 347(4):248–255.

Renal transplantation following donation after circulatory death is associated with increased rates of delayed graft function because of longer warm ischaemic periods, but the long-term outcome is comparable to DBD (EBM 25.3). An increasing number of liver transplants are being performed following DCD, and whilst concerns regarding increased risk of primary non-function have not been borne out, with careful selection of donors, the risk of biliary complications is higher than in DBD.

The extended criteria donor (ECD)

With the limited numbers of organs available for transplantation, donors who would have been previously declined are now being considered. Criteria include extremes of age, death from intracranial haemorrhage, organ-specific diseases such as excess alcohol intake or hepatitis, general co-morbidities such as diabetes, cerebrovascular accident or cardiovascular instability. The long-term outcomes of transplants performed from ECD are poorer than standard criteria donors, and the potential risks to the recipient must be weighed against the benefits. The risks of use of ECD are general and organ-specific. For liver transplants, the risk of primary non-function is increased in donors with severe fatty liver disease (steatosis). In kidney transplantation, there is in an increased risk of delayed graft function. Systemic risks from donors exist due to the possible transmission of infection and malignancy. The risk of transmission of blood-borne viral diseases such as hepatitis B, C or HIV is always present, and is minimized by predonation screening. Risk of malignancy is low, but there are documented cases of such.

Living donation

There has been an increase in the number of transplants being performed from living donors. These are mainly kidney transplants but increasing numbers of living donor liver transplants are being performed in the United Kingdom.

Living donor kidney transplantation

Donor selection

Each potential donor must go through a rigorous assessment process, always bearing in mind that the major operation they are planning to undergo will have no direct benefit to the individual, and so great care must be taken to minimize risk. The assessment is outlined in Table 25.6, and evidence of significant co-morbidity should halt the work-up. Uncontrolled hypertension or diabetes should be considered absolute contraindications to living donation, because of the risk of deterioration in donor renal function following nephrectomy. Obesity is not an absolute contraindication, but it does make the operation more technically challenging, and it increases the risk of postoperative complications such as atelectasis, pneumonia, venous thromboembolic disease and wound infections. For these reasons, most units within the United Kingdom set a maximum body mass index limit of $30\,kg/m^2$.

Operative approaches

Laparoscopic surgery has revolutionized living donor kidney transplantation in that it has made the operation more acceptable to the donor, when compared with

---

Table 25.6 Assessment of the potential living kidney donor

History
- General health: obesity, hypertension, diabetes
- Cardiovascular risk: past medical history, family history, smoking, obesity
- History of thromboembolic events or bleeding disorders
- Respiratory risk (for anaesthetic): past medical history of asthma, chronic obstructive pulmonary disease, smoking
- Risk of renal disease: family history, particularly if disease in recipient is familial; past history of renal infections, haematuria
- Psychiatric history

Examination
- General
- Cardiovascular
- Respiratory
- Abdominal

Investigations
Immunology
- Blood group; HLA type; T- and B-cell flow cytometric crossmatching

Haematology
- Full blood count; coagulation studies

Biochemistry
- Urea and electrolytes; creatinine clearance; liver function tests; blood glucose

Urinalysis
- Protein; blood; sugar culture; sensitivity and microscopy

Cardiovascular
- Serial blood pressure measurements; electrocardiogram

Virus screen
- Hepatitis B and C; human immunodeficiency virus (HIV); cytomegalovirus infection; Epstein–Barr virus; syphilis; *Toxoplasma*

Radiology
- Chest X-ray; isotope glomerular filtration rate; renal ultrasound; angiogram/spiral computerized tomography/magnetic resonance angiography

the traditional flank approach. The main benefits to the donor are improved cosmesis and shorter recovery time. Hospital stay can be reduced by several days. However, it is a technically demanding procedure. There are various options depending on the expertise of the surgeon: the full laparoscopic approach may be performed by a transperitoneal or retroperitoneal approach, or it may be undertaken hand-assisted. The benefits of the hand-assisted approach are the use of the hand for retraction and the ability to rapidly control intraoperative haemorrhage. Open techniques include the traditional flank approach which may be rib-sparing or rib-dividing, or it can be performed via a mini-incision, which may have similar benefits to laparoscopic approaches.

Procedure-related morbidity and mortality

The mortality of donor nephrectomy is low, estimated at 1 in 3000 for all surgical approaches. Life expectancy for living donors is probably higher than the general population due to bias in the selection process. The risk of major complications such as pneumothorax, vascular or splenic injury is approximately 5%, and is 15% for all complications.

SUMMARY BOX 25.2

Organ donation

- Shortage of organs for donation remains a significant challenge to the transplant community
- Strategies aimed at increasing use of organs for donation include use of marginal donors and donors without a heart beat
- Well-established programmes for living donor kidney transplants exist within the UK, with an increasing drive to establish living donor liver transplantation.

RENAL TRANSPLANTATION

The optimal management for patients with end stage renal failure is a kidney transplant; it both improves quality of life, releasing patients from the limitations of dialysis, and increases survival. However, not all patients will benefit from transplantation, and consideration must be given as to the best use of the scarce commodity of donated organs. Thus patients undergo rigorous assessment prior to being listed for transplantation.

Indications and patient assessment

Absolute contraindications to renal transplantation are active infection and malignancy; relative contraindications include advanced age, severe cardiovascular disease and likelihood of non-compliance with immunosuppressive therapy. In addition, heed must be paid to the likelihood of the underlying disease causing problems within the transplanted kidney (e.g. diabetes mellitus, glomerulo-sclerosis, amyloidosis and hypertension). Potential recipients need to undergo rigorous medical (Table 25.7), psychological and social evaluation. An important component of this is the education of the patient and their family about the benefits and risks of transplantation and of immunosuppression, so that fully informed written consent can be obtained.

Table 25.7 Assessment of the potential recipient for renal transplantation
General assessment
• History, clinical examination
Blood tests
• Haematology: full blood count, clotting screen
• Biochemistry: urea and electrolytes, liver function tests
• Virology: HIV, hepatitis B and C
• Immunology: ABO and HLA typing
Urinalysis and culture
• 24-hour urine collection for creatinine clearance
Other tests
• ECG, chest X-ray
Cardiovascular assessment
• Patients > 45 years, history of diabetes or of cardiovascular disease: exercise tolerance test, stress echocardiogram or stress radionuclide scan; if abnormal, proceed to coronary angiography
Gastrointestinal assessment
• Abnormal liver function tests, history of peptic ulcer disease: liver ultrasound scan, upper GI endoscopy
Assessment for infection
• Active bacterial infection: contraindication to transplantation
• Viral infections: cytomegalovirus status
Urological assessment
• Urine culture and renal ultrasound; if positive, require assessment of bladder emptying, e.g. postmicturition ultrasound, cystoscopy
Immunological assessment
• Blood group: for ABO compatibility
• HLA typing, anti-HLA antibodies: for HLA matching and organ allocation

Patient listing for transplantation

Once a decision has been made to list an individual for transplant, their blood group and tissue typing must be carefully documented, and this information is given to the central UK office, which has responsibility for kidney allocation. Several factors are taken into account in the national allocation scheme (EBM 25.4), but priority is given to HLA matching, as this has been shown to have a significant impact on outcome. Once the kidney has been allocated, a final cross-match test is undertaken in the majority of cases for anti-HLA antibodies that may have developed in response to blood transfusion, pregnancy or a previous transplant. An increasing number of transplants in which the risk of a positive cross-match is low are being performed prior to receiving the cross-match results. Patients that are eligible for this virtual cross-matching are carefully selected, and this is undertaken in an attempt to reduce the cold ischaemic time, which is a main contributor to delayed graft function.

The operative procedure

Back table preparation

Final preparation of the donor kidney is undertaken at the recipient centre. This involves careful dissection of the donor renal artery and vein, removal of perinephric fat, and careful inspection of the kidney to ensure that

25

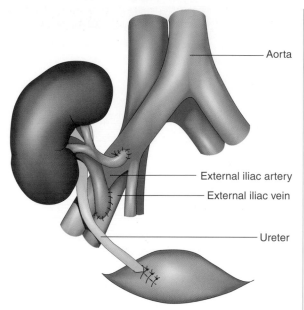

Fig. 25.5 Renal transplantation. The renal transplant is placed retroperitoneally on to the iliac vessels with the ureteric anastomosis as shown.

there is no damage to the renal capsule, to the vessels or donor ureter. It is imperative to identify any damage at this stage, and prior to reperfusion, when haemorrhage can ensue.

Recipient operation

The Rutherford Morris incision is made in the iliac fossa, and the iliac vessels are exposed by retroperitoneal dissection. Lymphatics overlying the iliac vessels must be ligated and divided with care, to avoid the development of a postoperative lymphocoele. Following careful preparation of the recipient vessels, the anastomosis is performed between donor renal vein and recipient external iliac vein. The arterial anastomosis may be performed onto the recipient's internal or external iliac artery, depending on the calibre of the donor renal artery and the positioning of the arteries (Fig. 25.5). If the internal iliac artery has been used on the contralateral side, this must not be used. The kidney is then reperfused, and the ureteric anastomosis performed between donor ureter and recipient bladder, over a double J stent. Insertion of the ureteric stent has been shown to reduce the risk of early ureteric complications such as urinary leak.

Postoperative management

The patient should be managed in a high dependency unit by nursing staff who are experienced in the management of transplant recipients. During the early postoperative period, careful attention must be paid to fluid management. Whether or not the kidney has primary function will depend in part on the source of the kidney, and it is important that this is carefully noted. Primary function is expected in a transplant from a living donor, and so, if this is not the case, rapid and thorough investigation into the cause of delay is necessary. A kidney from a DCD has a high chance of delayed graft function, and so the early postoperative management will be different.

The mainstay of early postoperative management is, rigorous assessment and maintenance of fluids. A brisk diuresis is common and careful assessment and maintenance of volume status, blood pressure and serum electrolytes is crucial to optimize renal function. Delayed graft function (DGF) is defined as the need for dialysis in the first postoperative week and occurs in approximately 30% of all cadaveric transplants.

Management of delayed graft function

If the patient is well-filled, with a central venous pressure of around 8–10mmHg, and there is no evidence of postoperative haemorrhage, an ultrasound scan is performed to exclude urinary leakage or obstruction, inadequate renal blood flow or the presence of a perinephric haematoma. If DGF is expected, the patient's fluids are carefully managed over the next few days and the patient is reassured that this is a common feature after transplant. If the kidney is still not functioning at day 5, a renal biopsy is performed to check that there is no evidence of rejection, expecting evidence of acute tubular necrosis (ATN).

Complications

Early complications following renal transplantation may be general complications of major surgery, technical or immunological. The main immunological complications have been dealt with elsewhere in the chapter. Technical complications involve the vascular or ureteric anastomoses. Acute renal artery thrombosis is rare (incidence of approximately 1%), venous thrombosis has an incidence of 6%. Both must be recognized rapidly, using Doppler ultrasound, and require the patient to be returned to theatre immediately, if there is to be any chance of salvaging the transplant.

Urinary leaks occur less commonly now that ureteric stenting is adopted more widely: they present with falling urine output and increasing pain. They may be managed conservatively with prolonged urinary catheterization, but may require surgical intervention. Urinary tract obstruction can occur early or late. The diagnosis is confirmed by a percutaneous antegrade nephrostogram, during which a nephrostomy tube may be placed for temporary decompression. Subsequent percutaneous dilatation and insertion of a double J stent will often treat the stricture, with open surgery reserved for cases in which percutaneous management has failed.

Late vascular complications include renal artery stenosis, which occurs in 3–5% of patients and usually presents several months post-transplantation with hypertension and deteriorating graft function. The diagnosis is confirmed by angiography and the treatment of choice is angioplasty.

Fluid collections (lymphocoeles) around the transplant are a common finding on ultrasound scan but are only relevant if they become symptomatic or are causing urinary obstruction. Percutaneous drainage gives temporary symptomatic relief. Definitive management involves drainage of the lymphocoele into the peritoneal cavity and this fenestration can be performed laparoscopically.

Outcome

The 1-year renal graft survival is approximately 90% and patient survival exceeds this. However, there remains 2–5% perioperative mortality, as many renal patients have severe co-morbidity. The 5-year graft survival is around 70%, and at this time graft losses are commonly due to chronic allograft damage or to cardiovascular death in a patient with a functioning graft.

Recent developments in renal transplantation

The significant benefits that arise from living donor renal transplantation and the ongoing shortage of organs for donation have led to an expansion in renal transplant programmes to undertake higher risk transplants than would previously have been considered. In the United Kingdom the paired exchange programme has developed following changes in legislation in 2006. This programme exists for donor–recipient pairs who are unable to directly donate due to incompatibility, be it due to blood group or HLA incompatability, or to the presence of donor specific antibodies. Pairs are entered into the national programme to determine whether a paired exchange transplant is possible. These transplants are then undertaken in the two transplant centres simultaneously, and the kidneys are transported between centres.

In addition, an increasing number of ABO incompatible transplants are being performed across the United Kingdom. Recipients undergo a period of desensitisation, involving treatment with the anti-CD20 antibody, rituximab, and several rounds of plasma exchange. Anti-A or B antibody titres are monitored throughout treatment, and the transplant is performed when the titres are low. Despite the fact that the majority of recipients develop recurrent anti-A or B antibodies, antibody-mediated rejection is uncommon and the long-term results of ABO incompatible transplants are comparable to those that are compatible.

SUMMARY BOX 25.3

Renal transplantation

- Renal transplant is the optimal treatment for patients with end-stage renal failure, improving quality of life and survival compared with dialysis
- Renal transplantation is associated with 90% 1-year and 70% 5-year survival
- Chronic rejection remains a significant cause of late graft loss.

LIVER TRANSPLANTATION

Indications and patient assessment

The most effective therapy for end stage liver failure is liver transplantation. Patients with chronic liver failure who show signs of hepatic decompensation despite optimal medical management, those with certain forms of liver tumours or patients with acute liver failure should be referred to specialist liver transplant units. Signs of decompensation in chronic liver failure include oesophageal varices, ascites, infection including spontaneous bacterial peritonitis, all of which may be combined with poor synthetic liver function as demonstrated by hypoalbuminaemia, hyperbilirubinaemia and prolonged clotting times where the prothrombin time is prolonged over control. Indications for liver transplant are demonstrated in Table 25.8.

Table 25.8 Indications for liver transplant

Common indications in adults
- Alcoholic liver disease
- Hepatitis C
- Primary biliary cirrhosis
- Primary sclerosing cholangitis
- Hepatocellular carcinoma
- Autoimmune hepatitis
- Non-alcoholic steatohepatitis (fatty liver)
- Cryptogenic cirrhosis
- Acute liver failure e.g. paracetamol toxicity, drug reaction or virus

Rarer indications in adults
- Haemochromatosis
- Wilson's disease
- Alpha 1-antytripsin deficiency
- Budd-Chiari syndrome
- Polycystic disease
- Metabolic diseases (such as hyperoxaluria)

Common indications in children
- Biliary atresia
- Metabolic disorders including Alpha 1-antytripsin deficiency
- Wilson's disease
- Crigler–Najjar Type 1

Patient assessment must be undertaken by a multidisciplinary team comprising surgeons, hepatologists, specialist anaesthetists and, where the patient demonstrates addictive behaviour, a specialist psychiatrist. In general patients should be expected to have at least a 50% chance of surviving 5 years post-transplantation. Table 25.9 demonstrates the criteria used to decide whether someone should receive a liver transplant in fulminant hepatic failure. To help assess priority for organ allocation, the model for end stage liver disease (MELD) was developed in the United States. This was originally developed to assess the prognosis of cirrhotic patients who underwent treatment for portal hypertension. It has also been shown to predict short-term outcome in patients awaiting liver transplantation and therefore is used both in the US and, sometimes with modification, in other countries for identifying those patients most in need of liver transplant (Table 25.10).

Table 25.9 Criteria for liver transplantation in acute liver failure

Paracetamol toxicity
- pH < 7.3
- Prothrombin time > 100 seconds and creatinine > 300 μmol/l in patients with encephalopathy

Non-paracetamol toxicity
- Prothrombin time > 100 seconds (with encephalopathy)
- Any 3 of the following:
  age < 10 or > 40 years
  non-A/non-B hepatitis
  drug reaction or halothane hepatitis
  jaundice for > 7 days prior to encephalopathy
  prothrombin time > 50 seconds
  serum bilirubin > 300 μmol/l

25

Table 25.10 Equation for determining MELD score

MELD score =
3.8 loge (bilirubin mg/dl)
+ 11.2 loge (International Normalized Ratio)
+ 9.6 loge (creatinine mg/dl)
+ 6.4 (aetiology: 0 if cholestatic or alcoholic, 1 if otherwise)

Living donation for liver transplantation

The liver is a remarkable organ which is able to regenerate if liver resection is performed. This property has allowed for a portion of liver to be removed either from an adult's liver for a child or a larger portion removed to allow transplant into a small recipient. The first successful live donor liver transplant was done nearly 20 years ago, however this still remains a very controversial and complex area. Mortality in the donor is approximately 0.5% and risk of significant complications around 20%. Although this procedure has been accepted in a number of countries around the world, the extra risks both for donor and recipient make any decision to go ahead a very difficult one.

The operative procedure

The operation begins with preparation of the donor liver during 'back-table' dissection. All vessels are prepared and the liver examined carefully for any damage or underlying abnormality.

The recipient's abdomen is opened either through a 'Mercedes-Benz' incision or through a midline incision which is curved to the right following the line of the costal margin (Fig. 25.6). There are many variations to the liver transplant operation and in the most common (Fig. 25.7) the liver from the recipient is removed but leaving the inferior vena cava intact. The new liver is attached to the recipient by joining together the inferior vena cava of the donor liver with the inferior vena cava of the recipient. This is called a 'piggyback procedure' and accomplished by performing a side-to-side anastomosis between the two vena cava. This is then followed by portal venous and hepatic arterial anastomoses (Fig. 25.8). The liver is reperfused with recipient blood and haemostasis carried out carefully. The donor gallbladder is then removed and an end-to-end common bile duct to common bile duct anastomosis performed unless there is a specific indication to perform

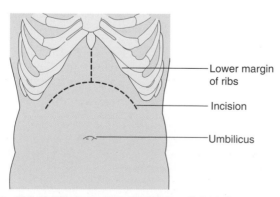

Fig. 25.6 The Mercedes-Benz incision for orthotopic liver transplantation.

Lower margin of ribs

Incision

Umbilicus

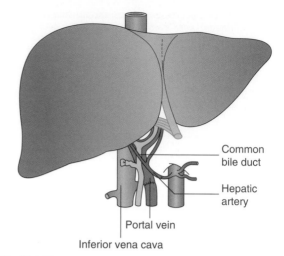

Fig. 25.7 Diagram demonstrating vascular and biliary anastomoses of a liver transplant.

Common bile duct

Hepatic artery

Portal vein

Inferior vena cava

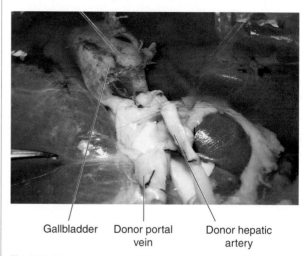

Gallbladder Donor portal vein Donor hepatic artery

Fig. 25.8 Hepatic artery anastomosis prior to reperfusion of liver.

a roux-en-Y hepaticojejunostomy (re-transplantation or primary sclerosing cholangitis in the recipient). Figure 25.9 shows a well-perfused liver following completion of the anastomoses.

Postoperative management and complications

Initially the patient tends to be managed in an intensive care setting and evidence of a functioning graft is based on the blood biochemistry of the recipient with falling blood lactate levels and return towards normal clotting signs of excellent function. Primary non-function or early dysfunction can occur and 2–5% of patients require urgent transplantation for non-function. As a liver transplant operation is a large procedure in patients with poor clotting, it is therefore very important to monitor the patients carefully for any evidence of bleeding. Re-exploration is often indicated. Vessel thrombosis, most commonly in the hepatic artery, can be detected on ultrasound and confirmed by arteriography. Suspicion of this serious complication necessitates re-exploration and it is possible that the patient may need a second transplant.

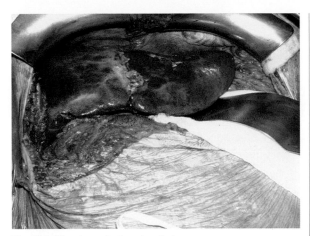

Fig. 25.9 Liver transplant postperfusion.

Rejection in the liver is much less common than with other organs for reasons which are not completely clear. Diagnosis of rejection is often made around day 7 with rising transaminases in the liver function tests. Biopsy may be performed to confirm the diagnosis and the rejection can be treated with daily boluses of methylprednisolone given over 3 days. It is rare, with modern immunosuppression, for acute rejection to cause complete failure of the graft.

Outcome

Many large single centre studies or information from registry data show that the 1-year survival for elective first liver transplant in adults is around 90%. European liver transplant registry data reports 5 years' survival post-liver transplantation in adults at 66%. In comparison patients with acute liver failure fare less well with approximately 70% surviving at 1 year. The vast majority of recipients report a very good quality of life but there remains the need, in most patients, to take immunosuppression in the long-term. In common with the recipients of other transplant organs, patients can experience nephrotoxicity and other side effects from immunosuppressive medication. However without the liver transplant procedure, the outcome would have been certain death and so this procedure remains one of the miracles of modern medicine.

SUMMARY BOX 25.4

Liver transplantation

- Liver transplantation is a potentially life-saving treatment for patients with acute or chronic liver failure
- Patients must undergo rigorous medical and psychosocial assessment prior to being listed for this major operation
- Outcome for patients following liver transplantation is excellent.

PANCREAS TRANSPLANTATION

Transplantation of the pancreas offers the only treatment that reliably offers insulin independence and normal glucose metabolism for patients with type I diabetes mellitus.

Islet cell transplantation may ultimately supersede solid-organ pancreas transplantation, but the latter remains the gold standard treatment.

Indications and patient assessment

Patients undergo pancreas transplant in three distinct clinical settings: simultaneous pancreas-kidney (SPK), pancreas after kidney (PAK) and pancreas transplant alone (PTA). SPK transplant is the most common, and will be considered in more detail here.

There is little doubt that diabetic patients with renal failure should be offered a kidney transplant if they are fit enough. The potential benefits of dual transplant include improved quality of life, with insulin independence, halting of the progress of diabetic complications and improved life expectancy. But this comes with significantly increased risk in terms of perioperative morbidity and mortality, with the potential for the pancreas transplant to adversely affect the outcome of the renal transplant.

Thus careful recipient selection is essential: cardiovascular co-morbidity is the most important factor leading to postoperative mortality, and may not be apparent in the history. Generally accepted indications for SPK transplant are inadequate glucose control by medical management alone, hypoglycaemic unawareness and 'brittle diabetes', where extremely high or low blood glucose levels are precipitated by minor dietary modifications. Contraindications are systemic sepsis, malignancy and significant medical co-morbidity. Significant aortoiliac disease is a relative contraindication.

Insulin resistance is a relative contraindication and should be suspected in obese patients, those with late-onset diabetes or those requiring high insulin doses. Thorough assessment of these patients is essential as the majority have ESRF.

It is important to counsel patients and relatives that a pancreas transplant is a major undertaking and one that is life-enhancing rather than life-saving, as in the case of a liver transplant. Most patients will require a simultaneous renal transplant and the results for such combined transplants are better than for solitary pancreas.

The operative procedure

Back table preparation

The pancreas is retrieved en bloc with the spleen, and this is carefully excised on the back table, paying careful attention to the ligation and division of the vessels. The c of duodenum is carefully reduced and the ends both stapled and oversewn to avoid leakage. An arterial conduit is created: a Y graft is formed using donor iliac vessels onto the donor splenic and superior mesenteric vessels (Fig. 25.10). Figure 25.11 illustrates a pancreas graft just before implantation and shows the vascular reconstruction that is performed on the back table.

Recipient operation

In SPK transplantation, the pancreas implantation is usually performed first due to the ischaemic intolerance of the pancreas relative to the kidney, and it is implanted intraperitoneally into the right side. The venous anastomosis is performed between donor portal vein and the distal inferior vena cava, and the arterial conduit constructed on the back table is anastomosed to the recipient common iliac artery.

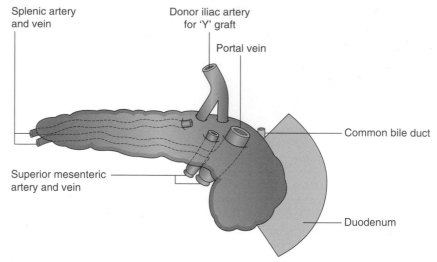

Fig. 25.10 Back table preparation of the pancreas graft. Showing arterial Y graft using donor iliac vessels onto superior mesenteric and splenic arteries to create a single arterial conduit for anastomosis.

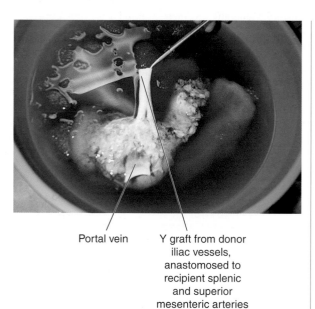

Fig. 25.11 Pancreas graft showing interposition Y graft prior to implantation.

Table 25.11 **Complications of pancreas transplantation**
Infective complications
Systemic infection (opportunistic infections)
Local infections (peritonitis, localized collections, fistulae)
Vascular complications
Haemorrhage: early or late
Thrombosis: arterial or venous thrmobosis
Allograft pancreatitis
Ischaemia-reperfusion injury
Reflux pancreatitis

Reperfusion of the pancreas usually results in some haemorrhage, which has to be controlled with careful suture ligation of the small pericapsular vessels. Drainage of the exocrine secretions is achieved by a simple entero-enterostomy between donor duodenum and recipient small bowel.

Postoperative management and complications

Patients are often managed in the Intensive Care Unit postoperatively, where close monitoring and early identification of postoperative complications are likely to improve early outcome.

Pancreas transplantation is associated with a higher incidence and a greater range of complications than kidney transplant, due to a requirement for greater immunosuppression, in a high-risk diabetic population who have impaired infection resistance, poor healing and high levels of co-morbidity. Between one-fifth and one-quarter of patients require relaparotomy in the early postoperative period. Complications of pancreas transplant are outlined in Table 25.11. Risk factors for complications include increasing donor age, prolonged preservation time and donor and recipient obesity.

Rejection of a pancreas transplant alone has been notoriously difficult to diagnose, with no reliable early markers available. In SPK transplants, the diagnosis of rejection relies on monitoring renal function and undertaking renal biopsy when indicated. Acute rejection of the pancreas affects exocrine function first and gives rise to an inflammatory response, which may well be masked by the immunosuppressive regimen. Dysfunction of islets occurs as a late sign of rejection, which may then be less amenable to treatment.

Outcome

There has been considerable improvement in the 1-year patient and graft survival following pancreas transplant over the last decade, with 95% patient survival, 82% survival of the pancreas grafts and 92% of kidney grafts. There is 89% patient survival at 5 years, making it comparable to other solid organ transplants, There is increasing evidence to suggest that pancreas transplantation has a favourable influence on diabetic complications and survival prospects.

Pancreas transplantation

- Combined kidney and pancreas transplantation is an excellent treatment for a carefully selected group of patients with type 1 diabetes mellitus
- Patients must undergo rigorous medical evaluation prior to being listed, as they have complicated diabetic disease
- Pancreas rejection is difficult to diagnose and this may lead to delay in initiating therapy for such episodes
- Despite this, combined kidney-pancreas transplant is associated with a 5-year survival of 70%.

PANCREATIC ISLET TRANSPLANTATION

Transplantation of islets alone offers an attractive alternative to whole pancreas transplantation and is associated with less serious morbidity. There is no doubt that islet transplantation can be effective. It has been shown to have led to long-term insulin independence in a small number of patients and in other patients, it renders their diabetic control more predictable to manage with reduced insulin requirements. One challenge that needs to be overcome is the requirement for several pancreata in order to isolate sufficient islets to treat one patient.

HEART AND LUNG TRANSPLANTATION

Indications and patient assessment

Heart

The reasons for undertaking heart transplants are to prolong life and improve its quality. The indications for heart transplant have not changed in recent years: the main indications are coronary-related heart failure (38%) and cardiomyopathies (45%). Other indications include valvular disease, adult congenital abnormalities and miscellaneous diagnoses account for the rest. Children can be treated as successfully as adults, although the shortage of suitable paediatric donors is limiting.

Potential candidates for heart transplant are patients with advanced heart failure who are on maximal medical therapy, including vasodilators, digoxin, diuretics and β-blockers. Patients should be considered if they have increasing medication requirements, frequent hospitalizations or overall deterioration in clinical status.

Contraindications to heart transplant include:

- factors that increase perioperative mortality, such as irreversible pulmonary hypertension, active sepsis, severe obesity
- factors affecting long-term prognosis, such as age > 65 years, severe renal impairment, active or recent malignancy, other major co-morbidity
- factors that impair compliance such as active mental illness, recent drug abuse refractory to treatment.

Lung

The lung has been the most challenging of the human organs to be transplanted in clinical practice. Lungs may be transplanted singly or sequentially as a bilateral lung transplant. Indications include chronic obstructive pulmonary disease (35%), cystic fibrosis (CF) (15%) and pulmonary fibrosis (16%). Bilateral lung transplant is indicated when all native lung must be removed, e.g. when it is a significant source of sepsis, as in CF. Single lung transplantation is an attractive option for the treatment of lung failure, as it can be performed with reduced risk of acute lung injury and without the requirement for cardiopulmonary bypass.

The operative procedure

Heart

Cold ischaemic time must be kept to a minimum in cardiac transplantation, such that the recipient operation may be commenced once the donor heart has been visualized and assessed for suitability. The operation is undertaken via a midline sternotomy. Cardiopulmonary bypass is established, the patient cooled to 32°C, and the heart is removed. The donor heart is prepared for implantation. Donor and recipient atria are anastomosed, followed by the aortic anastomosis. Heart reperfusion is a critical time. The heart usually starts to beat and if ventricular fibrillation occurs, the heart is promptly defibrillated. Reperfusion is followed by the pulmonary arterial, inferior and superior vena caval anastomoses. Once the implantation is complete the body temperature is brought back to 37°C. Cardioversion and temporary pacing may be required.

Lung

Lung transplantation similarly requires a short cold ischaemic time. For a single lung transplant, a lateral thoracotomy is performed and the native lung is excised with ligation of inferior and superior pulmonary veins and pulmonary artery. The bronchus is divided and the native organ removed. The pericardium is now incised and the pulmonary veins and artery are mobilized for subsequent anastomoses.

Implantation starts with the bronchial anastomosis, followed by the left atrial and pulmonary arterial anastomoses. Ventilation of the new lung commences.

Postoperative management and complications

Heart

The principles of early postoperative management of heart transplant recipients are to maintain graft function, specifically to recognize and manage right ventricular impairment, to establish adequate immunosuppression, to prevent and treat early infections and to allow the recovery of other organs, such as the kidneys.

Most patients have impaired myocardial function requiring inotropic support for the first 24–48 hours. Some patients develop ventricular dysfunction, which requires supportive management with inotropes.

Routine endocardial biopsies are taken from the right ventricle of heart transplant recipients using X-ray screening and right internal jugular venous access. If rejection is confirmed, augmentation of immunosuppression is carried out. Rejection can also cause rapidly progressive coronary artery disease, with thickening and narrowing of the coronary arteries. Because the donor heart is denervated, the patient will not experience angina, and therefore coronary angiography is performed annually from 2 years onwards.

25

The most common causes of 30-day mortality following heart transplant are graft failure (41%), non-CMV infection (14%) and multiorgan failure (14%). Beyond 5 years, cardiac allograft vasculopathy, and late graft failure are the commonest causes of death. Malignancies are increasingly common after 10 years.

Lungs

Apical and basal chest drains are placed perioperatively and patients are managed in the ITU for monitoring and care.

Infection is a major cause of postoperative morbidity in the lung transplant patient. Antibiotic prophylaxis with flucloxacillin and metronidazole is commenced and adjusted as microbiological results from donor and recipient samples become available.

Postoperative acute lung injury, occurring as a result of reperfusion injury, causes problems with ventilation, requiring meticulous supportive management of fluids, optimization of ventilation and microbiology. Another life threatening complication of lung transplantation is dehiscence of the tracheal or bronchial anastomosis, with prolonged air leak and mediastinitis.

Transbronchial biopsies are performed regularly in the weeks and months post-transplant to diagnose rejection, which can be treated in the standard fashion.

Combined heart and lung transplant

Combined heart and lung transplant was the commonest form of lung transplant, but its use has declined significantly over the last 15 years. Indications for the combined procedure are now confined to pulmonary hypertension without congenital heart disease. The operation is performed via a median sternotomy, and requires cardiopulmonary bypass. The results are similar to lung transplantation, with survival at 1 and 5 years of 60% and 40% respectively.

Outcome

Survival following heart transplant is approximately 65% at 5 years, 50% at 10 years and 30% at 15 years. The success of cardiac transplantation, as is the case with other solid organ transplants, has raised expectations that cannot be fulfilled, with the shortage of organs for donation and the death rate on the cardiac transplant waiting list is high. The 5-year survival of lung transplant recipients is close to 50%, and 25% after a decade.

SUMMARY

Solid organ transplantation provides excellent treatment for patients with end-stage organ failure, with 1-year graft survival exceeding 80% for most organs. The advantage of transplantation must be weighed against the price of immunosuppression and it is important that potential recipients are fully counselled. One of the greatest challenges facing transplantation is the shortage of organs for donation and this chapter has described specific strategies aimed at combating this: namely, use of marginal donors, living donors and donors after cardiac death.

SUMMARY BOX 25.6

Heart-lung transplantation

- Ischaemic heart disease and cardiomyopathy are the most common indications for heart transplant
- Both heart and lung transplantation require short cold ischaemic times in comparison with intra-abdominal organs
- Outcomes following heart and lung transplantation are similar to those seen following transplantation of intra-abdominal organs.

J.A. Wilson

26

Ear, nose and throat surgery

EAR

Anatomy

External ear

The pinna (Fig. 26.1) is made of fibroelastic cartilage. The external auditory meatus has an outer cartilage portion; the inner part is formed by the tympanic bone (Fig. 26.2). It is lined by squamous epithelium and contains ceruminous glands that produce wax. There is very little subcutaneous tissue and soft tissue swelling is very painful.

Middle ear

The vibrating tympanic membrane is conical and attached to the margin of the bony ear canal laterally and to the handle of the malleus, the first of the three ossicles, medially (Fig. 26.2). The head of the malleus is attached to the body of the incus in the space superior to the middle ear known as the attic. The long process of the incus attaches to the head of the stapes via its lenticular process. The stapes is joined to the oval window margin by the annular ligament. The middle ear is lined by simple cuboidal epithelium containing some mucus-secreting cells. The middle ear space is connected to the nasopharynx by the Eustachian tube, which maintains the middle ear at atmospheric pressure.

The inner ear

The inner ear membrane encloses a labyrinth filled by a fluid called endolymph. This is surrounded by a bony labyrinth, the otic capsule, which is filled with perilymph. The cochlea, the hearing component of the inner ear, is a tube linking the oval and round windows, coiled up like a shell. The vestibular (balance) portion of the inner ear consists of three semicircular canals, together with their vestibule, which contains the saccule and utricle, medial to the stapes footplate. The cochlear

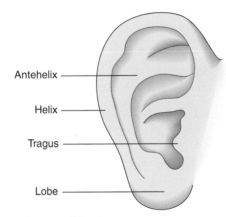

Fig. 26.1 Anatomy of the pinna.

Antehelix

Helix

Tragus

Lobe

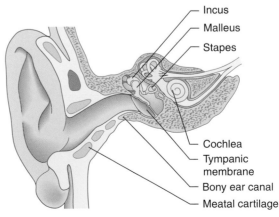

Fig. 26.2 Anatomy of the ear.

Incus

Malleus

Stapes

Cochlea

Tympanic membrane

Bony ear canal

Meatal cartilage

and vestibular nerves combine in the internal auditory meatus and pass medially to the brainstem. The facial nerve enters the temporal bone through the internal auditory meatus and passes laterally to the geniculate ganglion, where it turns posteriorly (the first genu). It passes through the middle ear above the oval window and turns inferiorly (the second genu) to exit at the stylomastoid foramen.

Physiology

The pinna funnels sound into the ear canal. The tympanic membrane lever mechanism, the ossicular lever mechanism and the large size of the drum relative to the stapes footplate act as an impedance-matching transformer. Vibrations in air are thus transferred to the cochlear fluids without excessive loss of energy. The cochlea converts these endolymph vibrations into electrical impulses in the auditory nerve, by stimulation of hair cells in the organ of Corti. The maximum response to high frequencies occurs in the basal turn of the cochlea. Low frequencies maximally stimulate the apex. Auditory neurons connect via the brainstem to the auditory cortex, where again different groups of cells are stimulated by nerve impulses coded for different frequencies. The hair cells in the ampullae of the semicircular canals are stimulated by angular acceleration. The saccule and utricle are stimulated by linear acceleration. Information from the labyrinths, eyes and limbs is combined within the brainstem. Connections from the vestibular nuclei pass to the cortex and the cerebellum (Fig. 26.3).

Assessment

Clinical features

Disorders of the external or middle ear can impair sound transmission to the inner ear and cause conductive deafness. Sensorineural deafness results from lesions of the cochlea or its nerve. Deafness is often associated with a noise in the ear (tinnitus). Ear pain (otalgia) may be due to ear disease but may also be referred from other sites (Table 26.1). Ear-related disorders of balance usually cause a sensation of movement (vertigo), most often rotation. 'Unsteadiness' however, typically has a non-otological cause. Patients with ear disease occasionally fall to the ground but never lose consciousness.

Table 26.1 Causes of referred otalgia
Pharynx and larynx   • Tonsillitis   • Tonsillectomy   • Tumours
Mouth   • Dental disease   • Tumour
Temporomandibular joints (TMJ)   • TMJ dysfunction   • Arthritis
Neck   • Cervical spondylosis   • Tumour
Paranasal sinuses   • Maxillary sinusitis

Examination

The ear canal and tympanic membrane are inspected with an otoscope, a rigid telescope or a microscope. Microscopy can assist in wax or discharge removal. Tuning fork tests differentiate between conductive and sensorineural hearing loss (Rinne's test). In health or sensorineural deafness, a tuning fork is heard better via the ear canal (air conduction) than via the mastoid process (bone conduction). When there is a conductive hearing loss, the tuning fork is heard better by bone conduction. When hearing is symmetrical, a tuning fork placed in the centre of the forehead is heard equally well in both ears (Weber's test). If a conductive hearing loss is present in one ear, the tuning fork is heard better in the deaf ear if the loss is conductive which can be easily shown by occluding one ear and applying the fork to your own head. Conversely, in a unilateral sensorineural deafness, the sound is louder in the good ear.

Audiometry

Hearing by air conduction can be assessed by pure tone audiometry, in which sounds of known pitch and loudness are presented to each ear in turn via headphones. Bone conduction (cochlear function) can be separately tested by applying sounds to the mastoid process. A masking tone is needed if the two cochleae are to be tested separately. The difference between the air and bone conduction gives the level of conductive hearing loss (Figures 26.4 and 26.5). The patient's ability to hear speech can be tested by presenting lists of words via headphones. The percentage correctly identified at different loudness levels allows derivation of a speech reception threshold (50% of words correct) and a discrimination score. Middle ear function (compliance) can be assessed by tympanometry. The amount of sound from a probe reflected back from the drum is measured while the pressure in the ear canal is made to vary. The compliance is maximal when the pressure in the ear canal equals the pressure in the middle ear, because when pressure is the same on both sides of the drum it is maximally mobile. Tympanometry is most often used to confirm the presence of fluid in the middle ear.

Temporal bone imaging

In patients with unilateral sensorineural hearing loss, MRI is used to detect an acoustic neuroma (Fig. 26.6). MRI also demonstrates the presence of normal fluid in the cochlea

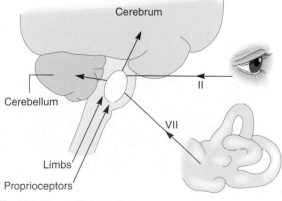

Fig. 26.3 The vestibular system.

Cerebrum

Cerebellum

II

VII

Limbs

Proprioceptors

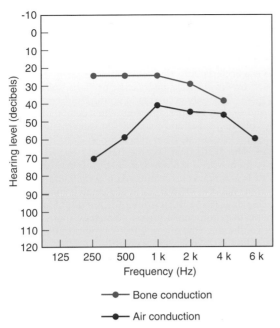

Fig. 26.4 Audiogram showing conductive deafness.

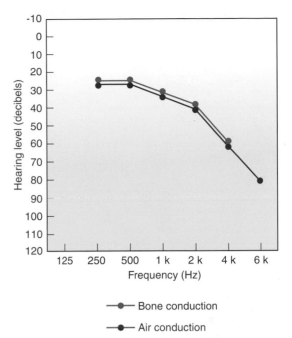

Fig. 26.5 Audiogram showing sensorineural deafness.

before attempting cochlear implantation. CT scans can be used to demonstrate temporal bone anatomy, congenital abnormalities and fractures or unusual pathology.

Diseases of the pinna

Bat ears

A developmental abnormality results in absence of the anti-helical fold (see Fig. 26.1). This produces prominent ears that cause embarrassment. The abnormality can be corrected surgically.

Trauma

Trauma to the ear may result in a haematoma, which strips the perichondrium off the underlying cartilage. Secondary infection may lead to loss of cartilage, resulting in a 'cauliflower ear'. Haematomas should therefore be drained under strict aseptic conditions.

Tumours

Basal cell and squamous carcinomas may occur on the pinna and require excision (Fig. 26.7).

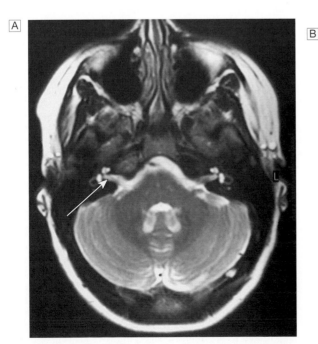

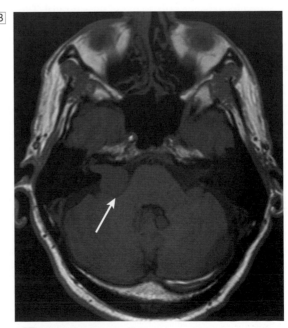

Fig. 26.6 Magnetic resonance imaging (MRI) of the cerebellopontine angle. [A] Normal MRI scan of cerebellopontine angle. Thin arrow = IAM (internal auditory meatus). [B] MRI showing an acoustic neuroma. Thick arrow = lesion compressing cerebellum.

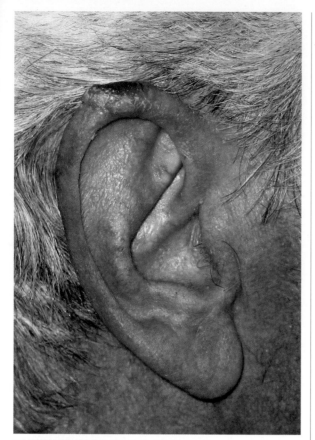

Fig. 26.7 Squamous carcinoma of the pinna.

Diseases of the external auditory meatus

Wax

Wax (cerumen) is normally found in the ear canal. The ear canal has a migratory epithelium that carries wax to the opening of the external auditory meatus. Wax seldom causes deafness, unless it becomes packed against the eardrum.

Otitis externa

This is an inflammatory condition of the ear canal skin. Secondary infection with bacteria or, less frequently, fungi may occur. It is managed by cleaning the ear, followed by local treatment with eardrops, sprays or ointment containing a steroid, with or without antiseptic, or a weak acid solution (which controls the typical causative anaerobic organisms). Adults tend to develop skin sensitivities to the components of topical antibiotic preparations – which are thus best avoided. Antibiotics also predispose to fungal superinfection. Both phenomena simply exacerbate the severity of this painful condition. Keeping water out of the ear with Vaseline-coated plugs helps prevent any recurrence. Uncommonly, chronic otitis externa causes stenosis of the ear canal.

Tumours

Squamous carcinoma of the ear canal occurs uncommonly. It is treated by a combination of surgery and radiotherapy.

Diseases of the middle ear

Acute suppurative otitis media

This is a bacterial infection of the middle ear space, usually caused by *Streptococcus pneumoniae* or *Haemophilus influenzae*, most commonly occurring in young children (3 years of age and under). Children present with a combination of ear pain (otalgia), fever and malaise. On examination, dilated blood vessels are seen on the drum surface in the early stages. The drum then becomes red and begins to bulge. Perforation with discharge frequently occurs, usually followed by spontaneous healing. Antibiotic therapy remains controversial: the majority of cases resolve spontaneously in a few days (EBM 26.1). Antibiotics are useful in high risk patients (e.g. immunosuppression) as they shorten the episodes and reduce the rate of infective complications such as mastoiditis, facial palsy or meningitis.

EBM 26.1 Antibiotics for acute otitis media in children

'Clinicians need to evaluate whether the minimal short-term benefit from longer treatment of antibiotics is worth exposing children to a longer course of antibiotics.'

Kozyrskyj et al. Short-course antibiotics for acute otitis media. Cochrane Database of Systematic Reviews 2010, Issue 9. Art. No.: CD001095. DOI: 10.1002/14651858.CD001095.pub2

For further information: www.cochrane.org

Otitis media with effusion (OME), or 'glue ear'

In this condition, fluid accumulates in the middle ear space, usually in children. A minority of adult cases are caused by nasopharyngeal tumours and systemic disease. Childhood OME causes hearing loss and may interfere with the acquisition of language and performance at school. Virtually all cases resolve spontaneously, but this may take as long as 10 years. Initial management involves documentation of the presence of effusion and the degree of hearing loss during a period of watchful waiting. If the effusions persist, hearing may be improved by drainage of the effusion (myringotomy) and insertion of a ventilation tube (Fig. 26.8). In children, removal of the adenoids leads to more effective resolution. Spontaneous resolution may also occur in adults, but often effusions persist. Ventilation tubes can also be of value, but some cases are better managed with a hearing aid.

Chronic suppurative otitis media

This causes aural discharge and deafness.

Tubotympanic or mucosal disease

This is characterized by the presence of a perforation of the tympanic membrane, which typically discharges. Swimming and other activities that involve water entering the ear may exacerbate the discharge. The hearing loss is worse when the ossicles are eroded, most commonly the incus long process. Discharge can be controlled by cleaning the ear and introducing eardrops. To minimize the risks of ototoxicity, drops should be used for a maximum of 2 weeks. Surgery is indicated to prevent discharge, improve hearing or allow the patient to swim. The operation to repair a perforation is called a myringoplasty. Defects of the ossicular chain can be repaired by removing the incus and repositioning it to bridge the gap between the malleus and stapes or by using a prosthesis (ossiculoplasty).

Atticoantral or squamous disease

A cholesteatoma forms as a retracted area of the drum in which keratin accumulates. The drum tissue at the periphery of the cholesteatoma produces a number of chemical mediators that stimulate osteoclast activity. Hence the cholesteatoma can erode surrounding bone and cause complications such as disruption of the ossicular chain, facial palsy and intracranial sepsis. The primary treatment goal is to eliminate the disease. Surgical treatment (mastoidectomy) is mandatory in all but the very elderly and those who are medically unfit.

SUMMARY BOX 26.1

Otitis media

- Acute otitis media is extremely common under the age of 3 years
- The child typically awakes crying at night with a painful ear. The diagnosis is confirmed by a red, inflamed bulging tympanic membrane on otoscopy
- Pain relief is important. Antibiotics should be given to prevent the development of complications
- Otitis media with effusion (glue ear) occurs transiently in many children and is manifested by temporary hearing impairment. Most cases settle spontaneously. Bilateral persistent hearing impairment may demand surgery (adenoidectomy, or insertion of a grommet)
- Chronic otitis media involves the middle ear and mastoid mucosa. There is permanent perforation of the tympanic membrane, hearing loss and a mucopurulent discharge. Inactive ears require closure of the perforated membrane (myringoplasty) and rebuilding of the ossicular chain. Ears with cholesteatoma may require surgical removal of the posterior canal wall to open the attic or mastoid cavity and so reduce the risk of meningitis, intracranial abscess and facial palsy.

Otosclerosis

This is a condition in which the stapes becomes fixed by new bone formation. It is more common in females and sometimes runs in families. It can be treated by an operation called stapedectomy, in which the stapes is replaced by a piston attached to the incus. This produces excellent hearing improvement in the majority of patients, but a minority suffer surgically-induced, permanent inner ear damage. The hearing loss can be managed with a hearing aid.

Diseases of the inner ear

Deafness

Deafness is most commonly due to changes in the cochlea. Ageing produces a gradual deterioration in hearing acuity (presbycusis). The cochlea may be damaged by chronic noise exposure, blast injuries and temporal bone fractures. Significant noise exposure may occur in heavy industry and agriculture, from playing in rock bands and shooting. Deafness may also be inherited or a manifestation of systemic disease. Some drugs, such as aminoglycosides and cytotoxic agents like cisplatinum, can damage the cochlea. Viral infections such as mumps and rubella can also cause sensorineural deafness. Unilateral hearing loss occurs in acoustic neuroma (Fig. 26.6B).

Most cases of inner ear deafness are managed with a hearing aid, but in cases of profound deafness, hearing may be restored by a cochlear implant. This consists of a series of electrodes surgically introduced into the cochlea. A speech processor converts sound into electrical energy, which stimulates the cochlear nerve.

Vertigo

In some cases, balance disorders may arise from abnormalities of the vestibular portion of the inner ear.

Benign paroxysmal positional vertigo is a very common condition in middle age and is due to debris floating in the posterior semicircular canal which stimulates the ampulla hair cells, producing vertigo. Episodes are triggered when the affected ear is down-most – as when the patient turns over in bed. Debris can be displaced therapeutically from the posterior canal by positioning the head so that it floats out of the canal into the vestibule (Epley's particle repositioning

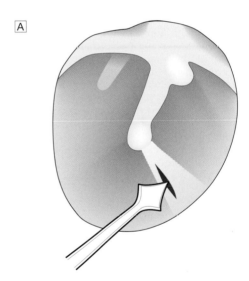

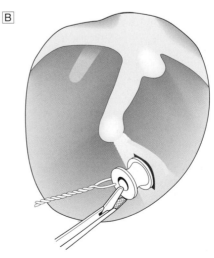

Fig. 26.8 Surgical treatment of otitis media with effusion.
A Myringotomy. B Grommet insertion.

26

manoeuvre). If this fails, division of the ampullary (singular) nerve or occlusion of the posterior semicircular canal is beneficial.

Vestibular neuronitis causes severe vertigo lasting for as long as several weeks. The hearing remains normal. It is due to severe temporary reduction of vestibular function in the affected ear. Patients are managed by bed rest and vestibular sedatives, such as prochlorperazine.

Abnormal fluctuations of fluid pressure within the inner ear (endolymphatic hydrops) produce a combination of fluctuating deafness, tinnitus and vertigo known as Ménière's disease. This uncommon condition is initially treated medically, using either a vasodilator agent (e.g. betahistine) or a diuretic. If medical treatment fails, the vestibular portion of the labyrinth may be destroyed by a middle ear injection of gentamicin. Procedures of last resort are surgical destruction of the labyrinth, or section of the vestibular nerve.

Disorders of the facial nerve

Facial palsy may result from temporal bone fractures or surgical trauma. When the nerve is divided, it may be repaired by end-to-end anastomosis or a cable graft derived from a sensory nerve of the right size, such as the sural nerve. Bell's palsy is an idiopathic (lower motor neuron) facial palsy that usually improves spontaneously. There is some evidence that it is caused by viral infection. Steroid therapy given soon after the onset is beneficial. Herpes zoster infection of the geniculate ganglion causes facial palsy, often associated with deafness and vertigo (Ramsay–Hunt syndrome). Vesicles may be seen on the palate and on the tympanic membrane. Antiviral treatment appears helpful for Ramsay–Hunt syndrome (unlike Bell's palsy). Intracranial disease and malignant tumours in the parotid area of the neck can also cause facial palsy.

NOSE

Anatomy

The nasal skeleton consists of two nasal bones superiorly and two pairs of cartilages inferiorly (Fig. 26.9). The nasal cavity is divided in two by a partition composed of cartilage anteriorly and bone posteriorly (the nasal septum). Three turbinate bones protrude from the lateral wall of the nose (Fig. 26.10). Between the inferior and middle turbinates is the middle meatus of the nose. Most of the paranasal sinuses open into this area under cover of a soft tissue flap known as the uncinate process. Obstruction of the sinus ostia in this area can cause sinus pain and may lead to sinus infection. Superior to the superior turbinate is an area of olfactory epithelium from which arise the nerve fibres of the olfactory nerve. The anterior portion of the nasal septum is called Little's area. Here prominent veins are often found, and nose bleeds most often arise from this part of the nose.

Physiology

The functions of the nose are to filter, warm and moisten inspired air. Olfaction is important in its own right and as an adjunct to taste.

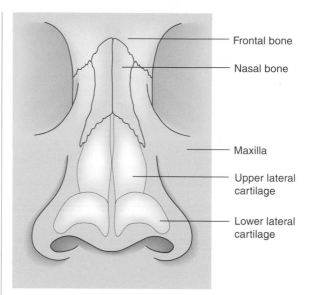

Fig. 26.9 Anatomy of the nasal skeleton.

Frontal bone

Nasal bone

Maxilla

Upper lateral cartilage

Lower lateral cartilage

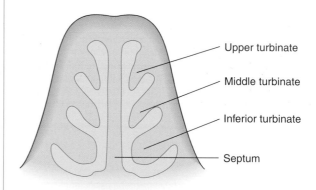

Fig. 26.10 Anatomy of the nasal cavity.

Upper turbinate

Middle turbinate

Inferior turbinate

Septum

Assessment

Clinical features

Nasal obstruction is a common symptom with a number of causes. Sneezing and rhinorrhoea are generally due to chronic rhinitis. Purulent nasal discharge and facial pain occur in sinusitis. Loss of smell may be due either to nasal blockage that prevents odours reaching the olfactory epithelium or to damage of the olfactory nerves. Smell is an important part of taste and reduced taste is therefore usually also reported by patients with anosmia.

Examination

The nasal cavity can be inspected using a nasal speculum or an otoscope. More detailed examination, particularly of the posterior part of the nose, is carried out with a rigid telescope.

Imaging

Imaging is not required if nasendoscopy is normal. Images are useful preoperatively to give the surgeon a guide as to individual variations especially in the areas of potential hazard – orbital wall, floor of the anterior cranial fossa (skull base) and to minimize the risk of complications.

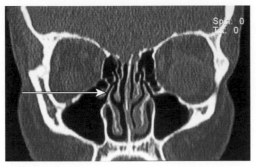

Fig. 26.11 Coronal CT scan sinuses. The narrow maxillary ostia and uncinate processes are seen on this cut (arrow), lateral to the middle turbinate.

Computed tomography (CT) is the best means of imaging the paranasal sinuses and also gives information about the middle meatus of the nose, where the sinus ostia are situated (Fig. 26.11). The sinuses can also be visualized by magnetic resonance imaging (MRI), but the bony anatomy is not shown and mucosal disease is exaggerated.

Diseases of the nose

Trauma

This may result in fracture and displacement of the nasal bones. If the fracture is not reduced within 14 days, it is usually fixed and hard to mobilize. There may also be displacement and fracture of the septal cartilage and bone (deviated nasal septum, Fig. 26.12). Corrective septoplasty surgery requires a post-trauma interval of 3 months to allow for soft tissue repair prior to surgery. Bleeding into the septum causes a septal haematoma, resulting in severe nasal obstruction. This should be drained under aseptic conditions, to prevent a septal abscess and collapse of the bridge.

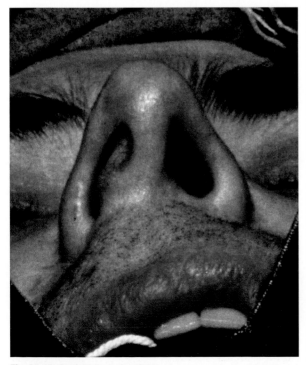

Fig. 26.12 Deviated nasal septum.

Chronic rhinitis

Some cases are due to allergy to aeroallergens (pollen or dust). Otherwise, it seems to be a reaction to environmental conditions such as temperature and humidity. It may be seasonal (usually summer) or perennial. Patients complain of nasal blockage that often switches from side to side, sneezing and rhinorrhoea. Most cases are best managed medically with a steroid nasal spray. In severe cases with nasal obstruction, reduction of the inferior or middle turbinates may provide relief.

Nasal polyps

Oedematous paranasal sinus mucosa extrudes through sinus ostia to produce nasal polyps. Most are multiple swellings from the ethmoid sinuses. Rarely, there is a single posterior protrusion from the maxillary sinus (antrochoanal polyp). Unilateral disease is usually defined by a prebiopsy CT (Fig. 26.13). Temporary improvement in the resulting nasal obstruction can be produced by topical or systemic steroids. As most polyps eventually recur following excision, many patients opt for periodic courses of steroid therapy, and only resort to surgery when symptoms get out of hand. Endoscopic clearance is facilitated by use of the microdebrider (Fig. 26.14).

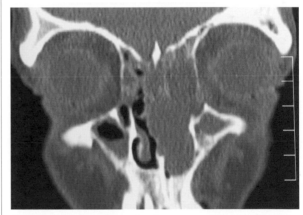

Fig. 26.13 Coronal CT scan showing gross unilateral (left) nasal 'polyp' (arrowed).

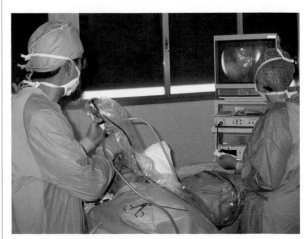

Fig. 26.14 Set-up for endoscopic sinus surgery, with the surgeon viewing the surgical field on a television monitor.

26

Epistaxis

Nose bleeds may be associated with a number of disease processes (Table 26.2). They are common in healthy children and young adults. Bleeding usually arises from Little's area and can be controlled by squeezing the nose (Fig. 26.15). In the elderly, more severe bleeding from further back in the nose may occur. In these cases, a nasal pack may be required to arrest the bleeding. Bleeding may be associated with the use of non-steroidal anti-inflammatory drugs (NSAIDs) or other antithrombotic therapy in this group. Severe bleeding not controlled by a pack can be arrested by clipping either the sphenopalatine, anterior ethmoid or maxillary artery.

Table 26.2 Diseases associated with epistaxis

Bleeding disorders
- Haemophilia
- Thrombocytopenia
- Von Willebrand's disease
- Excessive anticoagulation (e.g. with warfarin)

Systemic disease
- Liver disease
- Renal disease
- Hypertension
- Hereditary haemorrhagic telangiectasia

SUMMARY BOX 26.2

Epistaxis

- Epistaxis in young patients usually arises from a small blood vessel in Little's area; in older individuals, it arises from an arteriosclerotic vessel located more posteriorly
- Pressure on Little's area by compressing the anterior septum usually stops the bleeding, and topical 1 in 1000 adrenaline (epinephrine) on cotton wool may be helpful
- Bleeding more posteriorly may require balloon compression or packing
- Coagulation defects should always be excluded. Some of these will be caused by alcohol or non-steroidal analgesics
- In persistent epistaxis, it may be necessary to clip an artery e.g. the sphenopalatine.

PARANASAL SINUSES

Anatomy

The paranasal sinuses are air-filled cavities that open into the nasal cavity, mostly into the middle meatus of the nose. The maxillary sinuses occupy the cheeks (Fig. 26.16) and have ostia quite high in the sinus wall. The ethmoid labyrinth consists of a number of air cells lying between the orbit and the lateral wall of the nose. The frontal sinus is an ethmoid air cell that has migrated into the frontal bone, and it is connected to the nose via the frontonasal duct, which passes down to the middle meatus. The sphenoid sinus is posterior to the ethmoid labyrinth, inferior to the pituitary fossa.

Diseases of the paranasal sinuses

Sinusitis

Any of the sinuses may become infected, but the most commonly involved is the maxillary sinus. The site of the pain caused by sinusitis depends on which sinus it arises from. Pain arising from the maxillary sinus is felt in the cheek, that from the ethmoid labyrinth over the nasal bridge, and frontal sinus pain in the forehead. Sphenoid sinus pain is said to be maximal at the vertex. Acute sinusitis is most commonly caused by *Strep. pneumoniae* or *Haemophilus influenzae* and typically follows an upper respiratory infection. Gram-negative organisms may cause sinusitis related to a dental abscess. In some parts of the world, fungal infection is not uncommon.

Acute sinusitis is usually managed medically. Chronic sinusitis may result from failure of resolution of acute infection or may arise insidiously. Surgical treatment is frequently required and includes enlargement of the natural ostium of the maxillary sinus, often with clearance of infected ethmoid cells. Frontal and sphenoid sinusitis are much less common. Infection may spread from the sinuses, usually the ethmoid or frontal sinuses, to involve other areas such as the cranial cavity or orbit (Fig. 26.17).

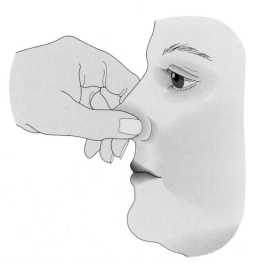

Fig. 26.15 Stopping epistaxis by squeezing the nose.

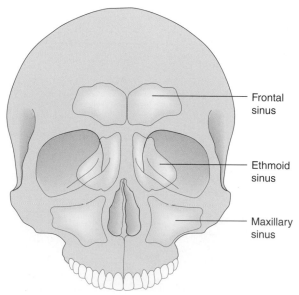

Frontal sinus

Ethmoid sinus

Maxillary sinus

Fig. 26.16 Anatomy of the paranasal sinuses.

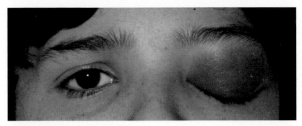

Fig. 26.17 Orbital cellulitis.

Tumours

The most common malignant neoplasm found in the paranasal sinuses is squamous carcinoma, but adenocarcinomas are seen in workers in the furniture industry, and numerous rare tumour types are also recognized. The most common sites of origin are the maxillary and ethmoid sinuses. Unfortunately, the disease has often spread beyond the primary site at presentation (Fig. 26.18). These relatively

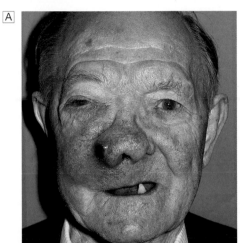

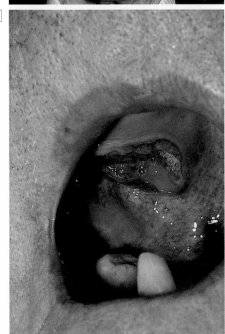

Fig. 26.18 Spread of sinus cancer. **A** There is evidence of spread into the cheek and orbit, with displacement of the eye. **B** There is ulceration of the hard palate, indicating spread into the mouth.

uncommon tumours are managed by a combination of surgery and radiotherapy, or by local surgery and topical chemotherapy.

NASOPHARYNX

Anatomy

The nasopharynx lies posterior to the nasal cavity and superior to the oropharynx. The skull base lies superiorly and the Eustachian tubes open into its lateral walls.

Diseases of the nasopharynx

Adenoids

The adenoids consist of B-cell predominant lymphoid tissue and in young children they occupy a significant proportion of the space within the nasopharynx. They increase in size until the age of 5 years and then become relatively smaller as the nasopharynx continues to grow. Few adults have significant amounts of residual adenoid tissue. Adenoid hypertrophy causes nasal obstruction in some children. They also have a role in the pathogenesis of childhood middle ear effusion and, increasingly in the West, sleep apnoea syndrome. Surgical removal may be indicated to improve the outcomes of glue ear treatment and in sleep apnoea.

Tumours

Carcinoma of the nasopharynx is very common in certain areas of the Far East such as South China. It is linked to the Epstein–Barr virus, male gender and there is a hereditary predisposition. Presentations include middle ear effusion, cervical lymph nodes, nasal obstruction or epistaxis. Skull base invasion may cause ophthalmoplegia. Treatment is by radiotherapy.

Male adolescents may rarely develop a benign but locally invasive angiofibroma of the nasopharynx. It presents with nasal obstruction and epistaxis and is treated by (open or transnasal endoscopic) surgical excision. A popular open approach is midfacial degloving, where the facial skin is elevated from a buccogingival sulcus incision.

MOUTH

Anatomy

The ducts of the submandibular salivary glands open into the anterior floor of mouth under cover of the tongue. The roof of the mouth is formed by the hard and soft palates. Laterally are the medial aspects of the cheeks. The parotid ducts open just above the second upper molar teeth.

Diseases of the mouth

Stomatitis and gingivitis

Inflammation of the oral mucosa and gums is often associated with poor oral hygiene. It may also be a manifestation of a systemic disorder, such as anaemia. Candida is an opportunist infection that may affect the oral cavity. It is characterized by white spots on the mucous membrane. Removal of the white material causes bleeding. Infection in the floor of the mouth may develop secondary to dental sepsis (Ludwig's angina). Pain, dysphagia, trismus and even airway obstruction may occur.

26

26

Mouth ulcers

Aphthous ulcers are the most common type. These have a punched-out appearance and are painful. They are thought to be due to a local failure of the mechanisms that protect the oral mucosa from damage. They resolve spontaneously, but this process can be speeded by the use of local treatment with steroid pellets. Oral ulceration is also seen in systemic disorders such as pemphigus and mucous membrane pemphigoid. Rarely, oral ulceration may be due to tuberculosis or syphilis.

Retention cysts

Mucous retention cysts may occur anywhere in the oral cavity. Those inferior to the tongue are called ranulas. They result from blockage of the openings into mucous and minor salivary glands. This may clear spontaneously, but otherwise excision may be required.

Leukoplakia

Leukoplakia (white patch) develops on the oral mucosa as a response to chronic irritation – for example, by a rough tooth, tobacco or alcohol (especially brown spirits) – causing hyperkeratosis (Fig. 26.19). This may progress to dysplasia and cellular atypia, thus leukoplakia is a pre-malignant condition. Removal of both the patches and the causative factors can prevent progression.

Tumours

Squamous carcinoma of the tongue is the most common neoplasm seen in the oral cavity. Lesions cause induration of the tongue, usually with ulceration (Fig. 26.20). Lymphatic spread occurs to the submental nodes and thence to other deep cervical nodes. Smoking and heavy spirit drinking are predisposing factors. Small lesions can be treated by local excision or radioactive implants (iridium wires), but more extensive tumours require excision with a margin of normal tissue. This often includes excision of part of the mandible.

OROPHARYNX

Anatomy

The oropharynx lies posterior to the oral cavity between the nasopharynx superiorly and the hypopharynx and larynx inferiorly. At the junction of the mouth and oropharynx are

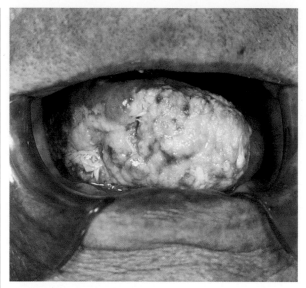

Fig. 26.20 Carcinoma of the tongue.

the tonsils, which consist of lymphoid tissue. Together with the adenoids (see above) and the lingual tonsil in the base of the tongue, they form a ring of lymphoid tissue. The system is important in the development of immunity during early infancy, but subsequently can be removed without ill effect. The pharynx itself is surrounded by three constrictor muscles arranged one inside the other like a stack of bottomless beakers.

Diseases of the oropharynx

Pharyngitis

Viral infection of the pharynx is common and often follows the common cold. Symptomatic relief can be obtained from analgesics with or without decongestants. Sore throat with exudate over the tonsils is a common manifestation of infectious mononucleosis (glandular fever). This disease is due to the Epstein–Barr virus which also causes cervical adenopathy and hepatosplenomegaly. Liver function should be tested, and patients with abnormal tests advised to refrain from alcohol for a period of time. Irritation of the pharynx may be due to tobacco smoke and acid reflux.

Tonsillitis

This is due to bacterial infection of the tonsils, usually with *Strep. pyogenes*. Patients present with episodic sore throat associated with dysphagia, lymph node enlargement, fever and malaise. Tonsillitis must be differentiated from viral sore throats, which are not usually associated with pyrexia and often form part of a more generalized upper respiratory tract infection. Infectious mononucleosis can easily be confused with tonsillitis (EBM 26.2). Tonsillitis may be complicated by the development of a peritonsillar abscess (quinsy). This may require incision and drainage. Recurrent tonsillitis can be treated successfully by tonsillectomy (EBM 26.3).

Snoring and sleep apnoea

Snoring arises because of obstruction within the pharynx during sleep or vibration of the soft palate. In some cases, it is associated with apnoeic episodes. These individuals tend

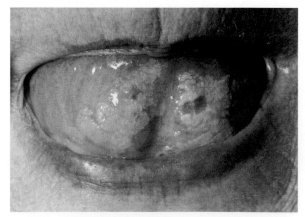

Fig. 26.19 Leukoplakia of the tongue.

'Antibiotics should not be used to secure symptomatic relief in sore throat.

In severe cases, where the practitioner is concerned about the clinical condition of the patient, antibiotics should not be withheld. Penicillin V 500mg 6-hourly for 10 days is the dosage used in the majority of studies.

Practitioners should be aware that infectious mononucleosis may present with severe sore throat. Ampicillin-based antibiotics should be avoided in infectious mononucleosis.

Sore throat should not be treated with antibiotics specifically to prevent development of rheumatic fever or acute glomerulonephritis.'

SIGN Guideline 117; 2010 Management of sore throat and indications for tonsillectomy.

For further information: www.sign.ac.uk

'The following are recommended as indications for consideration of tonsillectomy for recurrent acute sore throat in both children and adults:

- sore throats are due to acute tonsillitis
- the episodes of sore throat are disabling and prevent normal functioning
- seven or more well documented, clinically significant, adequately treated sore throats in the preceding year or
- five or more such episodes in each of the preceding two years or
- three or more such episodes in each of the preceding three years.'

SIGN Guideline 117; 2010 Management of sore throat and indications for tonsillectomy

For further information: www.sign.ac.uk

SUMMARY BOX 26.3

Tonsils and adenoids

- Adenoids are large in small children but become relatively smaller with age
- They may cause nasal obstruction and be involved in the pathogenesis of otitis media with effusion and childhood sleep apnoea
- Tonsils may require removal because of recurrent tonsillitis or peritonsillar abscess in adults and children. Children with sleep apnoea may also benefit from tonsillectomy
- Unilateral tonsillar enlargement may be due to squamous carcinoma or lymphoma.

to sleep poorly, wake unrefreshed and become drowsy during the day. If significant apnoea is confirmed by overnight monitoring, the use of nasal continuous positive airway pressure (CPAP) may be indicated. Simple snoring can be improved by weight loss and reduction of nocturnal alcohol intake. Sleep apnoea syndrome can also occur in children, in whom adenotonsillectomy will cure over 80%.

Tumours

B cell lymphomas occur mostly in adults (with a peak in those aged 50–60 years). There is a smooth enlargement of the affected tonsil. Squamous carcinoma usually presents with ulceration of the tonsil (Fig. 26.21). The traditional

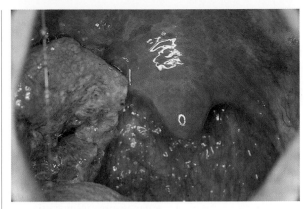

Fig. 26.21 Carcinoma of the tonsil.

association with cigarette smoking is less strong, as more now seem related to prior human papilloma virus exposure. Treatment is by (chemo) radiotherapy or surgery (including transoral laser resection).

HYPOPHARYNX

Anatomy

Below the oropharynx, the aerodigestive tract divides into an air passage (larynx/trachea) and an alimentary passage (oesophagus). The entrance to the air passage is protected by a purse string mechanism formed when the mobile cartilage of the epiglottis is drawn down over the laryngeal inlet as the aryepiglottic folds shorten. Closure of the false cords forms a second sphincteric layer to protect against aspiration. Glottic closure, conversely, serves chiefly to stop air escaping from the chest, as when sustaining a long note in phonation, straining or lifting (fixing the chest volume). The entry of material into the oesophagus is controlled by the cricopharyngeus ring of muscle. Lateral to the larynx, the pharynx continues inferiorly on both sides into a blind-ended pit known as the pyriform fossa (Fig. 26.22).

26

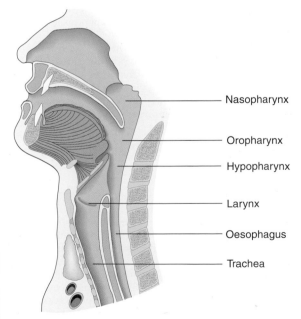

Fig. 26.22 Anatomy of the pharynx and larynx.

Physiology of swallowing

Swallowing is achieved by the coordinated contraction and relaxation of muscles. It is initiated by the tongue, which pushes the bolus to the back of the mouth. A solid bolus will then gather at the tongue base, until the tongue propels it off through the pharynx when the swallow reflex fires. The pharyngeal constrictor muscles follow the tail of the bolus – in particularly 'mopping up' any liquid pharyngeal residue. As the laryngeal inlet closes, the larynx itself moves upwards and forwards, widening the mouth of the oesophagus as the cricopharyngeal sphincter relaxes, and coming up over the now descending bolus. The entire sequence takes half a second, at the end of which respiration, which must pause during the swallow sequence, can resume. A much slower, smooth muscle peristaltic wave then carries the bolus down the tubular oesophagus to the stomach.

Assessment

Clinical features

Obstruction of the oesophagus and disorders that interfere with the muscle activity involved in swallowing cause dysphagia. Physical obstruction causes dysphagia that is worse for solids, whereas neurological disorders cause more difficulty with liquids. Hypopharyngeal pain may be felt locally or retrosternally, or may be referred to the ear (see Table 26.1). The level of obstructive dysphagia is always below the level at which the symptom is experienced. Hence dysphagia localized by the patient in the pharynx requires an assessment down to the gastro-oesophageal junction.

Examination

The pharynx can be assessed in the clinic using a flexible fibreoptic rhinolaryngoscope. Under general anaesthesia, the pharynx and oesophagus can be directly inspected using rigid endoscopes. A fibreoptic, ultra-thin, transnasal, digital video-oesophagoscope can be used to visualize the oesophagus under topical anaesthesia.

Imaging

A barium swallow will show structural abnormalities within the pharynx and oesophagus, and also gives some information about the dynamics of swallowing. Video recording (videofluoroscopy) can be used to provide additional information about the biomechanics of the swallow, aspiration and bolus transit. CT can be used to identify spread of oesophageal lesions into surrounding tissues and to demonstrate lesions causing external compression of the oesophagus.

Diseases of the hypopharynx

Pharyngeal pouch

This is formed by mucosal herniation through the weakest part of the pharyngeal musculature, the posterior midline between the two portions of the inferior constrictor of the pharynx. The cause may be muscular incoordination – it tends to occurs in men, in older age groups. The hall mark symptom is dysphagia for solids, as the pouch tends to fill and compress the tubular oesophagus. But there may also be regurgitation of food, sometimes hours or even days after it was swallowed. In most cases, it is possible to divide the wall between the pouch and the oesophagus anterior to it. A specially designed disposable staple gun is passed transorally via an adjustable endoscope (diverticuloscope). The jaws of the gun simultaneously cut and insert two rows of lateral staples. Once the bar is divided, there is usually only a low shelf between the pouch and the oesophagus, and food no longer builds up under pressure. If the endoscopic techniques are not possible, the pouch can be excised via a neck incision.

Tumours

Squamous carcinoma may arise from the pharyngeal walls, the epiglottis, the pyriform fossa or the upper oesophagus (postcricoid region). Postcricoid carcinoma is sometimes preceded by the development of a thin membrane in the upper oesophagus, a postcricoid web. This is associated with iron deficiency anaemia, glossitis and stomatitis (Paterson–Brown–Kelly syndrome). The web itself causes some dysphagia, and treatment of the anaemia can prevent progression to tumour. Other pharyngeal tumours are associated with smoking. Hypopharyngeal tumours are treated by radiotherapy or surgery.

LARYNX

Anatomy

The larynx has a cartilaginous framework. Superiorly, it is supported and protected anteriorly by the thyroid cartilage. Inferiorly lies the cricoid cartilage, which connects to the trachea (Fig. 26.23). Within the laryngeal lumen, two soft tissue folds pass from anterior to posterior. The upper folds are the ventricular bands or 'false cords'. The lower pair are the (true) vocal cords, which are responsible for phonation. These consist of a vocal ligament covered with mucosa. The vibrating free edge of the mucosa is important in achieving glottic closure and voice quality.

Physiology of voice

Voice production requires an air supply from the lungs, the presence of normally functioning vocal cords to create vibrations, and the tongue and mouth to articulate the vibrating air source into speech.

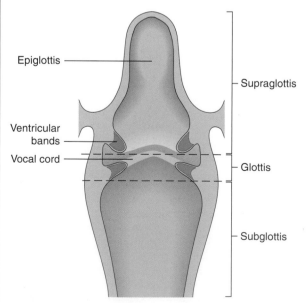

Epiglottis

Ventricular bands

Vocal cord

Supraglottis

Glottis

Subglottis

Fig. 26.23 Regions of the larynx.

Assessment

Clinical features

Hoarseness of the voice is the cardinal symptom of laryngeal dysfunction. Patients may also complain of pain locally or referred to the ear (see Table 26.1). The voice is weak and breathy in unilateral vocal cord palsy, but rough and husky in severe laryngitis and laryngeal cancer. Patients with psychogenic dysphonia often have a squeaky voice quality.

Examination

The larynx can be inspected in the clinic using a mirror, rigid telescope or flexible fibreoptic rhinolaryngoscope. Under general anaesthesia, a better view can be obtained using a rigid endoscope and operating microscope.

Imaging

CT can be used to assess the spread of laryngeal lesions to surrounding tissues.

Diseases of the larynx

Congenital disorders

Most congenital abnormalities of the larynx are rare. The commonest is laryngomalacia, where the laryngeal inlet – epiglottis and soft tissues which join it to the arytenoid cartilages (the aryepiglottic folds) – are high, soft and tend to collapse inwards. This causes inspiratory stridor and dyspnoea, which becomes worse during upper respiratory infections. Most children grow out of the problem by the age of 2 years and do not require active intervention. In severe cases, the CO_2 laser is used to divide or debulk the aryepiglottic folds.

Laryngitis

The commonest cause of hoarseness is acute inflammation of the vocal cords after an upper respiratory tract infection. Antibiotics are of no value but steam inhalations, voice rest and frequent drinking of small volumes of fluid may be helpful. The common predisposing factors for chronic laryngitis are smoking, acid reflux and excessive voice use. Women smokers with chronic laryngitis may have a fluid build up deep to the vocal cord epithelium (Reinke's oedema). This can be treated by surgical drainage of the submucosal space at microlaryngoscopy. Other morphological variants of chronic laryngitis include thickened red cords, or keratotic plaques (leukoplakia). In heavy voice abusers, vocal nodules at the junction of the anterior third and the posterior two-thirds of the vocal cords may develop. These may respond to speech therapy. If removal becomes necessary, patients must accept the risk of vocal cord scar and the need to undertake postoperative voice therapy to prevent recurrence.

Patients with hoarseness in the absence of a structural or movement disorder at laryngoscopy usually have functional dysphonia, which responds well in most cases to a programme of voice care and voice therapy. In many patients, the vocal cords appear normal and the problem is functional rather than structural. Speech therapy is often helpful in these cases.

Vocal cord palsy

The palsy is usually unilateral, more often on the left side, due to the intrathoracic course of the recurrent laryngeal nerve. The most commonly seen variant, left vocal cord palsy may be caused by invasion of the recurrent laryngeal nerve by a bronchial carcinoma. The right recurrent nerve does not pass down into the chest. Damage to the recurrent laryngeal nerves in the neck may occur as a result of surgery, trauma or neoplastic invasion. Unilateral palsy causes a weak breathy voice. The voice may be improved by the injection of fat, collagen or synthetic substances lateral to the vocal ligament under local or general anaesthetic. Bilateral cord palsy tends principally to cause stridor (airway obstruction). In high (vagal trunk) lesions, dysphagia may be pronounced.

Tumours

Carcinoma of the larynx is the most common single site of origin of head and neck cancer, and is almost always squamous. Over 90% of cases occur in smokers, many of whom also drink alcohol to excess. Tumours of the glottis (true vocal cords) tend to present earlier, due to the resulting hoarseness. As the glottis has very few lymphatics, regional nodes are involved late. Larger lesions may grow in the supraglottic space until they induce airway obstruction, haemoptysis or clinically apparent nodal disease. The treatment of early lesions may be by external beam radiotherapy or endolaryngeal laser resection. At least 90% of T_1 lesions of the vocal cord are cured, provided the patient gives up smoking. Early laryngeal tumours may also be treated by excision, using a laser. The outlook is less favourable in more advanced tumours. The treatment choices include more radical primary surgery or chemoradiotherapy with salvage surgery for treatment failures. Operative treatment of the more extensive lesions usually involves total removal of the larynx. Here, the trachea is brought out on to the surface of the neck as an end tracheostome. Patients can regain speech by generating a vibrating column of air in the pharynx. There are two ways of doing this: air swallowing, or valved speech through a surgically created tracheo-oesophageal puncture. Here, the patient has the advantage of lung-powered phonation. This valve diverts air from the trachea into the pharynx. Once the valve is closed, the air is expelled through the mouth where the articulators (teeth and tongue) use the airflow to generate the sounds of speech.

SUMMARY BOX 26.4

Carcinoma of the larynx

- Persistent hoarseness in smokers should be assumed to be carcinoma of the larynx until proved otherwise
- Up to 90% of T_1 glottic tumours can be cured by radiotherapy or transoral laser resection
- More extensive or recurrent disease may require removal of the larynx
- Following laryngectomy, the trachea is brought out on to the surface of the neck. Speech production is aided by a valve in a fistula between the trachea and the oesophagus.

Tracheostomy

Tracheostomy may be required to relieve acute upper airway obstruction (Table 26.3). It is carried out by creating a window in the anterior tracheal wall at the level of the second and third tracheal rings and introducing a suitable tube. When short-term airway support and the causative pathology allow, the situation is better managed by passing an endotracheal tube. Cricothyrotomy (Fig. 26.24) provides

Table 26.3 Causes of upper airway obstruction

Children
- Inhaled foreign body
- Acute epiglottitis
- Laryngotracheobronchitis

Adults
- Inhaled foreign body
- Acute epiglottitis
- Tumour
- Laryngeal trauma
- Bilateral vocal cord palsy

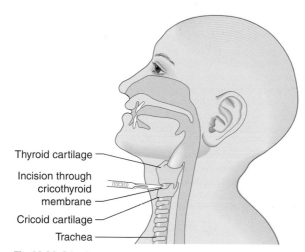

Thyroid cartilage

Incision through cricothyroid membrane

Cricoid cartilage

Trachea

Fig. 26.24 Cricothyrotomy.

a rapid short-term solution to airway obstruction and can be carried out with makeshift equipment. Foreign bodies in the upper airway can be displaced by turning a small child upside down. In a larger individual, a 'bear hug' around the chest and abdomen may expel the item (Heimlich's manoeuvre).

Tracheostomy may also be of value to reduce the dead space in patients with respiratory disease and to facilitate longer-term artificial ventilation.

NECK

Anatomy

Knowledge of the anatomy of the neck is essential if the likely origin of neck masses is to be determined (Fig. 26.25). In the midline lie the pharynx, larynx and trachea anteriorly. The oesophagus is deep to the trachea. The thyroid gland lies anterior and lateral to the trachea, low in the neck (i.e., confusingly, well below the thyroid cartilage). Laterally, the sternomastoid muscles link the sternum and clavicles inferiorly to the mastoid process superiorly. Between them and the midline, the anterior triangles contain the carotid arteries and jugular veins, with the related vagus nerve. Along the jugular vein is a chain of deep cervical lymph nodes (Fig. 26.26). In the submental region lie the submandibular and sublingual salivary glands. The parotid salivary glands lie posterior to the angle of the mandible and anterior to the external auditory meatus (Fig. 26.27). The facial nerve runs through the parotid gland and emerges as a number of branches. The submandibular salivary gland is the second largest major salivary gland and is situated in the floor of the mouth medial to the mandible (Fig. 26.28). Its duct passes anteriorly and opens just below the tip of the tongue. The sublingual salivary gland lies in the floor of the mouth anteriorly, close to the opening

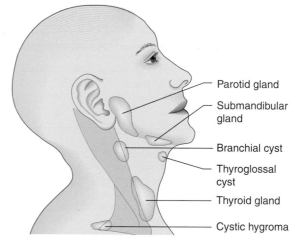

Parotid gland

Submandibular gland

Branchial cyst

Thyroglossal cyst

Thyroid gland

Cystic hygroma

Fig. 26.25 Key structures the head and neck.

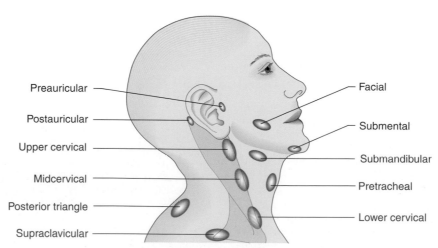

Preauricular

Postauricular

Upper cervical

Midcervical

Posterior triangle

Supraclavicular

Facial

Submental

Submandibular

Pretracheal

Lower cervical

Fig. 26.26 Lymph node groups in the head and neck.

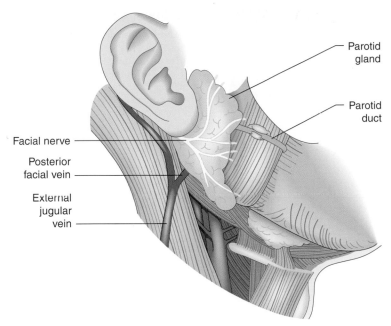

Fig. 26.27 Anatomy of the parotid gland.

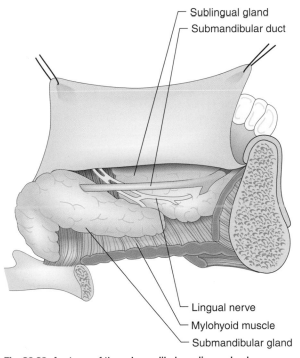

Fig. 26.28 Anatomy of the submandibular salivary gland.

of the submandibular duct. The mucosa of the mouth contains numerous small accessory salivary glands.

Assessment

Clinical features

Most neck masses are painless, but infection and malignant disease may cause pain. Rapid enlargement makes malignant disease more likely. Salivary gland swellings due to duct obstruction enlarge when the patient eats; there may also be a bad taste.

Examination

After inspection, assess the duct orifices and look for medial tonsil displacement, implying deep lobe parotid disease. Palpate the neck from behind to establish the site, size, shape and consistency of the swelling. Fixation to the skin or underlying structures should be established.

Imaging

CT can be used to assess most neck masses and will sometimes reveal lymph node swellings that have not been detected clinically. Cystic swellings can be differentiated from solid ones by ultrasound. Plain X-rays can be used to demonstrate salivary calculi (Fig. 26.29). Both CT and MRI are of value in assessing salivary gland swellings (Fig. 26.30).

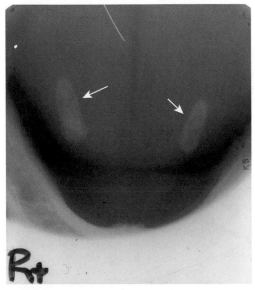

Fig. 26.29 Floor of mouth X-ray showing bilateral submandibular salivary calculi (arrowed).

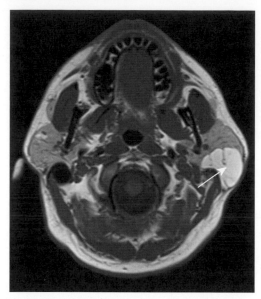

Fig. 26.30 MRI scan showing parotid lipoma (arrow).

The introduction of contrast into the duct of a salivary gland (sialogram) is occasionally used to confirm the presence of a calculus or to demonstrate inflammatory changes.

Diseases of the neck

Skin and subcutaneous swellings

Sebaceous cysts occur commonly in the head and neck and have a characteristic punctum. Furuncles or boils arise as a result of infection in hair follicles. Drainage may be required. When infection spreads to involve the dermis and subcutaneous tissue, a carbuncle is produced. It may have multiple discharging sinuses and may require wide excision. Remember the possibility of underlying diabetes mellitus. Kaposi's sarcoma occurs in patients with AIDS.

Thyroglossal cyst

The thyroid gland begins its embryological development in the tongue base. As it descends into the neck, it remains attached to the tongue by the thyroglossal duct. This duct should completely atrophy, otherwise a thyroglossal cyst may develop. This is a midline swelling usually situated just above the upper border of the thyroid cartilage. It moves on swallowing or tongue protrusion and can become infected. Occasionally, the thyroid gland fails to migrate as far as the lower neck. Thyroglossal cysts may be differentiated from aberrant thyroid tissue by an ultrasound scan – although the requirement for this appears more medicolegal than clinical. Treatment is by surgical excision. The centre of the hyoid bone and the persistent thyroglossal duct in continuity with a cuff of tongue base should also be excised with the cyst to reduce the recurrence rate (up to 10%).

Branchial cyst and fistula

Swellings lying laterally in the upper neck may be branchial cysts. They are thought to be remnants of the second and third branchial arches yet often present in young adults. The cysts contain opaque fluid with cholesterol crystals. Lymphoid tissue is found in their walls. They may become infected and usually require excision. Branchial fistulae may occur between the skin surface, low in the neck, and the tonsil or lower pharynx internally. Infection often occurs and excision is usually required.

Other cystic swellings

Cystic hygroma is a rare, benign lymphangioma of the neck, which usually presents in early life. Complete excision is difficult, leading to frequent recurrence. Dermoid cysts may also occur in the upper neck, usually in the midline or submandibular area, in younger children. They contain skin appendages unlike sebaceous cysts. Laryngocoeles occur as a result of herniation of laryngeal mucosa laterally into the neck. They distend with air during the Valsalva manoeuvre and may become infected. Excision is usually required.

 SUMMARY BOX 26.5

Lymphadenopathy

- Nodes become palpable when their diameter exceeds 1 cm, but impalpable nodes may contain tumour
- Tender nodes are usually inflammatory, whereas non-tender nodes may be malignant
- Painless neck nodes in patients over 45 years of age are often due to metastases from carcinoma. In most cases, the primary is within the head and neck. Such nodes must not be biopsied in the first instance; a thorough search for a primary lesion is the key to diagnosis
- Fine-needle aspiration cytology can be diagnostic for head and neck tumours or lymphoma
- CT defines the extent of the lymphadenopathy in cancer patients
- In lymphoma:
  ○ the nodes are often bilaterally enlarged, rubbery, firm and discrete
  ○ there may be is underlying immunosuppression
  ○ extranodal disease suggests non-Hodgkin's lymphoma
  ○ excision biopsy is diagnostic
  ○ bone marrow examination and CT are used in staging.

Lymph node swellings

Lymph nodes may become enlarged in response to infection in their area of drainage. Primary neoplasms (lymphomas) and secondary deposits, usually from squamous carcinomas of the head and neck must be considered among the wide differential (Table 26.4). Careful examination of the upper aerodigestive tract is therefore mandatory in assessing an undiagnosed neck node. Direct examination of the oral mucosa is followed by transnasal endoscopic examination of the nose, nasopharynx, hypopharynx, larynx and, increasingly, the oesophagus in centres offering transnasal oesophagoscopy. Supplementary palpation of the tonsils and tongue may reveal an occult tumour. If clinical findings are unhelpful the next step depends on the level of suspicion that there is a squamous cancer. PET CT scanning of the neck, fine needle aspiration cytology and rigid endoscopy under general anaesthetic with ipsilateral diagnostic tonsillectomy should all be considered. As a last resort, it may be necessary to excise the swelling for histological examination. However, small mobile lymph node swellings can be observed especially if ultrasound reveals a well preserved length to transverse ratio, i.e. a normal, oval shape. Tumour infiltrated nodes are more typically spherical.

Salivary gland disease

Submandibular salivary gland swelling is most often due to obstruction of the duct (by a stone or inflammation). Most submandibular calculi are radio-opaque. They

Table 26.4 Causes of lymphadenopathy
Infective
Bacterial
• Pyogenic infection in drainage area (e.g. streptococcal tonsillitis)
• Tuberculosis
• Brucellosis
Viral
• Infectious mononucleosis
• Cytomegalovirus
• Human immunodeficiency virus (HIV)
Protozoal
• Toxoplasmosis
Neoplasms
• Lymphoma
• Metastatic squamous carcinoma
• Other metastatic tumours
Systemic disease
• Collagen diseases
• Sarcoidosis
• Amyloidosis

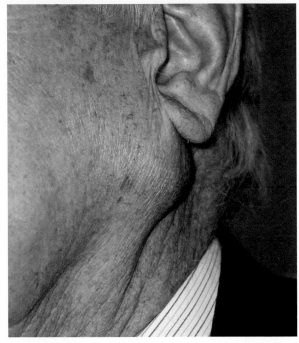

Fig. 26.31 Parotid tail swelling. The mass is statistically likely to be a benign tumour.

Table 26.5 Parotid neoplasms
Benign
• Pleomorphic adenoma
• Adenolymphoma
Intermediate
• Oncocytoma
• Mucoepidermoid tumour
Malignant
• Squamous carcinoma
• Adenoid cystic carcinoma
• Adenocarcinoma
• Lymphoma

sometimes pass spontaneously. Those in the main duct may be removed by opening the duct, endoscopy or basket retrieval. Those within the substance of the gland usually require gland excision. Inflammatory changes can occur in the absence of stone and are confirmed by ultrasound or sialography. Chronic sialadenitis may also be an indication for removal of the submandibular gland. By contrast, most swellings of the parotid gland are (benign) tumours. Since total removal of the parotid gland would be required to treat inflammation, this should thus be avoided if possible due to the risk of damage to the facial nerve.

Salivary gland tumours

Many different tumours arise in the salivary glands. Commonest are the pleomorphic adenoma (mixed salivary tumour, Fig. 26.31) and the adenolymphoma (Warthin's tumour). Malignant tumours and others of variable behaviour also occur (Table 26.5). Benign parotid tumours are excised with a cuff of normal tissue (superficial parotidectomy). Care must be taken to avoid damage to the facial nerve, which runs through the gland between the deep and superficial lobes. Submandibular gland tumours are treated by excision of the gland. Malignant tumours are treated by more radical surgery, with or without radiotherapy.

Carotid body tumours

These are rare tumours arising from chemoreceptor tissue in the carotid body, sometimes as a response to chronic hypoxia. A few are familial or bilateral. They present as pulsatile swellings in the upper neck at the level of the carotid bifurcation. Angiography is useful to define (and possibly embolize) the feeder vessels. Biopsy is hazardous because of the risk of bleeding. Surgical excision may be required.

 SUMMARY BOX 26.6

Salivary gland swellings

- Swellings in the submandibular gland are more often due to calculi, but those in the parotid gland are commonly benign neoplasms
- The most common salivary gland tumours are pleomorphic adenomas
- Parotid swellings generally require removal with a cuff of normal salivary tissue (superficial parotidectomy)
- The facial nerve runs through the parotid gland as a series of branches and is at risk during parotid surgery.

J.C. McKinley
I. Ahmed

Orthopaedic surgery

INTRODUCTION

Orthopaedic surgery involves the assessment and management of congenital, developmental (growing skeleton), traumatic and degenerative conditions of the bones and soft tissues. Assessment begins with history and examination, and is followed frequently by imaging. Management may be conservative or operative, and many conditions can be treated successfully by non-surgical means.

History

A diagnosis may often be made with a good history. Particular points in the orthopaedic history include the following.

Age

This will often help to distinguish degenerative conditions (elderly) from those related to an underlying congenital, birth-related or developmental problem (young).

Birth history

There may be a direct link between events around the time of birth and conditions such as upper limb weakness (traction injury to the brachial plexus), cerebral palsy (hypoxia) and dysplastic disease of the hip (more common in a breech delivery or first child).

Childhood

Abnormalities in the development of the growing skeleton may result in a range of conditions, some of which are associated with visible deformity. Sometimes, however, such apparent deformity is just a stage of normal development. For example, some children go through a phase of being bowlegged and anxious parents need to be reassured that this is a normal variation and not a disease.

Dominant hand

This is particularly relevant to upper limb conditions.

Occupation

Degenerative processes may be a consequence of, or at least exacerbated by, occupational use of the upper limb. The need to return a patient to employment may also affect the way and urgency with which a condition is treated.

Trauma

Many conditions follow a clearly defined episode of trauma, the nature and mechanism of which can help make the diagnosis. For example, sudden injury to the knee, with acute swelling followed by instability, is highly suggestive of anterior cruciate ligament (ACL) rupture.

Details of previous treatment

The condition may have been treated by means of physiotherapy, acupuncture, osteopathy, steroid injection and drugs over many years in primary care prior to referral to an orthopaedic surgeon. Previous operations performed on the same joint or limb may affect both the current options for surgery and the chance of success.

Past medical history

If operative intervention is planned, then general fitness for anaesthesia and surgery must be carefully assessed and the patient medically optimized. The consequences of other co-morbidity must also be considered. For example, the presence of open leg ulcers in a patient about to undergo a hip replacement will increase the risk of prosthetic joint infection and the ulcers should be healed, if possible, prior to surgery.

Drug history

With regard to analgesia, changing the dose or preparation may result in significant relief of symptoms. Other drugs, such as warfarin or clopidogrel, may need to be stopped prior to surgery. Some immunosupressive drugs increase the risk of infection; smoking and nonsteroidal anti-inflammatories can slow bone healing.

EXAMINATION

Examination should include all the other systems (cardiovascular, respiratory and neurological), as well as the specific limb and joint. It is important to assess other joints and limb alignment, for example hip pathology can present with knee pain; hindfoot pathology may be exacerbated by a varus or valgus knee. Musculoskeletal examination should always involve look, feel, and then assessing both passive and active movement.

Look

In lower limb conditions, observe gait, the use of a stick, and the ability to get out of a chair unaided and walk across the consulting room. Observe any joint or limb asymmetry or limb wasting, deformity, malalignment or shortening. Look for scars from previous operations or trauma, which may give clues to the cause of the current problem. Note any colour changes in the skin.

Feel

Palpate around the joint or limb. Establish areas of pain, and try to relate these to anatomical structures (e.g. tendons, joint lines etc.). Establish the presence of any swelling and whether this is fluctuant or solid (Table 27.1). Test the neurovascular status of the limb (sensation to light touch and pinprick, and peripheral pulses) and compare with this to the other side.

Move (active and passive)

Ask the patient to move the affected part (actively) through its full range of movement. Observe limitations of movement, pain, difficulty or apparent weakness. Then (passively) move the limb or joint, stopping in response to pain or stiffness. Test power in relevant muscles and apply stress tests to the ligaments looking for instability.

Table 27.1 Features describing a lump or swelling – three groups starting with SCTF			
S	Size	Shape	Surface
C	Colour	Consistency	Contour
T	Tenderness	Temperature	Transilluminable
F	Fluctuance	Fixity	Fields

There are specific provocative tests for most joints which are performed depending on the initial findings. Examples include testing for shoulder impingement (Hawkin's test), asking the patient to stand on one leg to test the power of the abductor muscles of the hip (Trendelenburg test) and stressing the anterior cruciate ligament of the knee to look for a rupture (anterior drawer test).

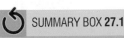

SUMMARY BOX 27.1

Orthopaedic examination

- Look
- Feel
- Move
- Special tests.

INVESTIGATIONS

Plain X-rays

Two views, in orthogonal planes including the joint above and below are generally used to evaluate almost all bone pathology and are performed weight-bearing whenever possible. Alignment (the degree of varus or valgus deformity), as well as true bone length, can be quantified. X-rays are also routinely used to confirm the correct position of bones, joints or prostheses after surgery.

Ultrasound

This is used frequently to evaluate soft tissue pathology (e.g. tendon ruptures, bleeds into soft tissues, other muscular or tendinous pathology) and to guide biopsy or injection. As a dynamic technique, it can be used to visualize the movements of tendons and muscles under direct vision.

Nerve conduction tests and electromyography (EMG)

These are used to evaluate nerve entrapment syndromes, nerve injuries, neuropathies and abnormalities of muscular contraction.

Computed tomography (CT)

CT provides excellent images of bone anatomy (Fig. 27.1) and can be used to supply three-dimensional images to help in the reconstruction of complex fractures. The thin axial slices are particularly useful as a guide for obtaining biopsy specimens

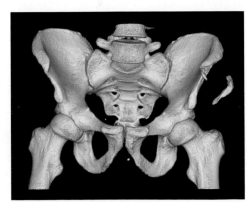

Fig. 27.1 A three dimensional CT showing a iliac wing fracture.

27

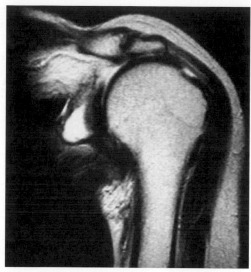

Fig. 27.2 An MRI scan of a shoulder through the level of the acromioclavicular joint and the glenohumeral joint.

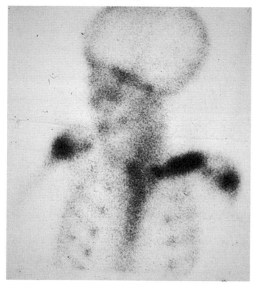

Fig. 27.3 An example of a bone scan showing increased uptake of radioactive tracer in the clavicle: in this case, indicative of infection. There are also increased areas of uptake in the shoulders and sternum.

Magnetic resonance imaging (MRI)

MRI (Fig. 27.2) provides excellent images of soft tissue, joint and bone pathology without exposure to radiation. It is widely used in virtually all branches of orthopaedics for diagnosis and preoperative planning.

Bone scans

These can be used to assess a number of bone conditions, including infection and tumours (Fig. 27.3).

DESCRIPTION OF DEFORMITY

With patients in the anatomical position (i.e. lying on their back with their palms pointing up to the ceiling), limb deformities are described relative to the midline (away = valgus, towards = varus) and to the alignment

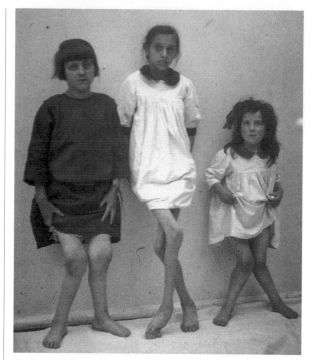

Fig. 27.4 Historical slide of children, showing deformities of the knees. All the children show valgus knee, i.e. knock-kneed, deformities.

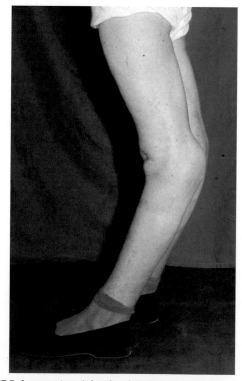

Fig. 27.5 A recurvatum deformity of the knees with hyperextension.

of the limb below the joint or deformity. For example, with respect to the knees, bowleggedness is a varus deformity, while knock-knees are a valgus deformity (Fig. 27.4). With the patient viewed from the side, there is a range of descriptive terms available. For example, hyperextension of the knee joint is known as recurvatum (Fig. 27.5). The three types of spinal deformity are:

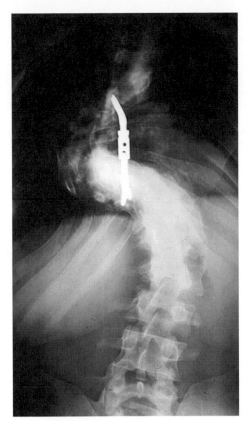

Fig. 27.6 An X-ray of the thoracic and lumbar spine, showing gross scoliosis of both.

- *kyphosis:* forward flexion ('the kyphotic kisses his knees').
- *lordosis:* the opposite, extension, or bent-over-backwards deformity; this represents the normal alignment of the lumbar and cervical spine.
- *scoliosis:* a sideward deformity that is normally associated with a degree of rotation (Fig. 27.6).

OSTEOARTHRITIS: DEGENERATIVE DISEASE OF THE JOINTS

Osteoarthritis (OA) of a joint may occur as a primary idiopathic condition or secondary to problems such as malalignment, intra-articular fractures or over-stressing (obesity, overuse). In some patients, there is a strong genetic component. OA may occur in any joint (shoulder, elbow, wrist and hands) but predominantly affects those that are weight-bearing (hip and knee) (Figs 27.7 and 27.8). Idiopathic OA is generally of slow onset and affects the elderly. Secondary OA can affect the young and may develop quite rapidly when a joint injury leads to loss of articular cartilage. On plain X-ray, OA is associated with:

- joint space loss due to thinning of articular cartilage
- sclerosis of the joint surface, with the development of increased density of the bone just under the joint space
- osteophytes
- cystic change.

The treatment of OA may be conservative or operative (Table 27.2). The former focuses on the use of drugs and physical methods of pain and stress relief to the joint.

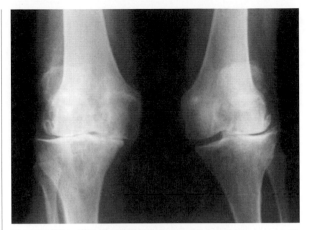

Fig. 27.7 Bilateral knee osteoarthritis. The left knee (on the right-hand side in the illustration) shows predominantly lateral wear and has a valgus deformity. The right knee has osteoarthritis of both medial and lateral compartments.

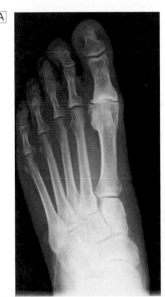

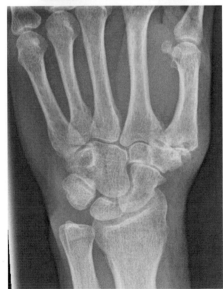

Fig. 27.8 Osteoarthritis can affect any joint. **A** Here, the first toe metatarsophalangeal joint is clearly arthritic. **B** Similarly, the carpometacarpal joint at the base of the thumb can also be affected.

Table 27.2 **Management options for osteoarthritis**	
Non-operative	**Operative**
Analgesia	Osteotomy
Physiotherapy	Joint debridement
Orthotics	Excisional osteotomy
Injections	Joint replacement (arthroplasty)
Lifestyle modifications	Joint fusion (arthroplasty)

Medical management of OA

Drug therapy

Simple analgesics, such as paracetamol, with or without the inclusion of nonsteroidal anti-inflammatory drugs (NSAIDs), are the mainstay of treatment. More powerful analgesic combinations may be introduced such as codeine or morphine, if simple analgesics prove inadequate.

Off-loading

This involves the use of aids, such as a walking stick and weight loss, aimed at reducing the forces passing through the joint. In the obese, weight loss is helpful as the load across a joint is three to six times body weight. Various insoles and splints are commonly used in orthopaedics to offload joints and are fitted by an orthotist.

Injections

Introducing a mix of a corticosteroid and local anaesthetic into the joint may reduce inflammation and ease pain. Injections of compounds of hyaluronic acid are increasingly used and are designed to supplement the natural joint levels of hyaluronic acid essential to normal functioning of articular cartilage. They work best in early OA but have little, if any, effect in late-stage disease.

Other conservative treatments

Physiotherapy and hydrotherapy both have a part to play in the control of symptoms, especially in early disease. Building up lost muscle bulk (frequently lost due to reduced activity) provides the joint with an increased degree of muscular control and may lead to considerable symptom improvement. Other treatment modalities, such as acupuncture, are recognized to have a role in the management of pain associated with OA. Failure of conservative methods normally leads to consideration of surgical intervention; in the patient unfit for surgery, benefit may be gained from referral to a pain therapist.

Surgical management of OA

The main operative interventions include osteotomy, replacement and fusion. Certain joints, particularly the knee, may benefit from a more minimal approach, such as arthroscopic debridement. This may help when a patient complains of physical symptoms indicative of underlying mechanical problems, such as locking or discomfort related to meniscal problems. However in well established OA this intervention can have a limited affect.

Osteotomy

This is useful in the younger patient, in whom joint replacement may not be advisable. The aim is to change the axis of the joint, so that a portion of the joint surface that has thus far been protected from wear and tear now forms the weight-bearing

area. For example, with respect to the knee, although there may be severe OA of the medial compartment in conjunction with a varus deformity, the lateral compartment may have well-preserved articular cartilage. Over-correcting the varus deformity by means of osteotomy (removing wedges of bone from the tibia), so that body weight is now largely transmitted through the lateral compartment, may lead to significant improvement in symptoms, thus delaying the need for joint replacement (Fig. 27.9). Osteotomies generally use opening wedges (adding bone), closing wedges (removing bone) or may be translational or rotational.

Joint replacement

The hip, knee, ankle and shoulder, and indeed almost any joint, can now be partially or completely replaced in a number of different ways with varying degrees of success.

Hemi-arthroplasty

In this operation, only one-half of the joint is replaced, leaving half of the joint intact. It is normally the natural socket – for example, the acetabulum – that is left untouched. The most

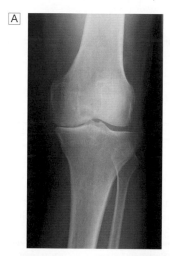

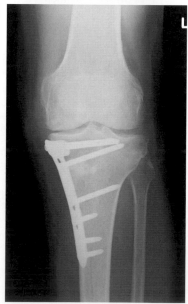

Fig. 27.9 An example of an osteotomy to the proximal tibia.
A The osteotomy site has been fixed by a plate and screws. **B** The cut of the osteotomy lies between the top two screws and the bottom three screws.

common example is following fracture of the femoral neck in the elderly. Such patients usually have low demand on the joint, and the hemi-arthroplasty (Fig. 27.10) gives adequate function without risking many of the complexities of a total hip replacement.

Total joint replacement

This entails resurfacing of both sides of a joint (Fig. 27.11). The choice of materials for the weight-bearing surfaces varies, depending on the joint and prosthesis in question. Currently, metal against a high-density polyethylene is the most common, although new prostheses involving metal and ceramics surfaces have been developed for use in young people (Fig. 27.12). Fixation of the implants may be with cement, or by encouraging bone to grow into or onto the surface of the implant. In small joints, such as those of the hand in patients with rheumatoid arthritis, silastic may be used as a buffer or spacer between the two joint surfaces.

Arthrodesis

Any residual cartilage is removed down to bleeding cancellous bone before the joint is rigidly fixed resulting in complete loss of movement (Fig. 27.13). Small joint fusions of toes and fingers are the most common examples. Fusion

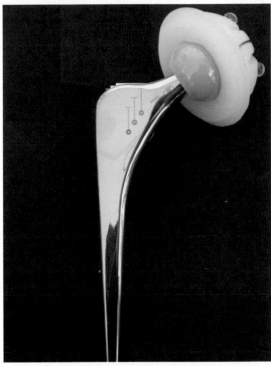

Fig. 27.12 A modern total hip replacement showing a cobalt chrome femoral stem, ceramic femoral head and a polyethlene acetabular cup. Courtesy of Stryker.

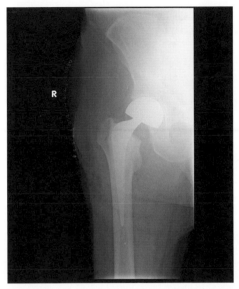

Fig. 27.10 An example of a hemi-arthroplasty of the hip, where only the femoral part of the hip joint has been replaced. This type of procedure is commonly used after a displaced intracapsular fracture of the hip.

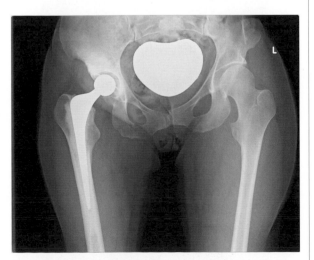

Fig. 27.11 A total hip replacement. The acetabulum contains a high-density polyethylene socket that is radiolucent, with a wire to give an indication of the sockets position within the acetabulum. The femur contains a metal prosthesis. Both acetabulum and femoral components are cemented in with polymethylmethacrylate cement.

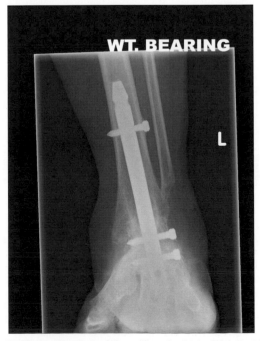

Fig. 27.13 An arthrodesis of the ankle and subtalar joint. The joint has been excised and the bone surfaces have been brought together. An intramedullary nail has been used to hold the position.

of a large joint, such as the hip or knee, will have a significant effect on mobility and will add additional stress on the joints above and below. Thus, pre-existing OA in the joints either proximal or distal to the joint being considered for fusion is a relative contraindication.

Interposition arthroplasty

The joint is excised and the residual space is filled with autogenous or allograft material. For example, the trapezium in the hand can be excised and the space filled with a rolled-up tendon, such as palmaris longus.

Excision arthroplasty

The joint surfaces are excised, giving a 'joint' formed of scar tissue. For example, in Keller's procedure, the first metatarsalphalangeal joint is excised to treat hallux rigidus; in a Girdlestone's operation, the femoral head is excised. The hip heals in a very shortened position and patients require a significant shoe raise to equalize the length of their legs, but the joint is relatively pain-free. Nowadays, this would be regarded as a salvage procedure after, for example, removal of an infected hip prosthesis.

RHEUMATOID ARTHRITIS AND INFLAMMATORY DISEASE OF JOINTS

Rheumatoid arthritis is a chronic systemic inflammatory disorder that can affect many tissues and organs, but principally attacks synovial joints leading to destruction of articular cartilage. Clinically RA can be differentiated from OA in that it presents with a symmetrical poly-arthropathy affecting the small joints of the hand, feet and cervical spine but affect larger joints such as the hip and knee.

Radiologically, there is often peri-articular osteopenia, soft tissue swelling, loss of joint space and as the disease advances, there may be bony erosions and subluxation of the joints.

The majority of patients with RA and other inflammatory disease of joints have been assessed and treated by a rheumatologist prior to orthopaedic referral. Often referral for surgical intervention is made when there has been a failure of medical treatment with disease modifying anti-rheumatic drugs (DMARDs). Orthopaedic treatment options range from synovectomy to joint fusion or replacement.

Other inflammatory disorders which can present to the orthopaedic surgeon include gout and pseudogout, Systemic Lupus erythematosus (SLE) and Ankylosing Spondylitis. Knowledge of these conditions and their management is essential for the practising orthopaedic surgeon.

BONE AND JOINT INFECTION

Primary infection

Primary infection of bones (osteomyelitis) or joints (septic arthritis) is rare and secondary to haematogenous transmission of microorganisms. Primarily a disease of childhood, these infections present with acute pain, swelling, loss of function (reluctance to use the limb), and often follow a bout of respiratory or skin infection. The most common sites are the long bones and joints of the lower limb. In children, 90% of cases are due to *Staphylococcus aureus*. By contrast, adults may present with rare and unexpected organisms as a result of other co-morbidity, immunosuppressant therapy, indwelling prosthetic material (e.g. renal dialysis catheters) or intravenous drug abuse. The importance of obtaining

positive microbiology from blood cultures, aspirations or bone samples prior to starting antibiotics cannot be overemphasized. Poorly treated acute osteomyelitis may lead to chronic osteomyelitis which is associated with a life-long risk of exacerbations or sinus formation and septic arthritis may lead to articular cartilage destruction and secondary osteoarthritis.

Secondary infection

Osteomyelitis secondary to trauma (open fracture) or operation (insertion of metalwork) is relatively more common than primary osteomyelitis. Dead bone (sequestrum) acts as a reservoir of infection and, although this may be walled off by new bone growth (involucrum), infection, once established, may lie dormant for many years before reactivating. Orthopaedic operations (without preceding trauma) are a relatively rare cause of true osteomyelitis (although any foreign prosthesis placed in bone may become infected). Infection of an implant or fracture fixation device may be very difficult to eradicate and is the most common reason for implant failure.

OVERVIEW OF JOINT REPLACEMENT SURGERY

Knee and hip replacements are the most common procedures, although shoulder, elbow, ankle, wrist and finger replacements may all be performed. With regard to the knee, there has also been a move away from traditional total joint replacement towards replacing that part of the joint affected by OA (Figs 27.14 and 27.15). These advances permit less invasive surgery and quicker recovery. Successful joint replacement surgery is associated with low infection and revision rates for prosthetic failure: ideally, less than 95% at 10–15 years (Figs 27.16 and 27.17). Revisional joint replacement surgery is more complex and associated with greater rates of complications and further device failure. Postoperative infection is divided

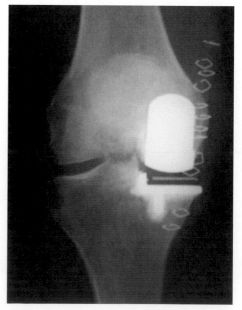

Fig. 27.14 This is a unicompartment joint replacement. A local resurfacing of the tibia and the femur for osteoarthritis of the medial compartment of the knee joint.

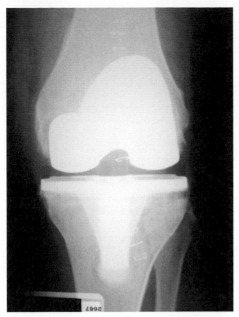

Fig. 27.15 A normal knee replacement, showing the resurfacing of the femur with a femur-shaped component. The tibial component can be seen as a metal base plate that holds the plastic bearing surface, which creates the gap between the femur and tibia.

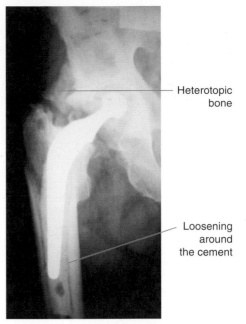

Heterotopic bone

Loosening around the cement

Fig. 27.17 Failure of a total hip replacement. The hip is surrounded by heterotopic ossification and the cement mantle (surrounding the femoral prosthesis) has started to come loose.

OVERVIEW OF ARTHROSCOPIC SURGERY

Arthroscopic techniques have been adopted in most areas of orthopaedics. The ability to repair soft tissues, place suture anchors into bone, and drill bone through the scope has permitted the development of arthroscopic-assisted:

- *repair:* menisci in the knee and the rotator cuff in the shoulder
- *stabilization of unstable joints:* the recurrently dislocating shoulder
- *joint fusion:* ankle, subtalar joint
- *ligament reconstruction:* anterior cruciate ligament.
- *debridement* – removal of infected tissue, loose or impinging bone.

PAEDIATRIC ORTHOPAEDIC SURGERY

The growing child presents particular challenges, and certain disease processes may only occur at certain stages of childhood. Surgery must be planned carefully so as not to interfere with the growth plates. Parents often require strong reassurance.

Dysplastic disease of the hip (DDH)

This is more common in breech deliveries, the first-born and females. It is due to inadequate development of the hip joint (Fig. 27.18), and presents with varying severity. When diagnosed in the newborn, milder forms in which the femoral head has a tendency to sublux from the acetabulum, are best treated using a 'harness device' that allows freedom of movement while holding the femoral head in the joint. More severe forms, where there is actually fixed dislocation, may require operative reduction and occasionally osteotomies.

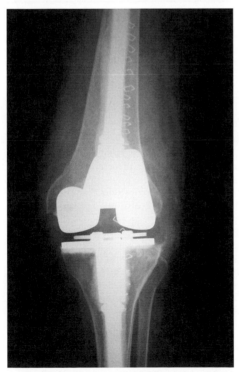

Fig. 27.16 A revision knee replacement. As can be seen when contrasted with the normal knee replacement in Figure 27.15, this is more complex and requires stems that go up the femur and down the tibia to create extra stability.

into early and late. Early infections are usually purulent, occur within the first few weeks, and may be eradicated with early debridement and appropriate antibiotics, but may necessitate removal of the prosthesis. Late infection is usually due to more indolent organisms such as *Staph. epidermidis,* may follow a bacteraemia or colonization at the time of implantation, and often presents as early loosening which leads frequently to revisional surgery.

27

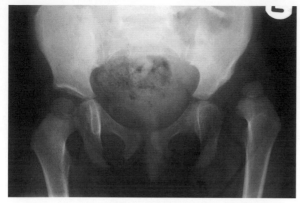

Fig. 27.18 Dysplastic disease of the hip, showing a dislocated left hip.

Perthes' disease

This is a self-limiting disease due to avascular necrosis of a portion of the developing femoral head. The cause is unknown but disease tends to occur between 4 and 10 years of age and is more common in males. An early stage of inflammation and synovitis is followed by a regenerative stage, in which the necrotic area is replaced by viable bone (reossification). Clinically, the onset is slow and the child complains of pain and limping. Treatment aims to relieve pain and prevent deformity while the femoral head is healing. Prognosis depends on the age of onset, degree of involvement of the femoral head, and adequacy of treatment; in general, the older the patient, the worse the outcome.

Cerebral palsy (CP)

This is a disorder of movement and posture due to a defect in the developing brain. CP is usually caused by adverse birth events, such as hypoxia and infection, and comes in a variety of forms (spastic, athetoid, ataxic, mixed) and extents: monoplegia (one limb – rare), hemiplegia (one side of the body affected), diplegia (both lower limbs affected), tetraplegia and quadriplegia. Contractures can be treated with regular stretching, botulinum toxin, tendon release or muscle transfer. Bony abnormalities may require osteotomy.

Slipped upper femoral epiphysis (SUFE)

The femoral head epiphysis weakens and the head slips, resulting in the upward and anterior displacement of the femoral neck. SUFE is of unknown aetiology. It usually develops between 10 and 16 years old, and is most common in boys at the time of their growth spurt; it is found more frequently in the short, fat, hypogonadal or hypothyroid child, suggesting a hormonal influence. It is a bilateral condition in 25% of cases. It frequently presents with referred pain to the knee and is thus commonly misdiagnosed as a knee problem. The condition may present as a chronic slip that occurs over a few months, or acutely after a seemingly minor episode of trauma. Treatment involves pinning of the slip, using a screw, together with corrective osteotomy if there is any significant residual deformity after healing. The contralateral side is generally fixed prophylactically and there is a risk of avascular necrosis in severe slips.

Congenital club foot (talipes equinovarus or ctev)

This is an idiopathic fixed deformity of the foot, which is frequently bilateral. There may be a genetic component and it is twice as common in males. Simple methods of treatment include strapping and splinting for minor deformities, and surgical correction where conservative methods have failed.

Scoliosis

This can be divided into structural and non-structural. 'Non-structural' scoliosis is secondary to some other problem (e.g. inequality of leg length, lumbar disc prolapse) and disappears when the underlying cause is removed. Structural scoliosis can be caused by a variety of conditions, although 90% of childhood cases are idiopathic. Unlike the non-structural form, there is an accompanying rotational deformity. The usual presentation is between 10 and 13 years of age, and the condition is more common in females. Usually, it is asymptomatic and, if there is pain, one should think of other reasons for the scoliosis (e.g. tumour). The treatment of scoliosis is complex but involves spinal bracing and surgical intervention.

Angular deformities

Genu varum (bowlegs) is often seen in very early childhood. It often corrects and tends to genu valgum (knock-knees) between 18 months and 3 years; this then corrects by 4–7 years. It is important not to forget alternative diagnoses, such as rickets and Blount's disease (idiopathic abnormality of the upper medial tibial epiphysis).

MUSCULOSKELETAL TUMOURS

Musculoskeletal tumours may arise from cartilage, skeletal muscle, synovium or bone, and may be benign or malignant. They are rare, and usually present with deep-seated pain that often continues into the night, or a soft tissue swelling. There may be a history of incidental trauma, to which the symptoms are frequently attributed. High-grade tumours may have a short history (of several months), whereas the more benign lesions have a prolonged course. Clues to malignancy include rapid growth, fracture through unusual bone, destruction of the bone cortex and invasion into the soft tissues. Primary bone tumours are rare; they occur largely in the second decade of life and frequently affect the metaphysis. The most common malignant tumour is osteosarcoma, 50% of which will occur around the knee. The next most common is Ewing's sarcoma. Once a bone tumour is suspected, the patient should be referred immediately to the regional specialist treatment centre for biopsy, staging and definitive treatment. Over the last decade, advances in adjuvant treatment (chemotherapy prior to and following surgery) have resulted in considerable improvements in long-term prognosis.

THE UPPER LIMB

The shoulder

Anterior dislocation

Anterior shoulder dislocation is the commonest form of dislocation, and can be associated with or without fracture

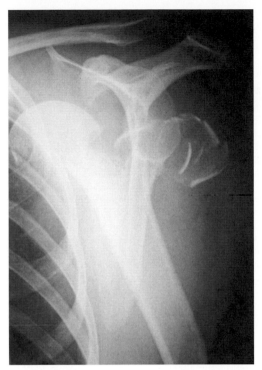

Fig. 27.19 A fracture dislocation of the humeral head, showing the humeral shaft and head as separate pieces, as well as portions of the greater tuberosity. All are separate from the normal anatomical position of the femoral head, and the glenoid can be clearly seen in the background of the X-ray.

(Fig. 27.19). The cause of an anterior dislocation is often traumatic. Treatment involves immediate reduction with analgesia and sedation using Kocher's, Milche's or Hippocratic methods. Patients require to be immobilized in a sling and a check radiograph is mandatory to confirm reduction and exclude a fracture. Instability following shoulder dislocation is common in young males and in this group of patients an arthroscopic examination and stabilization may be required if there is a high risk of recurrence.

Impingement syndrome

Weakness through disuse, degeneration and tearing of the rotator cuff muscles (supraspinatus, infraspinatus, subscapularis) predisposes to superior subluxation of the humeral head against the acromion, leading to so-called impingement pain. Steroid injections and physiotherapy may be effective. If there is a bony spur at the front of the acromion that is contributing to the impingement, this can be removed arthroscopically (subacromial decompression).

Rotator cuff disease

Rotator cuff disease is a degenerative process affecting the tendons that make up the rotator cuff (supraspinatus, infraspinatus, subscapularis and teres minor). In particular the avascular region near the insertion of the supraspinatus tendon can be affected. Complete or partial tears may be present in up to 50% of the population over 60 years of age but most are asymptomatic. Acute rotator cuff tears may occur as a result of trauma or chronic impingement. Patients most commonly present with pain around the shoulder and weakness particularly on shoulder abduction.

Treatment options include conservative management with physiotherapy and corticosteroid injections or surgical (arthroscopic repair with a subacromial decompression).

Osteoarthritis

Arthritic changes can affect the glenohumeral or the acromioclavicular joint (ACJ) and may give rise to prolonged pain associated with shoulder movements. ACJ OA is treated with either injection or excision of the joint. OA of the glenohumeral joint may be secondary to avascular necrosis of the humeral head or as result of previous fracture of the proximal humerus. If conservative methods fail, glenohumeral joint OA can be treated with either shoulder replacement or resurfacing.

The elbow

Tennis and golfers' elbow

The most common pathologies to affect the elbow are inflammation of the lateral (tennis) or medial (golfers') epicondyle at the point of insertion of the muscle mass. The mainstays of treatment are bracing and strapping, injections and physiotherapy. If these fail, operative release of the tendinous insertion may be warranted.

Rheumatoid elbow

Options include a synovectomy, with debridement of the joint and excision of the radial head; interposition and covering the joint surfaces of the elbow with fascia; and total elbow replacement.

The hand and wrist

Wrist disease

The cause of pain around the wrist can be a challenging diagnosis to make. Common causes include those secondary to trauma such as a distal radius fracture (Colles fracture) or a scaphoid fracture (see below); degenerative causes such as rheumatoid arthritis or osteoarthritis and those secondary to inflammation affecting the tendon sheaths such as De Quervain's disease which affects the abductor pollicis longus and extensor pollicis brevis tendons.

Carpal tunnel disease

The median nerve is compressed, either by the tunnel itself or by its contents: for example, by a synovial swelling. Symptoms include pins and needles or sensory loss in the territory of the median nerve (a variable area of supply normally including the palmar aspect of the thumb, index and middle fingers, with a variable amount of the ring finger involved). Treatment options include night splinting and injection or surgical decompression of the tunnel by releasing the flexor retinaculum overlying the median nerve.

Trigger finger

Thickening of the flexor tendon causes it to jam under the pulley system that would normally allow the tendon to slide backwards and forwards. Injection around the tendon or release of the first pulley results in a cure of the condition.

Dupuytren's disease

Thickening of the palmar fascia draws the fingers (predominantly the fourth followed by the fifth) into a flexed and deformed position, resulting in disability and loss of

27

function. It is more common in diabetics, epileptics and can often be associated with previous trauma to the area affected. The condition mainly affects men over the age of 40 years. Surgery is considered if there is significant disability affecting the fingers. This involves either dividing the thickened tissue (fasciotomy), dissecting and removing the thickened fascial bands alone (fasciectomy) or with the overlying skin (dermo-fasciectomy), taking great care to preserve the associated nerves and blood vessels. In severe cases, amputation of the little finger may be the best line of treatment.

THE LOWER LIMB

The hip joint

The main problems are the late complications of young persons' diseases of the hip and OA. Treatment ranges from conservative methods through osteotomy to joint replacement surgery. Where a remnant of articular surface remains intact, osteotomies may be extremely useful to realign usable portions of cartilage against each other.

Avascular necrosis of the femoral head

This typically presents with severe pain, often at night, and initial X-rays may appear normal. MRI is usually diagnostic. If the head has not collapsed, it is usually decompressed via a channel drilled up the femoral neck (core decompression). If the head has collapsed, then total joint arthroplasty may be the treatment of choice.

Hip arthroscopy

Recent developments in hip arthroscopy have led to a greater understanding of the nature of adolescent and adult hip pathologies and their management, particularly in athletes and other young individuals with hip injuries. It remains to be seen whether early diagnosis and treatment of acetabular labral tears or lesions of the cartilage using this technique will curb the progression of osteoarthritis.

The knee joint

History

The history often points to the likely diagnosis. Inability to carry on playing sport immediately after an injury hints at a ligament rupture. Rapid swelling within a few minutes or hours suggests a major injury within the knee. A large haemarthrosis occurring within the first few hours after an injury indicates a major ligament tear, a peripheral tear of the meniscus or an osteochondral fracture. All of these conditions require further evaluation. Ligament injuries may present in clinic with a history of preceding injury and subsequent instability. Often, this is a feeling of an inability to trust the knee on trying to move from side to side, although the knee may feel stable when the person is running in a straight line. Regular episodes of giving way are thought to accelerate the development of OA. Patterns of injury do tend to coexist and may be related to certain mechanisms of injury.

Meniscal injuries

These are relatively common and can be divided into two major groups. Younger patients are more likely to have a purely traumatic tear of the medial meniscus. As the patient gets older, degenerative tear of the lateral meniscus is more frequent. Symptoms may consist of swelling and localized pain in the knee, particularly around the joint line. If a fragment of meniscus is loose within the joint space, true locking may occur, with a loss of ability to extend the knee.

Osteoarthritis

This is very common and may affect the whole of the knee (tricompartmental OA), or just particular compartments such as the medial or patellofemoral. Symptoms may be precisely localized both to precipitating events and to an anatomical site; for example, pain going up and down stairs reflects patellofemoral disease, while in isolated medial OA the pain may be well localized to the medial side of the knee. The knee lends itself to surface replacements purely of the affected parts, and isolated medial and patellofemoral joint replacements exist, as well as total knee replacements. When patients are asked for consent for replacement knee joints, it is customary to warn them that the prosthesis will last for 10–15 years but, in fact, many prostheses continue to function well beyond this limit and there is no sudden dramatic increase in the rate of revision once 10 years have passed.

The foot and ankle

Sprains of the ankle are very common – most recover, but damage to the supporting lateral ligaments may lead to instability and recurrent 'giving way' of the ankle. This may be associated with damage to the cartilage in the ankle.

Arthritis may occur in any of the joints of the foot – ankle arthritis is increasingly treated with an ankle replacement, but other joints are generally fused or treated non-operatively.

Foot deformities frequently occur – the most common are pes planus (flat feet with loss of the medial arch) and pes cavus (excessive arching of the foot), leading to chronic foot pain and difficulty in walking. The most common forefoot deformity is hallux valgus (more commonly known as a bunion), in which the great toe is deviated in a valgus direction at the metatarsophalangeal joint. Treatment is generally with a metatarsal osteotomy to realign the toe. Hallux rigidus is OA of the first metatarsophalangeal joint and can be treated with insoles, a fusion or a joint replacement. Frequently, the lesser toes may be deformed and are straightened using tendon transfers or fusions. Nerve entrapments are sometimes seen – Morton's neuroma (compression of the digital plantar nerve) and tarsal tunnel syndrome (tibial nerve compression) are the most common.

TRAUMA AND FRACTURES

General approach

The initial assessment and resuscitation of the (multiply) injured patient follows the Advanced Trauma Life Support (ATLS) guidelines (Table 27.3) Management of the injured patient requires a team approach, and often entails joint care by a number of different specialties, from the time of initial resuscitation in the accident and emergency department right through to the definitive treatment of each injury. Certain patterns of injury can be anticipated. For example, patients who fall from a height and land on their feet may be expected to have sustained an injury to calcaneus, tibial plateau, hip and pelvis. At impact, patients tend to fall forward, often leading to spinal fractures.

Table 27.3 **Advanced trauma life support guidelines**

Primary survey	
A	Airway with C-spine control
B	Breathing and ventilation
C	Circulation and haemorrhage control
D	Disability (neurological evaluation)
E	Exposure and environment
Secondary survey	
Once the resuscitation efforts are well established and the vital signs are normalising, the secondary survey can begin. This involves a complete history and physical examination, including the reassessment of all vital signs.	

Examination

Careful examination of each injured limb includes:

- *Skin.* Ascertain whether any skin breaks communicate with any underlying fracture.
- *Circulation.* The most common cause of absent pulses is kinking or compression of the artery by the fracture. Often, a reduction of the fracture (realigning the fracture into the anatomical position) or application of traction results in the return of perfusion.
- *Nerves.* Certain injuries may have a high associated risk of neurological injury, manifest by loss of power and/or sensation. For example, the axillary nerve is at risk from shoulder fracture dislocation and its integrity should be documented prior to reduction (see Fig. 27.19).
- *Joint above and below.* Often fractures can involve the joint immediately above or below. A complete examination of these joints is required as it may influence definitive treatment of the injury.

Joint dislocation

Reduction of the joint must be performed as soon as possible, either in the accident and emergency department under sedation (e.g. anterior dislocation of the shoulder), or in the operating theatre under general anaesthesia. In some cases where closed reduction fails, open surgical reduction is performed.

Fracture management

Classification

Fractures are usually classified by:

- whether they are in communication with the skin surface (open or compound) or not (closed)
- their appearance on X-ray: for example, comminuted (in multiple pieces, Fig. 27.20), spiral (where the fracture curves in a large spiral around the long axis of the bone) or transverse (straight across the bone, Fig. 27.21) This appearance usually correlates with the mechanism of injury – a twisting injury tends to cause a spiral fracture for example.
- anatomical site: for example, intra-articular (involving the joint surface, Fig. 27.22), metaphyseal, epiphyseal or diaphyseal.

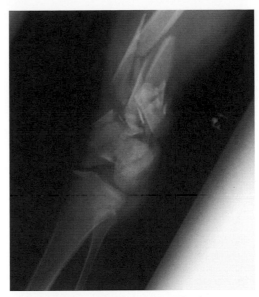

Fig. 27.20 **A comminuted fracture of the distal femur involving the knee joint as well.** The femur can be seen to have broken into multiple (comminuted) fragments.

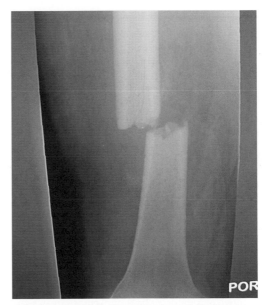

Fig. 27.21 A transverse fracture of the femoral shaft over 50% displacement.

Children

Fractures often behave differently in children. Because their bones are more pliable, children may suffer from greenstick fractures, in which the cortex of the bone does not break but bends instead. Fractures may also affect the growth plate (epiphysis) of the bone, leading to problems with slowing of the growth of the bone (growth arrest) or deformity of the growing bone (Fig. 27.23). Generally, fractures heal much more quickly in children.

Principles of fracture healing

There are many differing ways of treating fractures. However, they all have the same fundamental objectives: namely, the close approximation of uncontaminated, well-vascularized

27

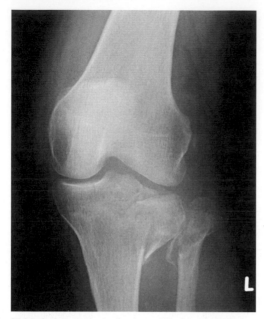

Fig. 27.22 An intra-articular fracture of the lateral tibial plateau of the knee.

bone ends in a stable configuration that will maximize bone and soft tissue healing without deformity or loss of function. In general, the fracture healing process takes approximately 8–10 weeks in adults but can take longer depending on the severity of the injury and whether it is an open fracture.

Compound fractures

These should be treated within 6 hours. However, new guidance from the combined orthopaedic and plastic surgery associations advises that these injuries can be left until the following morning (if admitted overnight and not grossly contaminated) when an experienced surgeon is available. Definitive treatment should involve:

• removal of all the damaged and dead tissue
• thorough cleaning of the wound, with at least 3 litres of fluid depending on the degree of contamination ('the solution to pollution is dilution')
• intravenous antibiotics
• stabilization of the fracture to realign the bones to their anatomical position. Depending on the degree of contamination and soft tissue coverage, this may be by definitive or temporary fixation. Temporary external

fixators are often attached by means of pins to the bones either side of the fracture site to allow access to the wound while imparting stability.

Intra-articular fractures

It is essential that the joint surface be reconstructed as accurately as possible to minimise the progression of secondary osteoarthritis. In certain fractures of the humeral and femoral heads, joint replacement may be the best option.

Conservative treatment

Closed fractures with good healing potential are usually treated with external stabilization using a simple bandage, plaster of Paris (POP) or a synthetic lightweight cast. In some cases where there is significant swelling the initial cast should not encircle the whole circumference of the limb. Use of a 'back slab' of plaster allows the limb to swell and avoids the potential risk of a compartment syndrome. Once the acute swelling has settled, the cast can be completed to become a circumferential (full) cast. Displaced fractures often require manipulation under some form of anaesthetic prior to immobilization in POP.

Compartment syndrome

The diagnosis of compartment syndrome must be considered in any patient with an injury to the limb who complains of increasing pain in the limb, out of proportion and worse on passive stretch, which is refractory to analgesia. Paralysis, paraethesia, and absent pulses are very late signs. If compartment syndrome is suspected or cannot be excluded, the POP must be split down to skin immediately, even if the fracture position is lost. A pressure transducer can be inserted into the muscle compartments to monitor the pressures (diagnostic if the opening intracompartmental pressure is >30 mmHg or if the difference in the diastolic blood pressure and intracompartmental pressure is <30 mmHg) Missed compartment syndrome has devastating consequences for the patient, and is a common cause of medicolegal litigation. If splitting the POP fails to relieve the symptoms of a compartment syndrome very quickly, then further urgent, possibly surgical, decompression will be required and senior help must be sought immediately.

Operative treatment

This involves the use of devices that are broadly divided into those that remain external to the skin (see above) and those that are internal (screws, plates and nails, Fig. 27.24).

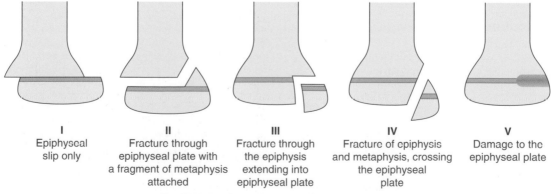

I	II	III	IV	V
Epiphyseal slip only	Fracture through epiphyseal plate with a fragment of metaphysis attached	Fracture through the epiphysis extending into epiphyseal plate	Fracture of epiphysis and metaphysis, crossing the epiphyseal plate	Damage to the epiphyseal plate

Fig. 27.23 The Salter-Harris classification of fractures.

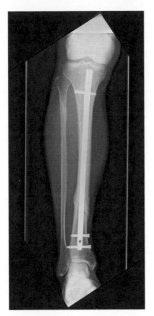

Fig. 27.24 The use of an intramedullary nail to fix a tibial fracture

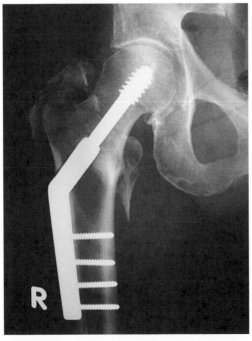

Fig. 27.25 A dynamic hip screw, a device used to secure hip fractures where the hip fracture is extracapsular as shown. The device is dynamic, as the screw can collapse down as the fracture heals.

The details of their use are beyond the scope of this book but depend on fracture type, site and morphology. Some devices are 'dynamic', in that they allow controlled collapse of the fracture, leading to compression of the bone ends and early weight bearing (Fig. 27.25).

Some specific fractures

Detailed treatment of individual fractures is beyond the scope of this book. However some common fractures and their management principles are discussed below.

Fractures of the femoral neck

These are generally seen in the elderly with osteoporotic bone, as a result of low-velocity falls on to the hip. They are extremely common and utilize very considerable health-service resources. Such fractures are divided into:

- *extracapsular,* occurring outside the margins of the joint capsule, particularly the metaphysis of the femur
- *intracapsular,* involving the femoral neck within the capsule.

This differentiation is important because blood reaches the femoral head via the capsule and runs along the femoral neck. Extracapsular fractures are normally reduced and stabilized using a pin and plate system, commonly known as a dynamic hip screw (DHS), which allows sliding and impaction of the fracture site as the patient walks. Without these there is the risk of a malunion occurring (Fig. 27.26).

Undisplaced intracapsular fractures are pinned commonly in the hope that the blood supply to the femoral head has been preserved and avascular necrosis of the femoral head will not develop. Displaced intracapsular fractures are treated frequently with joint replacement. In older, -less active patients, this is often a hemi-arthroplasty (see Fig. 27.11). In this operation, only one-half of the joint is replaced, leaving the natural socket(the acetabulum) untouched. Such patients usually have low demand on the joint, and the hemi-arthroplasty gives good function without risking many of the complexities and complications associated with a total hip replacement. Younger patients and those expected to rehabilitate to a higher level of activity usually receive a total hip replacement.

Colles' fractures

These are distal radial fractures, usually sustained as a result of falling forward onto an outstretched hand; they produce dorsally based (dinner fork) deformity of the distal fragment. This is most commonly seen in the osteoporotic elderly. Two well-described complications are compression of the median nerve and (usually delayed) rupture of the extensor pollicis longus tendon. A Smith's fracture is similar but has volar displacement of the distal fragment.

Forearm fractures

The principle behind all forearm fractures is that it is difficult to fracture one bone and have displacement and shortening without there being another injury to the other bone in the forearm or to the proximal or distal joint. The fracture(s) may occur at any point along the length of the radius and ulna. Although in the child it may be permissible to treat these conservatively, in the adult midshaft fractures are almost

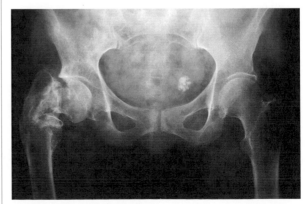

Fig. 27.26 This fracture has healed in a malunited position and would be called a malunion.

27

invariably fixed into anatomical alignment using open reduction and plate fixation. Correct anatomical alignment is essential to allow correct pronation and supination of the forearm.

Scaphoid fractures

These may present with subtle symptoms and signs: typically, pain and tenderness in the anatomical snuffbox following a fall on the outstretched hand. Initial X-rays may fail to demonstrate the fracture and, if clinical suspicion is high, it is wise to immobilize the wrist and repeat the X-ray at 2 weeks. If suspicion is still high but the X-rays appear normal, then further imaging (MRI scan or CT) should take place. The scaphoid gains its blood supply for the proximal portion through blood vessels that pass from the distal to proximal pole. Thus, a displaced fracture in the proximal portion of the scaphoid may disrupt the blood supply and lead to non-union or avascular necrosis leading to secondary arthritic change.

Ankle fractures

These can involve any portion of the distal tibia or fibula. Technically, the fractures involving the actual articular surface of the distal tibia are known as tibial plafond fractures, whereas fractures involving either the medial or lateral malleoli (and certain combinations of fibula injury) are ankle fractures. The types and classification of ankle fracture are complex, but, depending on the displacement or the threat to joint stability, will determine whether the fracture can be treated conservatively or requires internal fixation. Stable injuries have a good prognosis almost irrespective of treatment and are managed in plaster cast for around 6 weeks. Internal fixation of unstable fractures is carried out in those injuries that have a high suspicion of displacing in cast or leading to delayed or non-union.

Tibial plateau fractures

These are intra-articular fractures of the knee joint involving the tibial plateau in varying forms. Treatment depends on age, the patient's functional level and the degree of displacement. A large proportion of these fractures will require internal fixation to achieve the best clinical result. Complications include knee stiffness and development of OA. Non-union is unusual, as the tibia at this point is normally well vascularized.

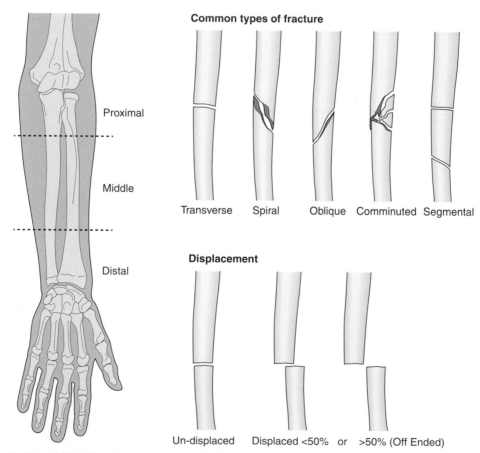

Fig. 27.27 The location and description of many common fracture types.

Note: Page numbers followed by *f* indicate figures, *t* indicate tables, and *b* indicate boxes.

Epidermis, 281, 283
  cancer of the, 297
  neoplasms, 295–300, 295t, 298b
Epididymis, 419–420
  cysts, 423
Epididymo-orchitis, 422
Epidural anaesthesia, 76–77, 77f, 77t
Epidural analgesia, 78
Epigastric hernia, 143–144, 144f
Epigastric pain, 176
Epilepsy, 441
  perioperative implications of, 75t
Epispadias, 420
Epistaxis, 466, 466b, 466f, 466t
Epithelial hyperplasia, breast, 309
Epley's particle repositioning manoeuvre, 463–464
Epstein-Barr virus, 468
Erb's sign, 334
Erection, penile, 420
  disorders of, 420
Erythema, burns, 291
Erythrocytes, 229
Erythrocyte sedimentation rate (ESR), 400
Eschar, 289
Escharotomy, 294
Escherichia coli
  antibiotics for, 51t
  peritonitis, 161
Estimated blood volume (EBV), 24t
Ethics, 56–60
  committees, 60
  principles, 56–57
  sources of further information on, 59t
  specific topics, 59–60
Eustachian tube, 459
Euthanasia, 59
Evaporative dressings, burns, 294
Evidence-based neurosurgery, 443
Excision arthroplasty, osteoarthritis, 482
Excision of lumps and swellings, 117
Exercise
  colorectal adenocarcinoma, 256
  lower limb ischaemia, 351
  preoperative, 62
Exercise electrocardiography, coronary artery disease assessment, 381
Exocrine function, pancreas, 215
Exophthalmos, 329, 329f
Explicit consent, 58
Extended Spectrum Beta Lactamase (ESBL)-producing Escherichia coli, 49
External abdominal hernia, 145
External auditory meatus, 459, 462
External beam radiotherapy (EBRT), prostate cancer, 413
External inguinal ring, 139, 139f
Extra-anatomic bypass, lower limb ischaemia, 353, 354f, 355f
Extracellular fluid, 10, 10f, 12f
Extracorporeal shock-wave lithotripsy (ESWL), 405
Extradural haematoma, 432, 433f

F

Facial nerve (CN VII), 425
  disorders of, 464
Facial palsy, 464
Factor II, 29
Factor VII, 29
Factor VIII, 29
Factor IX, 29
Factor X, 29
Factor XIII, 29

Faecal incontinence, 275–276, 275t, 276b
Faecal occult blood test (FOBT), 257
Fallot's tetralogy, 390
Falls, 93, 93f
Familial adenomatous polyposis (FAP), 242, 254, 254f
Fasciotomy, 362, 362f
FAST (Focused Abdominal Scans for Trauma), 160
Fasting, preoperative, 69, 69b
Fat metabolism, 8, 9b
Female incontinence, 417–418
Feminization, adrenal, 340
Femoral aneurysms, 366
Femoral canal, 142
Femoral head, avascular necrosis of the, 486
Femoral hernia, 142–143, 143f, 146
Femoral neck fractures, 489, 489f
Femoral ring, 142, 143f
FEV₁, 66t, 396
Fever, 3, 11
  abscesses, 53
  non-haemolytic transfusion reaction, 33t
  postoperative, 126, 126b
FEV₁/FVC ratio, 66t
Fibre, dietary, 256
Fibrinogen
  in cryoprecipitate, 29
  deficiency, 25
Fibrinolysis, 25
  pulmonary embolism, 125
Fibrin sealant, 36
Fibroadenoma, breast, 305f, 307, 307f
Fibroepithelial anal polyp, 272
Fibronectin, 29
Fibrosarcoma, 137, 301
Fibrotic lung disease, 62
Fine-bore nasogastric tubes, 110
Fine needle aspiration cytology, 306
Firearm injuries, 90
Fire services, 94
First aid, burns, 291–294, 291t
Fissure-in-ano, 267–268, 268b, 268f, 269b
Fistula
  branchial, 474
  colonic diverticular disease, 249
  in Crohn's disease, 237–238, 238f
  gastrointestinal, in pancreatitis, 222
  intestinal, 252
  mammary duct, 310
  urinary tract, 419
Fistula-in-ano, 270–271, 270f, 271b, 271f
Flail segment, 96
Flamazine, 294
Flame burns, 291
Flaps see Skin flaps
Flat feet, 486
Flavine adenine dinucleotide (FADH₂), 20
Fleming, Alexander, 45
Flora, normal, 46f
Florey, Howard, 45
Flow cytometry cross match (FC-XM), 446
Flow phase, 3
Fludrocortisone acetate, 342
Fluid
  balance, 10–17
    postoperative care, 121
    conserving measures, 5–6
    daily requirements, 10, 10t
    distribution, 10f

intravenous administration see Intravenous fluid administration
  loss
    assessing, 11
    in burns, 289
    following surgery and trauma, 5t
    insensible, 11, 11t
    normal daily, 10t
    sources of, 11, 11t
  management see also (Intravenous fluid administration)
    thoracic surgery, 397
2-Fluorodeoxy-D-glucose (2FDG), 118
5-Fluorouracil, 261
Foam cells, 345
Focal neurological deficit, 436
Focal nodular hyperplasia (FNH), 201, 202f
Follicle-stimulating hormone (FSH), 5t, 334
Follicular carcinoma, 330, 330f
Foot, 486
  diabetic see Diabetic foot
  warts, 295–296, 295f, 296f
Foot pump, 367
Foramenotomy, posterior, 442
Foraminal herniation, 426, 427f
Forced expiratory volume in one second (FEV₁), 66t, 396
Forced vital capacity (FVC), 66t
Forearm fractures, 489–490
Foreign bodies
  airway obstruction, 120
  oesophageal, 169, 170t
Foreskin, 420
Fournier's gangrene, 54
Fractures, 486–490
  in children, 487
  classification, 487, 487f, 488f
  compartment syndrome, 488
  compound, 488
  conservative treatment, 488
  healing, 487–488
  intra-articular, 488
  operative treatment, 488–489, 489f
  specific, 489–490
Frank-Starling curve, 24f
Frantz tumour of the pancreas, 225, 225f
Free fatty acids (FFAs), 8
Free-standing day units, 127
Fresh frozen plasma (FFP), 29, 34
Frozen section, breast, 306
Full blood count
  acute abdomen, 155
  preoperative, 64–65
Full-thickness burns, 290–291, 290f
Full-thickness rectal prolapse, 274–275, 274f
Full-thickness skin grafts, 287, 294
Fulminant Crohn's colitis, 237–238, 238f
Functional neurosurgery, 440–441
Fundoplication, 174–175, 175f
Fungal infections, 53
Funiculitis, 422
Furuncles, 474
FVC, 66t

G

Gadolinium, 118
Gallbladder, 204–214
  agenesis, 205
  cancer, 86f
  carcinoma, 214

congenital abnormalities, 205–206
  physiology, 204–205
  stones see Gallstones
  strawberry, 208
Gallstone ileus, 207
Gallstones, 206–213, 207b
  cholangitis, 213
  cholecystitis, 206, 207, 207b, 208, 213
  common clinical syndromes associated with, 207–208
  investigations, 208–209, 208f
  non-surgical treatment, 213
  pancreatitis, 217, 217f, 218, 220
  pathogenesis, 206
  pathological effects of, 206–207
  retained, 211–212, 211f, 212f
  surgical treatment, 209–211, 209b
Gamma glutamyl transferase (GGT), 155
Ganglioneuromas, 341
Gangrene
  in appendicitis, 163
  diabetic foot, 54f
  gas, 52t, 54
  ischaemic colitis, 250
  synergistic bacterial, 54
  venous, 374
Gardner's syndrome, 137, 254
Gas gangrene, 52t, 54
Gas transfer factor, 66t
Gastrectomy, 182, 182f, 187–188, 188f
Gastric banding, 191, 191f
Gastric bypass, 191, 191f
Gastric cancer, 185, 190b
  advanced, 186–187, 186f, 187f
  clinical features, 187
  diagnosis, 187
  early, 186
  factors affecting survival, 186–187
  hereditary diffuse, 186, 186b
  palliation, 188–189, 189f
  prognosis, 189, 189t
  staging, 187, 187t, 188f
  treatment, 187–188, 188f
Gastric dilatation, 97
Gastric dysplasia, 186
Gastric emptying, 169, 172
Gastric erosions, burns patients, 293
Gastric inhibitory peptide, 169
Gastric juice, 11t
Gastric lavage, 110
Gastric polyps, 185
Gastric secretions, 169
Gastric ulcers, 180
  complications, 183, 185
  management, 182, 182f
Gastrin, 169
Gastrinomas, 181, 227, 228, 228t
Gastritis, 186, 190
Gastroenteritis, 163
Gastroenterostomy, 186
Gastrografin, 117
Gastrointestinal bleeding, 184, 184t, 222, 222f
Gastrointestinal fistulae, 222
Gastrointestinal ischaemia, 222
Gastrointestinal stromal tumours (GISTs), 172–173, 173f, 185, 185f, 242, 262
Gastrointestinal tract
  effects of shock on, 22, 22b
  fluid loss from, 11, 11t
  investigation of the luminal, 235
  symptoms assessment, 233b
Gastro-oesophageal reflux disease (GORD), 173–175, 174b, 175b, 175f